Neural Tube Defects

NEURAL TUBE DEFECTS
From Origin to Treatment

Edited by

DIEGO F. WYSZYNSKI

Genetics Program
Department of Medicine
Boston University School of Medicine
and
Department of Epidemiology
Boston University School of Public Health
Boston, Massachusetts

OXFORD
UNIVERSITY PRESS
2006

OXFORD
UNIVERSITY PRESS

Oxford University Press, Inc., publishes works that further
Oxford University's objective of excellence
in research, scholarship, and education.

Oxford New York
Auckland Cape Town Dar es Salaam Hong Kong Karachi
Kuala Lumpur Madrid Melbourne Mexico City Nairobi
New Delhi Shanghai Taipei Toronto

With offices in
Argentina Austria Brazil Chile Czech Republic France Greece
Guatemala Hungary Italy Japan Poland Portugal Singapore
South Korea Switzerland Thailand Turkey Ukraine Vietnam

Published by Oxford University Press, Inc.
198 Madison Avenue, New York, New York 10016
www.oup.com

Library of Congress Cataloging-in-Publication Data
Neural tube defects : from origin to treatment / edited by Diego F. Wyszynski.
p.; cm.
Includes index.
ISBN-13: 978-0-19-516603-3
ISBN: 0-19-516603-5
1. Neural tube—Abnormalities.
[DNLM: 1. Neural Tube Defects. WL 101 N4918 2005] I. Wyszynski, Diego F.
QM695.N45N494 2005
618.92'80443—dc22 20040294777

2 4 6 8 9 7 5 3 1
Printed in the United States of America
on acid-free paper

Foreword

Imagine the day when all babies are born healthy, free of birth defects and developmental disabilities, or imagine the day, even sooner, when all babies born with a birth defect or a developmental disability live long, healthy, and productive lives. These visions may seem too idealistic, but they are not for neural tube defects (NTDs). This book is a testimonial to the significant advances in the management of spina bifida, the enormous progress in understanding the etiology of NTDs, and the successful translation of knowledge into primary prevention of NTDs. Many disciplines have contributed to the current understanding of the causes, prevention, and treatment of NTDs, and they represent a framework that can be emulated in advancing studies on the treatment, etiology, and prevention of other birth defects.

Anencephaly and spina bifida are two NTDs that result from failure of closure of the neural tube and have been known to occur for thousands of years. Some of the earliest accounts were summarized by Warkany (1971) in his monograph "Congenital Malformations," stating that mummies of infants with anencephaly were found in ancient Egypt in the tombs of pharaohs. Over the centuries, additional discussion of NTDs appeared in historic writings, but the major advances in their understanding occurred during the twentieth century, when epidemiologic data accumulated rapidly. Most of the available data were thoughtfully summarized in Elwood and Elwood's (1980) now classic book on the epidemiology of spina bifida and anencephaly.

Neural tube defects were considered to represent a classic example of multifactorial inheritance because the evidence pointed to both environmental and genetic factors. The epidemics of NTDs represented some of the strongest evidence suggesting environmental factors as the cause. The Irish potato famine, one of the best studied, led to the theory that the fungus that causes potato blight—*Phytophthora infestans*—was the culprit. Subsequent epidemiologic studies showed this not to be the case. In the United States, McMahon and Yen (1971) retrospectively documented in Massachusetts and Rhode Island an epidemic of NTDs in the 1930s, and Lian and colleagues (1987) described an epidemic in northern China in the early 1980s. Other factors pointing to environmental factors included the east-west (high to low) trend noted in the United States, the clustering in certain geographic areas, such as the high rate in the Appalachian Mountain chain documented by James (1993) at the Centers for Disease Control and Prevention (CDC), and the strong association between low socioeconomic status and high rates of NTDs in diverse populations.

The evidence for genetic factors was also quite strong. The 3%–5% recurrence risk for NTDs, well above the population birth prevalence, was documented in many studies. Twin studies showed a strong heritability index. High rates of NTDs among specific populations, such as the Irish, and low rates among African-Americans added to the evidence for genetic factors.

Smithells and his colleagues (1976) provided the initial evidence that deficiency of nutritional elements played a key role in the etiology of NTDs. His now classic observational study suggested the potential benefit of folic acid in preventing NTDs. He intended to conduct a randomized clinical trial, but his Institutional Review Board only approved the observational design. Although the findings of Smithells' study were compelling, most members of the scientific community considered it insufficient evidence on which to base a public health recommendation. Most subsequent epidemiologic studies pointed to a protective effect of multivitamins containing folic acid in reducing the risk for NTDs. It took over a decade to answer the question conclusively. In 1991 Nick Wald conducted a randomized clinical trial under the auspices of the United Kingdom Medical Research Council (MRC) (Wald et al., 1991). The study examined whether multivitamins alone, 4 mg folic acid daily, or a combination taken at least 1 month before conception reduced the risk of NTD recurrence. The study was stopped early because the findings were very clear: folic acid reduced the risk of recurrence of NTDs by about 70%. Learning about that finding was a memorable day in my life. Godfrey Oakley received a call from Nick Wald on June 24, 1991, at about 5 p.m. Eastern Standard Time while attending the meeting of the Teratology Society in Florida. Godfrey called Dave Erickson and me to strategize about the next steps. Although it was difficult to keep this exciting finding confidential until after the manuscript was published, the delay provided precious time to discuss the findings within our group and prepare for its publication. At long last, the evidence was sufficiently robust to lead to a public health recommendation. The first CDC recommendation appeared in CDC's *Morbidity and Mortality Weekly Report* right after publication of the MRC trial results (Centers for Disease Control and Prevention, 1991). It stated that women with a prior NTD-affected pregnancy should consume 4 mg folic acid daily beginning at least 1 month prior to conception and through the first 3 months of pregnancy to reduce the risk of NTD recurrence. At this time, no recommendation was made regarding the prevention of NTDs in women without a previously affected pregnancy (prevention of occurrence). Although evidence of the effectiveness of folic acid for occurrence prevention was available from published retrospective studies, it was the Hungarian randomized clinical trial led by Czeizel and Dudas (1992) that provided definitive evidence. That trial used 800 μg folic acid daily, so the question of the optimal dosage remained. Evidence for the effectiveness of 400 μg folic acid was later provided by the community intervention trial in China led by Berry et al (1999).

The first comprehensive U.S. Public Health Service recommendation for the use of folic acid to reduce the risk of NTDs was issued on September 11, 1992 (Centers for Disease Control and Prevention, 1992). It stated that all women who are capable of becoming pregnant should consume 400 μg folic acid daily to reduce their risk of an NTD-affected pregnancy. The recommendation for 4 mg daily for women with a prior NTD-affected pregnancy planning a pregnancy was emphasized. The guidelines offered three approaches to ensure sufficient folic acid consumption: (*1*) increasing consumption of foods high in naturally occurring folates (e.g., leafy green vegetables), (*2*) using folic acid–containing dietary supplements, and (*3*) fortification of the food supply with folic acid. Studies quickly showed that increasing consumption of dietary folate was difficult, costly, and complex. Increasing daily consumption of multivitamins or folic acid supplements among women of childbearing age also proved to be challenging, although some success has been documented for specific population groups.

By 1996, following lengthy discussions within the federal agencies concerned with food and nutrition issues, the U.S. Food and Drug Administration issued its recommendation, which required all cereal grains labeled "enriched" to contain 0.14 mg folic acid per 100 g cereal by January 1998. That level was estimated to deliver, on average, a daily folic acid consumption of 125 μg, or 30% of the recommended level daily. Although this was not enough to ensure that all women of reproductive age would consume the recommended 400 μg/day, it was a start. Canadian millers quickly adopted the same fortification recommendation for wheat flour since the United States is their largest international market. In the year 2000, Chile elected a fortification level that delivers an average of 400 μg folic acid daily.

The United States and Canada registered significant declines in NTDs following mandatory fortification of enriched cereals. During 1996 to 2001, the overall decline for NTDs in the United States reached nearly 25%—1000 fewer NTD-affected pregnancies per year (Mathews et al., 2002). That means that 1000 pregnancies per year that would have resulted in a fetal or infant death, pregnancy termination, or lifelong disability resulted in a healthy baby. The impact in terms of reduced health care and societal costs is staggering—about $500 million per yearly cohort. The intangible human cost is unmeasurable.

Although we should be pleased with the progress made so far, more can be done. We have not yet documented that the maximum benefit of folic acid in the United States has been reached. Reaching a percentage reduction similar to that observed in clinical trials could provide indirect evidence, although this method is complicated by differences in genetic risk factors in varying populations. A more direct method to answer this question is to determine for each pregnancy affected with an NTD whether it was a missed opportunity to consume folic acid or whether it followed consumption of the recommended folic acid dosage. When we reach the point of no missed opportunities to consume folic acid, then we will have achieved the maximum benefit of this intervention. At that time, it will be possible to determine the proportion of NTDs that are preventable by folic acid and provide further opportunity to expand our knowledge of other causes of NTDs.

Advances in molecular genetics have helped identify specific polymorphisms in genes in the folic acid pathway that are associated with an increased risk for NTDs. The best studied is the methylenetetrahydrofolate reductase (MTHFR) gene. Mothers homozygous for the *T* allele have increased homocysteine levels and a higher risk for NTDs than mothers who are not homozygous for the *T* allele. An excellent global collaboration led by Botto and Yang (2000) has shown wide variation in the frequency of the C677T polymorphism of MTHFR throughout diverse populations of the world. Other genes in the folic acid pathway have also been associated with an increased risk for NTDs. Now, thanks to the advances in molecular genetics, it is possible to better understand the interaction of the genetic and environmental factors leading to NTDs that are related to folic acid. In the future, we hope to be able to understand other gene–environment interactions.

Advances in clinical care have led to remarkable improvements in the survival and quality of life of individuals living with spina bifida. Wong and Paulozzi (2001) studied the survival of infants with spina bifida in metropolitan Atlanta and found that, for the cohort born during 1979–1994, overall survival to the first year of life was 87.2%, better than that in previous published reports. Survival to age 1 improved from 82.7% in the 1979–1983 cohort to 91.0% in the 1989–1994 birth cohort. Several factors contributed to the increased survival, including improvements in surgical procedures allowing early closure of the back and the development of ventriculoperitoneal shunts for treatment of the hydrocephalus often associated with spina bifida. On a long-term basis, better management of urinary tract infections has diminished the occurrence of chronic renal failure, resulting in improved survival and an enhanced quality of life of individuals living with spina bifida. In addition, better bowel management has led to fewer gastrointestinal complications and to an improved quality of life. Finally, research into the neuropsychological sequelae of spina bifida and hydrocephaly is improving early identification of interventions in learning problems affecting long-term educational and vocational pursuits.

The past three decades have seen significant societal change in the attitudes toward individuals with spina bifida, but much more needs to be done. There is more to learn to ensure optimal health and development for every child born with spina bifida. The Spina Bifida Association of America in collaboration with U.S. federal agencies recently developed a research agenda that, when implemented, will provide much needed data to inform the medical management of individuals with spina bifida.

This book offers an excellent compendium of currently available knowledge about the pathogenesis and etiology of NTDs, as well as the optimal management of individuals living with spina bifida. Let us hope that the framework used for NTDs will serve as a paradigm for finding causes and improved methods of treatment and prevention of other serious birth defects.

José F. Cordero, M.D., M.P.H.
Assistant Surgeon General
Director, National Center on Birth Defects and Developmental Disabilities
Centers for Disease Control and Prevention
Atlanta, Georgia

REFERENCES

Berry RJ, Li Z, Erickson JD, Li S, Moore CA, Wang H, et al. (1999). Prevention of neural-tube defects with folic acid in China. China-U.S. Collaborative Project for Neural Tube Defect Prevention. N Engl J Med 341:1485–1490.

Centers for Disease Control and Prevention (1991). Use of folic acid for prevention of spine bifida and other NTDs. 1983–1991. MMWR 40:513–516.

Centers for Disease Control and Prevention (1992). Recommendations for the use of folic acid to reduce the number of cases of spina bifida and other neural tube defects. MMWR 41:1–7.

Czeizel AE, Dudas I (1992). Prevention of the first occurrence of neural-tube defects by periconceptional vitamin supplementation. N Engl J Med 327:1832–1835.

Elwood JM, Elwood JH (1980). *Epidemiology of Anencephalus and Spina Bifida*. New York: Oxford University Press.

James LM (1993). Maps of birth defects occurrence in the U.S., Birth Defects Monitoring Program (BDMP)/CPHA, 1970–1987. Teratology 48:551–646.

Lian ZH, Yang HY, Li Z (1987). Neural tube defects in Beijing-Tianjin area of China. Urban-rural distribution and some other epidemiological characteristics. J Epidemiol Community Health 41:259–262.

MacMahon B, Yen S (1971). Unrecognised epidemic of anencephaly and spina bifida. Lancet 1:31–33.

Mathews TJ, Honein MA, Erickson JD (2002). Spina bifida and anencephaly prevalence—United States, 1991–2001. MMWR Recomm Rep 51:9–11.

Smithells RW, Sheppard S, Schorah CJ (1976). Vitamin deficiencies and neural tube defects. Arch Dis Child 51:944–950.

Wald N, Sneddon J, Densem J, Frost C, Stone R, MRC Vitamin Study Research Group (1991). Prevention of neural tube defects: results of the Medical Research Council Vitamin Study. MRC Vitamin Study Research Group. Lancet 338:131–137.

Warkany J (1971). *Congenital Malformations; Notes and Comments*. Chicago: Year Book Medical Publishers.

Wong LY, Paulozzi LJ (2001). Survival of infants with spina bifida: a population study, 1979–94. Paediatr Perinat Epidemiol 15:374–378.

Preface

Neural tube defects (NTDs) are birth defects that involve incomplete development of the neural tube, the structure that becomes the brain and spinal cord. There are several different types of NTDs. Spina bifida and anencephaly comprise 90% of all NTDs, and encephalocele accounts for the remaining 10%. In the United States, about 4000 pregnancies per year are affected by an NTD. Of these, about 1500 result in miscarriage or stillbirth. These numbers, however, are rapidly changing. It is now widely accepted that maternal dietary supplementation with folic acid results in a substantial decrease in the prevalence of NTDs at birth. The exact reason for this finding is still unknown.

Prenatal diagnosis can now be accomplished in more than 70% of all pregnancies with NTDs. For example, the alpha-fetoprotein test, which is performed between 16 and 18 weeks of pregnancy, can detect more than 90% of the cases of anencephaly and 64% to 80% of cases of spina bifida. However, this method also has false-positive results. When are prenatal tests for NTDs recommended?

Under specific circumstances, it is now possible to carry out prenatal surgery in fetuses with NTDs. The risks are considerable for both mother and fetus, and the long-term consequences of the surgery are unknown. However, if it is successful, individuals with NTDs can live a healthy, normal life. Is it worth the risk?

This book is intended to answer these and many other questions related to NTDs. Advanced graduate students, practitioners, and researchers interested in the field of birth defects will find its contents highly informative. The book is organized with a wide readership in mind, and many of the chapters will also be of interest to parents, siblings, and affected individuals.

The book includes a broad range of theoretical, experimental, and clinical topics written by experts in the fields of development, epidemiology, genetics, treatment and education, ethics, and public health. Following the format of a close "relative," *Cleft Lip and Palate: From Origin to Treatment* (Oxford University Press, 2002), the text is divided into three sections: Basic Principles, Treatment and Education, and Public Health Issues.

Section I has four parts: Clinical and Molecular Embryology of the Central Nervous System, Clinical Features of Neural Tube Defects, Epidemiology of Neural Tube Defects, and Genetics of Neural Tube Defects. This section will provide the reader with a deep understanding of the mechanisms involved in NTD formation, how to diagnose and classify the different types of NTDs, their worldwide geographical distribution, and the genetic and environmental factors involved in their etiology. These topics will be of great interest especially to basic scientists, researchers, and clinicians.

Section II describes in detail the methods used to assess and treat the needs of individuals with NTDs. These include prenatal and postnatal surgical techniques, orthopedic and urological management, genetic counseling and communication, the psychological adjustment and family relationships in children and adolescents with spina bifida, the transition to adulthood (including sexuality and toilet training), and education. Clinicians, family members, and individuals with NTDs will find this section highly informative.

Section III presents new areas of emerging interest to society at large, such as how and when to fortify foods to prevent NTDs, the costs of treatment of individuals with

NTDs, healthcare coverage, quality of life, and the ethics of contemporary medical management.

Rabbi Moses Chaim Luzzatto (1707–1746), a prominent Italian-Jewish mystic, introduced his ethical treatise *Path of the Just* in the following way: "I have written this work not to teach people what they do not know, but to remind them of what they already know and is very evident to them, for you will find in most of my words only things which most people know, and concerning which they entertain no doubts. But to the extent that they are well known and their truths revealed to all, so is forgetfulness in relation to them extremely prevalent. It follows, then, that the benefit to be obtained from this work is not derived from a single reading; for it is possible that the reader will find that he has learned little after having read it that he did not know before. Its benefit is to be derived, rather, through review and persistent study, by which one is reminded of those things which, by nature, he is prone to forget and through which he is caused to take to heart the duty that he tends to overlook." The quote applies well to this book. The vast majority of its content is available in the scientific literature, and much of it is generally known. However, although there is a large amount of information available on NTDs—from scientific journals, popular magazines, newsletters, books, television shows, and Web pages—it is difficult to sift through it all and know what is current and accurate. This book is intended to provide state-of-the-art review chapters to graduate students, researchers, practitioners, and family members interested in this condition. It is written with the collective knowledge of more than 55 experts in the field with the hope that it will help readers better understand the possibilities of prevention, diagnosis, treatment, and education of individuals with NTDs.

Acknowledgments

As the editor of this book, I wish to acknowledge with gratitude the contributors' investment of time and knowledge in the face of numerous competing demands for their attention. Drafts of each chapter were presented for formal review and comments to at least two anonymous experts in the respective field. I am grateful to the following individuals for engaging the contributors in challenging and incisive discussions and for supplying them with detailed comments about their work: William P. Allen, Robert T. Ammerman, Kristin Bruk Artinger, Juan Pablo Beca, Gregory D. Bennett, Robert G. Best, Susan Halloran Blanton, Philip R. Brauer, Timothy Brei, Mark P. Cain, Suzan Carmichael, Andres Carrasco, Suzanne B. Cassidy, Earl Y. Cheng, Nancy C. Chescheir, Anne Chiaramello, Adolfo Correa, Arthur J. DiPatri Jr., Peter Dirks, Helen Dolk, Charlotte M. Druschel, Rena E. Falk, Jack M. Fletcher, Joel E. Frader, Elena Gates, Michael R. Harrison, H. Eugene Hoyme, Louanne Hudgins, Laird G. Jackson, Marilyn C. Jones, Haresh Kirpalani, Arthur F. Kohrman, Carole LaBonne, J. Paul Leigh, Jim W. Loomis, Marlene Lutkenhoff, E. Mark Mahone, Pierpaolo Mastroiacovo, Roberto Mayor, Gavin V. McDonnell, Linnet McMahon, Molly McNulty, Elizabeth McPherson, Mark J. Merkens, Robert Meyer, Anne Molloy, M. Angela Nieto, Hope Northrup, W. Jerry Oakes, Michael D. Partington, Claudia Perandones, Joseph H. Piatt Jr., Ian Kenneth Pople, Christopher W. Reilly, Theodore S. Roberts, Leslie Rubin, Thomas Sadler, John Smulian, David A. Spiegel, Tsunenobu Tamura, Jeffrey D. Thomson, Helga Toriello, Naoto Ueno, Henny W. M. Van Straaten, Stein Emil Vollset, Deborah Klein Walker, Michael Wiley, Gordon Worley, Juan Yang, and Pamela C. Yelick. I owe special thanks to Marcia Liebman and Michelle Prince, who provided me with excellent comments on Chapter 13.

My involvement in the field of birth defects and this book are fruits of the warm support I received from many people in locations as diverse as Buenos Aires (Argentina), Baltimore, Bethesda, and Boston. Some of them deserve grateful recognition for inspiring me to fulfill this dream and for serving as role models: Elsa Muñoz de Suárez, Vicente Mazzáfero, Terri Beaty, Jon Samet, Joan Bailey-Wilson, Sakkubai Naidu, Laura Mitchell, Scott Diehl, Lewis Holmes, and Lindsay Farrer.

Deep appreciation is also expressed to Jeffrey House, formerly at Oxford University Press, who lent his support to this project from the very beginning; to William Lamsback, who masterfully expedited its production; and to Nancy J. Wolitzer, who was instrumental in shaping this final volume and who made my priorities and timelines hers. Finally, I acknowledge my loving parents, Drs. Enrique and Celia Wyszynski, for their constant support all these years; my lovely wife, Carolien, for her understanding and enduring belief in me; and my four children, Shoshana, Sara, Daniel, and Rena, who are my inspiration and the loves of my life.

Contents

Contributors

KELLY A. BENNETT, M.D., F.R.C.S.C.
Department of Obstetrics and Gynecology,
Division of Maternal Fetal Medicine
Vanderbilt University Medical Center
Nashville, Tennessee

MARK J. BLITON, PH.D.
Division of Medical Ethics
Department of Medicine
Clinical Ethics Consultation Service
Center for Clinical and Research Ethics
Vanderbilt University Medical Center
Nashville, Tennessee

MARIANNE BRONNER-FRASER, SC.B., PH.D.
Division of Biology
California Institute of Technology
Pasadena, California

JOSEPH P. BRUNER, M.D.
Department of Obstetrics and Gynecology,
Division of Maternal Fetal Medicine
Vanderbilt University Medical Center
Nashville, Tennessee

COLLEEN F. BUCK, B.A.
Psychology Department
Graduate Clinical Psychology Program
Loyola University Chicago
Chicago, Illinois

ELLEN M. CARPENTER, PH.D.
Department of Psychiatry and Biobehavioral Science
David Geffen School of Medicine at UCLA
Los Angeles, California

ALAN R. COHEN, M.D., F.A.C.S., F.A.A.P.
Pediatric Neurological Surgery
Rainbow Babies
and
Children's Hospital, Case Western Reserve University
Cleveland, Ohio

ANDREW J. COPP, M.B.B.S., D.PHIL., F.R.C.PATH.
Neural Development Unit
Institute of Child Health
University College London, United Kingdom

GEORGE H. DAVIS, D.O.
Department of Obstetrics and Gynecology,
Division of Maternal Fetal Medicine
Vanderbilt University Medical Center
Nashville, Tennessee

LUCIANO DIAS, M.D.
Department of Orthopaedic Surgery
Northwestern University Medical School
Chicago, Illinois

JAIME L. FRÍAS, M.D.
Department of Pediatrics
University of South Florida Birth Defects Center
University of South Florida
Tampa, Florida

GLENN J. GARDENER, M.B.B.S., F.R.A.N.Z.C.O.G.
Department of Obstetrics and Gynaecology
University College London, United Kingdom

HOLLY GRASON, M.A.
Department of Population and Family Health Sciences
Bloomberg School of Public Health
Johns Hopkins University
Baltimore, Maryland

NICHOLAS D.E. GREENE, PH.D.
Neural Development Unit
Institute of Child Health
University College London, United Kingdom

RACHEL NEFF GREENLEY, M.A.
Psychology Department
Graduate Clinical Psychology Program
Loyola University Chicago
Chicago, Illinois

SCOTT D. GROSSE, PH.D.
National Center on Birth Defects
and Developmental Disabilities
Centers for Disease Control and Prevention
Atlanta, Georgia

GRAYSON N. HOLMBECK, PH.D.
Psychology Department
Graduate Clinical Psychology Program
Loyola University Chicago
Chicago, Illinois

DAVID B. JOSEPH, M.D., F.A.A.P, F.A.C.S.
Department of Urology
University of Alabama at Birmingham
and
Children's Hospital
Birmingham, Alabama

HAKRYUL JO, PH.D.
Whitehead Institute for Biomedical Research
Cambridge, Massachusetts

RUSSELL S. KIRBY, PH.D., M.S., F.A.C.E.
Department of Maternal and Child Health
School of Public Health
University of Alabama at Birmingham
Birmingham, Alabama

ROLV T. LIE, PH.D.
Section for Epidemiology and Medical Statistics
Department of Public Health and Primary Health Care
University of Bergen
Bergen, Norway

GREGORY S. LIPTAK, M.D., M.P.H.
Department of Pediatrics
University of Rochester Medical Center
Rochester, New York

LAURA ANNE LOWERY
Whitehead Institute for Biomedical Research
and
Massachusetts Institute of Technology
Cambridge, Massachusetts

ELIZABETH C. MELVIN, M.S., C.G.C.
Center for Human Genetics
Duke University Medical Center
Durham, North Carolina

SERGIO A. MENDOZA, M.D.
Department of Orthopaedics and Rehabilitation
University of Iowa Hospitals and Clinics
Iowa City, Iowa

JONATHAN P. MILLER, M.D.
Neurological Surgery
Rainbow Babies
and
Children's Hospital
Case Western Reserve University
Cleveland, Ohio

CYNTHIA A. MOORE, M.D., PH.D.
Division of Birth Defects and Developmental Disabilities
National Center on Birth Defects
and Developmental Disabilities
Centers for Disease Control and Prevention
Atlanta, Georgia

JENNIFER N. MURDOCH, PH.D.
MRC Mammalian Genetics Unit
Harwell, Didcot
Oxon, United Kingdom

GODFREY P. OAKLEY, JR., M.D., M.S.P.M.
Department of Epidemiology
Rollins School of Public Health
Emory University
Atlanta, Georgia

SONYA G. OPPENHEIMER, M.D.
Division of Developmental Disabilities
and
University Affiliated Cincinnati Center
for Developmental Disorders
Cincinnati Children's Hospital Medical Center
Cincinnati, Ohio

JAMIE J. PERRY, M.D., M.P.H.
Kennedy Krieger Institute
Johns Hopkins University School of Medicine
Baltimore, Maryland

INEKE M. PIT-TEN CATE, PH.D.
Developmental Brain-Behaviour Unit
School of Psychology
University of Southampton
United Kingdom

EVADNIE RAMPERSAUD, M.S.P.H.
Center for Human Genetics
Duke University Medical Center
Durham, North Carolina

SONJA A. RASMUSSEN, M.D.
National Center on Birth Defects
and Developmental Disabilities
Centers for Disease Control and Prevention
Atlanta, Georgia

HAROLD L. REKATE, M.D.
Pediatric Neurosciences
Barrow Neurological Institute
Phoenix, Arizona

CHARLES H. RODECK, D.SC., F.R.C.O.G., F.R.C.PATH., F.MED.SCI.
Department of Obstetrics and Gynaecology
University College London, United Kingdom

PATRICK S. ROMANO, M.D., M.P.H.
Division of General Medicine and
Section of General Pediatrics
School of Medicine
University of California, Davis
Sacramento, California

RIMA ROZEN, PH.D., FCCMG
Departments of Human Genetics, Pediatrics and Biology
McGill University—Montreal Children's Hospital
Montreal, Canada

JOHN F. SARWARK, M.D.
Division of Pediatric Orthopaedic Surgery
Children's Memorial Hospital
and
Feinberg School of Medicine
Northwestern University
Chicago, Illinois

ROBERT A. SAUL, M.D.
Greenwood Genetic Center
Greenwood, South Carolina

LAURIE H. SEAVER, M.D.
Hawaii Community Genetics
Honolulu, Hawaii

LOWELL E. SEVER, PH.D.
Division of Epidemiology
University of Texas School of Public Health
Houston, Texas

DAVID B. SHURTLEFF, M.D.
Department of Pediatrics
University of Washington
Seattle, Washington

HAZEL SIVE, PH.D.
Whitehead Institute for Biomedical Research
and
Biology Department
Massachusetts Institute of Technology
Cambridge, Massachusetts

CAROLE A. SOBKOWIAK, F.C.S.P., S.R.P.
Society for Research into Hydrocephalus and Spina Bifida
Durham, United Kingdom

MARCY C. SPEER, PH.D.
Center for Human Genetics
Duke University Medical Center
Durham, North Carolina

JIM STEVENSON, PH.D.
Developmental Brain-Behaviour Unit
School of Psychology
University of Southampton
United Kingdom

ROGER E. STEVENSON, M.D.
Greenwood Genetic Center
Greenwood, South Carolina

CARY R. TEMPLIN, M.D.
Orthopaedic Surgery
Northwestern University Medical School
Chicago, Illinois

VINCENT TROPEPE, PH.D.
Whitehead Institute for Biomedical Research
Cambridge, Massachusetts
and
Department of Zoology
University of Toronto
Toronto, Ontario
Canada

NOEL TULIPAN, M.D.
Department of Neurosurgery
Vanderbilt University Medical Center
Nashville, Tennessee

NORMAN J. WAITZMAN, PH.D.
Department of Economics
University of Utah
Salt Lake City, Utah

WILLIAM WALKER, M.D.
Department of Pediatrics
University of Washington
Seattle, Washington

STUART L. WEINSTEIN, M.D.
University of Iowa Hospitals and Clinics
Iowa City, Iowa

DIEGO F. WYSZYNSKI, M.D., M.H.S., PH.D.
Genetics Program
Department of Medicine
Boston University School of Medicine
and
Department of Epidemiology
Boston University School of Public Health
Boston, Massachusetts

JILL ZUKERMAN, B.A.
Psychology Department
Graduate Clinical Psychology Program
Loyola University Chicago
Chicago, Illinois

I

BASIC PRINCIPLES

I

Clinical and Molecular Embryology of the Central Nervous System

1

Neural Crest Formation

MARIANNE BRONNER-FRASER

A central question in developmental biology is how a single cell, the fertilized egg, can give rise to multiple types of tissues in the complex adult organism. This is exemplified by the forming brain, where seemingly homogeneous neuroepithelial cells eventually differentiate into myriad of mature neurons and glia of the central nervous system. Equally intriguing is the neural crest, a population of cells that initially arises within the newly formed central nervous system. Subsequently, these cells undergo an epithelial-to-mesenchymal transition whereby they leave the neuroepithelium and transform into a migratory population that forms much of the peripheral nervous system. In addition, neural crest cells give rise to other diverse cell types as different as pigment cells, the craniofacial skeleton, adrenal chromaffin cells, and some vascular smooth muscle. This chapter serves as a general introduction to the formation, cell interactions, and migration pathways that are involved in generating this fascinating cell population. For more detailed information about neural crest induction, plasticity and formation of craniofacial structures, readers are referred to the following in-depth recent reviews: Knecht and Bronner-Fraser (2002), Dupin and LeDouarin (2003), Gammill and Bronner-Fraser (2003), Helms and Schneider (2003), Santagati and Rijli (2003), and Trainor and Nieto (2003).

INITIAL STEPS IN NEURAL CREST FORMATION

The neural crest was first recognized in the chick as a band of material lying between the presumptive epidermis and the neural tube (His, 1868; Hall and Hörstadius, 1988). Cells that will eventually give rise to the neural crest are induced at the border between the neural plate, which will form the central nervous system, and the non-neural ectoderm, which will form the epidermis. During neurulation (nervous system formation) the neural plate forms in the midline of the embryo as a thickening in the epithelium that results in the formation of a morphologically distinct set of neuroepithelial cells. The edges of the neural plate, termed *neural fold cells,* begin to elevate and eventually the neural plate folds inward on itself, transforming from a plate into a cylindrical neural tube that extends from the rostral to the caudal limits of the embryo. In most vertebrates, the neural tube initiates closure at the rostral end of the embryo and the tube completes closure in a rostral-to-caudal progression. The open ends form the anterior and posterior neuropores, respectively, that close later in development. Because the process of neural tube closure is initially tenuous, it is thought that the dorsal closure point is a site prone to secondary opening that can lead to neural tube defects.

As a consequence of neurulation, neural crest progenitors come to lie within the neural folds and, later, in the dorsal neural tube at most axial levels. However, in the mouse, neural crest cells at cranial levels initiate migration prior to neural tube closure. Following the process of emigration, they form a motile mesenchymal population that migrates to many distinct locations. Thus, the neural crest is a transitory embryonic structure composed of proliferating precursors that migrate away from the closing or closed neural tube to populate the periphery. Although many cells within this population will acquire a neuronal fate and form parts of the peripheral nervous system, others will give rise to a wide variety of structures ranging from the melanocytes of the skin to the craniofacial skeleton (Fig. 1.1).

During normal embryogenesis, neural crest cells form only at the most lateral edges of the neural plate (future dorsal region) at its border with prospective epidermis. The neural plate border from which neural crest progenitors arise does not, however, give rise exclusively to

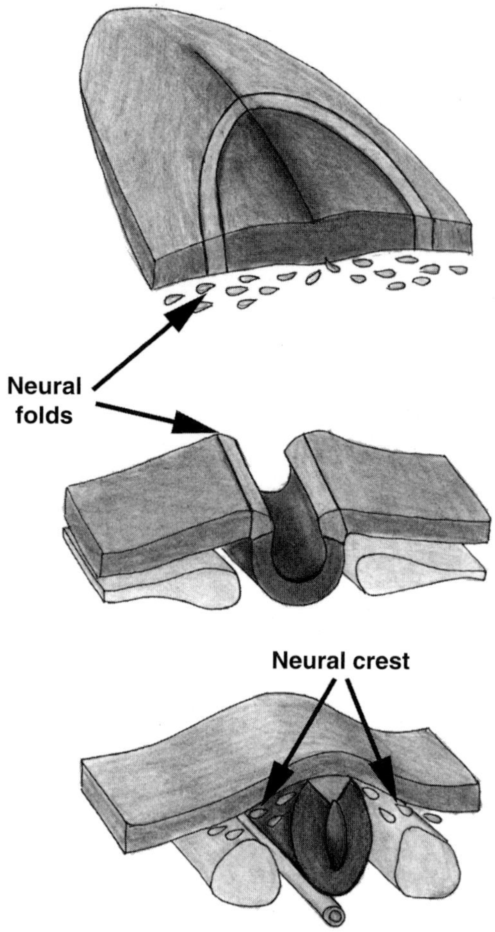

FIGURE 1.1. Localization of neural crest precursors during neurulation. When the neural plate is open, neural crest precursors (shaded region) lie at the border between the neural and nonneural ectoderm. As the neural tube closes, the presumptive neural crest cells come to lie within the dorsal neural tube and begin to migrate as individual cells at around the time of neural tube closure.
Source: Paige Fraser.

neural crest cells. Single-cell lineage labeling experiments have demonstrated that a single cell in the elevating neural folds can give rise to derivatives not only of the neural crest, but also of the neural tube and epidermis (Selleck and Bronner-Fraser, 1995). Even after neural tube closure, labeled dorsal neural tube cells can give rise to both neural tube and neural crest cells (Bronner-Fraser and Fraser, 1988). Thus, the term *premigratory neural crest cells,* referring to cells in the neural folds and dorsal neural tube, is really a misnomer since these cells have broad developmental potential. Furthermore, migrating neural crest cells labeled after they have left the neural tube have the capacity to contribute to multiple neural crest lineages (Bronner-Fraser and Fraser, 1988).

Once they have left the neural tube, neural crest cells do not normally contribute to the central nervous system; however, if challenged by injection into the ventral neural tube, even migrating neural crest cells can adopt the fates of their neighbors, forming floor plate and motor neurons (Ruffins et al., 1998). Similarly, some ventral neural tube cells from older embryos will migrate and differentiate into neural crest cell derivatives after transplantation onto neural crest cell migration pathways (Sharma et al., 1995; Korade and Frank, 1996). Thus, it seems that many neural plate–derived cells can become neural crest cells if given appropriate signals. These results demonstrate that neural fold and neural crest cells display remarkable flexibility in their fates.

TISSUE INTERACTIONS IMPLICATED IN NEURAL CREST CELL FORMATION

Although neural crest cells do not become morphologically identifiable until they leave the neural tube, there is increasing evidence suggesting that induction of this population occurs well before the process of neural tube closure and may likely begin during gastrulation. This induction appears to occur via a tissue interaction between the neural plate (presumptive central nervous system) and nonneural ectoderm (presumptive epidermis). This is not surprising given the close proximity of the neural plate and nonneural ectoderm, which makes likely the possibility of such an interaction between these two tissues.

The requirement for tissue interactions in neural crest induction was tested experimentally by Rollhäuser-ter-Horst (1980) and more recently by Moury and Jacobson (1989), who juxtaposed presumptive epidermis and neural plate in urodeles. They found that neural folds developed at the junction of the two tissues and neural crest cells were generated de novo. Additional experiments, in which epidermis and neural plate were taken from different pigmented species of urodeles, revealed that neural crest cells arose from both the epidermis and the neural plate (Moury and Jacobson, 1990). Interestingly, melanocytes arose primarily from the neural plate, whereas the epidermis gave rise to spinal and cranial ganglia.

In avian embryos, similar juxtaposition of nonneural ectoderm and early neural plate tissue also induces the formation of neural crest cells (Selleck and Bronner-Fraser, 1995). This can occur with neural plate tissue taken from early stages (stage 4) just after neural plate formation, as well as with later-stage intermediate neural plate derived from the closing neural plate (stage 10). The ability of the neural plate to respond to neural crest induction is restricted as a function of time, declining precipitously after the 10-somite stage (Basch et al., 2000). In addition to up-regulation of neural crest markers, neural plate from later but not earlier embryos expresses dorsal neural tube markers like *Wnt-1* and *Wnt-3a* after inductive interactions with epidermis (Dickinson et al., 1995).

MOLECULAR INTERACTIONS THAT GENERATE NEURAL CREST CELLS

Induction of the neural crest requires both a source of inducer (the ectoderm) and a competent receiving tissue (the neural plate). Several molecules have been implicated in neural crest cell formation. These include members of the TGF-β transforming growth factor-β (TGF-β) superfamily such as dorsalin and bone morphogenetic protein (BMP-4), as well as fibroblast growth factors (FGFs) and, more recently, *Wnt*'s.

The first molecular description of a molecule with neural crest–inducing ability was provided by Basler et al. (1993), who found that dorsalin-1, which is expressed transiently in the dorsal neural tube of the chick embryo, is able to induce neural crest cells from neural plates in vitro. However, its relatively late expression excludes the possibility that it is involved in initially inducing neural crest cells at the neural plate border. Subsequently, Liem et al. (1995) showed that BMP-4 can induce the formation of neural crest cells from chick neural plate explants in vitro in the presence of N2/F12 medium. Hence BMP-4 can substitute for nonneural ectoderm in the formation of neural crest cells from neural plate explants. Although the authors suggest that BMP-4 is expressed in the ectoderm flanking the neural plate, recent data show that it is expressed only very transiently in this location, then down-regulated from ectoderm and up-regulated in the neural folds and dorsal neural tube (Watanabe and LeDouarin, 1996; Garcia-Castro et al., 2002). Furthermore, blocking BMP signaling using the BMP inhibitor, Noggin, in vivo at the time that BMP is transiently expressed in the ectoderm has no effect on neural crest formation; in contrast, blocking when neural folds have elevated and when BMP is expressed in the neural folds does inhibit maintenance of neural crest markers (Selleck et al., 1998). These results suggest that BMPs are likely to function in the neural folds/dorsal neural tube, playing a secondary role in maintaining an already induced neural crest population rather than in the induction process itself. Interestingly, BMPs and other members of the TGF-β family have later roles in dorsoventral neural tube patterning, inducing different populations of dorsal sensory neurons in naive neural plate at stages when they have lost the ability to form neural crest cells (Liem et al., 1997).

Fibrolast growth factors also may factor into the induction cascade since they can induce neural crest cells from neuralized ectoderm. Mayor and colleagues (1995) treated *Xenopus* animal caps with various soluble factors and found that, when combined with Noggin, bFGF induced neural crest cells. Overexpression of a dominant negative FGF receptor (dnFGFR) in *Xenopus* seems to inhibit neural crest formation without affecting formation of the neural plate (Mayor et al., 1997). These experiments suggest that FGF can induce neural crest cells from neural ectoderm and may be involved in neural crest cell formation in vivo. However, neural crest markers are not up-regulated in bFGF-treated neural plates in vitro (Mayor et al., 1997), suggesting that the dnFGFR in the neural plate of the conjugate may be interfering with a non-FGF signal from the epidermis. Furthermore, embryos overexpressing a dnFGFR seem to have normal neural crest derivatives (Amaya et al., 1991; Godsave and Durston, 1997). However, a role for FGF cannot be ruled out at this point. Increasing evidence suggests that an FGF signal may be indirect and may function through the *Wnt* signals (LaBonne and Bronner-Fraser, 1998).

Members of the *Wnt* family have been implicated in neural crest cell formation in *Xenopus* embryos (Saint-Jeannet et al., 1997; LaBonne and Bronner-Fraser, 1998). Saint-Jeannet et al. (1997) demonstrated that GSK-3 overexpression led to neural crest defects in the absence of effects of rostrocaudal neural patterning. LaBonne and Bronner-Fraser (1998) demonstrated that overexpression of a dominant negative *Wnt* ligand led to a loss of the earliest steps in neural crest formation. Moreover, Deardorff et al. (2001) have used morpholino-mediated depletion to show that a specific *Wnt* receptor, *frizzled 3*, mediates this process in vivo. Saint-Jeannet and colleagues (1997) showed that neural crest cell markers were up-regulated in neuralized (Noggin-expressing) animal caps treated with *Wnt-1* and *Wnt-3a;* similarly, overexpressing *Wnt-1* or *Wnt-3a* in embryos dramatically increased the number of neural crest cells. A complication is that *Wnt-1* and *Wnt-3a* are expressed in the dorsal neural tube only after neural tube closure, suggesting that they are not involved in the initial induction of neural crest cells, which occurs when the neural plate is still open. This correlates with the results from recombinations of different stages of chick neural plate with nonneural ectoderm; whereas early neural plate plus ectoderm generates neural crest cells, as assayed by *Slug* expression, *Wnt-1* and *Wnt-3a* are only induced from ectoderm combined with late-stage neural plates (Dickinson et al., 1995) (Fig. 1.2). However, *Wnt*'s other than *Wnt-1* and *Wnt-3a* may be expressed in the mesoderm underlying the neural folds; for example, *Wnt8* is know to be present in the mesoderm at a time and place consistent with a role in neural crest induction in both zebrafish and *Xenopus,* and has been shown to be a positive effecter of neural crest formation both in vivo and in animal cap assays.

In avian embryos as well, there is recent evidence that neural crest induction requires *Wnt* signals in vivo. Expression of the neural crest marker, *Slug,* is inhibited

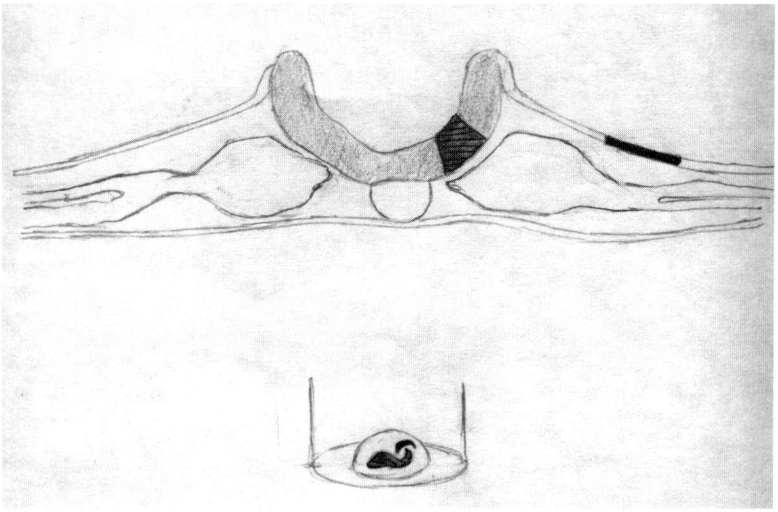

FIGURE 1.2. Neural crest cells can be induced by recombining naive intermediate neural plate and nonneural ectoderm. Naive intermediate neural plate (from stage 4 to 10 chick embryos) can be dissected from the newly formed neural plate or closing neural tube and combined in tissue culture with nonneural ectoderm. After 24–36 hours of coculture, this results in the production of neural crest cells.
Source: Paige Fraser.

when cells expressing a dominant negative *Wnt* (*dnWnt*) construct are introduced adjacent to the open neural plate at the site of epidermal–neural plate interactions. Similarly, injection into the closing neural tube also down-regulates *Slug* expression. This suggests that *Wnt*'s are necessary for neural crest formation. Interestingly, they are required both when the neural plate is open, when inhibition of BMP signaling by Noggin does not perturb *Slug* expression, as well as in the closing neural tube, when BMP inhibition does block *Slug* (Selleck et al., 1998). Furthermore, addition of a soluble form of *Wnt* is sufficient to induce neural crest cells in naive intermediate neural plate tissue in a defined saline medium with no other additives. In contrast, BMP-4 can only induce neural crest in a medium supplemented with other growth factors (N2/F12, which contains insulin-like growth factor [IGF] and other growth factors). Importantly, *Wnt6* has the correct spatial and temporal expression pattern in the ectoderm to mediate neural crest induction. These results strongly suggest that *Wnt* molecules are both necessary and sufficient to account for the early induction of neural crest in the avian embryo (Garcia-Castro et al., 2002).

GENE PROFILE OF NEWLY INDUCED NEURAL CREST CELLS

The molecular targets of the neural crest–inducing signals described above are not well understood. A small number of genes expressed in neural folds have been identified, and their requirement in neural crest formation has been shown using antisense and dominant negative approaches. These include *Slug, Sox9,* and *FoxD3* (Nieto et al., 1994; Spokony et al., 2002; Sasai et al., 2001). This, however, is not a comprehensive profile. To circumvent this problem, a complete collection of genes simultaneously expressed in those cell destined to form the neural crest has recently been performed (Gammill and Bronner-Fraser, 2002) using macroarray techniques (Rast et al., 2000).

Isolating neural crest precursors is complicated by the fact that this population is not segregated in the dorsal neural tube and is not distinguishable from other dorsal neural tube cells; thus, they cannot be isolated as a pure population. Furthermore, there are no known genes that specifically mark only neural crest precursors that will migrate. As a result, there is no way of defining a neural crest cell until it becomes migratory. To circumvent these problems, a chick cDNA library macroarray was prepared and screened with a subtracted probe generated from in vitro-induced neural crest. As described above, neural crest induction can be recapitulated in vitro by coculturing pieces of nonneural ectoderm and neural plate; this provides a powerful tool for producing neural crest precursors under defined conditions.

The combination of in vitro-induced neural crest with macroarray screening (Rast et al., 2000) and in situ hybridization made it possible to achieve novel neural crest gene expression profiling. First, genes common to neural plate and ectoderm were subtracted from those expressed in "induced" neural plate/ectoderm recombinants, thus leaving only those genes that were up-regulated by the induction process. These were identified by hybridization to the macroarrayed library. Then in situ hybridization was used as a secondary screen to verify the up-regulation and glean temporal expression information about individual clones. This allowed for the creation of a *molecular profile* that described the consequences of neural crest induction.

This screen revealed 83 genes that provide the first gene expression profile of a newly induced neural crest cell (Gammill and Bronner-Fraser, 2002). This profile contains numerous novel markers of neural crest precursors and reveals previously unrecognized similarities between neural crest cells and endothelial cells, another migratory cell population. Many of the genes fell into logical categories, which contained genes associated with the cytoskeleton, cell surface, receptors, signaling pathway, and extracellular matrix molecules (Gammill and Bronner-Fraser, 2002).

The data suggest a sequential activation of genes following neural crest induction. Precursor cells in the dorsal neural tube first change their state after induction by activating intermediate filaments, cell cycle components, and receptors/ligands, thus beginning the process of becoming a neural crest cell. Next, genes associated with migration are expressed, including those associated with changes in the actin cytoskeleton, rho pathway, and extracellular matrix; these may establish migratory potential. Finally, a subset of cells receives a signal that mobilizes their migratory potential so that they emigrate from the neural tube. Other cells remain in the neural tube and become part of the central nervous system, never accessing this migratory potential. This genomic approach provides a tool by which to characterize the molecular profile of neural crest cells at a variety of developmental stages at the genomic level. This, in turn, can be used to elucidate the complex molecular network regulating the development of this cell type.

NEURAL CREST AND DORSOVENTRAL NEURAL TUBE PATTERNING

Both during and after its closure, the neural tube develops a characteristic polarity along its dorsoventral axes, with different cell types arising from different portions of the neural tube. Dorsal structures include neural crest cells, roof plate cells, and commissural neurons (Kalcheim and LeDouarin, 1999). One characteristic ventral structure is the floor plate, which attracts commissural axons via production of netrins (Tessier-Lavigne et al., 1988; Placzek et al., 1990). Other ventral cell types are motor neuron pools, which form lateral to the floor plate and project their processes to targets in the periphery.

The notochord plays an important role in establishing the dorsoventral polarity of the neural tube. A notochord grafted lateral to the neural tube induces an extra floor plate and motor neuron pools (van Straaten et al., 1988; Smith and Schoenwolf, 1989; Yamada et al., 1991) via a *Sonic hedgehog*–mediated signal (Echelard et al., 1993; Roelink et al., 1995). *Sonic hedgehog* protein is expressed in the floor plate and notochord (Marti et al., 1995a), and application of either Shh-expressing cells or purified protein to intermediate neural plate explants leads to induction of floor plate and/or motor neuron differentiation in a dose-dependent fashion (Marti et al., 1995b).

Grafting a notochord into or lateral to the closing neural folds results in the juxtaposition of dorsal and ventral cells types by inducing floor plate cells and motor neurons dorsally. When single-cell lineage analysis using a vital dye was performed, both "dorsal" and "ventral" neural tube derivatives were found to arise from a single precursor in the dorsal neural tube adjacent to the grafted notochord derivatives (Artinger et al., 1995). Cells as diverse as sensory ganglion cells, presumptive pigment cells, roof plate cells, motor neurons, and floor plate cells have been observed emerging from the same clone. The presence of such diversity within single clones indicates that the responses to dorsal and ventral signals are not mutually exclusive; even in the closing neural tube, neuroepithelial cells are not restricted to the formation of only dorsal or ventral neural tube derivatives (Artinger and Bronner-Fraser, 1995) but are multipotent.

FACTORS INVOLVED IN NEURAL CREST DELAMINATION

An intriguing question is: what makes neural crest cells migrate from the neural tube, and what controls the timing of this emigration? Relatively little is known about what mediates these processes. Inhibition of BMP signaling appears to prevent neural crest emigration from the neural tube (Sela-Donenfeld and Kalcheim, 2000). RhoB is another molecule expressed by premigratory and early migrating neural crest cells (Liu and Jessell, 1998). It is an early response to a BMP signal and may be involved in the epithelial/mesenchymal transition occurring during neural crest emigration.

The zinc finger transcription factor *Slug* marks neural crest populations in the frog and chick (Nieto et al., 1994; Mayor, 1995) prior to emigration and during early stages of migration. Furthermore, *Slug* appears to be required for the process of leaving the neural tube and has been proposed to play a general role in epithelial-mesenchymal transitions and onset of cell motility. Antisense experiments in chick (Nieto et al., 1994) and in a mammalian cell line (Savagner et al., 1997) suggest that *Slug* is required for aspects of the epithelial/mesenchymal transition that precede migration in both neural crest cells and other mesenchymal cells. In the frog, *Slug* functions as a transcriptional repressor and plays an important role in formation of the neural crest as well as in emigration from the neural tube (LaBonne and Bronner-Fraser, 2000). However, *Slug* alone is not sufficient to induce neural crest development (LaBonne and Bronner-Fraser, 2000). Thus, this transcription factor is necessary but not sufficient to commit a cell to a neural crest fate.

Neural crest cells undergo a change in adhesion molecules as a function of their migration. While within the neuroepithelium, neural tube cells express high levels of N-cadherin and cadherin-6B (Nakagawa and Takeichi, 1998). After emigrating, N-cadherin is down-regulated as cadherin-6B is down-regulated in newly formed neural crest cells, and cadherin-7 expression increases in the migrating neural crest population. This suggests that a shift in cell surface and adhesive properties may accompany the onset of migratory behavior.

NEURAL CREST MIGRATION

Initiation of neural crest cell migration proceeds in a head-to-tailward (rostrocaudal) wave that follows closure of the neural tube. After emigration, these cells move in a highly patterned fashion through neighboring tissues. They localize in diverse but characteristic sites within the embryo, giving rise to diverse and numerous derivatives ranging from pigment cells and cranial cartilage to adrenal chromaffin cells and ganglia of the peripheral nervous system. At all axial levels, neural crest cells exhibit an orderly pattern in the timing of migration, contributing to their derivatives in a ventral-to-dorsal sequence (Serbedzija et al., 1989).

Several types of cell marking techniques, such as quail/chick chimera, molecular markers, and 1,1′-dioctadecyl-3,3,3′,3′-tetramethylindocarbocyanine perchlorate (DiI) labeling, have made it possible to identify the pathways followed by migrating neural crest cells. These migratory pathways and the derivatives formed by neural crest cells are regionalized according to their axial level of origin, such that cells from a given axial level give rise to a characteristic array of progeny and follow distinct pathways from those at other axial levels (Noden, 1975; Kalcheim and LeDouarin, 1999). The different populations of neural crest cells arising along the neural axis have been designated *cranial, vagal, trunk, and lumbosacral* (Fig. 1.3). Distinct cell types differentiate from these different populations.

At the cranial neural crest, cells arise from the forebrain, midbrain, and rostral hindbrain levels. These cells exhibit a wide range of developmental potential, with some cranial crest cells contributing to the cranial sensory ganglia and the parasympathetic ciliary ganglia of the eye, whereas others migrate ventrally to form many of the cartilaginous elements of the facial skeleton. Precise quail/chick grafting experiments have determined the regions of neural tube from which neural crest cells arise to contribute to cartilaginous elements. Cranial neural crest cells contribute to the quadrate, Meckel's cartilage and surrounding membrane bones, cartilage of the tongue, and membrane bones of the upper jaw and skull (Noden, 1978; Couly et al., 1992, 1993). Cranial neural crest cells can be subdivided further into regions designated *caudal forebrain, midbrain, rostral hindbrain,* and *caudal hindbrain* (which overlaps with rostral vagal) neural crest cells; each group has a somewhat different pattern of migration and prospective derivatives. For example, neural crest cells originating in the midbrain migrate as a broad, unsegmented sheet under the ectoderm; they contribute to derivatives ranging from the periocular skeleton, connective tissue, and membranous bones of the face to the ciliary and trigeminal ganglia (Kalcheim and LeDouarin, 1999). Neural crest cells arising in the hindbrain migrate ventrally and enter the branchial arches to form the bones of the jaw.

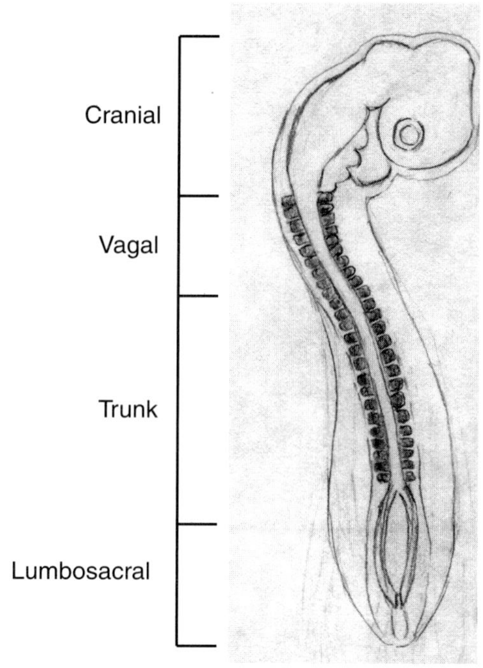

FIGURE 1.3. Different populations of neural crest cells arise at different levels of the embryonic axis. Neural crest cells that arise at different rostrocaudal levels follow different migratory pathways and give rise to different derivatives. From rostral to caudal, these are referred to as *cranial, vagal, trunk,* and *lumbosacral* populations.
Source: Paige Fraser.

Vagal neural crest cells migrate long distances to form the enteric nervous system of the gut, which also receives a contribution from the lumbosacral neural crest. Within the gut, the earliest-generated crest cells move as a wave from anterior to posterior to populate the bowel. In contrast to vagal neural crest cells that migrate long distances along the body axis to form the enteric ganglia, trunk neural crest cells fail to invade gut tissue immediately below their migratory pathways.

Trunk neural crest cells follow two primary migratory pathways (Weston, 1963): a dorsolateral pathway between the ectoderm and somite and a ventral pathway through the rostral half of the somitic sclerotome (Rickmann et al., 1985). The cells following the dorsolateral stream give rise to melanocytes. Those cells following the ventral pathway give rise to the peripheral nervous system of the trunk, including the chain of sympathetic ganglia and the dorsal root ganglia, as well as the chromaffin cells of the adrenal medulla. In addition to neurons, these cells generate glia of the peripheral ganglia and Schwann cells that ensheath and myelinate peripheral axons.

SEGMENTAL MIGRATION OF NEURAL CREST CELLS

Inherent segmentation is a hallmark of the developing peripheral nervous system. Accordingly, both cranial and trunk neural crest cells destined to form peripheral ganglia exhibit a segmental pattern of migration (Fig. 1.4). At trunk levels, after neural crest cells migrate from the neural tube and through the somites, they condense to form segmentally arranged sensory and sympathetic ganglia. For each somite, a single sensory ganglion and a sympathetic ganglion form. The relationship between neural crest cells and their surroundings tissues has been explored by manipulating the neural tube and/or somites in a series of grafting experiments. Removal of the somites results in the failure of segmentation of neural crest–derived ganglia, suggesting that somites are necessary for the segmentation of the neural crest. On the other hand, inversion of the segmental plate in the rostrocaudal dimension reverses the pattern of neural crest migration (Bronner-Fraser and Stern, 1991), such that neural crest cells migrate through the caudal (original rostral) halves of the rotated sclerotomes.

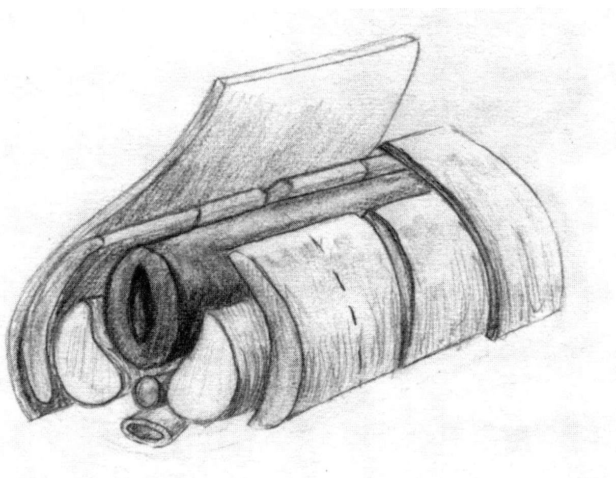

FIGURE 1.4. Neural crest cells migrate in a segmental pattern in the trunk. Neural crest cells migrate selectively through the anterior (A) portion of each somite but fail to migrate through the posterior (P) portion. These cells subsequently form dorsal root and sympathetic ganglion plus support cells. Other cells migrate over the somites in a nonsegmental pattern and form melanocytes

Other experimental manipulations demonstrate that the caudal-half somite is inhibitory, whereas the rostral-half somite is permissive for neural crest migration and motor axon guidance. Construction of somites with all rostral or all caudal-half sclerotomes results in the absence of segmentation or the absence of migration, respectively, for both neural crest cells and motor axons (Stern and Keynes, 1987). Taken together, these findings demonstrate that segmental migration of both neural crest cells and motor axons is due to cues inherent in the somite. These cues may be caused by attractive signals in the rostral-half sclerotome, inhibitory cues in the caudal-half sclerotome, or a combination of both.

Neural crest cell migration in the hindbrain is also segmented into three broad streams adjacent to rhombomere 2 (r2), r4, and r6, whereas no neural crest cells are apparent adjacent to r3 and r5. Focal injections of DiI at the levels of r3 and r5 and have demonstrated that both of these rhombomeres generate neural crest cells. The segmental distribution of neural crest cells resulted from the DiI-labeled cells that originated in r3 and r5 deviating rostrally or caudally and failing to enter the adjacent preotic mesoderm or otic vesicle region (Sechrist et al., 1993).

BOTH PERMISSIVE AND REPULSIVE CUES GUIDE NEURAL CREST CELL MIGRATION

After leaving the neural tube, neural crest cells encounter extracellular spaces that are rich in extracellular matrix molecules like fibronectin, laminin, collagens, and proteoglycans. These may serve as a good migratory substrate, and neural crest cells have abundant integrin receptors on their surfaces that mediate adhesion to these substrata. Microinjection of integrin antibodies (Bronner-Fraser, 1985, 1986) into embryos during cranial neural crest migration causes severe perturbations in neural crest development in the head. In addition, function-blocking antibodies that interfere with the α_4 subunit of integrin cause a number of interesting defects in neural crest cell movement in trunk explants (Kil et al., 1998). However, the segmental pattern of migration is unperturbed in these explants. These results suggest that perturbing integrin function alters the properties of migratory cells but not the overall metameric pattern of migration. Thus, cell–matrix interactions may play a permissive role in the segmental migration of neural crest cells through the somites, but they cannot play an instructive one.

Eph receptor tyrosine kinases and their ligands display intriguing patterns of expression in the developing nervous system. Their distributions are consistent with potentially important roles in early neural crest migration. Eph receptors are functionally divided into two subclasses: Eph A receptors, which interact primarily with a glycosylphosphatidylinositol (GPI)-linked subclass of ligands, and Eph B receptors, which interact primarily with a transmembrane subclass of ligands (Gale et al., 1996).

Neural crest cells migrate segmentally through the somites as described above. After differentiation, the sclerotomal compartment of the somite is subdivided into rostral and caudal halves. An Eph receptor, EphB3 in chick and EphB1 in rat, is expressed on neural crest cells as they migrate through the somites (Krull et al., 1997; Wang and Anderson, 1997). The cognate ephrin B1 ligand is expressed in a reciprocal pattern in the caudal portion of the sclerotome through which neural crest cells fail to migrate. Addition of exogenous ligand as a competitive inhibitor disrupts the segmental pattern of neural crest migration, demonstrating that the ligand is sufficient to inhibit neural crest migration (Krull et al., 1997). This suggests that interactions between Eph receptors and ephrin ligands restrict neural crest migration; this, in turn, leads to the subsequent metameric migration of neural crest cells and the subsequent organization of neural crest–derived sensory and sympathetic ganglia. These results raise the interesting possibility that much of neural crest cell guidance comes from negative cues that prevent this highly motile cell type from entering particular sites and thus constrain them to delimited pathways.

In the cranial region as well, interactions between Eph receptors and their ligands appear to provide patterning information. For example, the receptors EphA4 and EphB1 are expressed by migrating neural crest cells and mesodermal cells of the third and fourth branchial arches of *Xenopus* (Smith et al., 1997). In contrast, the ephrin B2 ligand is expressed in a complementary pattern in the adjacent second branchial arch neural crest and mesoderm. Inhibition of receptor/ligand signaling causes abnormal neural crest migration, with crest cells that normally populate the third branchial arch invading adjacent arches. These findings suggest that interactions between Eph receptors and ligands help segregate cranial neural crest cells into distinct streams that populate alternate branchial arches (Smith et al., 1997).

NEURAL CREST DIVERSIFICATION

Neural crest cells have been shown to have stem cell properties (Stemple and Anderson, 1992)—that is, the ability to form multiple differentiated cell types from a single precursor that can also renew itself. Both the environment and properties of neural crest cells themselves have been proposed to account for cell fate decisions. Timing is certainly a factor, since the latest migrating cells populate only the most dorsal neural crest derivatives such as dorsal root ganglia and melanocytes (Serbedzija et al., 1989). However, late-migrating neural crest–like cells travel along neural crest pathways and form sympathetic and sensory neurons after transplantation to younger embryos (Korade and Frank, 1996; Sharma et al., 1995), demonstrating that some neural crest stem-like-cells persist at later times. Thus, restriction in fate may sometimes reflect the available environment rather than the time of emigration from the neural tube. Further evidence that environmental factors can influence cell fate comes from experiments showing that clonal cultures of neural crest cells can form glia when cultured in glial growth factor, smooth muscle when cultured in the presence of TGF-β, sympathetic neurons when cultured in BMP-2, and pigment cells when cultured in endothelin (Shah et al., 1994, 1995, 1996, 1997; LeDouarin and Dupin, 2003). Thus, growth factors that have region-specific patterns of localization may influence the differentiation of multipotent neural crest precursors during and/or after their migration.

This does not, however, rule out the possibility of some fate restrictions that are intrinsic to the population. One example of this was demonstrated by Perez and colleagues (1999), who found that the basic helix-loop-helix transcription factors neurogenin 1 and neurogenin 2 are involved in early specification of sensory neurons. Ectopic expression of the molecules biases migrating neural crest cells to localize and express markers characteristic of the sensory neuron. Thus, there is evidence for both the influence timing of emigration and environmental cues in determining the neural crest cell fate.

CONCLUSIONS

The neural crest is a highly migratory population of cells that forms on the dorsal side of the closing neural tube. Its formation is mediated by complex inductive interactions that are likely to involve multiple factors working sequentially and/or in concert. *Wnt*'s play an important role in the early phase of neural crest induction by the nonneural ectoderm. Bone morphogenetic proteins are also involved in aspects of neural crest formation, which are likely to include maintenance of the newly formed cells and their emigration from the neural tube. In addition, FGF signaling has been implicated in neural crest formation. Once induced, neural crest precursors express a broad repertoire of new genes that aid their transition from a nonmotile to a motile cell type. They subsequently emigrate from the neural tube and migrate along defined pathways, where they appear to be guided by a combination of inhibitory and permissive cues. They differentiate into an array of cell types as diverse as neurons, glia, and craniofacial cartilage. This evolutionarily important cell type plays a key role in early formation of the vertebrate nervous system.

REFERENCES

Amaya E, Musci TJ, Kirschner MW (1991). Expression of a dominant negative mutant of the FGF receptor disrupts mesoderm formation in *Xenopus* embryos. Cell 66:257–270.

Artinger K, Fraser S, Bronner-Fraser M (1995). Dorsal and ventral cell types can arise from common neural tube progenitors. Dev Biol 172:591–601.

Basch ML, Selleck MA, Bronner-Fraser M (2000). Timing and competence of neural crest formation. Dev Neurosci 22:217–227.

Basler K, Edlund T, Jessell T, Yamada T (1993). Control of cell pattern in the neural tube: regulation of cell differentiation by *dorsalin-1,* a novel TGFβ family member. Cell 73:687–702.

Bronner-Fraser ME (1985). Alterations in neural crest migration by an antibody that affects cell adhesion. J Cell Biol 101:610–617.

Bronner-Fraser M (1986). An antibody to a receptor for fibronectin and laminin perturbs cranial neural crest development in vivo. Dev Biol 117:528–536.

Bronner-Fraser M, Fraser SE (1988). Cell lineage analysis reveals multipotentiality of some avian neural crest cells. Nature 335(8):161–164.

Bronner-Fraser M, Stern C (1991). Effects of mesodermal tissues on avian neural crest cell migration. Dev Biol 143:213–217.

Couly GF, Coltey PM, Le Douarin NM (1992). The developmental fate of the cephalic mesoderm in quail-chick chimeras. Development 114:1–15.

Couly GF, Coltey PM, Le Douarin NM (1993). The triple origin of the skull in higher vertebrates: a study in quail-chick chimeras. Development 117:409–429.

Deardorff MA, Tan C, Saint-Jeannet JP, Klein PS (2001). A role for frizzled 3 in neural crest development. Development 128:3655–3663.

Dickinson ME, Selleck MAJ, McMahon AP, Bronner-Fraser M (1995). Dorsalization of the neural tube by the non-neural ectoderm. Development 121:2099–2106.

Dupin E, Le Douarin NM (2003). Development of melanocyte precursors from the vertebrate neural crest. Oncogene 22:3016–3023.

Echelard Y, Epstein DJ, St-Jacques B, Shen L, Mohler J, McMahon JA, McMahon AP (1993). *Sonic hedgehog,* a member of a family of putative signaling molecules, is implicated in the regulation of CNS polarity. Cell 75:1417–1430.

Fraser SE, Bronner-Fraser M (1991). Migrating neural crest cells in the trunk of the avian embryo are multipotent. Development 112:913–920.

Gale NW, Holland S, Valenzuela, D, Flenniken A, Pan L, Henkemeyer M, Strebhardt K, Hirai H, Wilkinson DG, Pawson T, Davis S, Yancopoulos GD (1996). Eph receptors and ligands comprise two major specificity subclasses, and are reciprocally compartmentalized during embryogenesis. Neuron 17:9–19.

Gammill L, Bronner-Fraser M (2002). A genomic analysis of neural crest induction. Development 129:5731–5741.

Gammill L, Bronner-Fraser M (2003). Neural crest specification: migrating into genomics. Nat Rev Neurosci 4:795–805.

García-Castro M, Marcelle C, Bronner-Fraser M (2002). Ectodermal *Wnt* function as a neural crest inducer. Science 297:848–851.

Godsave SF, Durston AJ (1997). Neural induction and patterning in embryos deficient in FGF signaling. Int J Dev Biol 41:57–65.

Hall BK, and Hörstsadius S (1988). *The Neural Crest.* London: Oxford University Press.

Helms JA, Schneider RA (2003). Cranial skeletal biology. Nature 423:326–331.

His W (1868). *Untersuchungen über die erste Anlage des Wirbeltierleibes. Die erste Entwicklung des Hühnchens im Ei.* Leipzig: F. C. W. Vogel.

Kalcheim C, LeDouarin N (1999). New York: *The Neural Crest.* Cambridge University Press.

Kil S, Krull HCE, Cann G, Clegg D, Bronner-Fraser M (1998). The α_4 subunit of integrin is essential for neural crest migration Dev Biol 202:29–42.

Knecht A, Bronner-Fraser M (2002). Induction of the neural crest: a multigene process. Nat Rev Genet 3:453–461.

Korade Z, Frank E (1996). Restriction in cell fates of developing spinal cord cells transplanted to neural crest pathways. J Neurosci 16:7638–7648.

Krull CE, Lansford R, Gale NW, Marcelle C, Collazo A, Yancopoulos G, Fraser SE, Bronner-Fraser M (1997). Interactions between Eph-related receptors and ligands confer rostrocaudal polarity to trunk neural crest migration. Curr Biol 7:571–580.

LaBonne C, Bronner-Fraser M (1998). Neural crest cell induction in *Xenopus:* evidence for a two-signal model. Development 125:2403–2414.

LaBonne C, Bronner-Fraser M (2000). Snail-related transcriptional repressors are required in Xenopus for both the induction of the neural crest and its subsequent migration. Dev Biol 221:195–205.

Le Douarin NM, Dupin E (2003) Multipotentiality of the neural crest. Curr Opin Genet Dev 13:529–536.

Liem KF, Tremmi G, Jessell TM (1997). A role for the roof plate and its resident TGFbeta-related proteins in neuronal patterning in the dorsal spinal cord. Cell 91, 127–138.

Liem KF, Tremmi G, Roelink H, and Jessell TM (1995). Dorsal differentiation of neural plate cells induced by BMP-mediated signals from epidermal ectoderm. Cell 82:969–979.

Liu JP, Jessell TM (1998). A role for rhoB in the delamination of neural crest cells from the dorsal neural tube. Development 125:5055–5067

Marti E, Bumcrot DA, Takada R, McMahon AP (1995b). Requirement of 19K *sonic hedgehog* for induction of distinct ventral cell types in CNS explants. Nature 375:322–325.

Marti E, Takada R, Bumcrot DA, Sasaki H, McMahon AP (1995a). Distribution of *Sonic hedgehog* peptides in the developing chick and mouse embryo. Development 121:2537–2547.

Mayor R, Guerrero N, Martinez C (1997). Role of FGF and noggin in neural crest induction. Dev Biol 189:1–12.

Mayor TM, Morgan R, Sargent MG (1995). Induction of the prospective neural crest of *Xenopus.* Development 121:767–777.

Moury JD, Jacobson AG (1989). Neural fold formation at newly created boundaries between neural plate and epidermis in the axolotl. Dev Biol 133:44–57.

Moury JD, Jacobson AG (1990). The origins of neural crest cells in the axolotl. Dev Biol 141:243–253.

Nakagawa S, Takeichi M (1998). Neural crest emigration from the neural tube depends on regulated cadherin expression. Development 125:2963–2971.

Nieto AM, Sargent MG, Wilkinson DG, Cooke J (1994). Control of cell behavior during vertebrate development by *Slug,* a zinc finger gene. Science 264:835–839.

Noden DM (1975). An analysis of the migratory behavior of avian cephalic neural crest cells. Dev Biol 42:106–130.

Noden DM (1978). The control of avian cephalic neural crest cytodifferentiation. I. Skeletal and connective tissues. Dev Biol 67:296–312.

Perez SE, Rebelo S, Anderson DJ (1999). Early specification of sensory neuron fate revealed by expression and function of neurogenins in the chick embryo. Development 126:1715–1728.

Placzek M, Tessier-Levigne M, Jessell T, Dodd J (1990). Orientation of commissural axons in vitro in response to a floor plate derived chemoattractant. Dev Biol 110:19–30.

Rast JP, Amore G, Calestani C, Livi CB, Ransick A, Davidson EH (2000). Recovery of developmentally defined gene sets from high-density cDNA macroarrays. Dev Biol 228:270–286.

Rickmann M, Fawcett JW, Keynes RJ (1985). The migration of neural crest cells and growth cones of motor axons through the rostral half of the chick somite. J Embryo Exp Morphol 90:437–455.

Roelink H, Porter JA, Chiang C, Tanabe Y, Chang DT, Beachy PA, Jessell TM (1995). Floor plate and motor neuron induction by different concentrations of the amino-terminal cleavage product of sonic hedgehog autoproteolysis. Cell 81:445–455.

Rollhäuser-ter Horst J (1980). Neural crest replaced by gastrula ectoderm in Amphibia. Anat Embryol 160:203–211.

Ruffins S, Artinger KB, Bronner-Fraser M (1998). Early migrating neural crest cells can form ventral neural tube derivatives when challenged by transplantation. Dev Biol 203:295–304.

Saint-Jeannet JP, He X, Varmus HE, Dawid IB (1997). Regulation of dorsal fate in the neuraxis by Wnt-1 and Wnt-3a. Proc Natl Acad Sci USA. 94:13713–13718.

Santagati F, Rijli FM (2003). Cranial neural crest and the building of the vertebrate head. Nat Rev Neurosci 4:806–818.

Sasai N, Mizuseki K, Sasai Y (2001). Requirement of *FoxD3*-class signaling for neural crest determination in *Xenopus*. Development 128:2525–2536.

Savagner P, Yamada KM, Thiery JP (1997). The zinc-finger protein slug causes desmosome dissociation, an initial and necessary step for growth factor–induced epithelial-mesenchymal transition. J Cell Biol 137:1403–1419.

Sechrist J, Serbedzija G, Scherson T, Fraser S, Bronner-Fraser M (1993). Segmental migration of the hindbrain neural crest does not arise from segmental generation. Development 118:691–703.

Sela-Donenfeld D, Kalcheim C (2000). Inhibition of noggin expression in the dorsal neural tube by somitogenesis: a mechanism for coordinating the timing of neural crest emigration. Development 127:4845–4854.

Selleck MAJ, Bronner-Fraser M (1995). Origins of the avian neural crest: the role of neural plate-epidermal interactions. Development 121:525–538.

Selleck MAJ, Garcia-Castro M, Artinger KB, Bronner-Fraser M (1998). Effects of Shh and noggin on neural crest formation demonstrate that BMP is required in the neural tube but not ectoderm. Development 125:4919–4930.

Serbedzija G, Bronner-Fraser M, Fraser SE (1992). Vital dye analysis of cranial neural crest cell migration in the mouse embryo. Development 116:297–307.

Serbedzija GN, Fraser SE, Bronner-Fraser M (1989). A vital dye analysis of the timing and pathways of avian trunk neural crest cell migration. Development 106:809–816.

Shah NM, Anderson DA (1997). Integration of multiple instructive cues by neural crest stem cells reveals cell-intrinsic biases in relative growth factor responsiveness. Proc Natl Acad Sci USA 94:11369–11374.

Shah NM, Groves AK, Anderson DJ (1996). Alternative neural crest cell fates are instructively promoted by TGFb superfamily members. Cell 85:331–343.

Shah NM, Marchionni MA, Isaacs I, Stroobant PW, Anderson DJ (1994). Glial growth factor restricts mammalian neural crest stem cells to a glial fate. Cell 77:349–360.

Sharma K, Korade Z, Frank E (1995). Late-migrating neuroepithelial cells from the spinal cord differentiate into sensory ganglion cells and melanocytes. Neuron 14:143–152.

Smith A, Robinson V, Patel K, Wilkinson DG (1997). The EphA4 and EphB1 receptor tyrosine kinases and ephrin-B2 ligand regulate targeted migration of branchial neural crest cells. Curr Biol 7:561–570.

Smith J, Schoenwolf GC (1989). Notochordal induction of cell wedging in the chick neural plate and its role in neural tube formation. J Exp Zool 25:49–62.

Spokony RF, Aoki Y, Saint-Germain N, Magner-Fink E, Saint-Jeannet J-P (2002). The transcription factor Sox9 is required for canial neural crest development in Development 129:421–432.

Stemple DL Anderson DJ (1992). Isolation of a stem cell for neurons and glia derived from the mamalian neural crest. Cell 71:973–985.

Stern CD, Keynes RJ (1987). Interactions between somite cells: the formation and maintenance of segment boundaries in the chick embryo. Development 99:261–272.

Tessier-Lavigne M, Placzek M, Lumsden A, Dodd J, Jessell TM (1988). Chemotropic guidance of developing axons in the mammalian central nervous system. Nature 336:775–778.

Trainor P, Nieto MA (2003). Jawsfest: new perspectives on neural crest lineages and morphogenesis. Development 130:5059–5063.

van Straaten HWM, Hekking EJLM, Wiertz-Hoessels FT, Drukker J (1988). Effects of the notochord on the differentiation of a floor plate area in the neural tube of the chick embryo. Anat Embryol 177:317–324.

Vargesson N, Luria V, Messina I, Erskine L, Laufer E (2001). Expression patterns of Slit and Robo family members during vertebrate limb development. Mech Dev 106:175–180.

Wang HU, Anderson DJ (1997). Roles of Eph family transmembrane ligands in repulsive guidance of trunk neural crest migration and motor axon outgrowth. Neuron 18:383–396

Watanabe Y, Le Douarin NM (1996). A role for BMP-4 in the development of subcutaneous cartilage. Mech Dev 57:69–78.

Weston JA (1963). A radiographic analysis of the migration and localization of trunk neural crest cells in the chick. Dev Biol 6:279–310.

Yamada T, Placzek M, Tanaka H, Dodd J, Jessell TM (1991). Control of cell pattern in the developing nervous system: polarizing activity of the floor plate and notochord. Cell 64:635–647.

2

The Embryonic Basis of Neural Tube Defects

NICHOLAS D. E. GREENE
ANDREW J. COPP

Neural tube defects (NTDs) are severe abnormalities of the central nervous system (CNS) and are among the most common congenital malformations in humans. The clinical appearance of NTDs originates from failure of neurulation, the developmental process that results in formation of the neural tube, the primordium of the entire CNS. Therefore, in order to gain insight into the embryonic basis of NTDs, it is necessary to understand the morphologic processes and molecular mechanisms underlying neural tube closure. In this review, we will focus principally on the process of neurulation in mammals. The mouse is the most extensively studied mammalian experimental model, and findings from mice will be compared with human neurulation and NTDs wherever possible. Neural tube closure has also been described in detail in amphibia and birds, and these studies offer further insight into the pathogenesis of some aspects of neurulation and NTDs.

OVERVIEW OF THE PROCESS OF NEURULATION

Neurulation begins with formation of the neural plate, a thickening of the ectoderm on the dorsal surface of the early postgastrulation embryo. The neural plate, or neuroepithelium, is subsequently converted into the neural tube in a two-part process. Primary neurulation results in formation of the neural tube that will develop into the brain and most of the spinal cord. Although morphologic differences are observed between different classes of higher vertebrates, a unifying principle is that the neuroepithelium is subject to shaping and folding, with fusion in the midline to form the tube (Fig. 2.1). In contrast, the neural tube caudal to the midsacral region is formed by secondary neurulation (Schoenwolf, 1984; Copp and Brook, 1989). Instead of fusion of neural folds, the secondary neural tube is derived from a population of mesenchymal cells in the tail bud, which condenses to form an epithelial rod (Fig. 2.2). Canalization of this epithelium creates the secondary neural tube, the lumen of which is continuous with that of the primary neural tube (Schoenwolf, 1984). Secondary neurulation appears to be independent of primary neurulation since, in chick, it can occur when completion of primary closure is prevented experimentally (Costanzo et al., 1982). Although, the molecular mechanisms underlying neural tube closure are not completely understood, insights are being provided by the many (at least 80) mouse models in which NTDs occur as a result of genetic mutations (see Chapter 17).

Neural Tube Defects Result from Failure of Neurulation or Formation of the Axial Skeleton

The folding and fusion of the neural folds in primary neurulation occurs only in higher vertebrates, including amphibia, birds, and mammals. Open NTDs, in which the neural folds fail to appose and fuse, are therefore unique to these organisms and, moreover, occur only at levels of the body axis subject to primary neurulation. These defects (including spina bifida aperta/myelomeningocele and anencephaly in mammals) are characterized by exposure of the unfused neuroepithelium to the environment, with pathologic consequences including neuronal damage and degeneration (see Chapter 5). The majority of cases of open spina bifida are due to failure of primary neurulation. However, abnormalities in secondary neurulation can lead to closed forms of spina bifida in which the separation of the neural tube from surrounding tissues

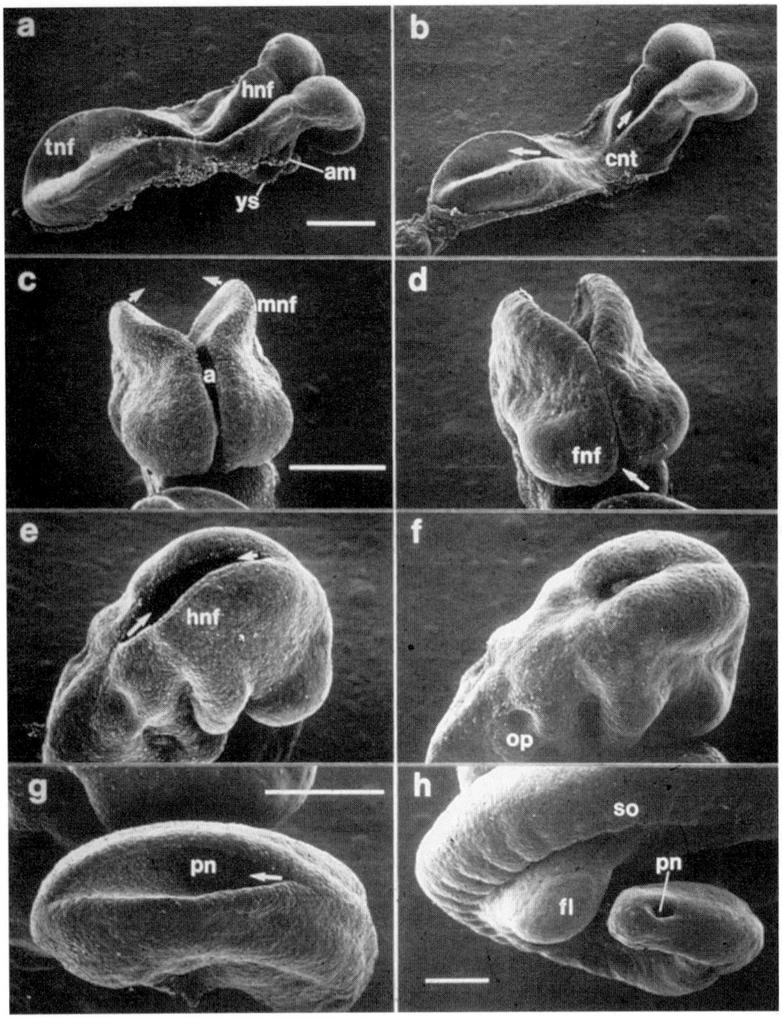

FIGURE 2.1. Morphological appearance of mouse embryos during primary neurulation. Scanning electron micrographs show the morphology of embryos immediately before (*a*) and after (*b*) initial fusion of the neural folds at the cervical/hindbrain boundary. Closure proceeds in cranial (*short arrow*) and caudal (*long arrow*) directions. A second site of initiation occurs at the forebrain/midbrain boundary, and the neural folds approach each other in the midline (*arrows* in *c*). Closure of the hindbrain occurs at E9.5 (*e,f*) due to progressive closure from the initiation sites in the cervical and cranial regions (*arrows* in *e*). Primary neurulation continues in a caudal direction (*arrow* in *g*) and is completed by closure of the posterior neuropore at E10.5 (*h*). Abbreviations: a, site of fusion at the forebrain/midbrain boundary; am, remaining fragment of the amnion; cnt, cervical neural tube; fl, forelimb bud; fnf, forebrain neural fold; hnf, hindbrain neural fold; mnf, midbrain neural fold; op, optic pit; pn, posterior neuropore; so, somites; tnf, thoracic neural fold; ys, torn edge of yolk sac. Scale bars represent 0.25 mm.

in the tail bud is abnormal. This commonly leads to *tethering* of the spinal cord to adjacent tissues, as also occurs in most cases of open spina bifida (Stiefel et al., 2003) (see Chapter 8). Tethering is associated with hydrocephaly and may lead to neuronal damage at the site of the defect due to differential rates of elongation of the spinal cord and vertebral column as the body axis lengthens during development.

The term *spina bifida* refers to the defects in the vertebral arches that obligatorily accompany open lesions. The vertebral arches form from the adjacent sclerotermal component of the axial mesoderm, which migrates to surround the closed neural tube and then differentiates to form the axial skeleton (and the skull vault at cranial levels). Where the neural folds remain open, the sclerotome is unable to cover the neuroepithelium and skeletogenesis occurs abnormally, such that the midline is exposed. In addition to open lesions that arise from failure of neural fold fusion (spina bifida aperta or myelomeningocele), another group of spina bifida malformations results from defects in development of the axial mesoderm such that the vertebral arches form abnormally, despite the completion of neural tube closure. Spina bifida occulta comprises "closed" defects in which vertebral arches are malformed but the lesion is skin-covered. Defects usually occur at the low lumbar and sacral regions and may be accompanied by tethering of the spinal cord (see above). Defects of the axial mesoderm that forms the vertebrae or cranium may also give rise to encephalocele or meningocele (spina bifida cystica) in which the closed neural tube herniates through the affected region of the skull or vertebral column, respectively (Harding and Copp, 2002). In the remainder of this chapter we will use the term *spina bifida* to refer to open defects unless specified.

Discontinuous Initiation of Neural Tube Closure

In mammals, unlike birds and amphibia, primary neural tube closure is initiated at several discrete points such that closure is a discontinuous process (Fig. 2.3). In mouse embryos the first site of closure (Closure 1) is located at the hindbrain/cervical boundary at embryonic

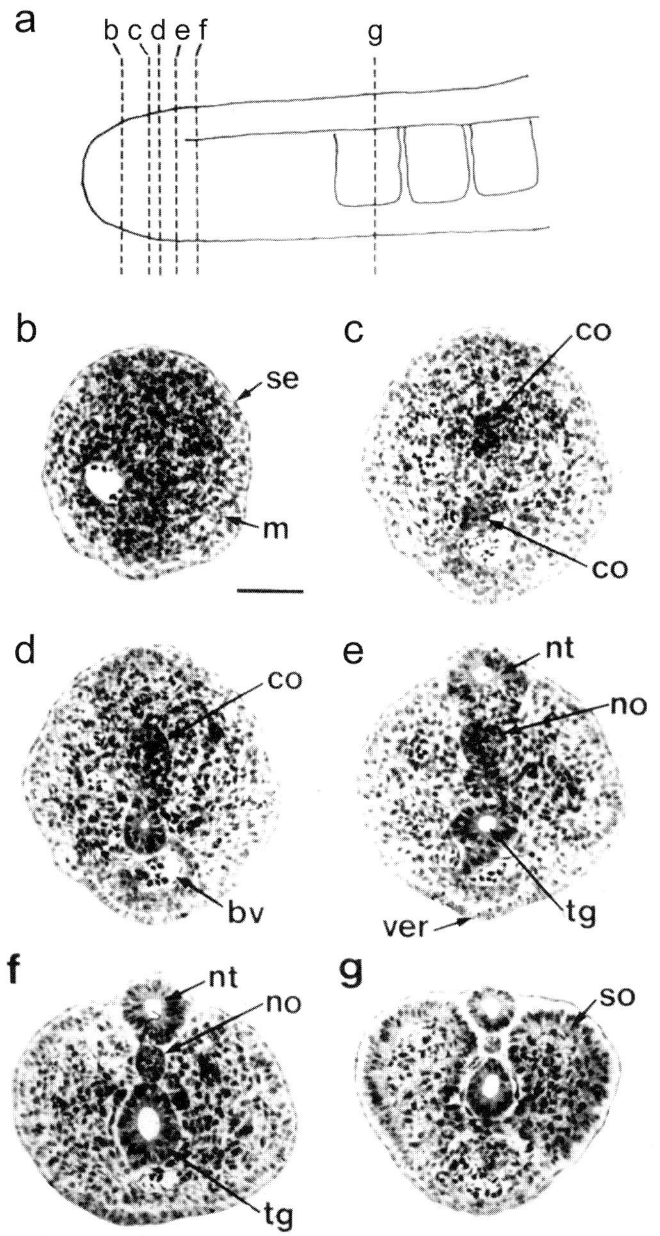

FIGURE 2.2. Secondary neurulation in the mouse embryo. The position of light microscopic sections through the caudal region of an E11.5 mouse embryo is shown diagrammatically (*a*). At the caudal extremity the tail bud consists of mesenchyme cells surrounded by surface ectoderm (*b*). Rostrally there is evidence of dorsally and ventrally located condensations (*c*), and further rostrally the mesenchymal condensations have enlarged and the ventral focus has cavitated to form tail gut (*d*). Cavitation of the dorsal condensation results in formation of the secondary neural tube (*e*). Ventral to the neural tube lies the notochord and roof of the tail gut. A typical cross section through the tail shows the neural tube, notochord, and tail gut (*f*), flanked at more cranial levels by epithelial somites (*g*). Abbreviations: bv, blood vessel; co, mesenchymal condensation; m, mesenchyme; no, notochord; nt, neural tube; se, surface ectoderm; so, somite; tg, tail gut; ver, ventral ectodermal ridge. Scale bar represents 0.1 mm.

day 8. Closure then progresses in both rostral and caudal directions into the regions of the future brain and spinal cord, respectively. In the cranial region, further sites of initiation occur at the forebrain/midbrain boundary (Closure 2) and at the rostral end of the forebrain (Closure 3). The open regions of neural folds between these discrete sites of initial closure are termed the *hindbrain neuropore* (between the sites of Closures 1 and 2) and *anterior neuropore* (between Closures 2 and 3). Cranial closure proceeds bidirectionally from the site of Closure 2 and in a caudal direction from Closure 3, causing the neuropores to shorten and finally close on embryonic day 9, although the exact timing of closure varies somewhat among mouse strains. Spinal neurulation occurs by progressive unidirectional closure, caudally from the site of Closure 1, and primary neurulation is completed by closure of the posterior neuropore on embryonic day 10.

In humans, neural plate bending begins at about 17–18 days after fertilization. It seems likely that discontinuous initiation of neural tube closure occurs in human embryos as in the mouse (Fig. 2.3). For example, events analogous to Closure 1 and 3 have been described in humans (Van Allen et al., 1993; O'Rahilly and Müller, 1994, 2002), although O'Rahilly and Müller (2002) suggest that the site of initial closure, equivalent to Closure 1, occurs at around 22 days postfertilization at a slightly more rostral level in humans than in mouse, being located in the rhomobencephalon as opposed to the rhombencephalon/cervical boundary. An event resembling Closure 3 certainly appears to occur at the extreme rostral end of the neural plate in human embryos, as in the mouse (O'Rahilly and Müller, 2002). The existence of an event equivalent to Closure 2 is more controversial. This has been described in some studies (Van Allen et al., 1993; Golden and Chernoff, 1995; Seller 1995a; Nakatsu et al., 2000) but not in others (O'Rahilly and Müller, 2002), suggesting that there may be variability in the position or occurrence of Closure 2. Primary neurulation is completed in human embryos with closure at the posterior neuropore 26–28 days after fertilization, following which secondary neurulation is a well-recognized feature of human development, leading to formation of the low sacral and coccygeal regions.

The Site of Closure 2 Is Polymorphic and Is a Risk Factor for Cranial Neural Tube Defects

Although the sites of Closure 1 and 3 are uniform among mouse strains, the site of Closure 2 varies. In some strains, such as DBA/2, Closure 2 occurs within the midbrain, caudal to the forebrain/midbrain boundary, whereas in others (e.g., NZW) Closure 2 occurs within the forebrain (Fleming and Copp, 2000). In extreme examples, Closure 2 occurs very rostrally, such that it is very close to Closure 3 and the two sites may even be indistinguishable,

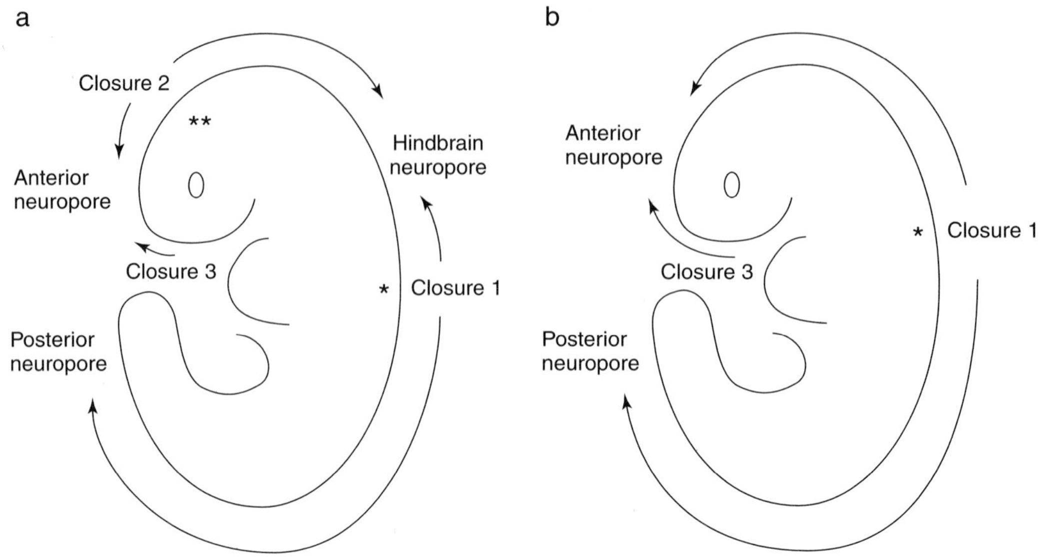

FIGURE 2.3. Schematic diagram of neural tube closure in mice (*a*) and humans (*b*). Neural tube closure is initiated by Closure 1 (single asterisk) at the hindbrain/cervical boundary in the mouse (*a*) and spreads caudally and rostrally from this site. Closure 1 in humans (*b*) may occur in the rhombencephalon, more rostrally than in the mouse. A second site of initial closure (Closure 2) occurs at the forebrain/midbrain boundary (double asterisks) in most mouse strains (*a*), although the position of the site of Closure 2 may vary among strains. This site may be absent in humans (*b*). Closure also initiates at the rostral limit of the forebrain (Closure 3) in the mouse, and an equivalent closure occurs in humans. Progress of neurulation from the initial sites of fusion results in shortening and closure of the anterior and hindbrain neuropores, indicated by arrows. Neurulation progresses caudally from the site of Closure 1 until fusion is finally completed by closure of the posterior neuropore. Secondary neurulation proceeds from the level of the closed posterior neuropore. *Source:* Modified from Copp et al. (1994).

as in the SELH/Bc strain (Gunn et al., 1993). The variation in the site of Closure 2 influences the susceptibility to development of NTDs. Crossing the *splotch* (Sp^{2H}) mutant allele onto the DBA/2 genetic background results in a caudal shift in the position of Closure 2 and a reduced incidence of exencephaly in homozygous embryos. In contrast, backcrossing Sp^{2H} onto the NZW background, which has a position of closure similar to that of the original Sp^{2H} strain, has no effect on the incidence of NTDs (Fleming and Copp, 2000). Similarly, the absence or extreme rostral position of Closure 2 in SELH/Bc mice is associated with a 10%–20% risk of exencephaly. This association appears to be causative since, in a cross of SELH/Bc with LM/Bc mice, in which Closure 2 occurs at the forebrain/midbrain boundary, the rostral Closure 2 location segregates with the increased susceptibility to NTDs (Gunn et al., 1992, 1995). Therefore, a rostral site of Closure 2 confers an increased risk of exencephaly, whereas a caudal site confers resistance to NTD. Since the position of Closure 2 seems also to vary in humans, this could be an important risk factor for NTDs.

Shaping and Folding of the Neuroepithelium

Conversion of the initially flat neural plate into the closed neural tube requires a complex sequence of shaping and bending that ultimately results in apposition of the neural folds. Shaping of the neuroepithelium ensures the subsequent formation of a tube as opposed to a spherical vesicle (Schoenwolf and Smith, 1990a). The rostrocaudal axis elongates as a result of growth of the caudal region of the embryo, which continues throughout the period of neural tube closure, as well as cellular convergent extension movements, which have recently been shown to be essential for initiation of closure (see below). Apicobasal elongation of cells as the neural plate forms is also predicted to contribute to narrowing (Colas and Schoenwolf, 2001).

Bending of the lateral edges of the neural plate produces folds that fuse in the midline to form the neural tube. In the cranial region the bending of the neural folds during closure is quite different from that in the spinal region. As they initially elevate, the neural folds assume a biconvex appearance in the midbrain with the tips of the folds facing away from the midline. In the second stage of cranial closure, the folds abruptly switch orientation to assume a biconcave shape in which the tips approach each other in the midline, allowing fusion to occur (Morriss-Kay, 1981; Morriss-Kay et al., 1994). The mechanisms controlling the complex bending of the neural folds during cranial neurulation are poorly understood, although there is evidence for roles of the underlying cranial mesenchyme and components of the actin cytoskeleton (see below).

Spinal neurulation contrasts with cranial closure in lacking a biconvex phase of neural fold elevation. Three differing closure morphologies (Fig. 2.4), termed *modes,* which differ in the number and location of the bending points in the neuroepithelium, have been described at varying axial levels and stages of spinal closure (Shum and Copp, 1996). Initial closure is characterized by the presence of a single bend in the midline above the notochord, the medial hinge point. The neural folds at the site of Closure 1 or subsequently at the posterior neuropore (PNP) are straight, resulting in a slit-shaped lumen once closure occurs. This morphology is observed at the PNP of embryos from the 6 to 15 somite stages. At the 16 to 23 somite stages PNP closure occurs at more caudal levels of the body axis, and here the neural folds exhibit additional lateral bending sites, the dorsolateral hinge points. At these levels the neural tube has a diamond-shaped lumen (mode 2). Finally, mode 3 closure occurs from the 24-somite stage on. At this stage and axial level, the PNP is characterized by the absence of a defined median hinge point but persistence of dorsal lateral hinge points such that the lumen of the closed neural tube is circular.

Variation in the Axial Level of Neural Tube Defects Reflects the Occurrence of Multiple Closure Sites

Open NTDs result from failure of primary neurulation and can occur at different levels of the body axis, both in humans and in mutant mouse strains (reviewed in Chapter 17). It has been proposed that all cases of anencephaly in humans result from failure of Closure 2, based on pathological analysis (Van Allen et al., 1993). However, incomplete closure of the cranial neural tube in mouse embryos may be caused by failure of one of the initiation events (Closure 2 or 3) or by a defect in the subsequent "zippering" and closure of the anterior or hindbrain neuropores following successful completion of Closures 2 and 3 (Fleming and Copp, 2000; Martinez-Barbera et al., 2002). While human anencephaly can be subdivided into those cases affecting predominantly the rostral brain and skull (mero-acrania) and those also affecting the posterior brain and skull (holo-acrania) (Seller, 1995b), there is no evidence to suggest that these NTD subtypes equate with failure of precise events of cranial neurulation during embryogenesis. It seems more likely that association of split face with anencephaly reflects failure of Closure 3. In the early stages of cranial NTDs the neural folds remain open and exposed to the environment, and the neuroepithelium characteristically appears to protrude from the developing brain, a phenotype known as *exencephaly.* The skull vault does not form over the open region, and subsequent degeneration of the exposed neural tissue gives rise to the typical appearance of anencephaly that is observed at birth (Wood and Smith, 1984).

Isolated defects may also occur at caudal levels of the body axis. Impairments of spinal neurulation delay the closure of the posterior neuropore, and in severe cases closure fails altogether, resulting in open spina bifida (myelomeningocele). The size of the lesion reflects the extent to which spinal neurulation is delayed. Spina bifida may occur either as an isolated defect or in combination with exencephaly. The occurrence of cranial NTDs or spina bifida as isolated defects or in combination is also reflected in the large number of mouse mutants that exhibit NTDs (reviewed in Chapter 17). The greater prevalence of cranial compared to spinal NTDs among mouse mutants perhaps indicates greater complexity in the

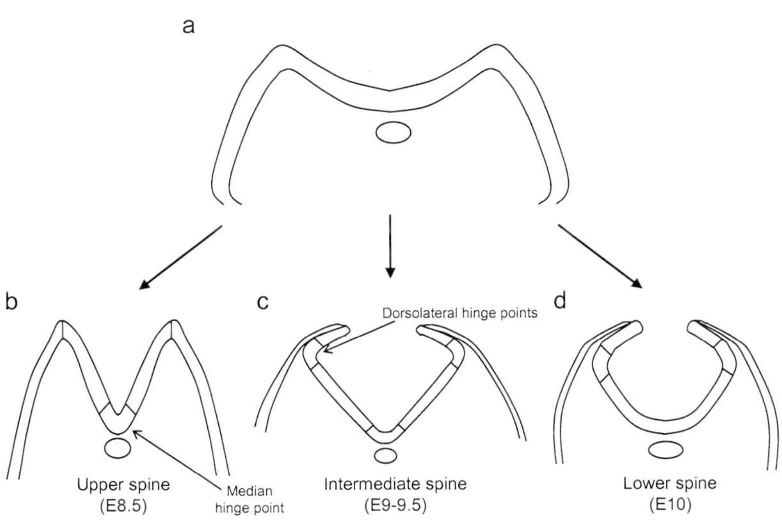

FIGURE 2.4. Differing morphology of spinal neurulation, as seen in a schematic transverse section. The posterior neuropore progresses along the body axis in a caudal direction during the developmental stages that encompass neural tube closure (E8.5–10.5). After initial neural fold bending (*a*), the morphology varies such that bending occurs only at the median hinge point (mode 1) at the upper spinal levels (*b*). At intermediate spinal levels (*c*), closure is characterized by the presence of median and dorsolateral hinge points (mode 2). In the lower spine at the final stages of posterior neuropore closure (*d*), dorsolateral hinge points are present but there is no median hinge point (mode 3). *Source:* Modified from Copp et al. (2003a).

process of cranial neurulation that results in sensitivity to a larger number of different genetic perturbations.

In addition to isolated lesions affecting the cranial or spinal neural tube, NTDs encompass defects, termed *craniorachischisis,* in which the entire neural tube from the midbrain to the low spine remains open. Craniorachischisis is the most severe form of NTD and, like anencephaly, is invariably lethal. Several genetic mutant models of craniorachischisis have been identified in the mouse (see Chapter 17), and NTDs in these mice closely resemble the corresponding human defects. Analysis of the embryonic development of craniorachischisis in mice indicates that the fundamental neurulation defect is failure of Closure 1, the initial closure event (Copp et al., 1994). In mouse craniorachischisis mutants, Closures 2 and 3 occur normally, so that the forebrain and rostral midbrain are generally unaffected (Greene et al., 1998; Murdoch et al., 2003). The relatively normal appearance of the forebrain in many human cases of craniorachischisis suggests that Closures 2 and 3 also occur normally in these individuals. Therefore, the genetic requirement for initial closure of the neural tube differs from that for subsequent closure sites.

The Mechanism of Neural Tube Closure Varies at Different Axial Levels

Several lines of evidence indicate that the mechanism of neural tube closure varies along the body axis. The morphologic appearance of the neuroepithelium differs during closure in the cranial region and at different axial levels of the future spine, suggesting that the shaping process differs. Moreover, the occurrence of isolated NTDs at cranial or caudal levels in humans and in different mouse mutants also suggests that there are region-specific mechanisms that are dependent on different gene products (Copp et al., 2003a). Similarly, several of the teratogens that cause NTD act specifically at either cranial or caudal levels. For instance, valproic acid causes spina bifida but not anencephaly in humans.

DRIVING FORCES IN NEURULATION

In the first part of this chapter we described the morphologic process of neural tube closure, involving shaping and fusion of the neural folds. We will now discuss the mechanisms underlying this process. These can be broadly classified as (*1*) forces that drive neurulation and (2) additional factors that are required for neural tube closure but are not necessarily directly responsible for the observed morphologic changes. The group of active processes required for closure includes convergent extension cell movements, expansion of the cranial mesenchyme, contraction of actin microfilaments, regulated bending of the neural plate, and adhesion of the neural folds. In different mouse models, cranial neurulation is more commonly perturbed than spinal neurulation, suggesting several different mechanisms that contribute to closure in the cranial region (summarized in Fig. 2.5). Processes that may be permissive rather than actively involved in the closure process include apoptosis and emigration of neural crest cells. However, it should be emphasized that the distinction between active and permissive processes is somewhat artificial since failure of any of these events can result in the development of NTDs.

The key forces driving the process of neurulation can also be considered as either intrinsic or extrinsic to the neuroepithelium. Intrinsic forces include convergent extension cell movements and the regulated formation of dorsolateral hinge points (Sections 1 and 4 below). Extrinsic forces that have been proposed include expansion of the cranial mesenchyme (Section 2) and, in birds, a requirement for the epidermal ectoderm that flanks the closing neural folds (Schoenwolf, 1988; Hackett et al., 1997).

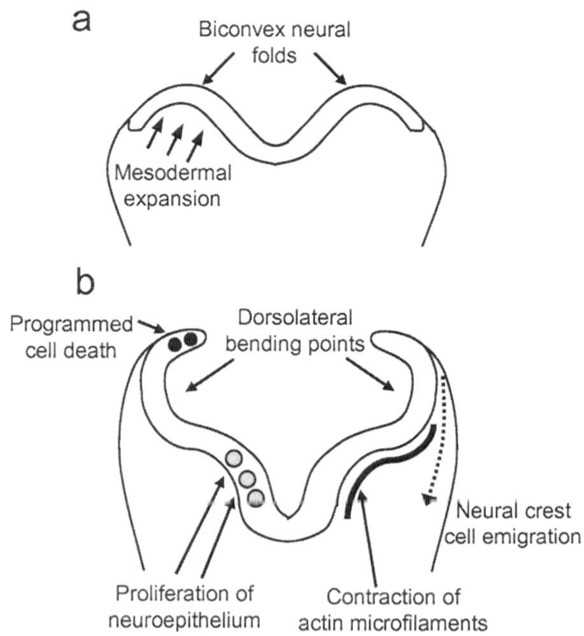

FIGURE 2.5. Potential contributory factors in cranial neurulation. The scheme shows the principal mechanisms required for midbrain cranial neural tube closure, as indicated by studies of mouse mutants. Mechanisms are depicted unilaterally for simplicity, although they occur bilaterally. Expansion of the cranial mesoderm assists the initial elevation of the neural folds with a biconvex morphology (*a*). The neural folds subsequently "flip around" and exhibit dorsolateral bending (*b*), assisted by contraction of subapical actin microfilaments, maintenance of a proliferative neuroepithelium, emigration of the neural crest, and localized apoptosis (programmed cell death). Apoptotic cell death at the tips of the neural folds is also involved in remodeling of the epithelia following closure. *Source:* Modified from Copp et al. (2003a).

Initiation of Neural Tube Closure Depends on Convergent Extension and Components of the Planar Cell Polarity Pathway

Recent research suggests that the embryonic process of convergent extension is one of the key requirements for initiation of neural tube closure (Copp et al., 2003b). Convergent extension was first described in amphibia as the process that accounts for the narrowing and lengthening of the neural plate during neurulation (Keller et al., 1985, 2000). The neural plate initially has a disc shape and then becomes longer and narrower concomitant with formation of neural folds at the lateral edges. Maps of cell position during neurulation based on time-lapse or video photography show that there is an overall movement of cells toward the midline. On cell trajectory maps, cells at the lateral edges of the neural plate exhibit principally mediolateral movement, whereas cells at the midline mainly move in an anterior direction. Intercalation of cells in the mediolateral direction, therefore, narrows the neural plate (convergence) and drives an increase in length (extension) along the anterior-posterior axis (Jacobson and Gordon, 1976; Keller et al., 1992). As convergent extension proceeds, the elevated neural folds approach the midline, and subsequently appose and fuse. In contrast, failure of this process gives rise to short, broad embryos in which the neural folds remain apart and do not close, leading to a spina bifida–like appearance (Wallingford and Harland, 2001; Goto and Keller, 2002; Wallingford et al., 2002; Takeuchi et al., 2003). In the chick embryo, closure of the neural tube in the brain is also coincident with rapid lengthening of the neural plate. Moreover, ultraviolet treatment that suppresses elongation of the neural plate also prevents neural tube closure, suggesting that elongation (or *extension*) may be necessary for closure (Jacobson, 1984).

At the molecular level, convergent extension in vertebrates appears to depend on the planar cell polarity signaling pathway that was first described in the fly, *Drosophila melanogaster,* as being responsible for the unidirectional array of bristles in the wing and ommatidia in the eye (Adler, 2002; Mlodzik, 2002). This pathway is commonly referred to as a *noncanonical Wnt signaling pathway* since it shares components of the *Wnt* signaling pathway, such as *Frizzled membrane* receptors, but does not involve downstream signaling via stabilization of beta-catenin. One of the key molecules in both canonical and noncanonical *Wnt* signaling is *dishevelled (dsh),* a cytoplasmic protein that contains DIX, DEP, and PDZ domains. Overexpression of mutant forms of *dsh* allows specific inhibition of noncanonical *Wnt* signaling in embryos of the frog, *Xenopus laevis,* and results in inhibition of convergent extension and failure of neural tube closure (Wallingford and Harland, 2002). Detailed discussion of the molecular pathway downstream of *dishevelled,* which appears to occur through the action of one or more kinases including Rho kinase, Jun kinase, and protein kinase C, is outside the scope of this chapter but is the subject of recent reviews (Mlodzik, 2002; Sheldahl et al., 2003). The function of other components of the PCP pathway, *strabismus, prickle,* and *glypican-4,* have also been experimentally disturbed in *Xenopus* embryos; in each case, convergent extension was inhibited (Darken et al., 2002; Goto and Keller, 2002; Ohkawara et al., 2003; Takeuchi et al., 2003). The role of convergent extension in neural tube closure appears to be most significant at the midline, since overexpression of mutant *dsh* in the *Xenopus* lateral neural plate does not inhibit neural tube closure (Wallingford and Harland, 2002). At the midline, cell movement is principally in an anterior direction, suggesting that extension, as opposed to convergence, may be the key driving force required for initiation of closure.

The recent identification of the mutant genes in several mouse models of craniorachischisis has also focused attention on the role of the planar cell polarity pathway in initiation of neural tube closure in mammals (see Chapter 17). Mouse embryos that are homozygous for mutations in *Dishevelled* (*Dsh* 1/2), *Vangl2* (homologous to *Drosophila Strabismus*), *Scribble,* or *Celsr1* (homologous to *Drosophila Flamingo*), genes that are implicated in the planar cell polarity pathway, all exhibit failure of Closure 1 (Murdoch et al., 2001a, 2001b; Hamblet et al., 2002; Curtin et al., 2003). An abnormality in convergent extension has yet to be conclusively demonstrated in these mutants, but the broad neural plate and reduced axial length observed in at least two of the mutants, *loop-tail* (*Vangl2* mutant) and *circle-tail* (*scribble* mutant), suggests that this is the primary defect (Greene et al., 1998; Murdoch et al., 2003). Planar cell polarity (PCP) pathway genes that play a role in convergent extension are thus good candidates as the causative genes for NTD, particularly craniorachischisis, in humans.

Cranial Neurulation Requires Expansion of the Cranial Mesenchyme

In the cranial region, elevation of the neural folds is preceded by an increase in extracellular space and in the rate of proliferation in the subjacent cranial mesenchyme (Morriss and Solursh, 1978b). These factors result in expansion of the cranial mesenchyme and are hence proposed to play a major role in determining the biconvex morphology that characterizes closure of the cranial neural folds (Fig. 2.3), as described above (Morriss-Kay, 1981). The increase in space within the cranial mesenchyme during neurulation is largely due to an increase in the abundance of highly hydrated extracellular matrix molecules, particularly hyaluronan, in addition to accumulation of other matrix constituents including heparan and chondroitin sulfate proteoglycans, fibronectin, and laminin (Solursh and Morriss, 1977; Morriss and Solursh, 1978a; Tuckett and Morriss-Kay, 1986). Evidence for a key role of mesenchymal expansion in neural fold elevation is provided by experimental disruption of the mesenchyme and by knockout mouse strains. Treatment of rat embryos in culture with hyaluronidase that digests extracellular matrix hyaluronan results in collapse of the cranial mesenchyme and causes delay of cranial neural tube closure (Morriss-Kay et al., 1986). In *Cart1* knockout mouse embryos, there is a more extreme depletion of forebrain mesenchyme resulting from an increased rate of apoptosis, and this is associated with failure of cranial closure and consequent exencephaly (Zhao et al., 1996). A deficit of cranial mesenchyme caused by reduced proliferation, as opposed to increased apoptosis, is also associated with cranial NTD in *Twist* knockout mice (Chen and Behringer, 1995).

Integrity of the Actin Cytoskeleton Is Essential for Cranial Neurulation

One of the long-standing questions in studies of neurulation concerns the potential role of the cytoskeleton in formation and movement of the neural folds (Nagele and Lee, 1980; Sadler et al., 1982; Schoenwolf et al., 1988). Actin microfilaments, and actin-associated proteins such as MARCKs, are localized circumferentially at the apical region of cells in the neural folds such that the future lumen is bordered by actin (Sadler et al., 1982; Ybot-Gonzalez and Copp, 1999; Zolessi and Arruti, 2001). An obvious implication of this asymmetric distribution in the neuroepithelium is that constriction of apically located microfilaments reduces the apical surface of neuroepithelial cells and contributes to bending and closure of the neural folds. Indeed, experimental disruption of the actin cytoskeleton by cytochalasins has reproducibly been found to cause exencephaly in cultured rodent embryos, indicating a role in neural tube closure (Morriss-Kay and Tuckett, 1985; Matsuda and Keino, 1994; Ybot-Gonzalez and Copp, 1999). However, treatment at different stages of neural tube closure suggests that there is a differential requirement for the cytoskeleton at different axial levels. Exposure of cultured mouse embryos to cytochalasin D inhibits not only cranial closure but also Closure 1, although at higher doses than those required to induce exencephaly (Ybot-Gonzalez and Copp, 1999). These observations suggest that elevation or apposition of the neural folds at the initial closure site and in the future brain depends on the integrity of the actin microfilaments. It remains unclear whether there is an active role of microfilament contraction or whether the cytoskeleton acts simply to stabilize the elevating folds. It is also likely that reorganization of the actin cytoskeleton plays a role in the polarized cell movements that are integral to convergent extension that is essential for Closure 1 (Wallingford et al., 2002; Copp et al., 2003a). The occurrence of exencephaly in several mouse mutants in which cytoskeletal function is disturbed (Chapter 17) provides further evidence for a critical role in cranial closure.

In contrast to the cranial region, spinal neurulation appears resistant to cytochalasin D since closure continues in treated embryos, although toxicity of this agent precludes analysis of closure throughout the entire period of spinal neurulation (Ybot-Gonzalez and Copp, 1999). Significantly, the characteristic hinge points at the posterior neuropore are maintained in cytochalasin D–treated embryos despite the disruption of the apical arrangement of actin in these embryos, whereas the nonbending regions lose their rigidity. Interestingly, however, targeted mutant mice that lack the F-actin-binding protein Shroom exhibit a low frequency of spina bifida in addition to the more prevalent phenotype of exencephaly (Hildebrand and Soriano, 1999). The reason for the failure of posterior neuropore closure in this mutant is not clear, but it appears likely that disruption of neuroepithelial apicobasal polarity is a critical factor.

Regulation of Hinge Point Formation in Spinal Neurulation

The defined bending of the neuroepithelium at the median hinge point (MHP) and dorsolateral hinge points (DLHP) is regulated by mutually antagonistic signals external to the neural folds. Experimental manipulation of chick embryos suggests that the MHP is induced by signals from the notochord since implantation of notochord fragments adjacent to the neural tube induces regions of bending with basally located nuclei, as at the MHP (Van Straaten et al., 1985; Van Straaten et al., 1988; Smith and Schoenwolf, 1989). Conversely, suppression of notochord development through ablation of the node results in the absence of an MHP in both chick and mouse embryos (Smith and Schoenwolf, 1989; Davidson et al., 1999; Ybot-Gonzalez et al., 2002). In contrast to the MHP, the presence of DLHP does not depend on signals from the notochord; rather, suppression of the notochord leads to the formation of DLHP at axial levels that are normally characterized by mode 1 (MHP only) closure (Ybot-Gonzalez et al., 2002). Therefore, spinal neural tube closure continues in the absence of the MHP by a "default" mechanism involving DLHPs only. However, the development of DLHP does depend on signals from the surface ectoderm, since unilateral removal of the surface ectoderm results in loss of dorsolateral bending of the subjacent neural fold (Ybot-Gonzalez et al., 2002). The specific molecular nature of the dorsal signals has not been determined. Dorsal bending appears to play a more active role in neural tube closure than midline bending since suppression of wedging at the DLHP inhibits closure in the chick, unlike suppression of the MHP (Schoenwolf and Smith, 1990b). The dependence of closure on DLHPs is yet to be proven in the mouse, although it is highly unlikely that closure can occur in the absence of both median and lateral bending.

Sonic hedgehog (Shh) has been implicated as the signal from the notochord that induces the floor plate of the neural tube, which differentiates at the same site as the MHP and has been regarded as synonomous with it (Placzek et al., 1990; Yamada et al., 1991; Chiang et al., 1996). The lack of requirement for an MHP in neural tube closure is supported by the fact that spinal NTDs do not arise in mouse embryos lacking *Shh,* HNF3β (Fox a2), Gli2, or Gli 1/2 (Ang and Rossant, 1994; Chiang et al., 1996; Weinstein et al., 1994; Ding et al., 1998; Matise et al., 1998; Park et al., 2000), all of which fail to form a floor plate. In these targeted mouse mutants the lumen of the neural tube is circular, suggesting that closure occurs by a DLHP-dependent mechanism. However, recent evidence suggests that, at least in the case of *Shh* null embryos, MHP formation occurs despite the fact that a floor plate is not formed. Therefore, induction of the floor plate and the MHP appear to be separable, with additional notochordal signals being required for induction of the MHP. *Shh* also appears to play a role in the regulation of dorsolateral bending. The DLHPs are most prominent at axial levels where *Shh* expression in the notochord is weak (mode 3), whereas they are absent from neuroepithelium (mode 1) overlying notochord that strongly expresses *Shh*. Indeed, *Shh* appears both necessary and sufficient to inhibit dorsolateral bending (Ybot-Gonzalez et al., 2002), and the phenotypes of mouse mutants for other components of the *Shh* pathway provide further support for a role of *Shh* signaling in regulation of neural tube closure (reviewed by Copp et al., 2003a).

Several different cellular mechanisms have been proposed to account for bending of the neuroepithelium at the hinge points (reviewed by Schoenwolf and Smith, 1990a, 1990b). At neural plate stages, the neuroepithelium is a pseudostratified epithelium of a single-cell thickness. A feature of the hinge points, particularly the MHP, compared to nonbending areas of the folds, is the predominance of cells that are wedge-shaped, with a wider basal (nonluminal) pole (Schoenwolf and Franks, 1984). Cell wedging appears to be essential for the formation of the MHP since the induction of both wedging and an MHP depends on the notochord (Smith and Schoenwolf 1989). A popular theory explaining cell wedging is based on localized apical constriction of neuroepithelial cells. Several studies have revealed the presence of circumferentially arranged, actin-containing microfilaments at the apical surface of the neuroepithelium of amphibia, birds, and mammals (reviewed by Schoenwolf and Smith, 1990b), raising the possibility that contraction of apical microfilaments may lead to cell wedging at hinge points. However, actin microfilaments are not concentrated at the hinge points but rather show an even distribution throughout the neuroepithelium. Moreover, the MHP and the DLHPs are resistant to cytochalasin D treatment (Ybot-Gonzalez and Copp, 1999; Ybot-Gonzalez et al., 2002), in contrast to the finding that cytochalasin prevents cranial neural tube closure (as described above). Interestingly, apical bands of microfilaments are present even during secondary neurulation, where there is no elevation or bending of the neuroepithelium. It seems most likely that microfilaments stabilize the shape of the neural folds or newly formed neural tube rather than driving the wedging of cells at hinge points (Schoenwolf and Smith, 1990b; Colas and Schoenwolf, 2001).

An alternative explanation for cell wedging at hinge points is based on the idea that cell cycle–dependent variations in the apicobasal position of nuclei within the pseudostratified neuroepithelium dictate the cell shape (Schoenwolf and Smith, 1990b). Each neuroepithelial cell extends from the luminal to the basal surface, but the apicobasal position of the nucleus varies with the stage of the cell cycle (so-called interkinetic nuclear migration) (Fig. 2.6). Nuclei migrate to the basal pole during S phase and to the apex during mitosis. The neuroepithlial cell is widest at the position of the nucleus, such that a basal location of the nucleus is associated with wedging of the cell. At the MHP there is an increased proportion of wedge-shaped cells, partly due to the fact that S phase is extended. In addition, the nuclei at this site appear to remain basal during the G_2 phase for a longer period than in nonbending regions. Therefore, it is proposed that regulation of the cell cycle and interkinetic nuclear migration results in production of the MHP (Smith and Schoenwolf, 1988). This is an attractive idea since, according to this model, hinge point formation is not microfilament-dependent, in keeping with the results of the cytochalasin experiments. A requirement for cell cycle regulation and interkinetic nuclear migration in formation of the DLHP has not been demonstrated to date.

Adhesion of Apposed Neural Folds Is Essential for Closure

Once the tips of the neural folds have achieved apposition at the dorsal midline, fusion must occur at the contact points in order to complete neural tube formation. Following adhesion and fusion, the neural fold apices remodel to create two continuous epithelial layers: the surface ectoderm and the neuroepithelium itself (Colas and Schoenwolf, 2001). The mechanisms of adhesion and fusion are poorly understood, but it is noteworthy that, following the initial closure event, the next region of open neural folds to close is immediately adjacent to

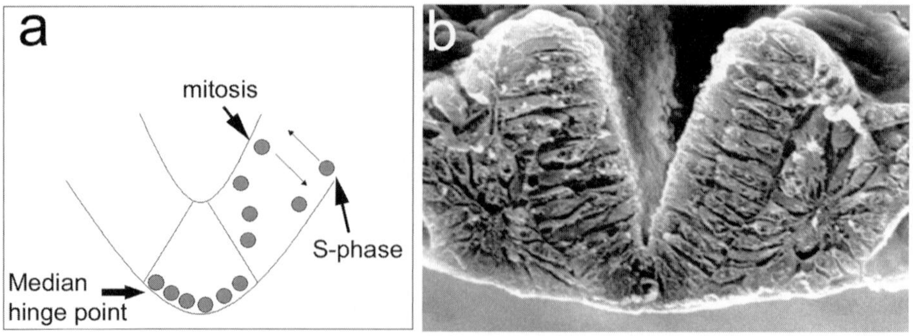

FIGURE 2.6. The cell cycle–dependent position of the nucleus contributes to bending of the neuroepithelium at the median hinge point. A transverse section through the neural folds is shown in a schematic diagram (*a*) and a scanning electron micrograph (*b*). In the neural folds, nuclei are located basally during S phase and apically during mitosis (*a*), moving between the cell poles during G1 and G2 phases (so-called interkinetic nuclear migration). Cells are widest at the site of the nucleus such that a basal location of the nucleus causes cell wedging. An increased proportion of cells at the midline are in S-phase with basally located nuclei (*a*), and this prevalence of wedge-shaped cells is associated with formation of the median hinge point (seen in *b*). *Source:* Modified from Greene et al. (1998) and Harding and Copp (2002).

a site where fusion has already been completed. It is possible, therefore, that adhesion of the neural folds is a major driving force in bringing the open neural folds into apposition in the immediately adjacent area. Failure of adhesion would be expected to result in NTD. In support of this idea, mice that lack the cell surface Eph ligand, ephrin-A5, exhibit exencephaly, as do mice that lack the EphA7 receptor, a potential ligand for ephrin-A5 (Holmberg et al., 2000). Cranial neural fold elevation and apposition appear to occur normally in these targeted mutant mice, suggesting that ephrin–Eph interactions may play a significant role specifically in adhesion of the neural folds. In addition to protein–protein interactions, it has been suggested that the abundance of extracellular carbohydrate material, including alpha-D-mannose, alpha-D-glucose, and *N*-acetyl-D-glucosamine, on the cell surfaces at the tips of the neural folds may be functionally related to the adhesive properties of these cells (Sadler, 1978; Smits et al., 1986). Significantly, the removal of carbohydrates by exposure of embryos to phospholipase C results in failure of closure (O'Shea and Kaufman, 1980). However, this treatment not only removes carbohydrates but also cleaves glycosylphosphatidylinositol-anchored proteins, including ephrin-A5, from the membrane. Hence, the specific requirement for carbohydrate-rich material at the site of neural fold fusion remains to be defined.

Although the progressive fusion of the apposed neural folds is commonly described as zipping up, the process may actually be discontinuous at the cellular level. Cellular protrusions, resembling filopodia, have been detected on the cells at the tips of the neural folds (Geelen and Langman, 1979). These appear to interdigitate as the bilateral folds come into apposition, providing an initial contact that facilitates subsequent cell adhesion. Microscopic examination of the site of posterior neuropore closure in chick embryos reveals interspersed regions of apposed, fused, and open neural folds such that initial contact between the folds is achieved by a series of bridging interactions (Van Straaten et al., 1993). It is possible, therefore, that adhesion occurs in a button-like fashion, with multiple initial closure sites, rather than by a continuous zipping action.

Most studies of the closure process assume that apposition and fusion occur at the tips of the neural folds. However, in the chick, an alternative mechanism has been proposed for closure in the mesencephalic region based on microscopic examination of living embryos and scanning electron microscopy (Van Straaten et al., 1997). In this model, the neural folds initially adhere deeply within the neural groove, with the area of contact increasing as adhesion spreads dorsally. Once the tips of the folds have been brought into contact, relatively late in the adhesion process, adhesion in the ventral region is released, enabling formation of the neural tube lumen. In this model, a sequence of cross sections of the neural folds during closure would appear as V, Y, I, and O shapes in comparison to a sequence of V, U, and O shapes. At present, there is little evidence for the occurrence of closure by this mechanism in mice or humans.

Apoptosis in Neural Tube Closure

Apoptotic cell death has been observed in the neuroepithelium at the tips of the neural folds, at the dorsolateral hinge points, and at the midline of the neural tube

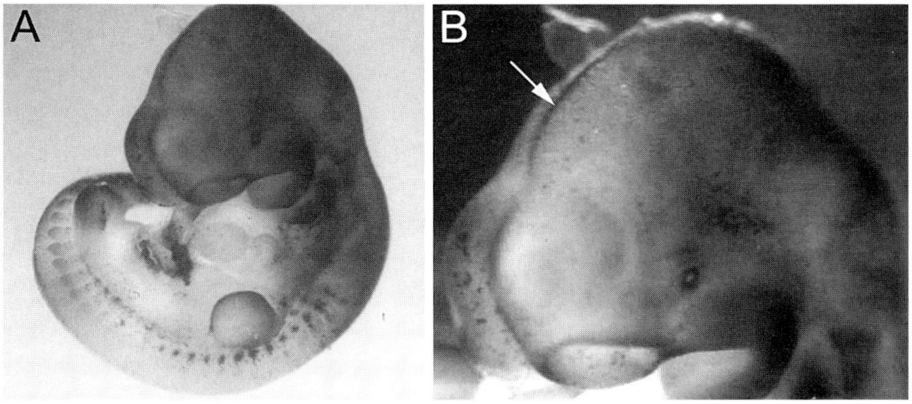

FIGURE 2.7. Apoptotic cells at the midline of the neural tube. Apoptotic cells are labeled by the TUNEL assay in a nonmutant mouse embryo at embryonic day 10.5 (*A*). Cranial neural tube closure is complete and apoptotic cells are apparent at the midline of the neuroepithelium after fusion (*arrow* in the enlarged view of cranial region in *B*).

after fusion (Fig. 2.7) (Schluter 1973; Lawson et al., 1999). Evidence from mouse mutants suggests that both excessive and insufficient apoptosis are potential causes of NTDs, most commonly exencephaly (Copp et al., 2003a). It is easy to see how excessive cell death could prevent cranial neural tube closure by causing insufficient cells to be present in the fusing neural folds or by disrupting the physical continuity of the dorsal midline, leading to reopening of recently closed folds.

The requirement for apoptosis in the normal process of neurulation is less easy to understand, however. Several mouse genetic mutants exhibit a reduction in neuroepithelial cell death in association with cranial NTD, while treatment of chick embryos with inhibitors of caspases, enzymes that act in a proteolytic cascade to bring about programmed cell death, prevents neural tube closure (Weil et al., 1997). It is possible that apoptosis at the DHLPs in the cranial region facilitates the abrupt change in bending from a biconvex to a biconcave morphology. Moreover, cell death at the site of fusion may be essential to allow remodeling of the epithelia at the tips of the neural folds to form the surface ectoderm and neuroepithlium. These possible functions of apoptosis in neurulation are not mutually exclusive and either, if disturbed, could generate NTDs.

Neural Crest Emigration and Neural Tube Closure

The relationship between neural crest migration and the development of NTDs is discussed in detail in Chapter 1. Briefly, the timing of neural crest emigration in relation to the progress of neural tube closure differs with the axial level. Thus, neural crest cells begin to emigrate from the tips of the neural folds prior to the onset of closure in the cranial region, whereas emigration in the spinal region occurs in regions where the neural tube has already closed (Morriss-Kay and Tan, 1987). Defects of neural crest derivatives (neurocristopathies) may occur in association with NTD (Nye et al., 1999), suggesting a possible link between timely neural crest emigration and neural tube closure. This relationship appears to be particularly important in the cranial region. For example, inhibition of cranial neural crest cell emigration by enzymatic removal of chondroitin sulfate or transgenic overexpression of connexin 43 results in exencephaly (Morriss-Kay and Tuckett, 1989; Ewart et al., 1997). It has been proposed that neural crest emigration may facilitate bending of the neural folds during cranial closure (Morriss-Kay and Tuckett, 1989; Morriss-Kay et al., 1994). Alternatively, loss of the neural crest from the tips of the neural folds may be a prerequisite for the cell rearrangements and neuroepithelial remodeling that occur upon fusion.

SUMMARY

Formation of the neural tube depends on a series of coordinated morphologic events that results in conversion of the flat neural plate into the neural tube. This process of neurulation varies along the body axis in terms of timing, morphology, and sensitivity to genetic or environmental insult. Failure of neurulation results in NTDs that may occur at the cranial and/or spinal levels and constitute a group of severe birth defects in humans. Evidence from careful observation, as well as genetic or experimental manipulation of model organisms, has contributed to an increasing understanding both of the normal processes of neurulation and of the mechanisms underlying the development of NTD.

REFERENCES

Adler PN (2002). Planar signalling and morphogenesis in *Drosophila*. Dev Cell 2:525–535.

Ang S-L, Rossant J (1994). *HNF*-3β is essential for node and notochord formation in mouse development. Cell 78:561–574.

Chen Z-F, Behringer RR (1995). *twist* is required in head mesenchyme for cranial neural tube morphogenesis. Genes Dev 9:686–699.

Chiang C, Litingtung Y, Lee E, Young KE, Corden JL, Westphal H, Beachy PA (1996). Cyclopia and defective axial patterning in mice lacking *Sonic hedgehog* gene function. Nature 383:407–413.

Colas JF, Schoenwolf GC (2001). Towards a cellular and molecular understanding of neurulation. Dev Dyn 221:117–145.

Copp AJ, Brook FA (1989). Does lumbosacral spina bifida arise by failure of neural folding or by defective canalisation? J Med Genet 26:160–166.

Copp AJ, Checiu I, Henson JN (1994). Developmental basis of severe neural tube defects in the *loop-tail* (*Lp*) mutant mouse: use of microsatellite DNA markers to identify embryonic genotype. Dev Biol 165:20–29.

Copp AJ, Greene ND, Murdoch JN (2003a). The genetic basis of mammalian neurulation. Nat Rev Genet 4:784–793.

Copp AJ, Greene NDE, Murdoch JN (2003b). Dishevelled: linking convergent extension with neural tube closure. Trends Neurosci 26:453–455.

Costanzo R, Watterson RL, Schoenwolf GC (1982). Evidence that secondary neurulation occurs autonomously in the chick embryo. J Exp Zool 219:233–240.

Curtin JA, Quint E, Tsipouri V, Arkell RM, Cattanach B, Copp AJ, Fisher EM, et al (2003). Mutation of *Celsr1* disrupts planar polarity of inner ear hair cells and causes severe neural tube defects in the mouse. Curr Biol 13:1–20.

Darken RS, Scola AM, Rakeman AS, Das G, Mlodzik M, Wilson PA (2002). The planar polarity gene *Strabismus* regulates convergent extension movements in *Xenopus*. EMBO J 21:976–985.

Davidson BP, Kinder SJ, Steiner K, Schoenwolf GC, Tam PPL (1999). Impact of node ablation on the morphogenesis of the body axis and the lateral asymmetry of the mouse embryo during early organogenesis. Dev Biol 211:11–26.

Ding Q, Motoyama J, Gasca S, Mo R, Sasaki H, Rossant J, Hui CC (1998). Diminished *Sonic hedgehog* signaling and lack of floor plate differentiation in Gli2 mutant mice. Development 125:2533–2543.

Ewart JL, Cohen MF, Meyer RA, Huang GY, Wessels A, Gourdie RG, Chin AJ, et al (1997). Heart and neural tube defects in transgenic mice overexpressing the Cx43 gap junction gene. Development 124:1281–1292.

Fleming A, Copp AJ (2000). A genetic risk factor for mouse neural tube defects: defining the embryonic basis. Hum Mol Genet 9:575–581.

Geelen JAG, Langman J (1979). Ultrastructural observations on closure of the neural tube in the mouse. Anat Embryol 156:73–88.

Golden JA, Chernoff GF (1995). Multiple sites of anterior neural tube closure in humans: evidence from anterior neural tube defects (anencephaly). Pediatrics 95:506–510.

Goto T, Keller R (2002). The planar cell polarity gene *Strabismus* regulates convergence and extension and neural fold closure in *Xenopus*. Dev Biol 247:165–181.

Greene NDE, Gerrelli D, Van Straaten HWM, Copp AJ (1998). Abnormalities of floor plate, notochord and somite differentiation in the *loop-tail* (*Lp*) mouse: a model of severe neural tube defects. Mech Dev 73:59–72.

Gunn TM, Juriloff DM, Harris MJ (1992). Further genetic studies of the cause of exencephaly in SELH mice. Teratology 45:679–686.

Gunn TM, Juriloff DM, Harris MJ (1995). Genetically determined absence of an initiation site of cranial neural tube closure is causally related to exencephaly in SELH/Bc mouse embryos. Teratology 52:101–108.

Gunn TM, Juriloff DM, Vogl W, Harris MJ, Miller JE (1993). Histological study of the cranial neural folds of mice genetically liable to exencephaly. Teratology 48:459–471.

Hackett DA, Smith JL, Schoenwolf GC (1997). Epidermal ectoderm is required for full elevation and for convergence during bending of the avian neural plate. Dev Dyn 201:397–406.

Hamblet NS, Lijam N, Ruiz-Lozano P, Wang J, Yang Y, Luo Z, Mei L, et al (2002). Dishevelled 2 is essential for cardiac outflow tract development, somite segmentation and neural tube closure. Development 129:5827–5838.

Harding BN, Copp AJ (2002) Congenital malformations. In Graham Dl, Lantos PL (eds): *Greenfield's Neuropathology*. London: Arnold, pp. 357–483.

Hildebrand JD, Soriano P (1999). Shroom, a PDZ domain-containing actin-binding protein, is required for neural tube morphogenesis in mice. Cell 99:485–497.

Holmberg J, Clarke DL, Frisén J (2000). Regulation of repulsion versus adhesion by different splice forms of an Eph receptor. Nature 408:203–206.

Jacobson AG (1984). Further evidence that formation of the neural tube requires elongation of the nervous system. J Exp Zool 230:23–28.

Jacobson AG, Gordon R (1976). Changes in the shape of the developing vertebrate nervous system analyzed experimentally, mathematically and by computer simulation. J Exp Zool 197:191–246.

Keller R, Davidson L, Edlund A, Elul T, Ezin M, Shook D, Skoglund P (2000). Mechanisms of convergence and extension by cell intercalation. Philoso Trans R Soc Lond B:Biol Sci 355:897–922.

Keller R, Shih J, Sater AK, Moreno C (1992). Planar induction of convergence and extension of the neural plate by the organizer of *Xenopus*. Dev Dyn 193:218–234.

Keller RE, Danilchik M, Gimlich R, Shih J (1985). The function and mechanism of convergent extension during gastrulation of *Xenopus laevis*. J Embryol Exp Morphol 89(Suppl):185–209.

Lawson A, Schoenwolf GC, England MA, Addai FK, Ahima RS (1999). Programmed cell death and the morphogenesis of the hindbrain roof plate in the chick embryo. Anat Embryol 200:509–519.

Martinez-Barbera JP, Rodriguez TA, Greene NDE, Weninger WJ, Simeone A, Copp AJ, Beddington R, Dunwoodie S (2002). Folic acid prevents exencephaly in *Cited2* deficient mice. Hum Mol Genet 11:283–293.

Matise MP, Epstein DJ, Park HL, Platt KA, Joyner AL (1998). *Gli2* is required for induction of floor plate and adjacent cells, but not most ventral neurons in the mouse central nervous system. Development 125:2759–2770.

Matsuda M, Keino H (1994). An open cephalic neural tube reproducibly induced by cytochalasin D in rat embryos *in vitro*. Zool Sci 11:547–553.

Mlodzik M (2002). Planar cell polarization: do the same mechanisms regulate *Drosophila* tissue polarity and vertebrate gastrulation? Trends Genet 18:564–571.

Morriss GM, Solursh M (1978a). Regional differences in mesenchymal cell morphology and glycosaminoglycans in early neural-fold stage rat embryos. J Embryol Exp Morphol 46:37–52.

Morriss GM, Solursh M (1978b). The role of primary mesenchyme in normal and abnormal morphogenesis of mammalian neural folds. Zoon 6:33–38.

Morriss-Kay G, Tan S-S (1987). Mapping cranial neural crest cell migration pathways in mammalian embryos. Trends Genet 3:257–261.

Morriss-Kay GM (1981). Growth and development of pattern in the cranial neural epithelium of rat embryos during neurulation. J Embryol Exp Morphol 65(Suppl):225–241.

Morriss-Kay GM, Tuckett F (1985). The role of microfilaments in cranial neurulation in rat embryos: effects of short-term exposure to cytochalasin D. J Embryol Exp Morphol 88:333–348.

Morriss-Kay GM, Tuckett F (1989). Immunohistochemical localization of chondroitin sulphate proteoglycans and the effects of chondroitinase ABC in 9- to 11-day rat embryos. Development 106:787–798.

Morriss-Kay GM, Tuckett F, Solursh M (1986). The effects of *Streptomyces* hyaluronidase on tissue organization and cell cycle time in rat embryos. J Embryol Exp Morphol 98:59–70.

Morriss-Kay G, Wood H, Chen W-H (1994). Normal neurulation in mammals. In Bock G, Marsh J (eds): *Neural Tube Defects*. Ciba Foundation Symposium 181. Wiley, Chichester: pp. 51–63.

Murdoch JN, Doudney K, Paternotte C, Copp AJ, Stanier P (2001a). Severe neural tube defects in the *loop-tail* mouse result from mutation of *Lpp1*, a novel gene involved in floor plate specification. Hum Mol Genet 10:2593–2601.

Murdoch JN, Henderson DJ, Doudney K, Gaston-Massuet C, Phillips HM, Paternotte C, Arkell R, et al (2003). Disruption of *scribble* (*Scrb1*) causes severe neural tube defects in the *circletail* mouse. Hum Mol Genet 12:87–98.

Murdoch JN, Rachel RA, Shah S, Beermann F, Stanier P, Mason CA, Copp AJ (2001b). *Circletail*, a new mouse mutant with severe neural tube defects: chromosomal localization and interaction with the *loop-tail* mutation. Genomics 78:55–63.

Nagele RG, Lee H (1980). Studies on the mechanisms of neurulation in the chick: microfilament-mediated changes in cell shape during uplifting of neural folds. J Exp Zool 213:391–398.

Nakatsu T, Uwabe C, Shiota K (2000). Neural tube closure in humans initiates at multiple sites: evidence from human embryos and implications for the pathogenesis of neural tube defects. Anat Embryol 201:455–466.

Nye JS, McLone DG, Charrow J, Hayes EA (1999). Neural crest anomaly syndromes in children with spina bifida. Teratology 60:179–189.

Ohkawara B, Yamamoto TS, Tada M, Ueno N (2003). Role of glypican 4 in the regulation of convergent extension movements during gastrulation in *Xenopus laevis*. Development 130:2129–2138.

O'Rahilly R, Müller F (1994). Neurulation in the normal human embryo. In Bock G, Marsh J (eds): *Neural Tube Defects*. Ciba Foundation Symposium 181. Chichester: Wiley, pp. 70–82.

O'Rahilly R, Müller F (2002). The two sites of fusion of the neural folds and the two neuropores in the human embryo. Teratology 65:162–170.

O'Shea KS, Kaufman MH (1980). Phospholipase C induced neural tube defects in the mouse embryo. Experientia 36:1217–1219.

Park HL, Bai C, Platt KA, Matise MP, Beeghly A, Hui CC, Nakashima M, Joyner AL (2000). Mouse *Gli1* mutants are viable but have defects in SHH signaling in combination with a *Gli2* mutation. Development 127:1593–1605.

Placzek M, Tessier-Lavigne M, Yamada T, Jessell T, Dodd J (1990). Mesodermal control of neural cell identity: floor plate induction by the notochord. Science 250:985–988.

Sadler TW (1978). Distribution of surface coat material on fusing neural folds of mouse embryos during neurulation. Anat Rec 191:345–350.

Sadler TW, Greenberg D, Coughlin P, Lessard JL (1982). Actin distribution patterns in the mouse neural tube during neurulation. Science 215:172–174.

Schluter G (1973). Ultrastructural observations on cell necrosis during formation of the neural tube in mouse embryos. Z Anat Entwickl-Gesch 141:251–264.

Schoenwolf GC (1984). Histological and ultrastructural studies of secondary neurulation of mouse embryos. Am J Anat 169:361–374.

Schoenwolf GC (1988). Microsurgical analyses of avian neurulation: separation of medial and lateral tissues. J Comp Neurol 276:498–507.

Schoenwolf GC, Folsom D, Moe A (1988). A reexamination of the role of microfilaments in neurulation in the chick embryo. Anat Rec 220:87–102.

Schoenwolf GC, Franks MV (1984). Quantitative analyses of changes in cell shapes during bending of the avian neural plate. Dev Biol 105:257–272.

Schoenwolf GC, Smith JL (1990a). Epithelial cell wedging: a fundamental cell behavior contributing to hinge point formation during epithelial morphogenesis. Semin Dev Biol 1:325–334.

Schoenwolf GC, Smith JL (1990b). Mechanisms of neurulation: traditional viewpoint and recent advances. Development 109:243–270.

Seller MJ (1995a). Further evidence for an intermittent pattern of neural tube closure in humans. J Med Genet 32:205–207.

Seller MJ (1995b). Sex, neural tube defects, and multisite closure of the human neural tube. Am J Med Genet 58:332–336.

Sheldahl LC, Slusarski DC, Pandur P, Miller JR, Kuhl M, Moon RT (2003). *Dishevelled* activates Ca^{2+} flux, PKC, and CamKII in vertebrate embryos. J Cell Biol 161:769–777.

Shum ASW, Copp AJ (1996). Regional differences in morphogenesis of the neuroepithelium suggest multiple mechanisms of spinal neurulation in the mouse. Anat Embryol 194:65–73.

Smith JL, Schoenwolf GC (1988). Role of cell-cycle in regulating neuroepithelial cell shape during bending of the chick neural plate. Cell Tissue Res 252:491–500.

Smith JL, Schoenwolf GC (1989). Notochordal induction of cell wedging in the chick neural plate and its role in neural tube formation. J Exp Zool 250:49–62.

Smits van PAE, Poelmann RE, Gesink AF, van Groeningen MJ, Vermeij Keers C (1986). The cell surface coat in neurulating mouse and rat embryos, studied with lectins. Anat Embryol 175:111–117.

Solursh M, Morriss GM (1977). Glycosaminoglycan synthesis in rat embryos during the formation of the primary mesenchyme and neural folds. Dev Biol 57:75–86.

Stiefel D, Shibata T, Meuli M, Duffy P, Copp AJ (2003). Tethering of the spinal cord in mouse fetuses and neonates with spina bifida. J Neurosurg 99:206–13.

Takeuchi M, Nakabayashi J, Sakaguchi T, Yamamoto TS, Takahashi H, Takeda H, Ueno N (2003). The prickle-related gene in vertebrates is essential for gastrulation cell movements. Curr Biol 13:674–679.

Tuckett F, Morriss-Kay GM (1986). The distribution of fibronectin, laminin and entactin in the neurulating rat embryo studied by indirect immunofluorescence. J Embryol Exp Morphol 94:95–112.

Van Allen MI, Kalousek DK, Chernoff GF, Juriloff D, Harris M, McGillivray BC, Yong S-L, et al (1993). Evidence for multi-site closure of the neural tube in humans. Am J Med Genet 47:723–743.

Van Straaten HWM, Hekking JWM, Thors F, Wiertz-Hoessels ELMJ, Drukker J (1985). Induction of an additional floor plate in the neural tube. Acta Morphol Neerl Scand 23:91–97.

Van Straaten HWM, Hekking JWM, Wiertz-Hoessels EJLM, Thors F, Drukker J (1988). Effect of the notochord on the differentiation of a floor plate area in the neural tube of the chick embryo. Anat Embryol 177:317–324.

Van Straaten HWM, Jaskoll T, Rousseau AMJ, Terwindt-Rouwenhorst EAW, Greenberg G, Shankar K, Melnick M (1993). Raphe of the posterior neural tube in the chick embryo: its closure and reopening as studied in living embryos with a high definition light microscope. Dev Dyn 198:65–76.

Van Straaten HWM, Peeters MCE, Szpak KFW, Hekking JWM (1997). Initial closure of the mesencephalic neural groove in the chick embryo involves a releasing zipping-up mechanism. Dev Dyn 209:333–341.

Wallingford JB, Fraser SE, Harland RM (2002). Convergent extension: the molecular control of polarized cell movement during embryonic development. Dev Cell 2:695–706.

Wallingford JB, Harland RM (2001). *Xenopus Dishevelled* signaling regulates both neural and mesodermal convergent extension: parallel forces elongating the body axis. Development 128:2581–2592.

Wallingford JB, Harland RM (2002). Neural tube closure requires *Dishevelled*-dependent convergent extension of the midline. Development 129:5815–5825.

Weil M, Jacobson MD, Raff MC (1997). Is programmed cell death required for neural tube closure? Curr Biol 7:281–284.

Weinstein DC, Ruiz i Altaba A, Chen WS, Hoodless P, Prezioso VR, Jessell TM, Darnell JE, Jr (1994). The winged-helix transcription factor *HNF-3β* is required for notochord development in the mouse embryo. Cell 78:575–588.

Wood LR, Smith MT (1984). Generation of anencephaly: 1. Aberrant neurulation and 2. Conversion of exencephaly to anencephaly. J Neuropathol Exp Neurol 43:620–633.

Yamada T, Placzek M, Tanaka H, Dodd J, Jessell TM (1991). Control of cell pattern in the developing nervous system: Polarizing activity of the floor plate and notochord. Cell 64:635–647.

Ybot-Gonzalez P, Cogram P, Gerrelli D, Copp AJ (2002). *Sonic hedgehog* and the molecular regulation of neural tube closure. Development 129:2507–2517.

Ybot-Gonzalez P, Copp AJ (1999). Bending of the neural plate during mouse spinal neurulation is independent of actin microfilaments. Dev Dyn 215:273–283.

Zhao Q, Behringer RR, De Crombrugghe B (1996). Prenatal folic acid treatment suppresses acrania and meroanencephaly in mice mutant for the *Cart1* homeobox gene. Nature Genet 13:275–283.

Zolessi FR, Arruti C (2001). Apical accumulation of MARCKS in neural plate cells during neurulation in the chick embryo. BMC Dev Biol 1:7.

3

The Zebrafish as a Model for Analyzing Neural Tube Defects

HAKRYUL JO
LAURA ANNE LOWERY
VINCENT TROPEPE
HAZEL SIVE

In this review, we consider whether the zebrafish, *Danio rerio*, is a useful model system for uncovering the genetic and molecular basis for human neural tube defects (NTDs) and conclude that the zebrafish is an excellent NTD model. This conclusion is based on the similarities in development and structure of human and zebrafish brains. It is also based on characteristics of the zebrafish as a model, including the accessibility of early embryos, and the ability to use both powerful genetic and molecular techniques to analyze the zebrafish nervous system.

Neural tube defects per se refer to incorrect formation of the neural tube—the precursor to the central nervous system. However, it is often not possible to determine whether neurological defects result from abnormalities in the specific morphogenetic processes by which the neural tube forms, or from other distinct processes that occur prior to neural tube formation (e.g., neural induction) or in the early stages after the tube has formed. We therefore define NTDs more broadly to include any abnormality of early nervous system formation. Most NTDs manifest at birth; however, late-onset neurological abnormalities may have their origins in early defects of the nervous system, and we include these in our definition.

ZEBRAFISH AS A MODEL SYSTEM

The zebrafish boasts an impressive record for providing insight into mechanisms that control vertebrate patterning, organogenesis, physiology, and behavior. Consequently, advances in these areas of basic research have made a great impact on our understanding of human biology and medicine. In the next sections we provide a general overview of the zebrafish as an experimental model. We outline the many genetic, molecular, and embryological techniques available to study this organism.

Basic Features of Zebrafish Biology

Several basic aspects of zebrafish biology make this organism an attractive genetic and molecular experimental model, particularly in the field of neural development. Fertilization of zebrafish eggs is external, which allows all embryonic stages to be easily observed. Zebrafish have a relatively short generation time (3 months), and clutch sizes from a single mating pair range between 100 and 200 embryos (Streisinger et al., 1981; Kimmel, 1989). Development is rapid, allowing rapid assays; for example, the neural plate is present by 6–7 hours postfertilization (hpf) and the first neurons form by 16 hpf. An important feature of zebrafish embryos is their optical transparency, resulting from the sequestration of yolk granules into a single giant yolk cell. Thus, easily accessible, transparent embryos offer an unprecedented advantage for visualizing molecular and cellular processes in live embryos. Furthermore, since zebrafish adults grow to an average size of only 3–4 cm, a rather large number of fish can be housed in a relatively small area. Therefore, the infrastructure and maintenance costs required for housing large numbers of animals for screening for morphological or behavioral mutants is far less than for equivalent assays in the mouse.

Genetic, Molecular, and Embryological Methods in Zebrafish Research

Experiments using zebrafish have proven to be very useful for studying fundamental embryological processes, including morphogenesis, lineage specification (what cells will become), timing of commitment (when cells decide to assume a certain fate), and the mechanism by which cell fate is acquired. As a consequence of embryonic transparency, the fate of individual cells across a broad range of developmental stages can be clearly resolved in vivo by labeling cells with lineage tracers such as fluorescent dyes. In addition, the external development of zebrafish embryos allows various embryological assays, including transplant and explant experiments (the latter developed in our lab) (Woo and Fraser, 1997; Grinblat et al., 1999), to determine the cell fate and the timing of tissue-specific inductive interactions.

Furthermore, assays have been developed to perform molecular *gain of function* experiments to determine what a gene can do and *loss of function* experiments to determine what it normally does. For example, microinjection of synthetic mRNA (Hyatt and Ekker, 1999) can be used during early embryogenesis in gain of function assays and to place genes in genetic pathways. More recently, chemically modified oligonucleotides (morpholinos), which target nascent mRNA and block translation, have been used in loss of function assays to ablate the function of specific genes, particularly early during development (Nasevicius and Ekker, 2000).

The attractive biological and economical aspects of zebrafish inspired the first large-scale chemical mutagenesis screens in a vertebrate species (Driever et al., 1996; Haffter et al., 1996), resulting in approximately 2000 mutations in developmental genes affecting a wide range of tissues. Subsequent approaches included viral insertional mutagenesis screens for developmental genes in diploid embryos (Amsterdam et al., 1999), for neural pattern formation genes in haploid gynogenotes (Wiellette et al., 2004), and for cocaine sensitivity based on behavioral phenotypes (Darland and Dowling, 2001). Although reverse genetics techniques (gene knockouts) have not been established, an alternative approach (termed *target-selected gene inactivation*) to isolating fish with a desired gene mutation has been described (Wienholds et al., 2002).

Together, these and other screens have generated thousands of mutant fish with a wide range of morphological, physiological, and behavioral phenotypes, many of which have been shown to recapitulate various human genetic and pathologic conditions (for review see Barut and Zon, 2000; Dodd et al., 2000). Therefore, studying these mutants is likely to uncover the key aspects of pathogenic processes of complex human disorders such as NTDs.

ONTOGENY OF THE ZEBRAFISH NERVOUS SYSTEM

Specializations in brain structure and function exist among vertebrates with distinct adaptations to specific environments. Despite these differences, however, the development and organization of the nervous system as a whole are highly conserved among all vertebrates (Fig. 3.1). In the next sections we discuss formation of the neural tube and brain ventricles, including a comparison between the zebrafish and mammalian systems (Fig. 3.2). We then compare zebrafish brain structure and function, highlighting the many similar organizational features that are shared with the mammalian brain. This discussion provides a conceptual foundation for our claim that the zebrafish is an excellent model of human brain ontogeny and NTDs.

Similar Mechanisms Underlying Zebrafish and Mammalian Neural Tube Formation

During the formation of the vertebrate nervous system, the initial neuroectoderm must form a tube that will become the future brain and spinal cord. This process is called *neurulation.* Later, the initial neural tube expands in several places to form the brain ventricles. There are many possible events during neurulation that can be perturbed, leading to NTDs of varying severity.

It is important to understand that there are actually two neural tubes that form independently and later merge to make up the complete neural tube in vertebrates. Anteriorly, in the brain and future trunk (cervicothoracic) region, tube formation is called *primary neurulation,* which is characterized by a pre-existing epithelial sheet undergoing folding, rolling, or bending to form a tube. These movements include epithelial columnarization, thickening of the neural plate edges to form the neural folds, folding of the plate, and fusion of the two sides to form a tube (Colas and Schoenwolf, 2001) (Fig. 3.3). While primary neurulation always begins with an epithelial substrate and ends with a tube, some of the steps involved can be quite variable among vertebrates and within one species at different levels of the anterior neural tube (Shum and Copp, 1996). Despite these variations, the underlying morphogenetic movements involved in reshaping the neuroepithelium appear to be conserved. Posteriorly, in the future lumbar and tail regions, the neural tube forms by *secondary neurulation,* in which a mesenchymal cell population condenses to form a rod that undergoes transformation to an epithelial tube (Criley, 1969). Neural tube defects might arise due to de-

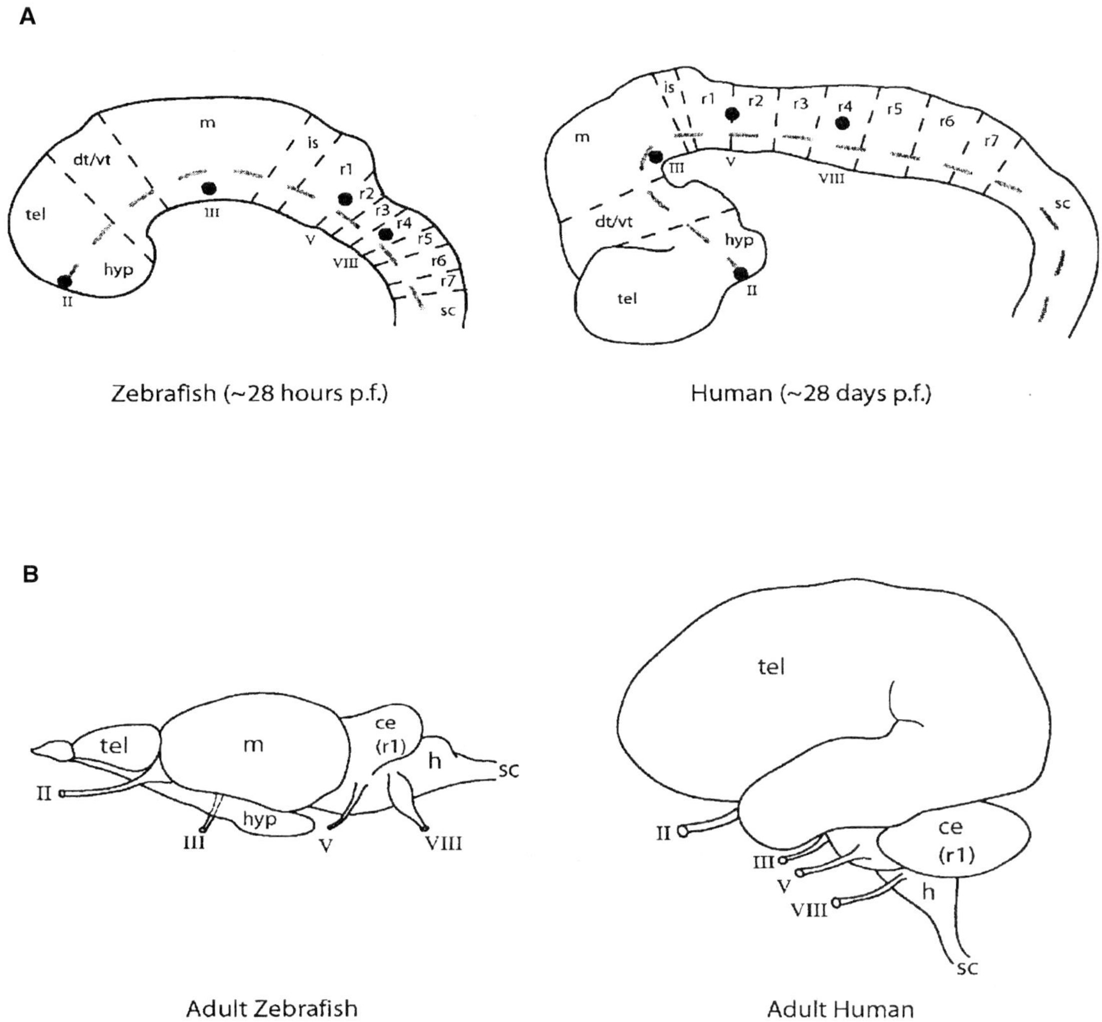

FIGURE 3.1. Brain development and structure are conserved between zebrafish and humans. The overall organization of the many parts of the vertebrate brain is similar among all vertebrates. (*A*) Here we provide a schematic representation of an embryonic and adult zebrafish brain and compare it to a schematic of the human embryonic and adult brain (anterior to the left, dorsal to the top). The figure depicts the segmental (neuromeric) organization of the embryonic brain, highlighting only a few of the proposed subdivisions (separated by black dashed lines). As a reference point, the boundary between the main alar (dorsal) and basal (ventral) subdivision of the brain and spinal cord is shown as a gray dashed line, and the locations of four cranial nerve primordia are depicted as black dots (II, optic nerve; III, oculomotor nerve; V, trigeminal nerve; VIII, octaval or vestibulocochlear nerve). (*B*) Despite the numerous morphological changes that occur during the course of development and the eventual size differences in a number of regions, the adult zebrafish and human brain share similar features. ce, cerebellum (a derivative of the dorsal r1); dt/vt, dorsal thalamus/ventral thalamus; h, hindbrain (the combined derivative of r2–r7); hyp, hypothalamus; is, isthmus; r1–r7, rhombomeres 1–7; m, midbrain; sc, spinal cord; tel, telencephalon.

fects in the steps to form either tube, by incorrect joining of the two tubes, or by failure to close the anterior or posterior neuropores to seal the tubes at either end. It is thought that the different brain and spinal cord regions use distinct yet overlapping spatial and temporal mechanisms to transform the epithelial sheet to the neural tube. The NTDs that result from improper neurulation include defects in localized regions of the neural tube such as anencephaly, spina bifida, rachischisis, or throughout its length, as in craniorachichisis (Harris and Juriloff, 1999; Juriloff and Harris, 2000).

Several lines of evidence indicate that zebrafish neurulation displays many similarities to mammalian neurulation (Fig. 3.3; Lowery and Sive, 2004). As in all primary neurulation, the zebrafish trunk neural tube begins as an epithelial sheet of cells, the neural plate. The lateral edges of the columnar epithelial thicken, akin to neural folds, and the plate sinks or rolls into the embryo (Geldmacher-

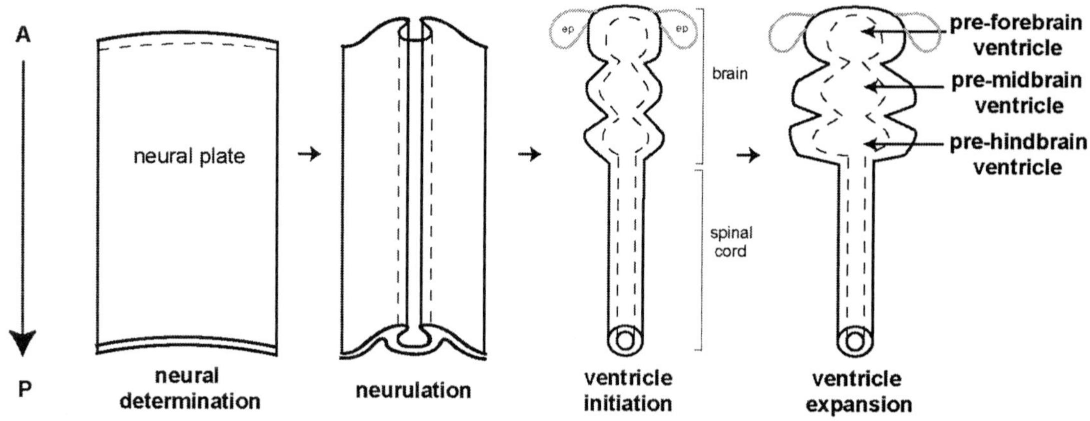

FIGURE 3.2. Steps in early brain development. The first step in brain development is neural determination, in which cells of the neural plate make the decision to form neural tissue but do not yet differentiate as neurons. The neural plate then undergoes neurulation, in which the epithelial neural plate rolls or bends to form the closed neural tube. During and after neural tube closure, the anterior portion of the tube dilates in three specific locations to form the future forebrain, midbrain, and hindbrain ventricles, which later undergo rapid expansion. ep, eye primordium. A, anterior, P, posterior.

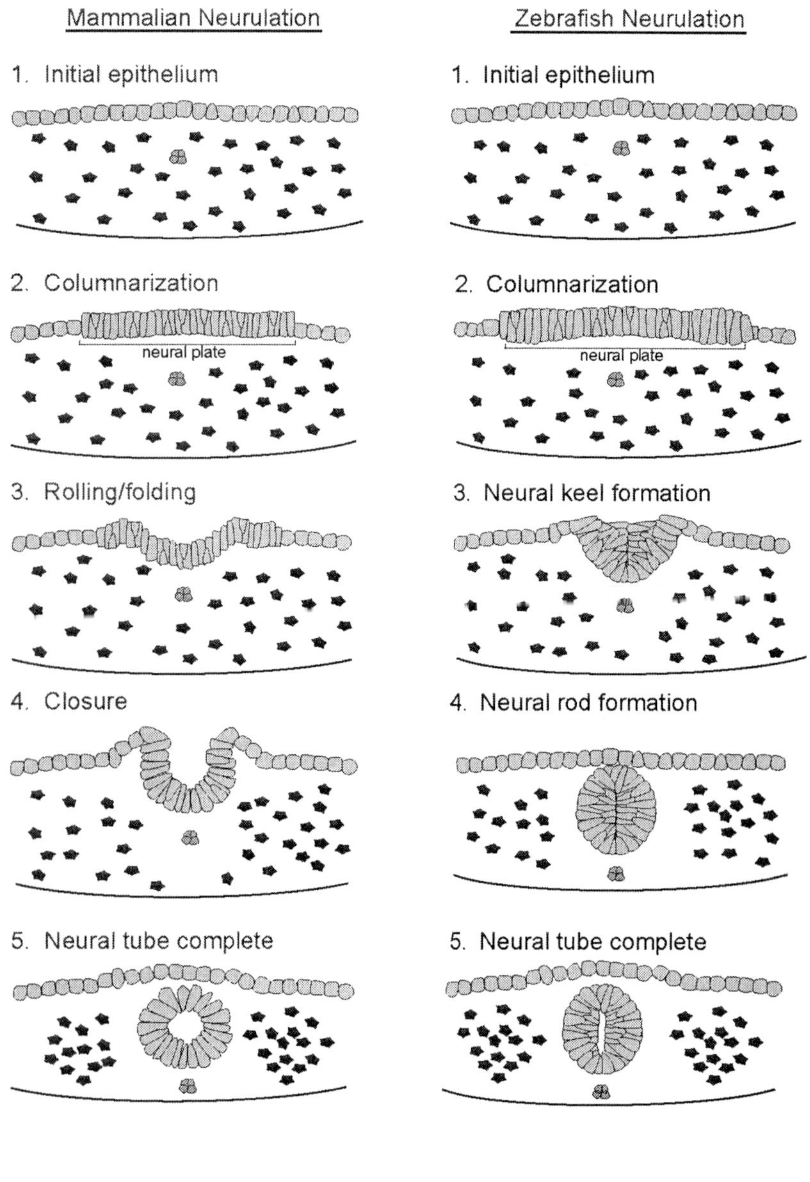

FIGURE 3.3. Comparison of mammalian and zebrafish neurulation. The morphogenetic steps are quite similar in both types of neurulation. Both begin with an initial epithelium sheet that columnarizes to form the neural plate. The mammalian neural plate then undergoes rolling or folding to bring the lateral edges to a more dorsal position, whereas the zebrafish neural plate undergoes a sinking movement (forming a *neural keel*) that is topologically similar to a rolling movement; the initial mediolateral position in the neural plate corresponds to the future dorsoventral position in the tube. The two sides of the mammalian neural folds then fuse to close the tube, while the two sides of the zebrafish neural keel come together to form the *neural rod,* and lumen opening occurs subsequently.

Voss et al., 2003). Fate mapping experiments indicate that these movements of the neural plate are similar to the neural plate movements in mammals, in which the initial mediolateral cell position corresponds to the later dorsoventral position in the neural tube (Papan and Campos-Ortega, 1994). This forms the neural keel, a solid rod of cells (Schmitz et al., 1993) in which the midline remains distinct (Geldmacher-Voss et al., 2003), with a pseudostratified columnar epithelium on either side. Subsequently, the lumen of the neural tube opens, beginning ventrally and moving dorsally (Schmitz et al., 1993). Lumen formation after initial primary neurulation is not zebrafish-specific, as there are regions in both the chick and *Xenopus* in which the trunk spinal cord is initially occluded, with a lumen developing after neural tube closure (Davidson and Keller, 1999). Thus, both the initial cell type and cell movements of the zebrafish are similar to those of other vertebrates.

Although it is not completely known how similar zebrafish and human neurulation is, it is known that many genes are conserved and the epithelial movements are similar. One question is whether the variations in primary neurulation between fish and mammals are reflected in the spectrum of NTDs that can be observed in the zebrafish. For example, does a very frequent human NTD such as spina bifida occur in the zebrafish, and if so, how frequently? The answer to the first question is clearly yes. In the zebrafish N-cadherin mutant *parachute*, the neural folds fail to fuse, as in human spina bifida. The frequency of such phenotypes has not been addressed, and it will take careful examination of existing mutants (Table 3.1) and further mutant screens to address this point. As indicated in Table 3.1 and discussed later, several zebrafish mutants have been identified that show defective neurulation. These will be important in connecting genes that affect mammalian neural tube formation with the underlying cellular defects.

Zebrafish as a Model for Brain Ventricle Formation

After neurulation is complete, the anterior region of the neural tube dilates in three specific locations to form the future forebrain, midbrain, and hindbrain ventricles (Fig. 3.2). During this process, the neural tube tissue must undergo proper morphogenesis to result in the positionally correct three-dimensional structure, which is thought to be necessary for normal brain function.

Like neurulation defects, defects in brain ventricle formation can have drastic effects on brain development and survival. Hydrocephaly, a defect in which increased cerebrospinal fluid and pressure within the brain lead to large increases in the brain ventricle space, is one of the most common brain ventricle defects in humans, and it can lead to death without treatment (Machado et al., 1991). Chiari malformation is a developmental defect in which part of the cerebellum protrudes into the spinal canal due to abnormal neurulation and subsequent ventricular abnormalities. This can lead to compression of the cerebellum and other regions, and a variety of neurological defects and nervous system damage can result (McLone and Knepper, 1989). In addition, a number of mental health disorders such as autism and schizophrenia display brain ventricle abnormalities (Hardan et al., 2001; Kurokawa et al., 2000). Although it is unknown whether the ventricular defects are primary or secondary to the mental health disorders, it is clear that more needs to be learned regarding how brain ventricle development is controlled at the genetic and molecular levels. This has been difficult due to lack of a good model system for studying brain ventricle morphogenesis.

Morphologically, brain ventricle development is highly conserved in all vertebrates from fish to humans. In previous mutagenesis screens, zebrafish mutants in brain ventricle formation were identified (Jiang et al., 1996; Schier et al., 1996). We have initiated a project to analyze brain ventricle formation using these and newly defined mutant lines (Table 3.1). This is likely to uncover mechanisms by which defects in ventricle formation arise and provide a means to interpret human neural tube defects that involve brain ventricle abnormalities.

Conserved Structure of the Adult Zebrafish and Human Brain

The conservation of overall adult brain structure in zebrafish, humans, and other vertebrates is also apparent after neural tube closure. As the simple neural tube structure takes shape and begins to grow, it forms a series of transverse bulges and constrictions giving rise to a segmented appearance, which in zebrafish occurs at ~16 hours postfertilization (Kimmel et al., 1995). Collectively, the segments are called *neuromeres*. This neuroanatomic topography was recognized in several vertebrate species well over a century ago, and today remains one of the most striking examples of conserved morphology in the developing vertebrate brain. Interestingly, pioneering studies in zebrafish were, in part, the first studies to demonstrate more convincingly that in the hindbrain and spinal cord, a serially repeated pattern of restricted neurogenesis exists (Eisen et al., 1986; Metcalfe et al., 1986; Hanneman et al., 1988; Trevarrow et al., 1990). Analyses of early differentiation and axonogenesis (Chitnis and Kuwada, 1990; Wilson et al., 1990; Ross et al., 1992), cell proliferation (Wullimann and Puelles, 1999), and early regionalized gene expression patterns (Hauptmann and Gerster, 2000; Hauptmann et al., 2002b) have firmly established that the formation of the zebrafish forebrain, midbrain, and hindbrain follows the principles of the neuromeric model (reviewed in Puelles, 1995; Rubenstein et al., 1998). Thus, the neuromeric organization of the neural tube defines the fundamental subdivisions of the embryonic brain in all vertebrates and

TABLE 3.1. *Zebrafish Mutants, Selected Genes, and Their Function or Phenotype*

Mutant	Gene	Function/Phenotype (Reference)
Planar Cell Polarity Pathway		
knypek	kny	Heparan sulfate proteoglycan, craniofacial defects (Topczewski et al., 2001)
trilobite*	vangl2	Transmembrane protein, associated with PCP, NTD in mouse (loop tail) knockout (Kibar et al., 2001; Jessen et al., 2002)
pipe tail	wnt5a	Impaired development of head skeleton (Rauch et al., 1997)
silberblick	wnt11	Cyclopia and midline defects in the head (Heisenberg et al., 2000)
Cell Polarity and Adhesion		
grumpy	lamb1	Laminin beta 1, notochord, and brain defects (Parsons et al., 2002)
heart and soul	aPKC l	Defects in the polarized epithelia of the retina/neural tube (Horne-Badovinac et al., 2001; Peterson et al., 2001)
nagie oko	nok	MAGUK, abnormal brain, retinal cell patterning defects (Wei and Malicki, 2002)
parachute/glass onion	n-cad	Cell adhesion, defects in neural tube and eye (Lele et al., 2002; Malicki et al., 2003)
sleepy	lamc1	Laminin gamma 1, irregular brain shape (Parsons et al., 2002)
Hedgehog Signaling		
detour	gli1	Zinc finger TF, defects in ventral neuroectoderm (Karlstrom et al., 2003)
slow muscle omitted	smoothened	Lateral floor plate and subpopulation of hypothalamic cells (Varga et al., 2001)
sonic you*	shh	Motorneuron axons and ganglion cells, NTD in mouse knockout (Harris and Juriloff, 1997; Schauerte et al., 1998)
you too	gli2	Zinc finger TF, midline development, retinal axon guidance, ectopic lens, interference with *Hh* signaling (Karlstrom et al., 2003)
Nodal Signaling		
bonnie and clyde	mixer	Paired-class homeodomain TF, abnormal brain shape (Kikuchi et al., 2000)
cyclops	ndr2	Nodal related 2, ventral midline patterning (Rebagliati et al., 1998; Sampath et al., 1998)
schmalspur	foxh1/fast1	Winged-helix transcription factor, prechordal plate, and ventral neuroectoderm (Pogoda et al., 2000; Sirotkin et al., 2000)
squint	ndr1	Nodal related 1, mild eye cyclopia (Feldman et al., 1998)
one-eyed pinhead	oep	EGF-CFC member and a coreceptor for nodal, cyclopia, mutation in human holoprosencephaly (Zhang et al., 1998)
Neuroectoderm Specification and Patterning		
acerebellar	fgf8	Defects in MHB and cerebellum (Reifers et al., 1998)
bozozok	dharma	Homeodomain TF, loss of neural fate anterior to MHB (Fekany et al., 1999)
chokh	rx3	Homeodomain TF, loss of eye (Loosli et al., 2003)
dino	chordin	BMP antagonist, reduced brain size (Schulte-Merker et al., 1997)
headless	tcf3	Truncation of forebrain structures (Kim et al., 2000)
lazarus	pbx	Segmental patterning of hindbrain and anterior trunk (Popperl et al., 2000)
masterblind*	axin1	Reduced eye and forebrain, NTD in mouse knockout (Zeng et al., 1997; Heisenberg et al., 2001)
neckless*	aldh1a2	Retinaldehydrogenase type 2, defects in neural tube and paraxial mesoderm, NTD in mouse knockout (Niederreither et al., 1999; Begemann et al., 2001)
no isthmus	pax2.1	No MHB, abnormal dorsal and ventral midbrain (Brand et al., 1996)
snailhouse	bmp7	Expansion of neuroectoderm (Dick et al., 2000; Schmid et al., 2000)
somitabun*	smad5	Expansion of neuroectoderm, NTD in mouse knockout (Chang et al., 1999; Hild et al., 1999)
spiel ohne grenzen	pou2	POU-domain transcription factor, MHB midbrain size and patterning of hind brain (Hauptmann et al., 2002a; Reim and Brand, 2002)
swirl	bmp2b	Expansion of neuroectoderm (Kishimoto et al., 1997)
too few	fezl	Zinc finger TF, defects in hypothalamic DA and 5-HT neurons (Levkowitz et al., 2003)
valentino	val	bZip transcription factor, required for r5 and r6, defects in inner ear (Moens et al., 1998)
Neural Crest		
lockjaw/mont blanc*	tfap2a	Hindbrain and sympathetic noradrenergic neurons, neural crest development, NTD in knockout (Harris and Juriloff, 1997; Holzschuh et al., 2003; Knight et al., 2003)
van gogh	tbx1	T-box gene, pharyngeal mesoderm, neural crest–derived cartilages, Di George syndrome (Piotrowski et al., 2003)

TABLE 3.1. *(continued)*

Mutant	Gene	Function/Phenotype (Reference)
Neurogenesis		
foggy	spt5	Transcription elongation factor, reduction of DA neurons and surplus of 5-HT neurons, notochord defects (Guo et al., 2000)
mind bomb	mib	Ring ubiquitin ligase, *Notch* signaling, excessive neuronal differentiation (Itoh et al., 2003)
pandora	spt6	Transcription elongation factor, defects in brain ventricle, eye, and ear (Keegan et al., 2002)
Subtle Neural Function		
ache	ache	Acetylcholinesterase; muscle fiber formation and innervation, death of primary sensory neurons (Behra et al., 2002)
astray	robo2	Roundabout homolog 2, defects in axon path finding (Fricke et al., 2001)
lakritz	ath5	Basic helix-loop-helix TF, retinal ganglion cell determination (Kay et al., 2001)
mariner	myosin 7a	Hair bundles, Usher 1B syndrome (Ernest et al., 2000)
nicotinic	chrna1	Cholinergic receptor nicotinic alpha polypeptide 1, nonmotile receptor, no clustering of acetylcholine receptors (Sepich et al., 1998)
no optokientic response *f*	gnat2	G protein alpha transducing activity polypeptide 2 defects in cone photoreceptor, mutation in human achromatopsia (color blindness) (Brockerhoff et al., 2003)
soulless	phox2a	Homeodomain TF, reduction in locus coeruleus noradrenergic neurons (Guo et al., 1999)
twich once	rapsyn	Inhibition of formation of acetylcholine receptor clusters, reduced synaptic strength (Ono et al., 2002)
young	smarca4	Chromatin remodeling complex, retinal cell differentiation (Gregg et al., 2003)

*Zebrafish mutants carrying mutations in zebrafish orthologs of mouse NTD genes (Juriloff and Harris, 2000)

BMP, bone morphogenetic protein; DA, dopamine; EGF-CFC, epidermal growth factor-like domain and mouse Cripto, Xenopus FRL-1, mouse Cryptic domain; 5-HT, 5-hydroxytriptamine; MHB, midbrain-hindbrain boundary; NTD, neural tube defect; PCP, planar cell polarity; POU, *PIT1* and *OCT1* of mammals and *Unc-86* of C. elegans; TF, transcription factor.

prefigures the major functional subdivisions of the adult brain (Fig. 3.1).

Functional Conservation of the Zebrafish Nervous System

There are differences in neuroanatomy between teleosts and mammals. Perhaps the most obvious difference is that the teleost telencephalon is rather small relative to the rest of the brain and lacks the characteristic structure of the cerebral cortex, with its highly folded appearance (resulting in the formation of gyri and sulci). Clearly, these specializations that are found in mammals reflect the specializations in the function of the telencephalon, especially in humans. Despite these differences, all teleosts retain the basic neural circuitry for sensory and motor functions that are characteristic of a vertebrate nervous system.

Zebrafish possess all of the classical sense modalities (vision, olfaction, taste, touch, balance, and hearing), and their sensory pathways share an overall homology with humans. For example, axons of sensory neurons expressing the same odorant receptor in the nasal epithelium project to a common glomerulus in the olfactory bulb (Byrd et al., 1996), a phenomenon that occurs in the mammalian primary olfactory pathway (Mombaerts, 2001). Similar to the mammalian olfactory system, neurons in the olfactory bulb project to secondary and tertiary targets in the telencephalon and diencephalon (Wullimann, 1998). In the visual system, the topographical projection of the retinotectal pathway for visual processing is highly conserved among all vertebrates. Interestingly, second-order motion perception, which in humans involves processing of relatively complex visual information in the visual cortex, can be observed in larval zebrafish, suggesting that higher-level cortical-like visual processing capacities are similarly inherent in teleosts (Orger et al., 2000). Although the neuroanatomical substrates for this complex behavior are currently unresolved, the ability to test this behavior in the zebrafish may facilitate the discovery of novel genetic pathways that are involved in mediating the function of this visual related cognitive process. With some exceptions, the descending motor and premotor pathways in the teleostean brain are conserved with those of mammals, including the reticulospinal, rubrospinal, and vestibulospinal projections, as well as the projections from the midbrain tectum and cerebellum to brainstem targets (Butler and Hodos, 1996).

Evidence for neuroanatomical and functional homology of integrative brain regions, such as the cerebellum, tectum, and telencephalon, between teleosts and other vertebrates offers a broader perspective of the evolution of cognitive processing. For example, spatial memory in mammals is critically dependent on the hippocampus (Eichenbaum et al., 1999), a structure that is developmentally derived from the medial part of the dorsal telencephalon (the medial pallium). In mammals, the central lumen of the telencephalic neural tube expands to form the lateral ventricles as the dorsal part of the neural tube bulges out in a process of evagination. However, in teleosts the telencephalon is everted such that the roof of the neural tube over the telencephalic central lumen thins and elongates, causing the dorsal part of the tube on either side to bend back on itself. Thus, the lateral pallium of teleosts appears to be structurally homologous to the mammaliam hippocampus–medial pallium (Butler, 2000; Rodríguez et al., 2002a). Although the theory of simple eversion accounting for the peculiar anatomy of the teleostean telencephalon is still controversial (Bradford, 1995), evidence from goldfish (a cyprinid cousin to the zebrafish) suggests that lesions of the lateral pallium do in fact selectively impair spatial memory representations, as hippocampal lesions do in mammals (Rodríguez et al., 2002b). This is a striking example of functional conservation between the brains of teleosts and mammals despite a rather distinct process of telencephalic morphogenesis.

These observations indicate that the neural circuitry and function of the teleost and mammalian nervous system are highly conserved. Thus, identifying the molecular and cellular determinants that govern the formation of the nervous system in zebrafish will provide us with a fundamental understanding of human brain formation and of the mechanisms by which NTDs have devastating consequences on nervous system function (see Tropepe and Sive, 2003).

LESSONS FROM ZEBRAFISH MUTANTS

The formation of the neural tube is a complex cellular process subjected to perturbation by many genetic components. Thus, any defects at the cellular level, including aberrant cell death, proliferation, differentiation, migration, and adhesion during neurulation, may result in NTDs. Various studies in animal models, mouse knockouts in particular, have proven useful for revealing the critical steps and providing candidate genes for human NTDs. However, these mouse models have three major obstacles that discourage systematic investigations for identifying the genetic and cellular pathways underlying human NTDs. First, in most cases, the precise molecular mechanisms by which the loss of a particular gene function leads to NTDs are not known. Second, the intrauterine development of mouse embryos prevents analysis of the developmental time course of NTDs. Third, many NTDs may be caused by mutations in multiple genes (Harris and Juriloff, 1997; Juriloff and Harris, 2000; Colas and Schoenwolf, 2001), and their phenotypic characterization may therefore require compound genetic analyses, such as identification of genetic modifiers. A relatively small litter size and expensive housing costs make it difficult to carry out such analyses in the mouse. In the next sections, we discuss the advantages of using zebrafish as a complementary genetic model system to study NTDs. We first discuss results of zebrafish mutant screens that have yielded brain mutants, highlighting those that may include NTD candidates. We then discuss feasible experimental strategies in zebrafish that could help elucidate the molecular mechanisms underlying human NTDs.

Zebrafish Mutants That Include Some with Putative Neural Tube Defects

Forward genetic screens in zebrafish have yielded a large number of mutants reflecting the key aspects of various developmental problems. Table 3.1 lists zebrafish mutants defective in brain morphology and neural function. These mutants are grouped into several categories according to the cellular function of the corresponding genes. These categories include mutants defective in major signaling pathways and those that alter cell polarity and adhesion, neuroectoderm specification and patterning, development of the neural crest, and neurogenesis. Importantly, some of these mutants encode zebrafish orthologs of mouse NTD genes, allowing phenotypes to be compared among species (Table 3.1). Many other zebrafish mutants with putative NTDs have been isolated for which the corresponding gene has not been identified (Schier et al., 1996; Schilling et al., 1996).

One interesting example that lends itself to comparison is the mouse *loop-tail* mutant, which corresponds to a homolog of *Drosophila Strabismus* (Wolff and Rubin, 1998; Kibar et al., 2001a, 2001b), a PSD95-DLG-Z01 (PDZ) domain transmembrane protein involved in the planar cell polarity (PCP) pathway. The *loop-tail* mutant exhibits craniorachischisis, a failure of neural tube closure from the midbrain to the lower spinal cord. However, the mechanisms by which loss of gene function gives rise to NTDs has not been investigated, partly due to the relatively inaccessible nature of mouse embryos. Recently, the zebrafish *trilobite* mutant has been cloned, and the gene encodes a fish ortholog of this protein (Jessen et al., 2002). In contrast to the mouse, analysis of the fish mutant was relatively simple, and the use of cell transplantation coupled with time-lapse imaging has revealed the mechanism by which the *trilobite* gene product controls cell shape changes and movements during gastrulation and neuronal migration (Jessen et al., 2002).

Further emphasizing the importance of the PCP pathway in vertebrate neurulation, disruption of mouse orthologs of other fly PCP components also leads to NTDs. Further, genetic interactions between these components have been shown (Kibar et al., 2001; Hamblet et al., 2002; Curtin et al., 2003; Montcouquiol et al., 2003; Murdoch et al., 2003). Similarly, zebrafish mutants defective in PCP components produce varying degrees of brain and crainiofacial defects (Rauch et al., 1997; Heisenberg et al., 2000; Topczewski et al., 2001; Jessen et al., 2002), and these phenotypes are enhanced by inhibition of other PCP components (Topczewski et al., 2001; Carreira-Barbosa et al., 2003).

Another appealing attribute of zebrafish is the ability to isolate multiple mutant alleles, allowing detailed analyses of gene dosage and structure–function relationships leading to brain phenotypes. For example, the zebrafish *foggy* encodes transcription elongation factor Spt5, and three alleles (*m806, sk8,* and *s30*) have been reported (Guo et al., 2000; Keegan et al., 2002a). The *m806* allele contains a missense mutation (*V1012D*), still leaving significant aspects of Spt5 function, whereas both the *sk8* and *s30* alleles are thought to be null. The differences in the nature of the molecular lesion correlate with the phenotypic strength of mutant alleles: *m806* exhibits neurogenetic defects without significant abnormalities in brain shape (Guo et al., 2000), whereas both *sk8* and *s30* manifest some degree of the altered brain morphology (Keegan et al., 2002b). In a striking example, 12 alleles of zebrafish *grumpy* mutants and 19 alleles of zebrafish *sleepy* mutants have been isolated, encoding laminin beta 1 and gamma 1, respectively, components of basal laminae (see http://zfin.org).

Relatively inexpensive maintenance of zebrafish mutant stocks and a large clutch size facilitate compound genetic analyses to determine genetic interactions (i.e., epistatic, synergistic, or antagonistic relationships) between NTD genes. For example, the zebrafish *knypek,* encoding a heparan sulfate proteoglycan, shows craniofacial defects with no cyclopic phenotype (Topczewski et al., 2001). Double mutants of *knypek* and *silberlick,* which encodes *wnt11* (involved in PCP signaling [Heisenberg et al., 2000]), manifests strong cyclopic phenotypes, identifying *Kny* as a component of the PCP pathway. Such analyses can either be performed by making classical double mutants or by using reverse genetics tools, such as antisense morpholino oligomers (as discussed in the section "Genetic, Molecular, and Embryological Methods in Zebrafish Research").

Epithelial cells display apical-basal cell polarization by a mechanism conserved between vertebrates and invertebrates. In the fly, localization of apical determinants, such as *Crumb,* is controlled by *Scribble* (Bilder and Perrimon, 2000). A mouse ortholog of the fly *Scribble* is a component of PCP (Montcouquiol et al., 2003), indicating a direct link between apical-basal polarization and PCP pathways. The zebrafish mutants in apical-basal polarity have been isolated and include *nagie oko, heart and soul,* and *parachute* (*glass onion*) (Horne-Badovinac et al., 2001; Peterson et al., 2001; Lele et al., 2002a; Wei and Malicki, 2002; Malicki et al., 2003a). These mutants exhibit a certain degree of NTDs, suggesting that genetic components involved in apical-basal cell polarity are candidates for NTDs and that phenotypic analyses of these mutants may provide new insights into cellular defects of NTDs.

Strategies Used to Study Neural Tube Defects in Zebrafish

What experimental strategies in zebrafish would help us better understand the molecular etiology of human NTDs? First, a *candidate* gene approach can be employed in the zebrafish, where the function of genes correlating with human NTD candidates is analyzed in the fish. Reverse genetic approaches will be very useful in this regard, as it is possible to generate partial loss of function phenotypes that may correspond to the situation in the human NTD. Partial loss of function phenotypes can be generated by injecting varying amounts of antisense morpholino or via target-selected gene inactivation (Wienholds et al., 2002, 2003), which allows isolation of multiple alleles of a single gene that may display different severity. Multiple alleles will also facilitate structure–function analysis of a given protein.

Neural tube defect phenotypes could be due either to direct effects of a given gene on the neural tube or to secondary effects of its early function. In situ hybridization and immunocytochemistry to determine where the protein is expressed are clearly essential. However, for ubiquitously expressed gene products, asking when the gene product is required will help narrow down the target of the gene. Temporally controlled expression can be effected using a heat shock–inducible promoter driving the gene of interest, allowing its controlled expression in a mutant line and assaying for rescue of the phenotype (Halloran et al., 2000; Yeo et al., 2001). Another mechanism to address the target of a gene product is to ask where this is required. Spatially restricted expression is possible using tissue-specific promoters and deriving lines of such fish that can be used to attempt rescue mutant lines.

Second, a forward genetics approach (random mutagenesis) will lead to identification of potential NTD genes in a relatively unbiased manner. Several forward genetic screens have yielded mutants affecting brain morphology and neural function (Table 3.1); however, a directed screen for mutants displaying NTDs has not been performed. Such a screen will be extremely useful in expanding the collection of potential NTD risk genes in human. Some NTDs may be caused by mutations in multiple genes, perhaps in association with environmental factors. Mutation in one NTD risk gene therefore may not cause an obvious phenotype. A crucial issue, then, is how to define genes that must act in concert with others to cause an NTD. One promising method is the use of genetic modifier screens. These start with a weak allele of a locus that gives an NTD when null. Forward genetic approaches could then be used to isolate other genes that strengthen or further weaken the phenotype.

Another approach, with potential therapeutic ramifications, uses small molecules of defined or unknown specificity that could be applied to mutant embryos in an effort to strengthen or weaken the phenotype. Such an approach has been taken with wild-type zebrafish embryos (Peterson et al., 2000). For example, in the zebrafish *heart and soul* mutant, neuroepithelial polarity is disrupted due to loss of protein kinase C (αPKC) lambda. A chemical inhibitor of this kinase has been identified and shown to cause phenotypes in wild-type embryos (Peterson et al., 2001a). Since αPKC lambda is a good candidate for NTD, genetic screens could be designed to look for suppressors (or enhancers) of the chemical inhibitor. This chemical approach could not only be used to define pathways that alter the NTD phenotype, but could also provide potential therapeutic agents that may abrogate neonatal NTD phenotypes.

CONCLUSION

In summary, we have discussed the utility of the zebrafish as a model for identifying and analyzing genes that cause human NTDs. Multiple zebrafish mutants that give NTDs have already been isolated, and some show defects similar to those of the mouse model. The powerful forward and reverse genetic approaches available in the zebrafish make this a highly promising model for clarifying the mechanisms underlying human NTDs.

ACKNOWLEDGMENTS

Our consideration of these topics was supported by grants from the NIH (MH59942 and MH070926).

REFERENCES

Amsterdam A, Burgess S, Golling G, Chen W, Sun Z, Townsend K, Farrington S, et al (1999). A large-scale insertional mutagenesis screen in zebrafish. Genes Dev 13:2713–2724.

Barut BA, Zon LI (2000). Realizing the potential of zebrafish as a model for human disease. Physiol Genomics 2:49–51.

Begemann G, Schilling TF, Rauch GJ, Geisler R, Ingham PW (2001). The zebrafish *neckless* mutation reveals a requirement for raldh2 in mesodermal signals that pattern the hindbrain. Development 128:3081–3094.

Behra M, Cousin X, Bertrand C, Vonesch JL, Biellmann D, Chatonnet A, Strahle U (2002). Acetylcholinesterase is required for neuronal and muscular development in the zebrafish embryo. Nat Neurosci 5:111–118.

Bilder D, Perrimon N (2000). Localization of apical epithelial determinants by the basolateral PDZ protein *Scribble*. Nature 403:676–680.

Bradford MR Jr (1995). Comparative aspects of forebrain organization in the ray-finned fishes: touchstones or not? Brain Behav Evol 46:259–274.

Brand M, Heisenberg CP, Jiang YJ, Beuchle D, Lun K, Furutani-Seiki M, Granato M, et al (1996). Mutations in zebrafish genes affecting the formation of the boundary between midbrain and hindbrain. Development 123:179–190.

Brockerhoff SE, Rieke F, Matthews HR, Taylor MR, Kennedy B, Ankoudinova I, Niemi GA, et al (2003). Light stimulates a transducin-independent increase of cytoplasmic Ca^{2+} and suppression of current in cones from the zebrafish mutant *nof*. J Neurosci 23:470–480.

Butler AB (2000). Topography and topology of the teleost telencephalon: a paradox resolved. Neurosci Lett 293:95–98.

Butler AB, Hodos W (1996). *Comparative Vertebrate Neuroanatomy: Evolution and Adaptation.* New York: Wiley-Liss.

Byrd CA, Jones JT, Quattro JM, Rogers ME, Brunjes PC, Vogt RG (1996). Ontogeny of odorant receptor gene expression in zebrafish, *Danio rerio*. J Neurobiol 29:445–458.

Carreira-Barbosa F, Concha ML, Takeuchi M, Ueno N, Wilson SW, Tada M (2003). *Prickle 1* regulates cell movements during gastrulation and neuronal migration in zebrafish. Development 130:4037–4046.

Chang H, Huylebroeck D, Verschueren K, Guo Q, Matzuk MM, Zwijsen A (1999). *Smad5* knockout mice die at mid-gestation due to multiple embryonic and extraembryonic defects. Development 126:1631–1642.

Chitnis AB, Kuwada JY (1990). Axonogenesis in the brain of zebrafish embryos. J Neurosci 10:1892–1905.

Colas JF, Schoenwolf GC (2001). Towards a cellular and molecular understanding of neurulation. Dev Dyn 221:117–145.

Criley BB (1969). Analysis of embryonic sources and mechanisms of development of posterior levels of chick neural tubes. J Morphol 128:465–501.

Curtin JA, Quint E, Tsipouri V, Arkell RM, Cattanach B, Copp AJ, Henderson DJ, et al (2003). Mutation of *Celsr1* disrupts planar polarity of inner ear hair cells and causes severe neural tube defects in the mouse. Curr Biol 13:1129–1133.

Darland T, Dowling JE (2001). Behavioral screening for cocaine sensitivity in mutagenized zebrafish. Proc Natl Acad Sci USA 98:11691–11696.

Davidson LA, Keller RE (1999). Neural tube closure in *Xenopus laevis* involves medial migration, directed protrusive activity, cell intercalation and convergent extension. Development 126:4547–4556.

Dick A, Hild M, Bauer H, Imai Y, Maifeld H, Schier AF, Talbot WS, et al (2000). Essential role of *Bmp7* (*snailhouse*) and its prodomain in dorsoventral patterning of the zebrafish embryo. Gene 127:343–354.

Dodd A, Curtis PM, Williams LC, Love DR (2000). Zebrafish: bridging the gap between development and disease. Hum Mol Genet 9:2443–2449.

Driever W, Solnica-Krezel L, Schier AF, Neuhauss SCF, Malicki J, Stemple DL, Stainier DYR, et al (1996). A genetic screen for mutations affecting embryogenesis in zebrafish. Development 123:37–46.

Eichenbaum H, Dudchenko P, Wood E, Shapiro M, Tanila H (1999). The hippocampus, memory, and place cells: is it spatial memory or a memory space? Neuron 23:209–226.

Eisen JS, Myers PZ, Westerfield M (1986). Pathway selection by growth cones of identified motoneurones in live zebrafish embryos. Nature 320:269–271.

Ernest S, Rauch GJ, Haffter P, Geisler R, Petit C, Nicolson T (2000). *Mariner* is defective in myosin VIIA: a zebrafish model for human hereditary deafness. Hum Mol Genet 9:2189–2196.

Fekany K, Yamanaka Y, Leung T, Sirotkin HI, Topczewski J, Gates MA, Hibi M, et al (1999). The zebrafish *bozozok* locus encodes *Dharma,* a homeodomain protein essential for induction of gastrula organizer and dorsoanterior embryonic structures. Development 126:1427–1438.

Feldman B, Gates MA, Egan ES, Dougan ST, Rennebeck G, Sirotkin HI, Schier AF, et al (1998). Zebrafish organizer development and germlayer formation require nodal-related signals. Nature 395:181–185.

Fricke C, Lee JS, Geiger-Rudolph S, Bonhoeffer F, Chien CB (2001). *astray,* a zebrafish roundabout homolog required for retinal axon guidance. Science 292:507–510.

Geldmacher-Voss B, Reugels AM, Pauls S, Campos-Ortega JA (2003). A 90 degrees rotation of the mitotic spindle changes the orientation of mitoses of zebrafish neuroepithelial cells. Development 130:3767–3780.

Gregg RG, Willer GB, Fadool JM, Dowling JE, Link BA (2003). Positional cloning of the young mutation identifies an essential role for the Brahma chromatin remodeling complex in mediating retinal cell differentiation. Proc Natl Acad Sci USA 100:6535–6540.

Grinblat Y, Lane ME, Sagerström C, Sive H (1999). Analysis of zebrafish development using explant culture assays. In Detrich HW, Westerfield M, Zon LI (eds): *Methods in Cell Biology,* Vol 59. *The Zebrafish: Biology.* Boston: Academic Press, pp. 128–156.

Guo S, Brush J, Teraoka H, Goddard A, Wilson SW, Mullins MC, Rosenthal A (1999). Development of noradrenergic neurons in the zebrafish hindbrain requires BMP, FGF8, and the homeodomain protein *soulless/Phox2a.* Neuron 24:555–566.

Guo S, Yamaguchi Y, Schilbach S, Wada T, Lee J, Goddard A, French D, et al (2000). A regulator of transcriptional elongation controls vertebrate neuronal development. Nature 408:366–369.

Haffter P, Granato M, Brand M, Mullins MC, Hammerschmidt M, Kane DA, Odenthal J, van Eeden FJM, Jiang YJ, Heisenberg CP, Kelsh RN, Furutani-Seiki M, Vogelsang E, Beuchle D, Schach U, Fabian C, Nüsslein-Volhard C (1996). The identification of genes with unique and essential functions in the development of the zebrafish, *Danio rerio.* Development 123:1–36.

Halloran MC, Sato-Maeda M, Warren JT, Su F, Lele Z, Krone PH, Kuwada JY, et al (2000). Laser-induced gene expression in specific cells of transgenic zebrafish. Development 127:1953–1960.

Hamblet NS, Lijam N, Ruiz-Lozano P, Wang J, Yang Y, Luo Z, Mei L, et al (2002). *Dishevelled 2* is essential for cardiac outflow tract development, somite segmentation and neural tube closure. Development 129:5827–5838.

Hanneman E, Trevarrow B, Metcalfe WK, Kimmel CB, Westerfield M (1988). Segmental pattern of development of the hindbrain and spinal cord of the zebrafish embryo. Development 103:49–58.

Hardan AY, Minshew NJ, Mallikarjuhn M, Keshavan MS (2001). Brain volume in autism. J Child Neurol 16:421–424.

Harris MJ, Juriloff DM (1997). Genetic landmarks for defects in mouse neural tube closure. Teratology 56:177–187.

Harris MJ, Juriloff DM (1999). Mini-review: toward understanding mechanisms of genetic neural tube defects in mice. Teratology 60:292–305.

Hauptmann G, Belting HG, Wolke U, Lunde K, Soll I, Abdelilah-Seyfried S, Prince V, et al (2002a). *spiel ohne grenzen/pou2* is required for zebrafish hindbrain segmentation. Development 129:1645–1655.

Hauptmann G, Gerster T (2000). Regulatory gene expression patterns reveal transverse and longitudinal subdivisions of the embryonic zebrafish forebrain. Mech Dev 91:105–118.

Hauptmann G, Söll I, Gerster T (2002b). The early embryonic zebrafish forebrain is subdivided into molecularly distinct transverse and longitudinal domains. Brain Res Bull 57:371–375.

Heisenberg CP, Houart C, Take-Uchi M, Rauch GJ, Young N, Coutinho P, Masai I, et al (2001). A mutation in the Gsk3-binding domain of zebrafish *Masterblind/Axin1* leads to a fate transformation of telencephalon and eyes to diencephalon. Genes Dev 15:1427–1434.

Heisenberg CP, Tada M, Rauch GJ, Saude L, Concha ML, Geisler R, Stemple DL, et al (2000). *Silberblick/Wnt11* mediates convergent extension movements during zebrafish gastrulation. Nature 405:76–81.

Hild M, Dick A, Rauch GJ, Meier A, Bouwmeester T, Haffter P, Hammerschmidt M (1999). The *smad5* mutation somitabun blocks *Bmp2b* signaling during early dorsoventral patterning of the zebrafish embryo. Development 126:2149–2159.

Holzschuh J, Barrallo-Gimeno A, Ettl AK, Durr K, Knapik EW, Driever W (2003). Noradrenergic neurons in the zebrafish hindbrain are induced by retinoic acid and require *tfap2a* for expression of the neurotransmitter phenotype. Development 130:5741–5754.

Horne-Badovinac S, Lin D, Waldron S, Schwarz M, Mbamalu G, Pawson T, Jan Y, et al (2001). Positional cloning of heart and soul reveals multiple roles for PKC lambda in zebrafish organogenesis. Curr Biol 11:1492–1502.

Hyatt TM, Ekker SC (1999). Vectors and techniques for ectopic gene expression in zebrafish. In Detrich HW, Westerfield M, Zon LI (eds): *Methods in Cell Biology,* Vol 59. *The Zebrafish: Biology.* Boston: Academic Press, pp. 117–126.

Itoh M, Kim CH, Palardy G, Oda T, Jiang YJ, Maust D, Yeo SY, et al (2003). Mind bomb is a ubiquitin ligase that is essential for efficient activation of *Notch* signaling by *Delta.* Dev Cell 4:67–82.

Jessen JR, Topczewski J, Bingham S, Sepich DS, Marlow F, Chandrasekhar A, Solnica-Krezel, L (2002). Zebrafish trilobite identifies new roles for *Strabismus* in gastrulation and neuronal movements. Nat Cell Biol 4:610–615.

Jiang YJ, Brand M, Heisenberg CP, Beuchle D, Furutani-Seiki M, Kelsh RN, Warga RM, et al (1996). Mutations affecting neurogenesis and brain morphology in the zebrafish, *Danio rerio.* Development 123:205–216.

Juriloff DM, Harris MJ (2000). Mouse models for neural tube closure defects. Hum Mol Genet 9:993–1000.

Karlstrom RO, Tyurina OV, Kawakami A, Nishioka N, Talbot WS, Sasaki H, Schier AF (2003a). Genetic analysis of zebrafish *gli1* and *gli2* reveals divergent requirements for *gli* genes in vertebrate development. Development 130:1549–1564.

Kay JN, Finger-Baier KC, Roeser T, Staub W, Baier H (2001). Retinal ganglion cell genesis requires *lakritz,* a zebrafish atonal homolog. Neuron 30:725–736.

Keegan BR, Feldman JL, Lee DH, Koos DS, Ho RK, Stainier DY, Yelon D (2002). The elongation factors *Pandora/Spt6* and *Foggy/Spt5* promote transcription in the zebrafish embryo. Development 129:1623–1632.

Kibar Z, Vogan KJ, Groulx N, Justice MJ, Underhill DA, Gros P (2001a). *Ltap,* a mammalian homolog of *Drosophila Strabismus/Van Gogh,* is altered in the mouse neural tube mutant *Loop-tail.* Nat Genet 28:251–255.

Kikuchi Y, Trinh LA, Reiter JF, Alexander J, Yelon D, Stainier DY (2000). The zebrafish *bonnie and clyde* gene encodes a Mix family homeodomain protein that regulates the generation of endodermal precursors. Genes Dev 14:1279–1289.

Kim CH, Oda T, Itoh M, Jiang D, Artinger KB, Chandrasekharappa SC, Driever W, et al (2000). Repressor activity of *Headless/Tcf3* is essential for vertebrate head formation. Nature 407:913–916.

Kimmel CB (1989). Genetics and early development of zebrafish. Trends Genet 5:283–288.

Kimmel CB, Ballard WW, Kimmel SR, Ullmann B, Schilling TF (1995). Stages of embryonic development of the zebrafish. Dev Dyn 203:253–310.

Kimmel CB, Warga RM, Kane DA (1994). Cell cycles and clonal strings during formation of the zebrafish central nervous system. Development 120:265–276.

Kishimoto Y, Lee KH, Zon L, Hammerschmidt M, Schulte-Merker, S (1997). The molecular nature of zebrafish swirl: BMP2 function is essential during early dorsoventral patterning. Development 124:4457–4466.

Knight RD, Nair S, Nelson SS, Afshar A, Javidan Y, Geisler R, Rauch GJ, et al (2003). *lockjaw* encodes a zebrafish *tfap2a* required for early neural crest development. Development 130:5755–5768.

Kurokawa K, Nakamura K, Sumiyoshi T, Hagino H, Yotsutsuji T, Yamashita I, Suzuki M, et al (2000). Ventricular enlargement in schizophrenia spectrum patients with prodromal symptoms of obsessive-compulsive disorder. Psychiatry Res 99:83–91.

Lele Z, Folchert A, Concha M, Rauch GJ, Geisler R, Rosa F, Wilson SW, et al (2002). *parachute/n-cadherin* is required for morphogenesis and maintained integrity of the zebrafish neural tube. Development 129:3281–3294.

Levkowitz G, Zeller J, Sirotkin HI, French D, Schilbach S, Hashimoto H, Hibi M, Talbot WS, Rosenthal A (2003). Zinc finger protein *too few* controls the development of monoaminergic neurons. Nat Neurosci 6:28–33.

Loosli F, Staub W, Finger-Baier KC, Ober EA, Verkade H, Wittbrodt J, Baier H (2003). Loss of eyes in zebrafish caused by mutation of *chokh/rx3*. EMBO Rep 4:894–899.

Lowery LA, Sive H (2004). Strategies of vertebrate neurulation and a re-evaluation of teleost neural tube formation. Mech Dev 121:1189–1197.

Ma C, Fan L, Ganassin R, Bols N, Collodi P (2001). Production of zebrafish germ-line chimeras from embryo cell cultures. Proc Natl Acad Sci USA 98:2461–2466.

Machado HR, Martelli N, Assirati JA, Jr, and Colli BO (1991). Infantile hydrocephalus: brain sonography as an effective tool for diagnosis and follow-up. Childs Nerv Syst 7:205–210.

Malicki J, Jo H, Pujic Z (2003). Zebrafish N-cadherin, encoded by the *glass onion* locus, plays an essential role in retinal patterning. Dev Biol 259:95–108.

McLone DG, Knepper PA (1989). The cause of Chiari II malformation: a unified theory. Pediatr Neurosci 15:1–12.

Metcalfe WK, Mendelson B, Kimmel CB (1986). Segmental homologies among reticulospinal neurons in the hindbrain of the zebrafish larva. J Comp Neurol 251:147–159.

Moens CB, Cordes SP, Giorgianni MW, Barsh GS, Kimmel CB (1998). Equivalence in the genetic control of hindbrain segmentation in fish and mouse. Development 125:381–391.

Mombaerts P (2001). How smell develops. Nat Neurosci 4(Suppl:)1192–1198.

Montcouquiol M, Rachel RA, Lanford PJ, Copeland NG, Jenkins NA, Kelley MW (2003). Identification of *Vangl2* and *Scrb1* as planar polarity genes in mammals. Nature 423:173–177.

Murdoch JN, Henderson DJ, Doudney K, Gaston-Massuet C, Phillips HM, Paternotte C, Arkell R, et al (2003). Disruption of *scribble* (*Scrb1*) causes severe neural tube defects in the circletail mouse. Hum Mol Genet 12:87–98.

Nasevicius A, Ekker SC (2000). Effective targeted gene *knockdown* in zebrafish. Nat Genet 26:216–220.

Niederreither K, Subbarayan V, Dolle P, Chambon P (1999). Embryonic retinoic acid synthesis is essential for early mouse post-implantation development. Nat Genet 21:444–448.

Ono F, Shcherbatko A, Higashijima S, Mandel G, Brehm P (2002). The zebrafish motility mutant twitch once reveals new roles for rapsyn in synaptic function. J Neurosci 22:6491–6498.

Orger MB, Smear MC, Anstis SM, Baier H (2000). Perception of Fourier and non-Fourier motion by larval zebrafish. Nat Neurosci 3:1128–1133.

Papan C, Campos-Ortega JA (1994). On the formation of the neural keel and neural tube in the zebrafish *Danio* (*Brachydanio*) *rerio*. Roux's Arch Dev Biol 203:178–186.

Parsons MJ, Pollard SM, Saude L, Feldman B, Coutinho P, Hirst EM, Stemple DL (2002). Zebrafish mutants identify an essential role for laminins in notochord formation. Development 129:3137–3146.

Peterson RT, Link BA, Dowling JE, Schreiber SL (2000). Small molecule developmental screens reveal the logic and timing of vertebrate development. Proc Natl Acad Sci USA 97:12965–1269.

Peterson RT, Mably JD, Chen JN, Fishman MC (2001). Convergence of distinct pathways to heart patterning revealed by the small molecule concentramide and the mutation *heart-and-soul*. Curr Biol 11:1481–1491.

Piotrowski T, Ahn DG, Schilling TF, Nair S, Ruvinsky I, Geisler R, Rauch GJ, et al (2003). The zebrafish *van gogh* mutation disrupts *tbx1*, which is involved in the DiGeorge deletion syndrome in humans. Development 130:5043–5052.

Pogoda HM, Solnica-Krezel L, Driever W, Meyer D (2000). The zebrafish forkhead transcription factor FoxH1/Fast1 is a modulator of nodal signaling required for organizer formation. Curr Biol 10:1041–1049.

Popperl H, Rikhof H, Chang H, Haffter P, Kimmel CB, Moens CB (2000). *lazarus* is a novel *pbx* gene that globally mediates *hox* gene function in zebrafish. Mol Cell 6:255–267.

Puelles, L (1995). A segmental morphological paradigm for understanding vertebrate forebrains. Brain Behav Evol 46:319–337.

Rauch GJ, Hammerschmidt M, Blader P, Schauerte HE, Strahle U, Ingham PW, McMahon AP, et al (1997). *Wnt5* is required for tail formation in the zebrafish embryo. Cold Spring Harb Symp Quant Biol 62:227–234.

Rebagliati MR, Toyama R, Haffter P, Dawid IB (1998). *cyclops* encodes a nodal-related factor involved in midline signaling. Proc Natl Acad Sci USA 95:9932–9937.

Reifers F, Bohli H, Walsh EC, Crossley PH, Stainier DY, Brand M (1998). *Fgf8* is mutated in zebrafish acerebellar (ace) mutants and is required for maintenance of midbrain-hindbrain boundary development and somitogenesis. Development 125:2381–2395.

Reim G, Brand M (2002). *Spiel-ohne-grenzen/pou2* mediates regional competence to respond to *Fgf8* during zebrafish early neural development. Development 129:917–933.

Rodríguez F, López JC, Vargas JP, Broglio C, Gómez Y, Salas C (2002a). Spatial memory and hippocampal pallium through vertebrate evolution: insights from retiles and teleost fish. Brain Res Bull 57:499–503.

Rodríguez F, López JC, Vargas JP, Gómez Y, Broglio C, Salas C (2002b). Conservation of spatial memory function in the pallial forebrain of reptiles and ray-finned fishes. J Neurosci 22:2894–2903.

Ross LS, Parrett T, Easter SS Jr (1992). Axonogenesis and morphogenesis in the embryonic zebrafish brain. J Neurosci 12:467–482.

Rubenstein JLR, Shimamura K, Martinez S, Puelles L (1998). Regionalization of the prosencephalic neural plate. Annu Rev Neurosci 21:445–477.

Sampath K, Rubinstein AL, Cheng AM, Liang JO, Fekany K, Solnica-Krezel L, Korzh V, et al (1998). Induction of the zebrafish ventral brain and floorplate requires *cyclops*/nodal signalling. Nature 395:185–189.

Schauerte HE, van Eeden FJ, Fricke C, Odenthal J, Strahle U, Haffter P (1998). *Sonic hedgehog* is not required for the induction of medial floor plate cells in the zebrafish. Development 125:2983–2993.

Schier AF, Neuhauss SC, Harvey M, Malicki J, Solnica-Krezel L, Stainier DY, Zwartkruis F, et al (1996). Mutations affecting the development of the embryonic zebrafish brain. Development 123:165–178.

Schilling TF, Piotrowski T, Grandel H, Brand M, Heisenberg CP, Jiang YJ, Beuchle D, et al (1996). Jaw and branchial arch mutants in zebrafish I: branchial arches. Development 123:329–344.

Schmid B, Furthauer M, Connors SA, Trout J, Thisse B, Thisse C, Mullins MC (2000). Equivalent genetic roles for *bmp7/snailhouse* and *bmp2b/swirl* in dorsoventral pattern formation. Development 127:957–967.

Schmitz B, Papan C, Campos-Ortega JA (1993). Neurulation in the anterior trunk region of the zebrafish *Brachydanio rerio*. Roux's Arch Dev Biol 202:250–259.

Schulte-Merker S, Lee KJ, McMahon AP, Hammerschmidt M (1997). The zebrafish organizer requires chordino. Nature 387:862–863.

Sepich DS, Wegner J, O'Shea S, Westerfield M (1998). An altered intron inhibits synthesis of the acetylcholine receptor alpha-subunit in the paralyzed zebrafish mutant *nic1*. Genetics 148:361–372.

Shastry BS (2001). Parkinson disease: etiology, pathogenesis and future of gene therapy. Neurosci Res 41:5–12.

Shum AS, Copp AJ (1996). Regional differences in morphogenesis of the neuroepithelium suggest multiple mechanisms of spinal neurulation in the mouse. Anat Embryol (Berl) 194:65–73.

Sirotkin HI, Gates MA, Kelly PD, Schier AF, Talbot WS (2000). *Fast1* is required for the development of dorsal axial structures in zebrafish. Curr Biol 10:1051–1054.

Streisinger G, Walker C, Dower N, Knauber D, Singer F (1981). Production of clones of homozygous diploid zebra fish (*Brachydario rerio*). Nature 291:293–296.

Streit A, Berliner A, Papanayotou C, Sirulnik A, Stern CD (2000). Initiation of neural induction by FGF signaling before gastrulation. Nature 406:74–78.

Sun Z, Hopkins N (2001). *vhnf1*, the MODY5 and familial GCKD-associated gene, regulates regional specification in the zebrafish gut, pronephros, and hindbrain. Genes Dev 15:3217–3229.

Thermes V, Grabher C, Ristorante F, Bourrat F, Choulika A, Wittbrodt J, Joly JS (2002). I-Sce meganuclease mediates highly efficient transgenesis in fish. Mech Dev 118:91–98.

Topczewski J, Sepich DS, Myers DC, Walker C, Amores A, Lele Z, Hammerschmidt M, et al (2001). The zebrafish *glypican knypek* controls cell polarity during gastrulation movements of convergent extension. Dev Cell 1:251–64.

Trevarrow B, Marks DL, Kimmel CB (1990). Organization of hindbrain segments in the zebrafish embryo. Neuron 4:669–679.

Tropepe V, Sive HL (2003) Can zebrafish be used to study the neurodevelopmental causes of autism? Genes Brain Behav 2: 268–281.

Varga ZM, Amores A, Lewis KE, Yan YL, Postlethwait JH, Eisen JS, Westerfield M (2001). Zebrafish *smoothened* functions in ventral neural tube specification and axon tract formation. Development 128:3497–509.

Wei X, Malicki J (2002). *nagie oko*, encoding a MAGUK-family protein, is essential for cellular patterning of the retina. Nat Genet 31:150–157.

Wienholds E, Schulte-Merker S, Walderich B, Plasterk RH (2002). Target-selected inactivation of the zebrafish *rag1* gene. Science 297:99–102.

Wienholds E, Van Eeden F, Kosters M, Mudde J, Plasterk RH, Cuppen E (2003). Efficient target-selected mutagenesis in zebrafish. Genome Res 13:2700–2707.

Wiellette E, Grinblat Y, Austen M, Hirsinger E, Amsterdam A, Walker C, Westerfield M, Sive H (2004). Combined haploid and insertional mutation screen in the zebrafish. Genesis 40:231–240.

Wilson SW, Ross LS, Parrett T, Easter SS Jr (1990). The development of a simple scaffold of axon tracts in the brain of the embryonic zebrafish, *Brachydanio rerio*. Development 108:121–145.

Wolff T, Rubin GM (1998). *Strabismus,* a novel gene that regulates tissue polarity and cell fate decisions in *Drosophila*. Development 125:1149–1159.

Woo K, Fraser SE (1997). Specification of the zebrafish nervous system by nonaxial signals. Science 277:254–257.

Wullimann MF (1998). The central nervous system. In Evans DH (ed): *The Physiology of Fishes,* 2nd ed. New York: CRC Press pp. 245–281.

Wullimann MF, Puelles L (1999). Postembryonic neural proliferation in the zebrafish forebrain and its relationship to prosomeric domains. Anat Embryol 329:329–348.

Yeo SY, Little MH, Yamada T, Miyashita T, Halloran MC, Kuwada JY, Huh TL, et al (2001). Overexpression of a *slit* homologue impairs convergent extension of the mesoderm and causes cyclopia in embryonic zebrafish. Dev Biol 230:1–17.

Zeng L, Fagotto F, Zhang T, Hsu W, Vasicek TJ, Perry WL 3rd, Lee JJ, et al (1997). The mouse *Fused* locus encodes *Axin,* an inhibitor of the *Wnt* signaling pathway that regulates embryonic axis formation. Cell 90:181–192.

Zhang J, Talbot WS, Schier AF (1998). Positional cloning identifies zebrafish *one-eyed pinhead* as a permissive EGF-related ligand required during gastrulation. Cell 92:241–251.

4

Genetic Regulation of Early Nervous System Development

ELLEN M. CARPENTER

The primordium of the central nervous system, the neural tube, appears by the end of the fourth week of human gestation. The neural tube develops through the process of neurulation, a set of morphogenetic movements that transform part of the embryonic ectoderm into the three-dimensional neural tube. In the first step of this process, the neural plate is induced from the dorsal ectoderm by the underlying mesoderm, while in subsequent steps the neural plate becomes shaped and folded into the neural tube.

The initial signal for neural plate formation stems from the secretion of inducing molecules from the axial mesoderm. These signals establish neural competence in the overlying ectoderm and initiate the shape changes characteristic of the transition from ectoderm to neural plate. Three secreted molecules, noggin, chordin, and follistatin, have this capability. Noggin, chordin, and follistatin all function by blocking local signaling by bone morphogenetic proteins (BMPs) within the ectoderm, thereby allowing the ectodermal cells to enter a neural pathway of development (Fig. 4.1) (Tanabe and Jessell, 1996; Sasai and De Robertis, 1997). Ectodermal cells outside of the neural plate that retain BMP signaling develop as epidermis. In response to neural inducing signals, ectodermal cells lengthen along their apicobasal axis and begin to express molecular markers characteristic of neural rather than ectodermal cells.

Once induced, the neural plate elongates rostrocaudally along the dorsal midline and narrows along the mediolateral axis, initiating the process of neurulation (Fig. 4.1) (reviewed in Smith and Schoenwolf, 1997). Cell at the midline of the neural plate are anchored to the underlying notochord and become wedge-shaped, forming the floorplate. This shape change starts a set of bending and folding movements that transform the flattened neural plate into a rounded neural tube. Neural folds are raised at the edges of the neural plate; neural crest cells arise at the junction between the neural folds and the ectoderm and migrate into the periphery. Neural tube fusion begins at the level of the hindbrain with the dorsal apposition of the neural folds and continues rostrally and caudally along the length of the embryo. With the completion of neural tube fusion, typically by 28 days of gestation in human embryos, the precursor of the central nervous system is formed.

Experiments in tissue culture have suggested that isolated embryonic ectoderm induced to form neural tissue will develop an anterior character; that is, the tissue expresses markers such as *Otx2* that are characteristic of anterior brain structures such as the forebrain (Lamb and Harland, 1995). Addition of a second, or transforming, signal in a gradient has been postulated as a requirement for the development of more posterior structures (Nieuwkoop et al., 1952). Under this model, "anterior" is the default fate of differentiated neural plate without the superposition of a transforming signal. Several candidates for transforming factors have been identified, including basic fibroblast growth factor (bFGF) and retinoic acid (RA). Addition of bFGF to neural plate tissue induces expression of more posterior neural markers in a concentration-dependent manner (Cox and Hemmati-Brivanlou, 1995; Kengaku and Okamoto, 1995; reviewed in Doniach, 1995), while RA treatment of whole embryos suppresses anterior development and increases posterior development (Ruiz i Altaba and Jessell, 1991; Maden and Holder, 1992; Papalopulu and Kintner, 1996). By themselves, neither bFGF nor RA appear to have the capacity for direct neural induction, but their

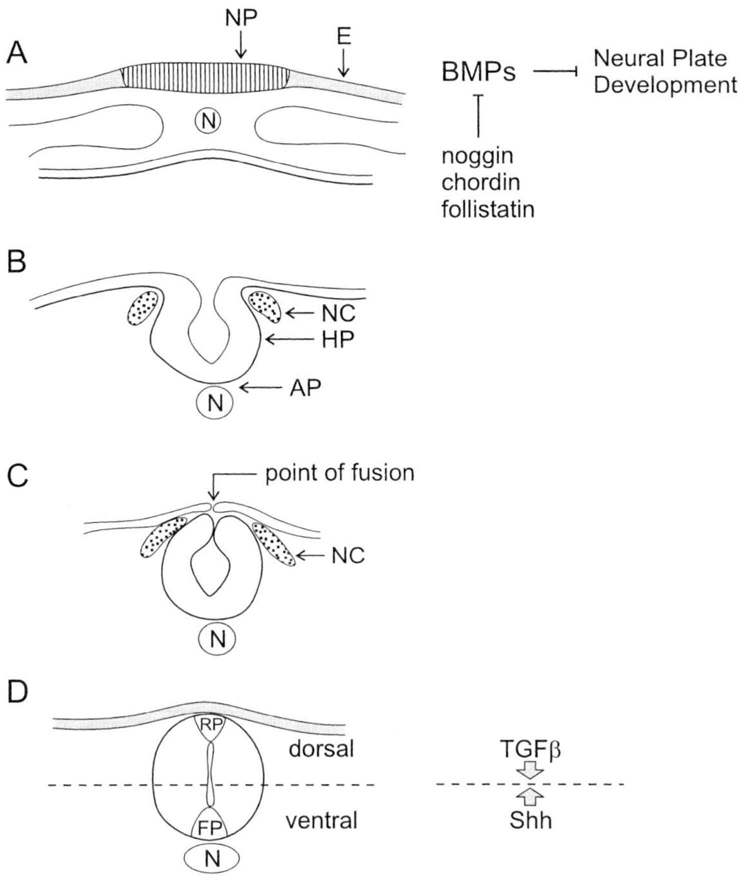

FIGURE 4.1. Neurulation. (*A*) Schematic representation of a transverse section through a vertebrate embryo at the neural plate stage and the molecular cascade involved in neural plate development. Inducing signals including noggin, chordin, and follistatin inhibit the activity of bone morphogenetic proteins (BMPs) in the ectoderm (E), allowing the induction of the neural plate (NP). N, notochord. (*B*) During neurulation, the neural plate becomes anchored to the underlying notochord at the anchor point (AP) and bends at lateral hinge points (HP). Neural folds are raised at the edges of the neural plate. Neural crest (NC) cells migrate from the edges of the neural folds to colonize the peripheral nervous system. (*C*) The folding neural plate fuses along the dorsal midline to form the neural tube. Neural crest cells continue to migrate away from the neural tube at this stage. (*D*) Schematic representation of the neural tube and dorsal and ventral signaling systems involved in neural tube patterning. Dorsal and ventral specification of the neural tube is achieved through signals arising from the roofplate (RP) and floorplate (FP), respectively. Dorsal patterning relies on the combinatorial expression of transforming growth factor β (TGFβ) family members, while ventral patterning is established through the expression of sonic hedgehog (Shh).

effects on neuralized tissue suggests that they may serve as transformers, triggering the generation of more posterior structures from differentiated neural plate. Additional evidence also supports Wnt signaling molecules and transforming growth factor β (TGFβ) proteins of the Nodal family as possible transformers (Wilson and Rubenstein, 2000).

THE DORSOVENTRAL AXIS

Patterning along the dorsoventral axis is initiated during the earliest stages of neural plate formation. As a result of neurulation, structures established along the midline of the neural plate are incorporated as the ventral elements of the neural tube, while more lateral neural plate regions become the dorsal elements of the neural tube. Regional identity along the dorsoventral axis of the developing neural tube appears to be established through the activity of complementary signaling systems that individually pattern the dorsal and ventral halves of the neural tube. These systems have been extensively examined in the development of the caudal neural tube, the precursor of the spinal cord. During neurulation, the notochord, a midline mesodermal structure, begins to express the sonic hedgehog protein (Shh). Shh is secreted by the notochord and induces the midline cells of the adjacent neural plate to differentiate into floorplate cells. Floorplate cells then themselves begin to express Shh, which regulates the development of several ventral neural tube cell types, including motor neurons, in a concentration-dependent fashion (Fig. 4.2) (Ericson et al., 1996; reviewed in Marti and Bovolenta, 2002). Signaling by this gradient of Shh establishes distinct progenitor domains within the ventral neural tube by regulating a set of homeodomain proteins including Pax, Nkx, Dbx, and Irx family members. These proteins have been subdivided into two classes based on their differential response to Shh signaling (Briscoe et al., 2000). The expression of class I proteins is repressed by Shh, while production of class II proteins requires the presence of Shh. Class I and class II proteins are induced or repressed at distinct Shh thresholds, allowing each protein to be expressed in a domain that reflects a specific sensitivity to Shh signaling. Induction or repression of these transcription factors defines five progenitor domains within the ventral neural tube, which give rise to five different classes of ventral neurons (Fig. 4.2). Boundaries between domains are stabilized due to repressive interactions between class I and class II proteins expressed within adjacent domains (reviewed in Jessell, 2000). Loss of Shh in mice deletes some ventral classes of cells in the spinal cord, including motor neurons, and

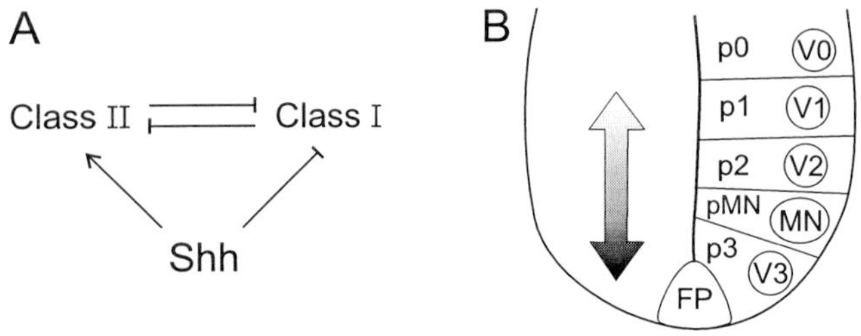

FIGURE 4.2. Ventral neural tube patterning. (*A*) Sonic hedgehog (Shh), initially secreted by the notochord and subsequently by the floorplate, activates class II and inhibits class I homeodomain proteins. Inhibitory interactions between various class I and class II proteins establish five ventral progenitor domains. (*B*) Schematic representation of the position of five ventral progenitor domains (p0, p1, p2, pMN, p3) and the resulting ventral classes of neurons (V0, V1, V2, MN, V3) in the developing neural tube. The Shh gradient that leads to the formation of these domains is represented by the double-headed arrow on the left side of the figure. FP, floor plate.
Source: Adapted from Jessell (2000).

shifts expression of markers for more lateral and dorsal cell types ventrally (Chiang et al., 1996). These observations suggest that Shh function is critical for the specification of ventral cell types in the developing spinal cord.

Shh also likely functions at more rostral neural tube levels because mutations in the *Shh* gene or in components of the Shh signaling pathway have been implicated in telencephalic development and in holoprosencephaly (Belloni et al., 1996; reviewed in Hayhurst and McConnell, 2003). Human gene mutations in *Shh,* in its receptor, *Patched* (*Ptc*), and in *DispatchedA* (*DispA*), which is required for the release and extracellular accumulation of Shh protein, have all been linked to holoprosencephaly. Mice carrying a mutation in the *Shh* gene lose ventral structures along the entire length of the neural tube, including ventrally positioned *Nkx2.1*-expressing cells in the forebrain (Ohkubo et al., 2002). In these animals, dorsally expressed genes become expressed more ventrally, encompassing regions that would have otherwise developed into ventral structures. For example, the dorsal telencephalic markers *Emx1* and *Otx1* are expressed in the entire anterior brain vesicle, and *Pax6* and *Otx2* expression expands ventrally into frontoventral regions (Chiang et al., 1996). More lateral markers, such as *Dlx2* and *Gsh2,* continue to be expressed, but their expression domains are shifted in position, suggesting that lateral structures become displaced ventrally toward the midline. Recent evidence also suggests that *Shh* plays a role in dorsal brain patterning, because *Shh* mutant mice show a failure in dorsal midline invagination and in the subsequent formation of dorsal midline structures such as the choroid plexus and hippocampus (reviewed in Hayhurst and McConnell, 2003). These types of failures may provide the basis for some of the morphological changes evident in holoprosencephaly.

Mice carrying a mutation in the *nodal* gene also show severe holoprosencephaly. Although human *nodal* mutations linked to holoprosencephaly have yet to be identified, mutations in both mice and zebrafish suggest the involvement of nodal signaling in ventral brain formation (reviewed in Hayhurst and McConnell, 2003). *Nodal* serves to establish the domain of *Shh* expression in rostral regions of the embryo because *nodal* mutant mice fail to express *Shh* rostral to the hindbrain (Lowe et al., 2001).

Dorsal neural tube development relies on a second set of signals emanating from the roofplate, which forms at the dorsal midline of the neural tube. Both roofplate ablation and neural tube explant cultures show that several classes of dorsal interneurons develop in response to signals derived from the roof plate (Liem et al., 1997; Lee et al., 2000). Many secreted factors are expressed in the roofplate, including BMPs, Wnt signaling molecules, and fibroblast growth factors (FGFs). Rather than differential responses to a single graded signal, as seen in ventral neural tube development, dorsal neural tube progenitors appear to be specified by the combinatorial activity of several different signaling molecules. These signals establish six different classes of dorsal progenitors that give rise to at least eight different types of dorsal interneurons (Gross et al., 2002; Müller et al., 2002; Helms and Johnson, 2003). Dorsal progenitor cells appear to express basis helix-loop-helix transcription factors including mammalian atonal homolog 1 (Math1), neurogenin 1 (Ngn1), and mammalian achaete-scute homolog 1 (Mash1) rather than the homedomain factors that characterize ventral progenitor populations.

REGIONAL PATTERNING ALONG THE ROSTROCAUDAL AXIS OF THE NEURAL TUBE

At its rostral extent, the neural tube expands to form three primary brain vesicles, the prosencephalon, mesencephalon, and rhombencephalon, or the forebrain, midbrain, and hindbrain (Fig. 4.3). The three primary brain vesicles subdivide to form five secondary vesicles, the telencephalon, diencephalon, mesencephalon, metencephalon, and myelencephalon. These five vesicles constitute the rudiments of all brain structures. The spinal cord develops from the remainder of the neural tube, caudal to the brain vesicles. Structures derived from these different vesicles appear to develop in substantially different ways; the rest of this chapter will focus on the regional differences in embryonic development and patterning in the forebrain, midbrain, hindbrain, and spinal cord.

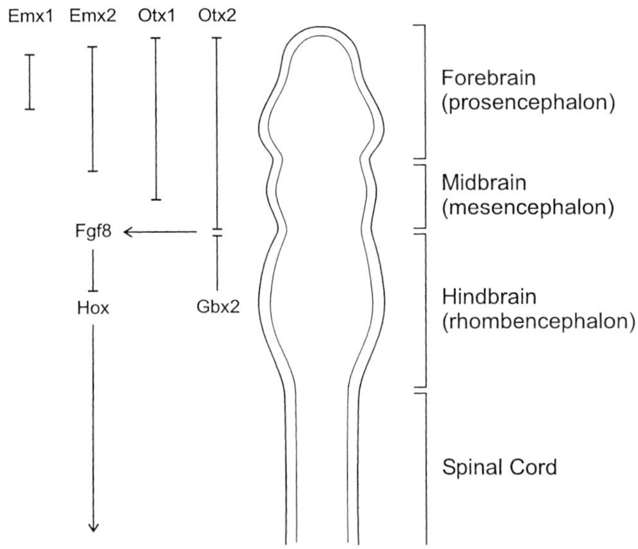

FIGURE 4.3. Early subdivisions of the developing brain are established through regional gene expression. The positions of the three primary brain vesicles and spinal cord are illustrated schematically. Expression domains for *Emx, Otx, Gbx, Fgf8,* and *Hox* genes are graphically depicted on the left side of the figure. Early forebrain patterning is established through the nested expression of *Otx2, Otx1, Emx2,* and *Emx1* within the developing forebrain. The boundary between *Otx2* and *Gbx2* expression establishes the position of the isthmus dividing the midbrain and hindbrain and regulates the domain of *Fgf8* expression. *Fgf8,* in turn, inhibits *Hox* gene expression in the rostral hindbrain, establishing the hindbrain territory that will give rise to the cerebellum.

Regional Patterning of the Forebrain

The forebrain develops at the most rostral extent of the neural tube and further subdivides into the telencephalon, the precursor of pallial and subpallial structures, and the diencephalon, the precursor for ventral forebrain structures including the thalamus. The vertebrate retina also develops from an outpocketing of the diencephalic wall. Nieuwkoop's two-signal model proposes that induced neural tissue possesses forebrain or anterior character and that a second transforming signal acts in a graded way to specify more posterior fates (Niewkoop et al., 1952). In this model, forebrain tissue would be the default state of development of the neural tube; however, evidence also exists for factors that actively promote forebrain development. For example, mutations that affect the embryonic organizer also disturb the anterior-posterior patterning of the neural plate and can lead to changes in forebrain fate specification (Wilson and Rubenstein, 2000). Inactivation of the *bozozok* gene in zebrafish produces phenotypes in which anterior neural plate fates are reduced or lost (Fekany et al., 1999; Koos and Ho, 1999), while overactivation of the Wnt signaling pathway appears to delete the telencephalon. Inactivation of the Nodal family of TGFβ proteins also suppresses telencephalic development. These observations suggest that in addition to forebrain development as a default state, there may be active signals encouraging forebrain development. The primary role for these signals may be to antagonize or negatively regulate factors that would posteriorize the neural plate. In mammals, a possible source of these antagonists is the anterior visceral endoderm (AVE) (Kiecker and Niehrs, 2001). Animals carrying mutations in genes required for AVE development are missing anterior tissues including the telencephalon. The AVE may function by the production of molecular signals including Cerberus, an antagonist of Wnt, BMP, and Nodal proteins, and Dickkopf, an antagonist of Wnt signaling (Glinka et al., 1998; Piccolo et al., 1999).

Another embryonic structure with a marked role in establishing the telencephalon is the anterior neural ridge. Telencephalic gene expression, such as the expression of *bf1,* a forebrain-restricted winged helix transcription factor (Xuan et al., 1995), is reduced or absent following removal of the anterior neural ridge, while telencephalic genes can be ectopically expressed following transplantation of the anterior neural ridge to more caudal regions of the developing neural plate. *Bf1* induction in the developing telencephalon may be regulated by Fgf8. Fgf8 can restore *bf1* expression to mouse neural tube explants in the absence of the anterior neural ridge (Shimamura and Rubenstein, 1997); however, Fgf8 is expressed too late in embryonic development to be the primary inducer of the telencephalon. One possible role for the anterior neural ridge may be to regulate the development of the anterior neural plate into telencephalic, optic, and diencephalic domains. Regional subdivision of the forebrain is disrupted in the zebrafish *masterblind* mutation (Heisenberg et al., 1996) and gain- and loss-of-function studies have identified a number of homeobox-containing transcription factors, including those encoded by the *Hesx, Rx, Six3,* and *Pax6* genes, that have roles in mediating the regional subdivision of the forebrain into its respective domains (Wilson and Rubenstein, 2000).

Once the forebrain territory has been established, this part of the brain is divided into distinct domains by the expression of several classes of transcription factors. The mechanisms that initially establish these domains are poorly understood but may stem from the early overlapping expression patterns of genes in the *Otx* and *Emx* families. *Otx* and *Emx* genes are related to the *Drosophila orthodenticle* and *empty spiracles* genes that are important for head development in flies. *Otx2* shows the largest domain of expression in the rostral neural tube, encompassing most of the developing forebrain and midbrain, with *Otx1, Emx2,* and *Emx1* all expressed in progressively smaller domains contained within the overall domain of *Otx2* expression (Fig. 4.3) (Boncinelli et al., 1993). Inactivation of some of these genes severely disrupts forebrain development, affecting both regional specification and cell proliferation and producing schizencephaly in humans (Ang et al., 1996; Brunelli et al., 1996; Qiu et al., 1996).

Fate-mapping studies in a variety of vertebrate embryos have defined the embryonic origins of many rostral brain structures and show that most homologous structures arise from similar embryonic territories. These mapping studies demonstrate that the organization of the embryonic anterior neural plate is essentially a flattened two-dimensional representation of the structural relationships seen in mature brains (Rubenstein et al., 1998). Embryonic primordia for the different brain regions may arise through the division of the anterior neural plate into longitudinal and transverse domains, each specified by a unique set of expressed transcription factors. Longitudinal domains may correspond mediolaterally to floor, basal, and alar plates and can be differentiated through their expression of *Shh* in the floorplate along with genes that are induced by *Shh* activity, including *HNF3*β and *Nkx2.2* in the medial basal plate. More laterally, the *Xash3* transcription factor may demarcate early alar plate. Superimposed on these longitudinal domains are transverse domains also defined by the expression of transcription factors. *Nkx2.1*, for example, is expressed to a caudal boundary between the developing telencephalon and diencephalon, while *bf1* expression defines the most rostral domain of the telencephalon (reviewed in Rubenstein et al., 1998).

During later stages of development, the different territories become linked with each other through the migration and intermixing of cells. For example, GABAergic cortical interneurons arise from cells proliferating in the medial and lateral ganglionic eminences. These cells are generated in a ventral forebrain territory defined by the expression of the transcription factors *Dlx1* and *Dlx2*. These cells undergo tangential migration from their origin to enter a dorsal neocortical domain defined by the expression of *Gli3* and *Ngn1/2*. Inactivation of *Dlx1* and *Dlx2* in mice does not affect the production of the GABAergic interneurons but does affect their ability to migrate dorsally into the neocortex (Anderson et al., 2001).

Regional Patterning of the Midbrain/Hindbrain Junction

Posterior to the diencephalon, cells in the mesencephalon develop into the colliculi, while the metencephalon contributes to the cerebellum. Patterning information for this region arises from the isthmus, the constriction that marks the junction between the developing midbrain and hindbrain. Quail-chick transplantation experiments demonstrated that the development of the mid/hindbrain junction could be regulated by a set of organizer cells located in the isthmus (reviewed in Alvarado-Mallart, 1993). Transplantation of isthmus tissue to ectopic locations in the developing brain induced the formation of morphologically distinct midbrain tissue and the expression of midbrain-specific markers in close proximity to the transplanted tissue, suggesting that the isthmus is the source of signaling information required for midbrain/hindbrain patterning. Early in development, the midbrain and hindbrain are differentiated from each other by the expression of *Otx2* rostral to the midbrain/hindbrain boundary and by *Gbx2* caudal to this boundary (Fig. 4.3). Apposition between tissues expressing these different transcription factors may serve to establish the boundary between the midbrain and hindbrain. Recent studies have demonstrated the importance of *Otx* and *Gbx* genes in establishing the position of this boundary. Examination of $Otx1^{-/-}/Otx2^{+/-}$ mice shows an enlargement of the metencephalon at the expense of more rostral tissue (Acampora et al., 2001), while inactivation of *Gbx2* deletes anterior hindbrain derivatives and allows expansion of the *Otx2* expression domain caudally (Wassarman et al., 1997). The expression domains of two secreted signaling molecules, FGF8 and Wnt1, become highly restricted to narrow bands of tissue surrounding the border between *Otx2* and *Gbx2* expression, while the transcription factors Engrailed-1 (*En-1*) and *En-2* are expressed in a wider domain across the *Otx2/Gbx2* boundary (Joyner et al., 2000; Liu and Joyner, 2001).

Transplantation of the isthmus repatterns the surrounding tissue in ways that suggest that the isthmus serves as an organizing center. Transplanting isthmus tissue into the diencephalon induces development of ectopic midbrain structures, while transplantation into the myelencephalon induces the development of ectopic cerebellar tissue. In both types of transplants, *En-1* expression is induced in the region surrounding the transplant before the ectopic structures develop, while ectopic *Wnt1* expression is seen only in the diencephalon. These experiments demonstrate that both rostral and caudal tissues are capable of responding to signals provided by the isthmus, but that the response differs depending on the recipient tissue. This differential competence may be induced through the earlier expression of genes such as *Otx2* and *Gbx2* that establish regional differences across the midbrain/hindbrain junction.

The role of FGF8 in midbrain/hindbrain induction has been examined in mutant mice and following transplantation of ectopic sources of FGF8. Fibroblast growth factor 8 is one of 19 FGF family members. The FGFs were initially identified as secreted proteins from transformed tumor cells, though FGF expression has also been described in many signaling centers in developing embryos. The *Fgf8* gene generates at least seven differentially spliced transcripts encoding proteins with a common core but variable N-terminal regions (Crossley and Martin, 1995). Mice homozygous for an *Fgf8* null allele die during gastrulation, suggesting that *Fgf8* provides critical signaling information prior to the development of the nervous system, while hypomorphic alleles show alterations in midbrain/hindbrain patterning including deletion of the posterior midbrain and cerebellar tissue (Meyers et al., 1998). Transplanting an ectopic source of FGF8 mimicked isthmus transplantations and induced the development of ectopic midbrain structures. Implanting an FGF8-soaked bead into the diencephalon induced the formation of midbrain tissue, in some cases producing mirror-image duplications of the midbrain around the bead (Fig. 4.4). Bead transplantation also induced the expression of the midbrain/hindbrain junction markers *En-2* and *Wnt1,* in addition to inducing FGF8 expression in tissue surrounding the bead. Interestingly, transplanting an FGF8-coated bead into the rhombencephalon did not induce ectopic gene expression or the formation of ectopic cerebellar tissue (Crossley et al., 1996).

Several other genes expressed in and around the isthmus region are required for midbrain/hindbrain patterning. Inactivation of both *Wnt1* and *En-1* leads to deletion of mesencephalic structures and part of the cerebellum in mice (Thomas and Capecchi, 1990; Wurst et al., 1994). *En-1* is initially expressed normally in *Wnt1* mutants, but its expression is subsequently lost. Driving *En-1* expression using a *Wnt1* promoter in a *Wnt1*$^{-/-}$ background rescues the *Wnt1* mutant phenotype, suggesting that *Wnt1* serves to maintain but not initiate *En-1* expression (Danielian and McMahon, 1996). Two members of the *Pax* family of transcription regulators, *Pax2* and *Pax5,* have also been implicated in the development of the midbrain/hindbrain junction. Both spontaneous and targeted mutant alleles of *Pax2* have deletions of the mesencephalic/metencephalic region, while *Pax5* mutants have a partial deletion of the inferior colliculus and a concomitent cerebellar expansion (Urbanek et al., 1997). *Pax2* and *Pax5* appear to have overlapping functions, as double mutant animals show much more severe defects (Schwarz et al., 1997). Pax2 and Pax5 proteins, along with Pax8 protein, can bind to *En-2* enhancer sites, suggesting that these genes may be involved in the regulation of *En-2* expression. However, mutation of these binding sites in vivo disrupts the initiation but not the maintenance of *En-2* expression (Song and Joyner, 2000).

The overlapping expression patterns and complicated interplay between genes in the midbrain/hindbrain junction suggest that many genes interact to pattern this region.

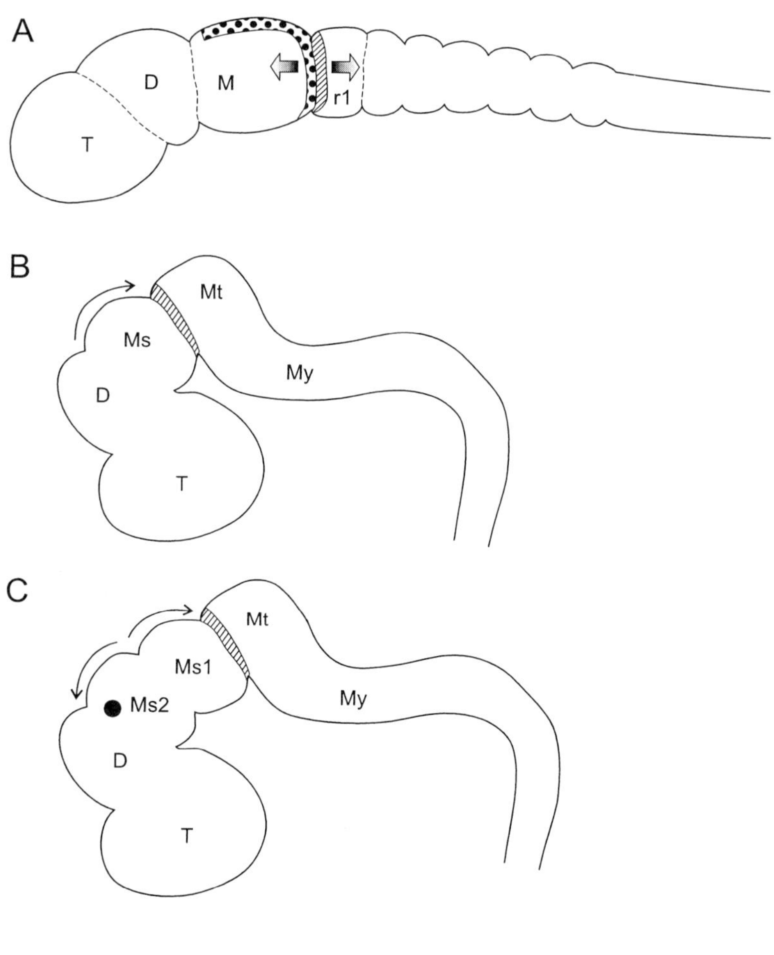

FIGURE 4.4. Patterning around the midbrain/hindbrain junction. (*A*) FGF8 (diagonal hatching) and Wnt-1 (dotted region) proteins are both expressed in discrete domains around the isthmus, the constriction marking the separation between the mesencephalon (M) and the first rhombomere (r1) during early stages of neural tube development. Engrailed-1 and engrailed-2 are also expressed in this region in a gradient, with levels of expression decreasing with increasing distance from the isthmus, as indicated by the shaded arrows. (*B*) At a later stage of development, FGF8 signals arising from the isthmus (diagonal hatching) have established the orientation of the mesencephalon (*curved arrow*). (C) Transplantation of an ectopic source of FGF8 (black dot) induces the development of a second mesencephalon (Ms2) with which it is oriented in response to the position of the ectopic source of the signal. The normal mesencephalon (Ms1) also develops in its appropriate location with the proper orientation in relation to the isthmus (diagonal hatching). D, diencephalon; Mt, metencephalon; My, myelencephalon; T, telencephalon.

Regional Patterning of the Hindbrain

The vertebrate hindbrain develops from the rhombencephalon. This part of the brain provides some of the strongest evidence supporting segmentation as a principle of neural patterning and development. At around the time of neural tube closure, a set of transient swellings called *rhombomeres* appear in the walls of the fourth ventricle at the level of the hindbrain. The most rostral rhombomere abuts the midbrain at the isthmus, and the most caudal rhombomere is continuous with the spinal cord. Rhombomeres (r) 1 and r2 contribute to the metencephalon, while r3–r8 form the myelencephalon. Each rhombomere represents an individual segment within the hindbrain and gives rise to a set of neurons that is repeated in surrounding segments. Reticular formation neurons are repeated with a one-segment periodicity, while branchiomotor neurons show a two-segment periodicity, with neurons from two adjacent rhombomeres exiting the hindbrain through the same cranial nerve (Lumsden, 1990). Dye labeling studies have demonstrated that once formed, cells from adjacent rhombomeres do not intermix (Fraser et al., 1990), suggesting that rhombomeres function as compartments analogous to the restricted developmental units present in *Drosophila*. Despite their initial similarities and repeated neuronal patterns, rhombomeres are not identical, as each one must innervate a specific set of peripheral structures. Differences between adjacent rhombomeres may be established through the segment-specific expression of several classes of genes.

The position and specification of r3–r8, the rhombomeres of the myelencephalon, is likely dependent on RA-mediated signaling. Retinoic acid is the biologically active metabolite of vitamin A. Changing the RA concentration during development through vitamin A deficiency or through application of exogenous RA alters rhombomere formation, with a decrease in RA increasing the territories occupied by more rostral rhombomeres (Maden et al., 1996) and an increase in RA inducing a posterior transformation of more anterior rhombomeres (Marshall et al., 1992). These observations suggest that an RA concentration–dependent mechanism establishes rhombomere identity. Retinoic acid is required early in development for the correct positioning of r3 and r4; later, RA is required for specification of more posterior rhombomeres (Begemann and Meyer, 2001; Gavalas, 2002).

A number of studies have demonstrated the rhombomere-specific expression patterns of different classes of genes. Early-expressed transcription factors such as *Krox20* and *MafB/kreisler*, *Hox* transcription factors, and *Eph* receptor genes all show expression patterns restricted to subsets of the rhombomeres. Retinoic acid signaling may activate expression of some of these genes, as *Hoxa1* and *MafB/kreisler* are both induced by RA (Begemann and Meyer, 2001; Dupe and Lumsden, 2001). Interestingly, the expression boundaries of all of these markers correspond closely to the position of rhombomere boundaries. These patterns suggest that gene expression in the hindbrain may serve to generate a unique identity for each of the rhombomeres. In turn, inactivating these genes through natural or targeted mutations in mice disrupts hindbrain patterning in ways that reflect the activity of the genes under observation. *Krox20*, which encodes a zinc finger transcription factor, is expressed in two stripes corresponding to the position of r3 and r5. Inactivation of *Krox20* eliminates these two rhombomeres but does not affect the overall segmentation of the hindbrain (Schneider-Maunoury et al., 1997). *MafB/kreisler* is expressed in r4 and r5; mice carrying a naturally occurring mutation in this gene have smooth hindbrains with no visible rhombomere boundaries. *MafB/kreisler* mutant mice also show rostral displacement in the expression of a number of markers for different rhombomeres, suggesting a disturbance in patterning along the rostrocaudal axis (Frohman et al., 1993).

Hox genes have been studied extensively for their role in hindbrain patterning. These genes share sequences and organization with the *Drosophila homeotic* genes that confer segmental identity in the developing fly. The similar expression of related genes in a segmented structure of the vertebrate brain suggested that *Hox* genes might also regulate segmental identity in vertebrates. The 39 members of the vertebrate *Hox* gene family encode transcription factors expressed in overlapping domains along the length of the hindbrain and spinal cord (Fig. 4.5) (reviewed in Carpenter, 2002). *Hox* genes are linked into four groups designated *Hox A, B, C, and D*. Paralogous genes within the four clusters occupy the same relative position and show overlapping patterns of expression, with *Hox* genes at the 3′ end of the complex expressed more rostrally than more *5′ Hox* genes. Inactivation studies in mice have demonstrated that *Hox* genes are essential for normal hindbrain patterning. Inactivation of *Hoxa1* eliminates r5 (Carpenter et al., 1993; Mark et al., 1993), while inactivation of a paralogous gene, *Hoxb1*, affects the formation of the somatic component of the seventh cranial nerve (Goddard et al., 1996). Inactivation of both genes together produces more severe hindbrain disruptions (Gavalas et al., 1998; Studer et al., 1998), suggesting that *Hox* genes interact to pattern the hindbrain. Inactivating a neighboring gene, *Hoxb2*, also affects formation of the somatic component of the facial nerve and alters *Hoxb1* expression in r4 (Barrow and Capecchi, 1996). This observation suggests that *Hox* genes might serve to regulate each other, providing a mechanism for their interaction in regulating development of a single rhombomere or patterning the same groups of cells. Extensive analysis of the promoters of

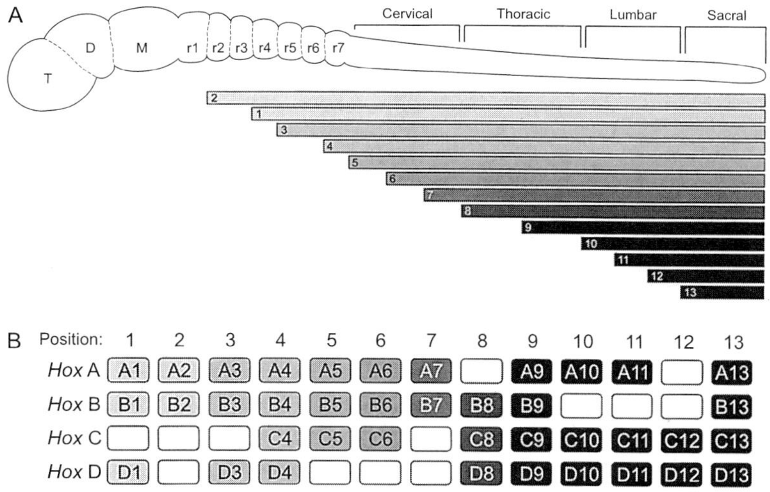

FIGURE 4.5. *Hox* gene expression in the developing neural tube. (*A*) Schematic representation of the organization of the developing neural tube and the overlapping expression domains of *Hox* genes along its length. Paralogous families of *Hox* genes, indicated numerically, show sharp rostral boundaries and broad domains of expression extending caudally along the length of the neural tube. In the hindbrain, rostral limits of expression are correlated with the position of boundaries between rhombomeres (r). In the spinal cord, the rostral extent of some expression domains correlates with the boundaries between cervical, thoracic, lumbar, and sacral spinal regions, while others show rostral limits of expression within a region. D, diencephalon; M, mesencephalon; T, telencephalon. (*B*) Mammalian *Hox* genes are partitioned into four families, designated *Hox A, Hox B, Hox C,* and *Hox D*. Numbered boxes indicate the location of *Hox* genes; empty boxes illustrate the absence of a gene at that position. Paralogous genes within each family occupy the same relative position and share the same numeric designation. Shading in *B* correlates with expression domains illustrated in *A*.

some of the *Hox* genes has demonstrated the presence of Hox protein binding sites and has shown that *Hox* genes have both autoregulatory and cross-regulatory activity (e.g., Di Rocco et al., 1997; Manzanares et al., 2001; reviewed in Tümpel et al., 2002). *Hox* genes can also be regulated by *Krox20* and *MafB/kreisler* (Manzanares et al., 2002), suggesting that several classes of genes interact in hindbrain patterning.

The development of more rostral rhombomeres may be regulated differently from more caudal segments. For example, *Hox* genes are not normally expressed in r1. Instead, r1-derived cells respond to signals generated in the isthmus and develop into the cerebellum, while more caudal rhombomeres do not participate in cerebellar development. Fibroblast growth factor 8, secreted by the isthmus, inhibits *Hox* gene expression in r1 (Irving and Mason, 2000). The presence or absence of *Hox* gene expression within the rhombencephalon might therefore distinguish tissues that will contribute to metencephalic versus myelencephalic structures.

The development of boundaries between adjacent rhombomeres stabilizes the segmental pattern of the developing hindbrain and inhibits mixing of cells between adjacent rhombomeres. Boundaries between rhombomeres may be established through the expression of Eph receptors and ephrins on cells in adjacent rhombomeres. Eph receptors constitute a large subset of receptor tyrosine kinases, with almost all Eph receptors expressed in the developing or adult nervous system. Eph receptors bind ephrin ligands expressed on neighboring cells and may mediate repulsive interactions between cells (reviewed in Flanagan and Vanderhaegen, 1998). Eph receptors and ephrins also show a segmental pattern of expression in relation to the developing rhombomeres, with Eph receptors expressed in some segments and their ephrin ligands expressed in adjacent rhombomeres. Binding between Eph receptors in one segment and ligands in the adjacent segment might then mediate the formation of a boundary between adjacent rhombomeres through repulsive interactions.

Regional Patterning of the Spinal Cord

Caudal to the hindbrain, the posterior extent of the neural tube develops into the spinal cord. Based on morphology, the spinal cord appears segmented, with spinal nerves emerging at regular intervals along the length of the spinal cord. Regional distinctions are superimposed on this segmented pattern, dividing the spinal cord along the rostrocaudal axis into cervical, thoracic, lumbar, and sacral domains. While each of these areas is continuous with adjacent domains, regional distinctions are reflected in the position and projection of different cell types from the different regions, so each domain may be identified by the targets innervated by each region and by the distribution of cholinergic efferent neurons. Somatic motor neurons at cervical and lumbar levels provide motor innervation for the musculature of the limbs, while sympathetic and parasympathetic preganglionic neurons appear at thoracic and sacral levels.

Spinal cord segmentation appears similar to that seen in the hindbrain, with efferent neurons projecting into spinal nerves at regular intervals along the length of the spinal cord. However, manipulations in developing embryos have suggested that spinal cord segmentation arises from interactions with the adjacent somites and is not established through gene expression domains, as with hindbrain segmentation (Detweiler, 1934; Phelan and Hollyday, 1990). Cervical, thoracic, lumbar, and sacral domains have largely been defined by the gross anatomy of the spinal cord based on the position and projection of efferent neurons from each area. Experimental manipulations in chickens have suggested that the positions of efferent neurons may be determined by signals from limb buds or paraxial mesoderm (Hollyday and Hamburger, 1976; Ensini et al., 1998). However, more recent studies have also argued for intrinsic patterning within the spinal cord that serves to establish regional identity (Lance-Jones et al., 2001).

Hox genes are expressed along the length of the spinal cord in broad overlapping domains with sharp anterior limits (Fig. 4.5), suggesting that these genes may regulate regional identity in the spinal cord. Most members of the *Hox* 6–9 gene families are expressed to anterior limits at cervical levels, while most members of the *Hox* 10–13 families have anterior limits at lumbar levels (reviewed in Carpenter, 2002). Few *Hox* genes have anterior limits at thoracic levels, suggesting that thoracic spinal cord may not rely on positional signals derived from the differential expression of *Hox* genes. While spinal cord expression patterns have been defined for many *Hox* genes, relatively few gain- or loss-of-function studies have demonstrated changes in spinal cord patterning. Because of the overlapping expression patterns of many *Hox* genes, loss of function of one gene may be compensated for by other *Hox* genes. Alternatively, because spinal cord organization is relatively uniform and readily plastic at early developmental stages, alterations in patterning caused by *Hox* gene inactivation may be functionally compensated for by changes in cell specification or projection; these phenotypes are difficult to detect without extensive anatomical analysis. Combinatorial interactions between *Hox* genes have been demonstrated through examination of animals carrying mutations in two or more *Hox* genes. For example, animals carrying mutations in both *Hoxa10* and *Hoxd10* have significant alterations in the number and position of lateral motor column motor neurons, substantially different from the phenotype of animals carrying either a *Hoxa10* or a *Hoxd10* mutation alone (Lin and Carpenter, 2003).

Once regional identity is established, the proper complement of cells must be generated within each region of the spinal cord. Progenitor domains distributed along the dorsoventral axis are established through complementary signaling systems mediated through the ventral expression of shh and the dorsal expression of members of the TGFβ superfamily, as described above. These domains can be identified through the expression of specific sets of transcription factors. Cell proliferation within these domains produces different classes of cells (Fig. 4.2). As proliferating cells become postmitotic, they shift from the expression of progenitor-specific transcription factors to the expression of markers for early-differentiating cells.

SUMMARY

The development of the human central nervous system is complex and multifaceted. Patterning along the dorsoventral axis relies on two complementary signaling systems to establish the identity of dorsal and ventral cell types, while patterning along the rostrocaudal axis appears in response to several different signaling centers and mechanisms along the length of the developing neural tube. The outcome of these different patterning activities is the production of the regionally specific cells and structures required for the formation of the mature central nervous system. Central nervous system development requires the expression and activity of a vast collection of genes, many of which encode transcription factors or signaling molecules. Although a comprehensive picture of the network of genes required for nervous system development has yet to be drawn, many genes have been identified that regulate nervous system patterning and development. Mutations in these genes, while devastating to central nervous system development, have been instructive in identifying the functions of these genes. Continued study of the genetics of neural tube development will allow the identification of many other genes and their roles in neural development and patterning, and will provide a biological and mechanistic understanding of the underpinnings of neural tube defects.

REFERENCES

Acampora D, Gulisano M, Broccoli V, Simeone A (2001). *Otx* genes in brain morphogenesis. Prog Neurobiol 64:69–95.

Alvarado-Mallart RM (1993). Fate and potentialities of the avian mesencephalic/metencephalic neuroepithelium. J Neurobiol 24:1341–1355.

Anderson SA, Marín O, Horn C, Jennings K, Rubenstein JLR (2001). Distinct cortical migrations from the medial and lateral ganglionic eminences. Development 128:353–363.

Ang, S-L, Jin O, Rhinn M, Daigle N, Stevenson L, Rossant J (1996). A targeted mouse *Otx2* mutation leads to severe defects in gastrulation and formation of axial mesoderm and to deletion of rostral brain. Development 122:243–252.

Barrow JR, Capecchi, MR (1996). Targeted disruption of the *Hoxb-2* locus in mice interferes with expression of *Hoxb-1* and *Hoxb-4*. Development 122:3817–3828.

Begemann G, Meyer A (2001). Hindbrain patterning revisited: timing and effects of retinoic acid signaling. BioEssays 23:981–986.

Belloni E, Muenke M, Roessler E, Traverso G, Siegel-Bartelt J, Frumkin A, Mitchell HF, Donis-Keller H, Helms C, Hing AV, Heng HHQ, Koop B, Martindale D, Rommens JM, Tsui L-C, Scherer SW (1996). Identification of *Sonic hedgehog* as a candidate gene responsible for holoprosencephaly. Nature Genet 14:353–356.

Boncinelli E, Gulisano M, Broccoli V (1993). *Emx* and *Otx* homeobox genes in the developing mouse brain. J Neurobiol 24:1356–1366.

Briscoe J, Pierani A, Jessell TM, Ericson J (2000). A homeodomain protein code specifies progenitor cell identity and neuronal fate in the ventral neural tube. Cell 101:435–445.

Brunelli S, Faiella A, Capra V, Nigro V, Simeone A, Cama A, Boncinelli E (1996). Germline mutatins in the homeobox gene *EMX2* in patients with severe schizencephaly. Nature Genet 12:94–96.

Carpenter EM (2002). *Hox* genes and spinal cord development. Dev Neurosci 24:24–34.

Carpenter EM, Goddard JM, Chisaka O, Manley NR, Capecchi MR (1993). Loss of *Hox-A1 (Hox-1.6)* function results in the reorganization of the murine hindbrain. Development 118:1063–1075.

Chiang C, Litingtung Y, Lee E, Young KE, Corden JL, Westphal H, Beachy PA (1996). Cyclopia and defective axial patterning in mice lacking *Sonic hedgehog* gene function. Nature 383:407–417.

Cox WG, Hemmati-Brivanlou A (1995). Caudalization of neural fate by tissue recombination and bFGF. Development 121:4349–4358.

Crossley PH, Martin GR (1995). The mouse *Fgf8* gene encodes a family of polypeptides and is expressed in regions that direct outgrowth and patterning in the developing embryo. Development 121:439–451.

Crossley PH, Martinez S, Martin GR (1996). Midbrain development induced by FGF8 in the chick embryo. Nature 380:66–68.

Danielian PS, McMahon AP (1996). *Engrailed-1* as a target of the Wnt-1 signaling pathway in vertebrate midbrain development. Nature 383:332–334.

Detweiler SR (1934). An experimental study of spinal nerve segmentation in *Amblystoma* with reference to the plurisegmental contribution to the brachial plexus. J Exp Zool 67:395–441.

Di Rocco G, Gavalas A, Pöpperl H, Krumlauf R, Mavilio F, Zappavigna V (1997). The recruitment of SOX/OCT complexes and the differential activity of HOXA1 and HOXB1 modulate the *Hoxb1* auto-regulatory enhancer function. J Biol Chem 276:20506–20515.

Doniach T (1995). Basic FGF as an inducer of anteroposterior neural pattern. Cell 83:1067–1070.

Dupé V, Lumsden A (2001). Hindbrain patterning involves graded responses to retinoic acid signaling. Development 128:2199–2208.

Ensini M, Tsuchida TM, Helting H-G, Jessell TM (1998). The control of rostrocaudal pattern in the developing spinal cord: specification of motor neuron subtype identity is initiated by signals from paraxial mesoderm. Development 125:969–982.

Ericson J, Morton S, Kawakami A, Roelink H, Jessell TM (1996). Two critical periods of *Sonic Hedgehog* signaling required for the specification of motor neuron identity. Cell 87:661–673.

Fekany K, Yamanaka Y, Leung T, Sirotkin HI, Topczewski J, Gates MA, Hibi M, Renucci A, Stemple D, Radbill A, Schier AF, Driever W, Hirano T, Talbot WS, Solnica-Krezel L (1999). The zebrafish *bozozok* locus encodes Dharma, a homeodomain protein essential for induction of gastrula organizer and dorsoanterior embryonic structures. Development 126:1427–1438.

Flanagan JG, Vanderhaeghen P (1998). The ephrins and Eph receptors in neural development. Annu Rev Neurosci 21:309–345.

Fraser S, Keynes R, Lumsden A (1990). Segmentation in the chick embryo hindbrain is defined by cell lineage restrictions. Nature 344:431–435.

Frohman MA, Martin GR, Cordes SP, Halamek LP, Barsh GS (1993). Altered rhombomere-specific gene expression and hyoid bone differentiation in the mouse segmentatin mutant, *kreisler* (*kr*). Development 177:925–936.

Gavalas A (2002). ArRAnging the hindbrain. Trends Neurosci 25:61–64.

Gavalas A, Studer M, Lumsden A, Rijli F, Krumlauf R, Chambon P (1998). *Hoxa1* and *Hoxb1* synergize in patterning the hindbrain, cranial nerves and second pharyngeal arch. Development 125:1123–1136.

Glinka A, Wu W, Delius H, Monaghan AP, Blumenstock C, Niehrs C (1998). Dickkopf-1 is a member of a new family of secreted proteins and functions in head induction. Nature 391:357–362.

Goddard JM, Rossel M, Manley NR, Capecchi MR (1996). Mice with targeted disruption of *Hoxb-1* fail to form the motor nucleus of the VIIth nerve. Development 122:3217–3228.

Gross MK, Dottori M, Goulding M (2002). *Lbx1* specifies somatosensory association interneurons in the dorsal spinal cord. Neuron 34:535–549.

Hayhurst M, McConnell SK (2003). Mouse models of holoprosencephaly. Curr Opin Neurol 16:135–141.

Heisenberg CP, Brand M, Jiang YJ, Warga R, Beuchle D, van Eeden FJ, Furutani-Seiki M, Granato M, Haffter P, Hammerschmidt M, Kane DA, Kelsh RN, Mullins MC, Odenthal J, Nusslein-Volhard C (1996). Genes involved in forebrain development in the zebrafish, *Danio rerio*. Development 123:191–203.

Helms AW, Johnson JE (2003). Specification of dorsal spinal cord interneurons. Curr Opin Neurobiol 13:42–49.

Hollyday M, Hamburger V (1976). Reduction of the naturally occurring motor neuron loss by enlargement of the periphery. J Comp Neurol 170:311–320.

Irving C, Mason I (2000). Signalling by FGF8 from the isthmus patterns anterior hindbrain and establishes the anterior limit of *Hox* gene expression. Development 127:177–186.

Jessell TM (2000). Neuronal specification in the spinal cord: inductive signals and transcriptional codes. Nat Rev Genet 1:20–29.

Joyner AL, Liu A, Millet S (2000). *Otx2, Gbx2,* and *Fgf8* interact to position and maintain a mid-hindbrain organizer. Curr Opin Cell Biol 12:736–741.

Kengaku M, Okamoto H (1995). bFGF as a possible morphogen for the anteroposterior axis of the central nervous system in *Xenopus*. Development 121:3121–3130.

Kiecker C, Niehrs C (2001). The role of prechordal mesendoderm in neural patterning. Curr Opin Neurobiol 11:27–33.

Koos DS, Ho RK (1999). The *nieuwkoid/dharma* homeobox gene is essential for bmp2b repression in the zebrafish pregastrula. Dev Biol 215:190–207.

Lamb TM, Harland RM (1995). Fibroblast growth factor is a direct neural inducer, which combined with noggin generates anterior-posterior neural pattern. Development 121:3627–3636.

Lance-Jones C, Omelchenko N, Bailis A, Lynch S, Sharma K (2001). *Hoxd10* induction and regionalization in the developing lumbosacral spinal cord. Development 128:2255–2268.

Lee KJ, Dietrich P, Jessell TM (2000). Genetic ablation reveals that the roof plate is essential for dorsal interneuron specification. Nature 403:734–740.

Liem KF, Tremml G, Jessell TM (1997). A role for the roof plate and its resident TGFβ-related proteins in neuronal patterning. Cell 91:127–138.

Lin A, Carpenter EM (2003). *Hoxa10* and *Hoxd10* coordinately regulate lumbar motor neuron patterning. J Neurobiol 56:328–337.

Liu A, Joyner AL (2001). Early anterior/posterior patterning of the midbrain and cerebellum. Annu Rev Neurosci 24:869–896.

Lowe LA, Yamada S, Kuehn MR (2001). Genetic dissection of nodal function in patterning the mouse embryo. Development 128:1831–1843.

Lumsden A (1990). The cellular basis of segmentation in the developing hindbrain. Trends Neurosci 13:329–339.

Maden M, Gale E, Kostetskii I, Zile M (1996). Vitamin A–deficient quail embryos have half a hindbrain and other neural defects. Curr Biol 6:417–426.

Maden M, Holder N (1992). Retinoic acid and development of the central nervous system. Bioessays 14:431–438.

Manzanares M, Bel-Vialar S, Ariza-McNaughton L, Ferretti E, Marshall H, Maconochie MM, Blasi F, Krumlauf R (2001). Independent regulation of initiation and maintenance phases of *Hoxa3* expression in the vertebrate hindbrain involve auto- and cross-regulatory mechanisms. Development 128:3595–3607.

Manzanares M, Nardelli J, Gilardi-Hebenstreit P, Marshall H, Giudicelli F, Martinez-Pastor MT, Krumlauf R, Charnay P (2002). *Krox20* and *kreisler* co-operate in the transcriptional control of segmental expression of *Hoxb3* in the developing hindbrain. EMBO J 21:365–376.

Mark M, Lufkin T, Vonesch J-L, Ruberte E, Olivo J-C, Dollé P, Gorry P, Lumsden A, Chambon P (1993). Two rhombomeres are altered in *Hoxa-1* mutant mice. Development 119:319–338.

Marshall H, Nonchev S, Sham MH, Muchamore I, Lumsden A, Krumlauf R (1992). Retinoic acid alters hindbrain *Hox* code and induces transformation of rhombomeres 2/3 into a 4/5 identity. Nature 360:737–741.

Marti E, Bovolenta P (2002). *Sonic hedgehog* in CNS development: one signal, multiple outcomes. Trends Neurosci 25:89–96.

Meyers EN, Lewandowski M, Martin GR (1998). An *Fgf8* mutant allelic series generated by Cre- and Flp-mediated recombination. Nature Genet 18:136–141.

Müller T, Brohmann H, Pierani A, Heppenstall PA, Lewin GR, Jessell TM, Birchmeier C (2002). The homeodomain factor Lbx1 distinguishes two major programs of neuronal differentiation in the dorsal spinal cord. Neuron 34:551–562.

Nieuwkoop PD, Boterenbrood EC, Kremer A, Bloesma FFSN, Hoessels ELMJ, Meyer G, Verheyen FJ (1952). Activation and organization of the central nervous system in amphibians. J Exp Zool 120:1–108.

Ohkubo Y, Chiang C, Rubenstein JL (2002). Coordinate regulation and synergistic actions of BMP4, SHH, and FGF8 in the rostral prosencephalon regulate morphogenesis of the telencephalic and optic vesicles. Neuroscience 111:1–17.

Papalopulu N, Kintner C (1996). A posteriorising factor, retinoic acid, reveals that anteroposterior patterning controls the timing of neuronal differentiation in *Xenopus* neuroectoderm. Development 122:3409–3418.

Phelan KA, Hollyday M (1990). Axon guidance in muscleless chick wings: the role of muscle cells in motoneuronal pathway selection and muscle nerve formation. J Neurosci 10:2699–2716.

Piccolo S, Agius E, Leyns L, Bhattacharyya S, Grunz H, Bouwmeester T, De Robertis EM (1999). The head inducer Cerberus is a multifunctional antagonist of Nodal, BMP, and Wnt signals. Nature 397:707–710.

Qiu M, Anderson S, Chen S, Meneses JJ, Hevner R, Kuwana E, Pedersen RA, Rubenstein JLR (1996). Mutation of the *Emx-1* homeobox gene disrupts the corpus callosum. Dev Biol 178:174–178.

Rubenstein JLR, Shimamura K, Martinez S, Puelles L (1998). Regionalization of the prosencephalic neural plate. Annu Rev Neurosci 21:445–477.

Ruiz i Altaba A, Jessell TM (1991). Retinoic acid modifies the pattern of cell differentiation in the central nervous system of neurula stage *Xenopus* embryos. Development 112:945–958.

Sasai Y, De Robertis EM (1997). Ectodermal patterning in vertebrate embryos. Dev Biol 182:5–20.

Schneider-Maunoury S, Seitaridou T, Charnay P, Lumsden A (1997). Segmental and neuronal architecture of the hindbrain of *Krox-20* mouse mutants. Development 124:1215–1226.

Schwarz M, Alvarez-Bolado G, Urbanek P, Busslinger M, Gruss P (1997). Conserved biological function between *Pax-2* and *Pax-5* in midbrain and cerebellum development: evidence from targeted mutations. Proc Natl Acad Sci USA 94:14518–14523.

Shimamura K, Rubenstein JLR (1997). Inductive interactions direct early regionalization of the mouse forebrain. Development 124:2709–2718.

Smith JL, Schoenwolf GC (1997). Neurulation: coming to closure. Trends Neurosci 20:510–517.

Song DL, Joyner AL (2000). Two *Pax2/5/8*-binding sites in *Engrailed-2* are required for proper initiation of endogenous mid-hindbrain expression. Mech Dev 90:155–165.

Studer M, Gavalas A, Marshall H, Ariza-McNaughton L, Rijli FM, Chambon P, Krumlauf R (1998). Genetic interactions between *Hoxa1* and *Hoxb1* reveal new roles in regulation of early hindbrain patterning. Development 125:1025–1036.

Tanabe Y, Jessell TM (1996). Diversity and pattern in the developing spinal cord. Science 274:1115–1123.

Thomas KR, Capecchi MR (1990). Targeted disruption of the murine *int-1* proto-oncogene resulting in severe abnormalities in midbrain and cerebellar development. Nature 346:847–850.

Tümpel S, Maconochie M, Wiedemann LM, Krumlauf R (2002). Conservation and diversity in the cis-regulatory networks that integrate information controlling expression of *Hoxa2* in hindbrain and cranial neural crest cells in vertebrates. Dev Biol 246:45–56.

Urbanek P, Fetka I, Meisler MH, Busslinger M (1997). Cooperation of *Pax2* and *Pax5* in midbrain and cerebellum development. Proc Natl Acad Sci USA 94:5703–5708.

Wassarman KM, Lewandowski M, Campbell K, Joyner AL, Rubenstein JL, Martinez S, Martin GR (1997). Specification of the anterior hindbrain and establishment of a normal mid/hindbrain organizer is dependent on *Gbx2* gene function. Development 124:2923–2934.

Wilson SW, Rubenstein JLR (2000). Induction and dorsoventral patterning of the telencephalon. Neuron 28:641–651.

Wurst W, Auerbach AB, Joyner AL (1994). Multiple developmental defects in *Engrailed-1* mutant mice: an early mid-hindbrain deletion and patterning defects in forelimbs and sternum. Development 120:2065–2075.

Xuan S, Baptista CA, Balas G, Tao W, Soares VC, Lai E (1995). Winged helix transcription factor BF-1 is essential for the development of the cerebral hemispheres. Neuron 14:1141–1152.

II

Clinical Features of Neural Tube Defects

5

Physical Examination of the Spine

SERGIO A. MENDOZA
STUART L. WEINSTEIN

Orthopedic problems frequently affect children with myelomeningocele. According to Swank and Dias (1992), 64% of these children require at least one orthopedic procedure before they turn 18, with an average of 5.4 procedures per patient. Spinal deformities affect children with myelomeningocele (MMC), regardless of their level of paralysis. Scoliosis has been described in 20% of patients with sacral-level compromise and in 94% of those with thoracic-level involvement (Christoferson and Brooks, 1985). These deformities may affect posture and sitting comfort, ultimately reducing self-sufficiency and, hence, social and academic development. For this reason, it is mandatory to carry out routine physical examination of the spine, including periodic radiographic screening.

The anatomical characteristics of the posterior element defect of MMC consist of widely separated, splayed pedicles, which are virtually oriented in the coronal plane, and completely inverted laminas with the normally anterior-facing surface oriented posterior and lateral (Fig. 5.1). The dural sac is exposed, with anterior-exiting nerve roots, and anterior-displaced paraspinal musculature, which function as flexors of the spine rather than extensors (Mueller and Nordwall, 1992). The muscles are markedly attenuated due to lack of innervation from the central nervous system.

Of special consideration is the isolated dysplasia of spinous processes and laminae, which is termed *spina bifida occulta* and most commonly affects the S1 level. According to Boone et al. (1985), 30% of the general population may have this presentation. The underlying neurological structures are intact; for this reason, it is believed that this condition is unrelated pathogenetically to MMC (Mueller and Nordwall, 1992). Other occult forms of spinal dysraphism may also present with occult neural tube anomalies, such as diastematomyelia and lipomeningocele. Their only external manifestations may be cutaneous stigmata lying on the midline of the back, such as hairy patches, nevi, hemangiomas, and midline lipomas (Fig. 5.2). Subtle abnormalities revealed by the neurological examination may also provide evidence of their presence.

Spinal deformities in MMC may have either a congenital or an acquired origin (Carman et al., 1990). Congenital anomalies include kyphosis related to dysplastic posterior spinal elements, scoliosis secondary to failure of formation and/or segmentation, and intrathecal anomalies such as diastematomyelia. Acquired deformities include idiopathic-like scoliosis, neuromuscular curves, and curves secondary to pelvic obliquity. The neurosegmental level of compromise determines the development of spinal deformity. In a low thoracic level of involvement, kyphosis of the spine consistently develops, whereas lower lumbar defects generally tend to be associated with scoliosis.

SPINAL DEFORMITIES IN MYELOMENINGOCELE

To understand spinal deformities, we will commence by defining some of the basic characteristics of the normal spine. The spine serves three basic functions: structural support, trunk motion, and protection of neural structures. The normal spine is straight in the frontal (coronal) plane. In the lateral (sagittal) plane, it presents with 30° to 40° of thoracic kyphosis and 50° to 60° of lumbar lordosis. In a well-balanced spine, the center of gravity falls from the center of the C7 vertebral body through the superior endplate of the sacrum in the lateral (sagittal)

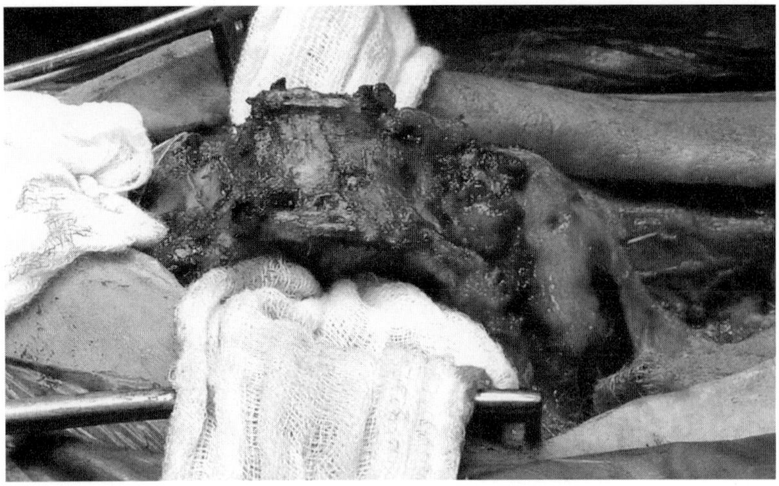

FIGURE 5.1. Intraoperative photography of kyphosis in myelomeningocele. The dura has been sectioned. Note the flattened vertebrae, splayed pedicles, and inverted laminas.

plane of space and through the midline of the sacrum in the frontal (coronal) plane of space. The basic mechanisms of neuromuscular control provide balance within a polygon of equilibrium, minimizing the amount of energy required to maintain posture. When the spine is unbalanced, the energy required to keep the body upright, as well as for ambulation, increases significantly. Ambulation may deteriorate, and to achieve balance while sitting, these children may require a third point of support (usually one of the hands or elbows) to keep an upright posture. If one of the hands is used to support the trunk, then it is not helping to accomplish social and academic chores (see Fig. 5.10).

We recommend clinical follow-up examinations of the spine from birth until skeletal maturity is reached: at birth, following surgery for closure of the neural placode, at 3 months, 6 months, 12 months, 18 months, and on a yearly basis until skeletal maturity occurs. Beyond that point, we continue to follow only those patients who have been diagnosed with spinal deformities. The visits consist of an interview, clinical examination, and upright posteroanterior (PA) and lateral films of the entire spinal column.

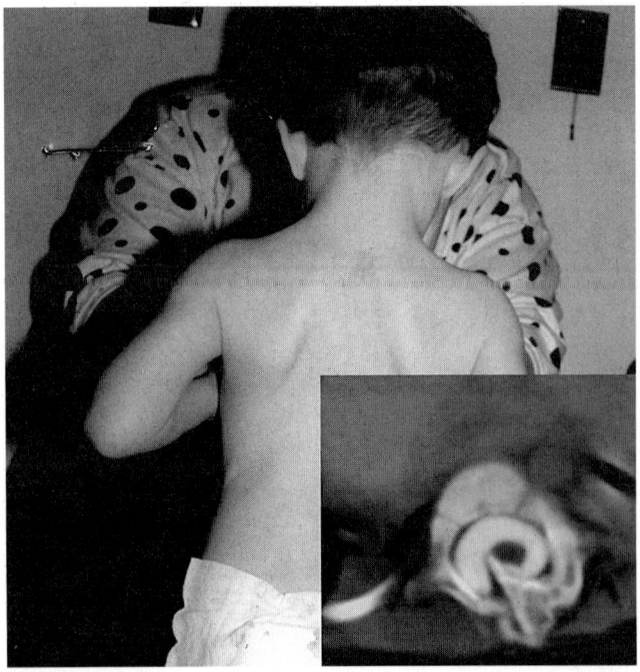

FIGURE 5.2. A 3-year-old girl with diastematomyelia at T3–T5. She presents with a midline hemangioma suggestive of occult spinal dysraphism. The insert shows a bony spur tethering the spinal cord.

Scoliosis

Scoliosis is defined as a curvature of the spine in the coronal plane of space of more than 10°, as measured by the Cobb method. For the purpose of clinical evaluation and follow-up, a two-dimensional approach is appropriate. Beyond this universal working definition, scoliosis is conceived today as a three-dimensional rotational deformity with vertebrae rotated maximally at the apex of the curvature. The apex is the point of maximal deflection from the midline. In the thoracic spine, as scoliosis develops in the coronal plane, the normal thoracic kyphosis decreases in the sagittal plane. The vertebral rotation is conveyed to the attached ribs, producing a characteristic chest wall deformity. This gibbous deformity gives a kyphotic appearance; nevertheless, the thoracic spine is actually lordotic.

Scoliosis is present in up to 90% of all patients with MMC and in 70% of children under 6 (Christoferson and Brooks, 1985). It is more likely to appear in nonambulatory children, who are usually those with higher neurosegmental involvement (Carman et al., 1990). Scoliosis has been described in 20% of patients with sacral-level compromise and in 94% of those with thoracic-level involvement (Christoferson and Brooks, 1985). Once scoliosis develops, it is consistently progressive. After diagnosis, the rate of progression may reach 5° per year (Mueller and Nordwall, 1992), especially in children younger than 15.

Possible etiologies for spinal deformity have been outlined in previous chapters. Scoliosis may develop as a consequence of the neuromuscular nature of MMC. The most common factor is paralysis, and due to its asymmetric nature, it may induce paravertebral muscle imbalance and deformity. In addition, brainstem and spinal cord abnormalities are frequent causes of spasticity and increased muscle tone. When rapidly progressive curves are encountered, other underlying neuromuscular conditions must be suspected, such as the progression of a tethered cord, Chiari II malformation, and expanding syringomyelia (Christoferson and Brooks, 1985). Shunt malfunction and progressive hydromyelia must always be considered, and neurosurgical consultation is warranted when a rapidly increasing curve develops.

Congenital malformations, which potentially induce scoliosis, include defects of formation (hemivertebrae) as well as defects of segmentation (unsegmented bars). A hemivertebra is a triangular vertebra that forms only on one side of the spine, with varying degrees of asymmetric growth potential (Fig. 5.3). In the thoracic spine, there may be concomitant rib deficiencies or fused ribs in the concavity. Progression of scoliosis depends on the degree of unbalanced growth. The convexity has higher potential than the concavity, with one or more additional growth plates. Defects due to failure of segmentation may inhibit longitudinal growth of the spine, and when these defects occur unilaterally, they can produce a growth tether resulting in scoliosis (Fig. 5.4). Remaining growth is a key factor when considering the prognosis and treatment. This may be estimated by the age at diagnosis, the onset of menses in girls, and the Risser grade. It must also be remembered that these children have abnormal growth patterns secondary to growth hormone deficiency and reach maturity at an earlier age.

Kyphosis

Kyphosis is found in 12% of these children at birth (Christoferson and Brooks, 1985) and in 20% (Carstens et al., 1991) to 46% (Morrisy et al., 1990) of MMC patients. It appears most frequently in thoracic or high lumbar of neurosegmental level patients, with the apex of the deformity most commonly found at L2 (T12–L5). This deformity is associated with both paralytic and congenital etiologies. The anteriorly displaced paravertebral musculature, sometimes also accompanied by innervated psoas, forces the spine into kyphosis. The paravertebral muscles as well as the psoas act as flexors, without extensor antagonists. Also, due to the absence of a posterior tension band, the incomplete posterior spinal architecture does not prevent the spine from falling into kyphosis (Figs. 5.5*A*, and 5.5*B*). Finally, there may be formation and/or segmentation defects associated with this deformity.

The kyphotic deformity progresses at a rate of 2°–5° per year (Carstens et al., 1991). In children more than 1 year of age who have curves of more than 90°, progression occurs at a rate of 6°–7° per year, but if a curve of this magnitude develops before 1 year of age, the rate of progression is >12° per year (Mueller and Nordwall, 1992).

With increasing deformity, the trunk height becomes significantly affected. The rib cage and abdomen rest on the child's thighs, forcing the rib cage to flare out (Fig. 5.6). The increased pressure on the diaphragm and horizontally flared-out ribs interfere with respiratory mechanics, and the collapsing trunk pushes the abdom-

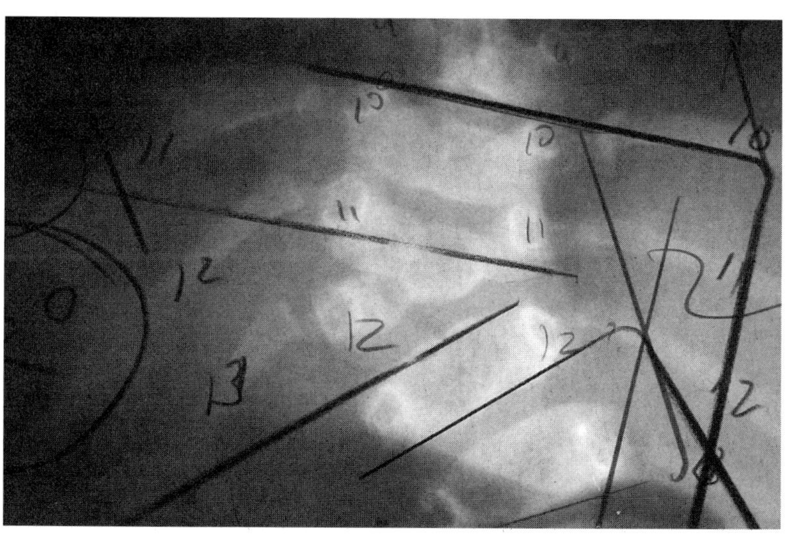

FIGURE 5.3. This X-ray shows a T12 left-sided hemivertebra. This represents two additional growth plates that are not present on the concave side. Note that the hemivertebra also presents with a 13th rib.

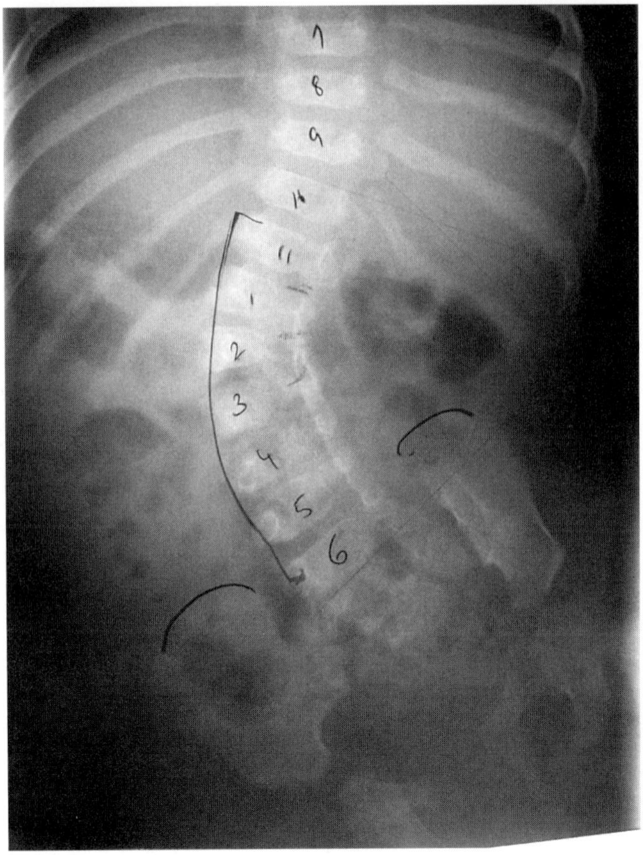

FIGURE 5.4. This X-ray of a 3-year-old child shows a unilateral segmentation defect affecting L1 through L6 on the right side. This is producing an asymmetric growth tether, with development of deformity.

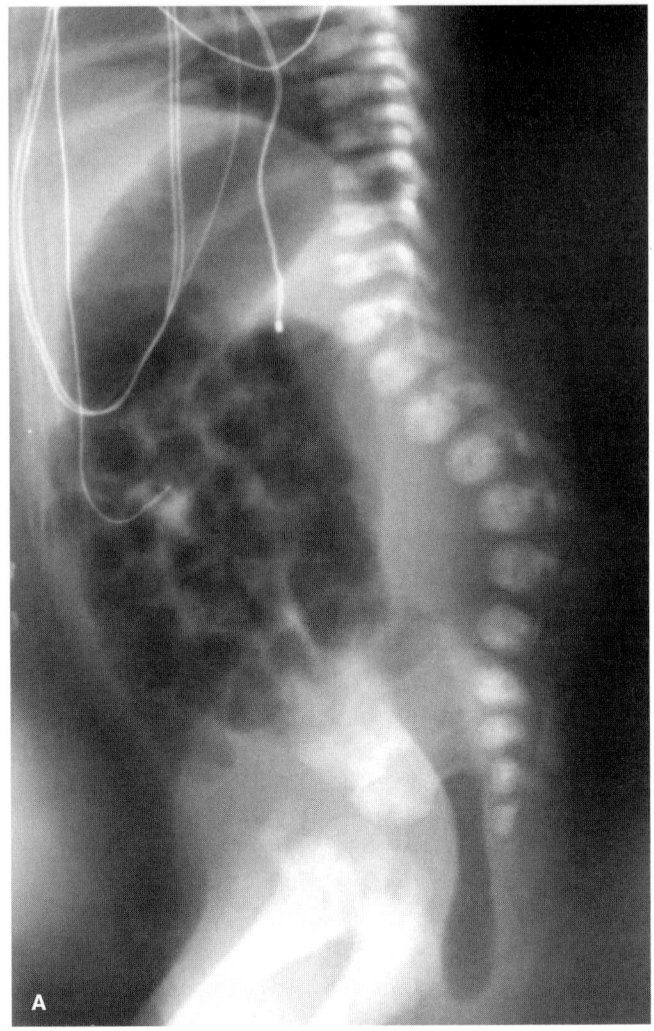

FIGURE 5.5. A 14-month-old girl with T9-level myelomeningocele and kyphosis. Upright lateral (*A*).

inal viscerae against the diaphragm, decreasing gastric compliance. Eating becomes increasingly difficult, leading to weight loss and malnutrition. This affects longitudinal growth and reduces wound-healing capacity, osteogenesis, and the immune response. Finally, the severe sagittal imbalance makes sitting upright a continuous effort, requiring almost permanent support from the arms. This reduces independence and, without adequate seating support, prevents the child from engaging in academic and social activities.

The effort to sit upright forces the thoracic spine into compensatory lordosis (Christoferson and Brooks, 1985), which becomes progressively rigid. This compensatory deformity affects ventilatory mechanics, as well as self-catheterization and perineal care.

INITIAL EXAMINATION OF THE SPINE

Ideally, the initial examination should be carried out in the nursery prior to surgery for closure of the neural placode. The examiner must try to determine the neurosegmental level of involvement and screen for associated musculoskeletal anomalies, including spinal deformity. Determining the neurosegmental level of involvement will provide fundamental baseline information, which will be reviewed and compared in every follow-up examination. Subtle changes may represent worsening hydrocephalus, hydromyelia, or tethered cord, for which early diagnosis is warranted.

With all the above said, the initial examination may be extremely difficult. First, the child is limited to the prone or lateral decubitus position because of the presence of the posterior defect (Fig. 5.7). Second, often the child will be lethargic and noncooperative as a result of fatigue, maternal anesthesia, and hydrocephalus. Examination of the infant after surgery for closure of the neural placode may be somewhat easier. By carefully observing the crying infant, it may be possible to determine its voluntary lower extremity muscular function. This may be spontaneous or occur in response to prox-

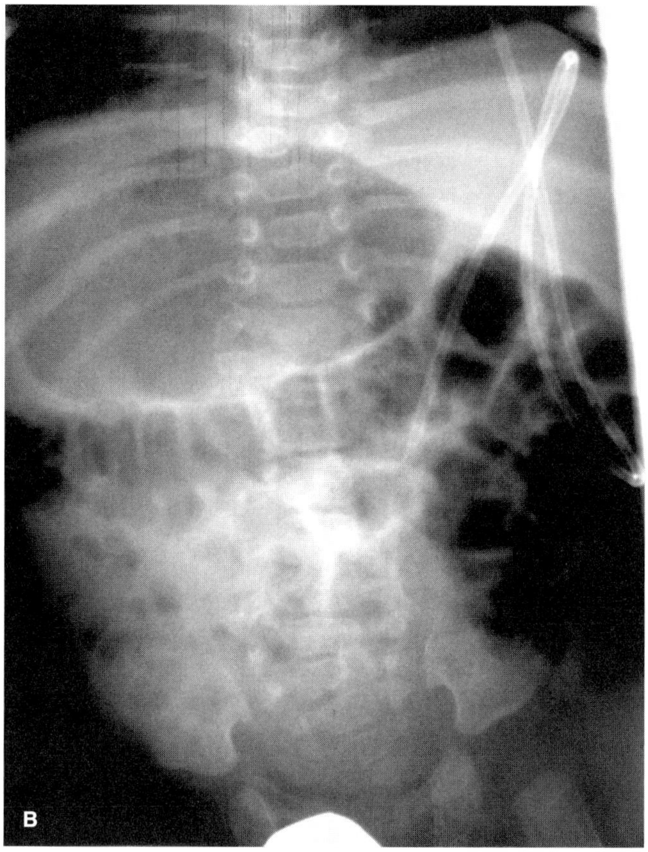

FIGURE 5.5. (*continued*) postero-anterior (*B*) X-rays show developing kyphosis in the lumbar spine. Note the widened vertebral bodies, splayed-out pedicles, and laminas at L1.

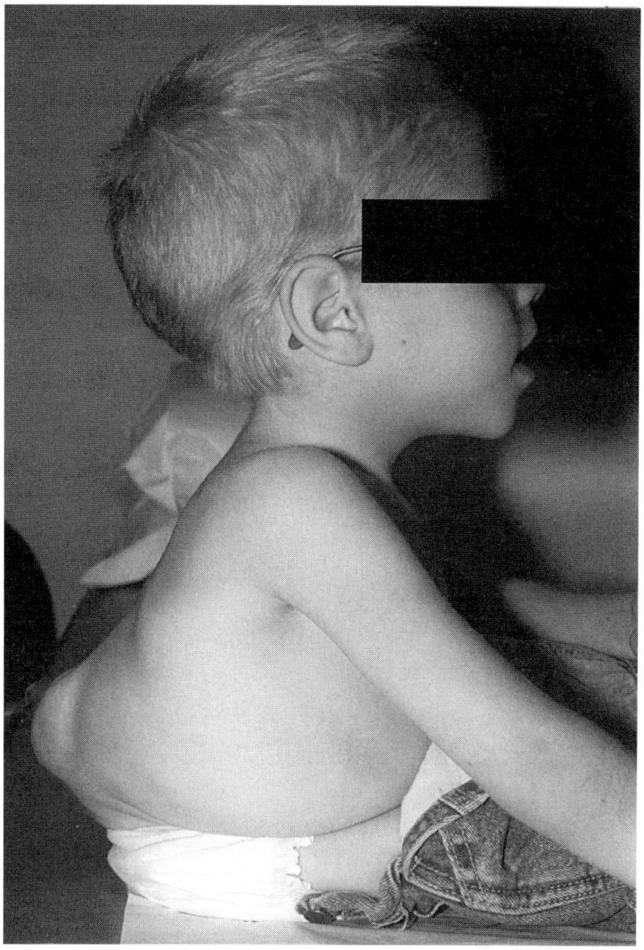

FIGURE 5.6. A 5-year-old boy with T10-level myelomeningocele and sharp-angled kyphosis. The abdomen and rib cage are completely resting on his thighs.

imal stimulation. The resting posture of the lower extremities may also help define coarsely the level of the paralysis. For example, children with a thoracic neurosegmental level of involvement will assume a "frog-leg" position and show no spontaneous motion of the lower extremities. Children with upper lumbar involvement may present with hyperextended knees and fixed heels at birth. The lowest functional myotomes are then correlated with the lowest responsive dermatomes; subsequently, the clinical findings can be correlated with ultrasound scans to identify the level of the spinal cord lesion. Identification of the neurosegmental level of involvement is also important because it helps predict physical function. A useful classification scheme is that proposed by Sharrard (1967), which categorizes patients according to the most caudal normally functioning motor level into four groups:

1. *Thoracic-level MMC* presents with paraplegia with a variable level of trunk involvement and, hence, variable sitting ability and posture control. These children have abducted and externally rotated hips as well as fixed knee flexion.
2. *Upper lumbar-level MMC* presents with hip and knee flexion deformity.
3. *Lower lumbar-level MMC* presents with active knee extension and foot dorsiflexion.
4. *Sacral MMC* presents with variable plantar and toe flexion, but may compromise sacral sensation, bowel/bladder control, and erectile function in males.

Although this scheme may help categorize children on the initial approach, it is not specific enough to allow for neurological screening or for prognostic purposes. For this reason, the International Myelodysplasia Study Group recommends a classification system based on manual motor testing. Specific myotomes are tested and classified into the following six categories:

0 No contraction

1 Voluntary muscle flickers that are inadequate for mobilizing joints

2 Muscle contraction that mobilizes joints in the absence of the effect of gravity

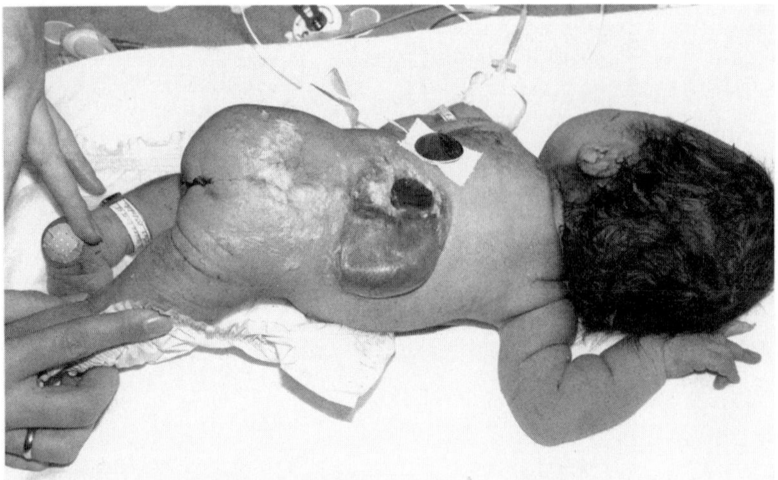

FIGURE 5.7. Newborn with a myelomeningocele that has been ruptured during delivery, exposing the neural placode. A patulous anus suggests bowel incontinence.

3 Muscle contraction that mobilizes the joint against the effect of gravity, throughout the complete range of motion, but is completely impaired by minimal resistance
4 Muscle contraction with partially impaired resistance
5 Normal muscle contraction with resistance

The neurosegmental level is designated as the most caudal segment, which demonstrates motor function of 3 or higher. Specific neurosegmental levels of inervation are described in Table 5.1 and represented by myotomes. This level of examination requires significant patient cooperation, which is obtained only after age 5 or 6. Hence, it is practical only for follow-up examinations.

TABLE 5.1. *Criteria for Determining Neurosegmental Level of Compromise*

Neurosegmental Level	Myotome
T10 or above	Sensory level; palpation of rectus abdominis segments; Beevor sign is present
T11	Exceeds T10 but does not meet criteria for T12
T12	Pelvis is partially controlled in the sitting position
L1	Weak iliopsoas (grade 2)
L2	Iliopsoas, adductors (grade 3 or higher)
L3	Quadriceps (grade 3 or higher)
L4	Tibialis anterior, medial hamstrings (grade 3 or higher)
L5	Tibialis posterior, lateral hamstring (grade 3 or higher), gluteus medius (grade 2 or higher)
S1	Gluteus medius (grade 3 or higher), gastrocnemius-soleus complex, gluteus maximus (grade 2 or higher)
S2	Gastrocnemius-soleus complex (grade 3 or higher), gluteus medius and maximus (grade 4 or higher)
S2–S3	One or two muscle groups may be grade 4. Bladder and/or bowel compromise will be missed in young infants

Source: Adapted from Wright (2001).

Following determination of the neurosegmental level of compromise, the entire spinal column is palpated, with a search for curvatures or defects. While the infant is prone, subtle evidence of occult dysraphism must be sought, especially at more cephalad levels. Hairy patches, midline dimples, and hemangiomas may be the only suggestions (Figs. 5.2 and 5.8).

Important points in the examination for musculoskeletal deformities are (*1*) obvious foot deformities, such as clubfoot or vertical talus, (*2*) reduced range of motion of the knees, (*3*) reduced range of motion of the hips, as well as reduced concentricity and stability, (*4*) reduced upper extremity function, and (*5*) reduced range of motion of the neck.

The initial assessment should be completed with PA and lateral views of the entire spine. The most caudal complete posterior elements should be correlated with the neurosegmental level of involvement. If a discrepancy exists between these two, ultrasound or magnetic resonance imaging (MRI) is warranted to rule out other central nervous system malformations.

FOLLOW-UP EXAMINATIONS OF THE SPINE

For follow-up visits, we recommend the following examinations: (*1*) characteristics of trunk shape and balance, (*2*) roentgenographic examination of the spine, (*3*) skin coverage, (*4*) neurological examination, and (*5*) musculoskeletal examination of the lower extremities.

Characteristics of Trunk Shape and Balance

The alignment of the spine must be evaluated at every follow-up visit, with the child standing or sitting unsup-

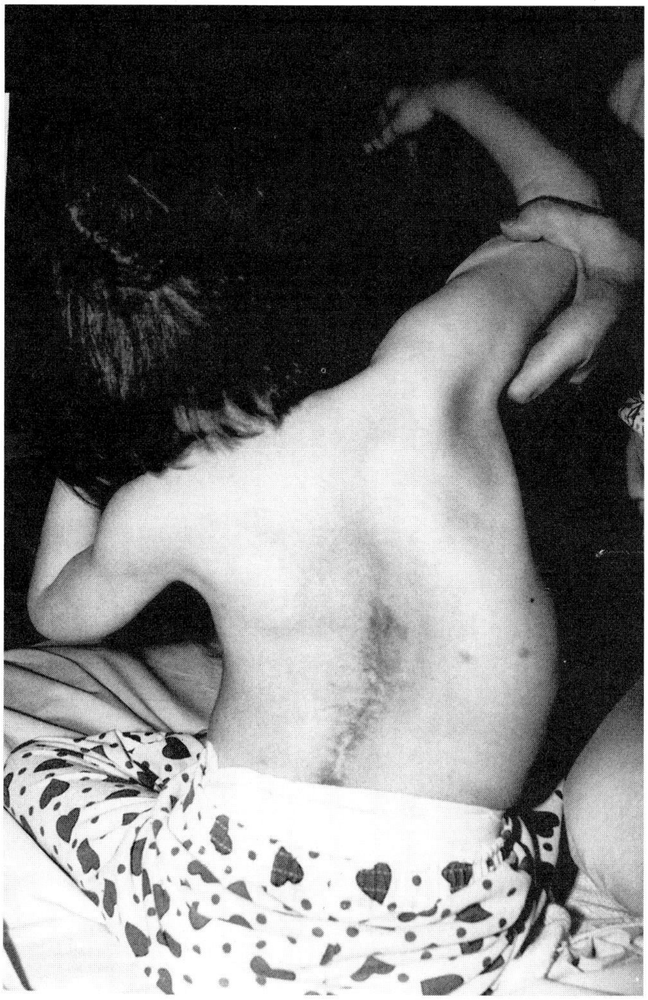

FIGURE 5.8. A 5-year-old girl with T10-level myelomeningocele. A hairy patch is noted in the lower thoracic region.

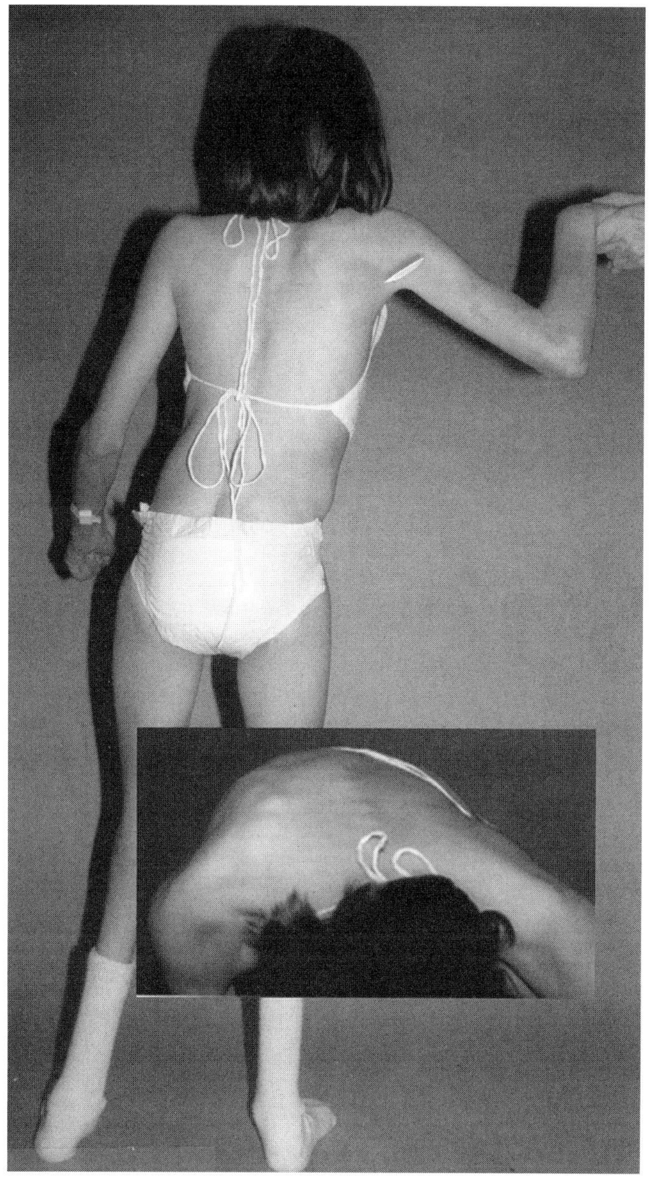

FIGURE 5.9. An 11-year-old girl with an L4-level myelomeningocele and a 40° T6–L1 right-sided curve, which had increased 14° in the last 6-month follow-up interval. On standing, there is right-sided trunk imbalance and noticeable asymmetry on the Adams forward-bending test (insert).

ported (according to the level of development). Hip contractures, as well as asymmetric weakness of the lower extremities in ambulatory children, may affect spinopelvic balance and alter the alignment of the spine. The coronal balance must be evaluated and the contours of the back carefully observed, including the shoulder height, waistline, scapular prominence, and pelvis. This will provide information on the appearance or progression of deformities.

In ambulatory children, the forward-bending (Adams) test is then performed, and the profile of the trunk is observed with the patient bending forward at the waist, with the knees straight and the palms together in front. High thoracic curves may be better appreciated when observing the patient from the front (Fig. 5.9 insert), and thoraco-lumbar or lumbar curves may be best appreciated when observing the patient from behind. With the use of a ruler, the height of the prominence is quantified and may be used as a follow-up measure. In the forward-bending position, the patient is then asked to turn to the right and left sides. Curves derotate toward the ipsilateral side of the convexity, and the extent to which this happens helps the clinician appreciate the relative flexibility or rigidity of the curve. In nonambulatory children, flexibility may also be assessed by supporting the trunk by the arms. This will force gravity to improve trunk alignment. Alternatively, the trunk is forced toward the convexity of the curve with a hand supporting the apex. In a similar manner, sagittal balance must also be evaluated. Special attention is paid to evaluating for kyphotic deformities of the thoraco-lumbar spine, as well as compensatory lordosis of the thoracic spine.

Pelvic obliquity with regard to the long axis of the trunk must be characterized as either supra- or infrapelvic and is also closely related to scoliosis (Locke, 2001). Infrapelvic obliquity is caused by pelvic-femoral muscle contractures. In the examination, this may be eliminated by abduction or adduction of the hips (Carman et al., 1990). Suprapelvic obliquity reflects a fixed spino-pelvic deformity and may not be eliminated by abduction or adduction of the hips (Fig. 5.10). Hip flexion contractures or "wideswept" hips (one side in abduction-contracture deformity and the other side in adduction) directly affect spino-pelvic balance and must be addressed as such.

The ability to walk depends on the neurosegmental level of involvement (Carman et al., 1990), as well as on trunk balance. In broad terms, 60% of all children with MMC are community ambulators at least during their childhood years. Children with thoracic level involvement are paraplegic, and 50% of them will stand during varying periods of their childhood with the aid of orthoses (Wright, 2001). Nevertheless, as their body size increases, it finally becomes more energy efficient to use a wheelchair (Locke et al., 2001). The same is true of children with upper lumbar level involvement, with 10% to 54% continuing to ambulate into adulthood. From 31% to 95% of those with lower lumbar level involvement continue to ambulate as young adults (Wright, 2001). Finally, 53%–100% of children with sacral level involvement become community ambulators in adult life with the use of simple orthotics.

Roentgenographic Examination of the Spine

Following clinical examination, lateral and PA X-rays of the spine should be taken during the first year of life and thereafter on a yearly basis. Obviously, closer scrutiny is needed if rapidly progressive deformities are identified. In the young infant, before sitting control is achieved, these films may be taken supine, but thereafter, they should be taken in the upright position, either standing or sitting, according to the neurosegmental level of compromise.

The technique is standardized and must include the entire spine on a single 36-inch film cassette. Positioning is also essential. For PA films, the arms must hang down on the corresponding sides. For lateral films, the patient should place the fists on the supraclavicular notch.

These X-rays will provide evidence of the levels of posterior element dysplasia, as well as the presence or absence of formation and/or segmentation defects (see Figs. 5.5*A* and 5.5*B*). Because of the cartilaginous nature of the growing spine in infants, these defects may not become apparent until the first or second year of life. The X-rays will also allow the examiner to evaluate the presence or absence of spinal deformity, as well as its magnitude, and the characteristics of trunk balance in both the frontal (coronal) and lateral (sagittal) planes of space.

The magnitude of the spinal curvatures is measured by the Cobb method (Cobb, 1948). This technique uses a protractor with single-degree demarcations, and the curvature is measured as the angle perpendicular to the cranial and caudal end vertebrae. The end vertebrae are defined as those most tilted into the curvature. A line is drawn perpendicular to the superior endplate of the proximal (cranial) end vertebra and perpendicular to the inferior endplate of the distal (caudal) end vertebra, and the angle between these two lines is measured (Fig. 5.11). In double or multiple curves, the caudal end vertebra of the proximal curve may also correspond to the cranial end vertebra of the distal curve. The Cobb method is also suitable for the quantification of deformities in the sagittal plane. As with many other anthropometric measures,

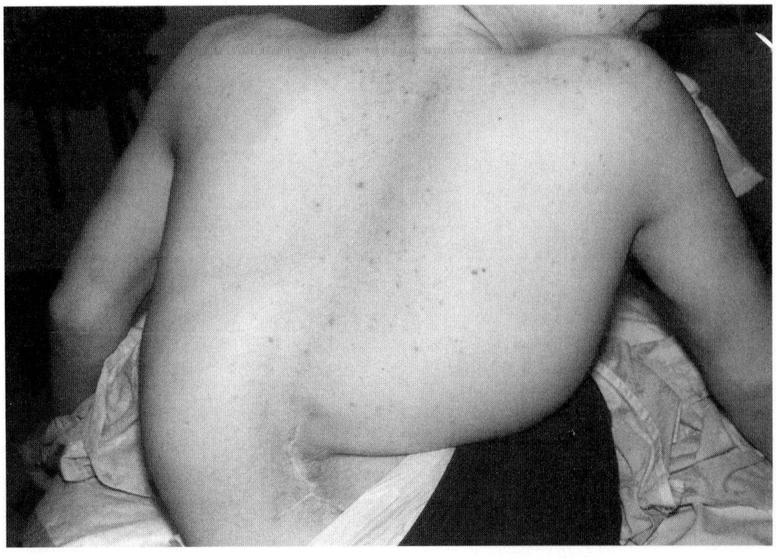

FIGURE 5.10. A 15-year-old boy with T12-level myelomeningocele and a 107° left-sided lumbar curve. The severe pelvic obliquity and coronal imbalance require constant support of both of his upper extremities to maintain an upright posture.

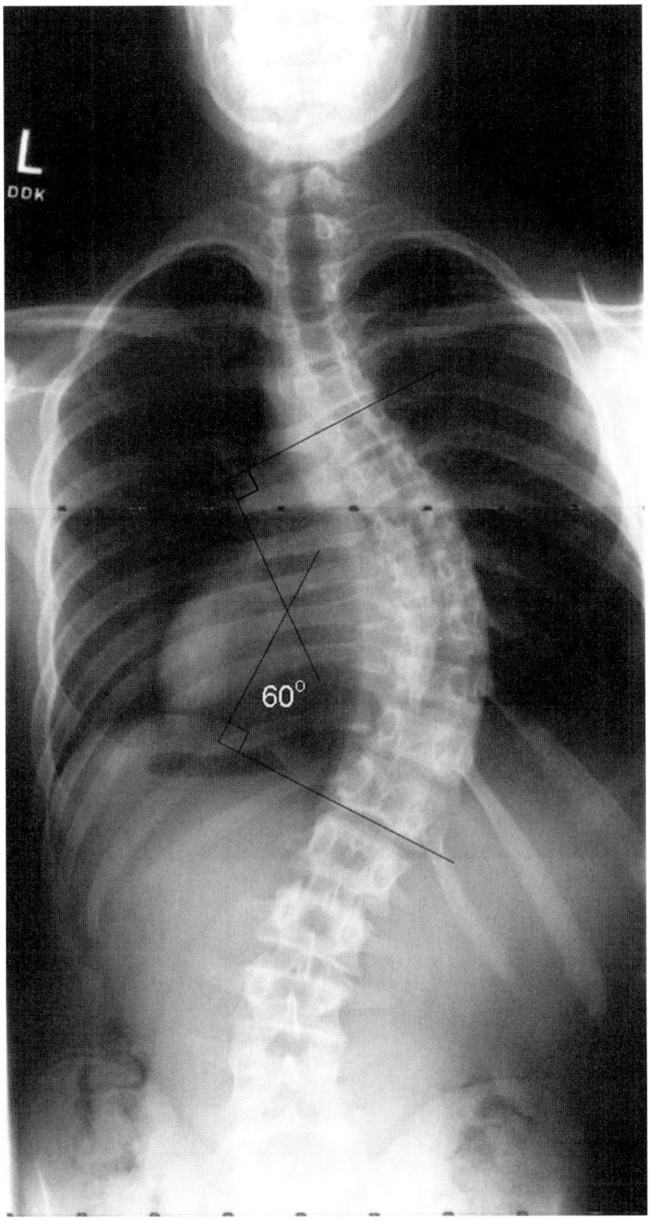

FIGURE 5.11. Measurement of the Cobb angle between T5 and T12.

inter- and intraobserver variability must be considered when comparing measurements, and there is a 5° error for any Cobb angle measurement (Morrisy et al., 1990). Two measurements can be considered truly different with a 95% CI if they differ by 10° or more (Carman et al., 1990). This is very important to keep in mind when defining the progression of a curve.

Helpful in the assessment of skeletal maturity is the degree of ossification of the iliac apophysis (Fig. 5.12). The amount of ossification is visible in the PA X-ray of the spine. Risser (1958) devised a classification of skeletal maturity as follows: 0 (no ossification), 1 (25% ossification), 2 (50% ossification), 3 (75% ossification), and

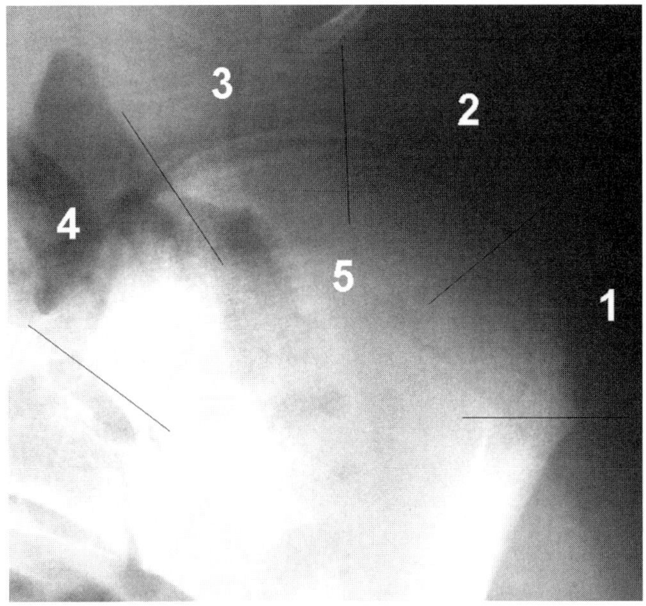

FIGURE 5.12. Ossification of the iliac apophysis in zones 1 through 4, described as a Risser grade 4.

4 (100% ossification). When this fuses to the rest of the iliac wing, it is classified as Risser 5. Risser 0–2 indicates that a significant amount of growth potential remains. The examiner must always remember that many of these children present with precocious puberty and that the remaining growth can be difficult to estimate.

Skin Coverage

Examination of the skin is also important for both diagnostic and therapeutic purposes. When neurological deterioration is found, cutaneous stigmata may be the only key to more proximal anomalies of the spinal cord or spinal canal. These have been previously enumerated (Figs. 5.2 and 5.8). The skin must also be examined for pressure sores over the spinal gibbus in patients with kyphotic deformity, which may be a precipitating factor for osteomyelitis. Recurrent skin breakdown is not uncommon and may be explained by multiple factors, including the pressure of the deformity, developmentally abnormal skin, scar tissue with decreased vascularity, insensitivity, malnourishment, and a decreased immune response (Fig. 5.13). The dura may also suffer from pressure ulcer, potentially leading to meningitis (Mueller et al., 1994), which under these circumstances may be a life-threatening event.

Pressure sores in sitting weight-bearing areas must be carefully monitored. They are prone to occur in nonambulators with rigid spino-pelvic deformities, pelvic obliquity, and asymmetric hip deformity. These sores may occur in the sacro-coccygeal area, ischial tuberosities, or greater trochanters. Patients who do not stay dry and

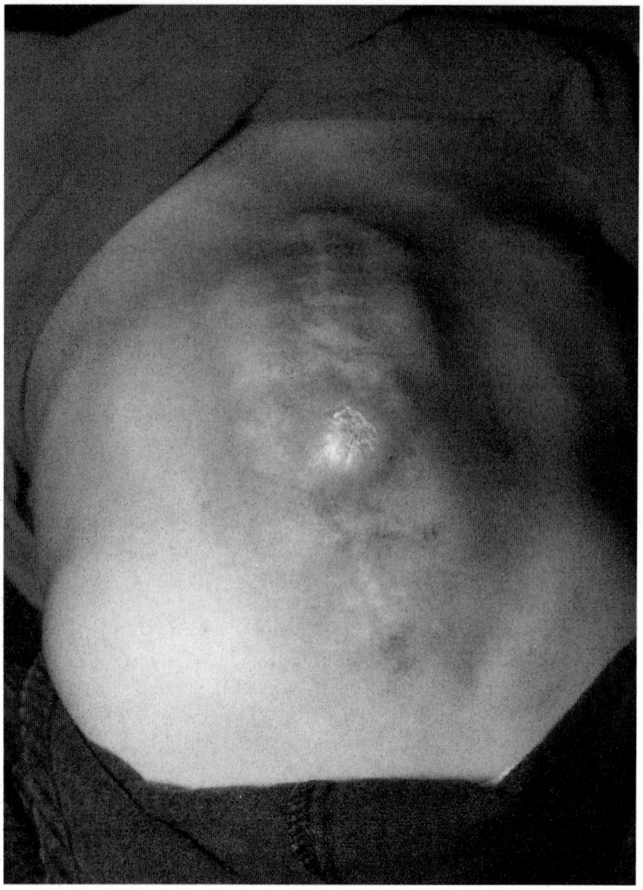

FIGURE 5.13. A 5-year-old boy with T11-level myelomeningocele and a sharp-angled kyphosis. The skin on the apex of the deformity is irritated and prone to breakdown. There are no protective soft tissues, and the paraspinal musculature has migrated anteriorly.

clean of urine are also more prone to develop recalcitrant pressure sores.

Neurological Assessment

A thorough neurological examination must be carried out at every follow-up visit. The neurosegmental level of involvement is reassessed and must be carefully correlated with the documented findings from previous visits. A pattern of nonprogression or progression must be established.

Neurological deterioration in children with MMC does not represent the natural history of this disorder but instead reflects progressive injury. The two most significant differential diagnoses are: spinal cord tethering (Martin et al., 1994), and shunt malfunction (Bowman et al., 2001). As these children grow, the cord may be tethered at the site of neural placode repair. Spinal cord tethering may also be attributed to other forms of occult spinal dysraphism. If the cause is unknown, it must be sought by an MRI study. Suggestive symptoms are (*1*) back pain and or vague lower extremity pain, (*2*) progressive lower extremity weakness or increased spasticity, (*3*) rapidly progressive scoliosis, (*4*) changes in bladder/bowel habits, and (*5*) progressive and or asymmetric lower extremity deformities. The diagnosis of a tethered cord is made solely on clinical grounds, provided that other causes of neurological deterioration have been ruled out.

Musculoskeletal Examination of the Lower Extremities

Joint range of motion and stability must be assessed in every visit. Children with thoracic-level involvement frequently present with hip and knee flexion contractures. Hip dislocation may develop and is frequently associated with the development of scoliosis. In patients with upper lumbar level involvement, hip and knee flexion contractures are also present. In contrast, children with lower lumbar level involvement may present with hyperextended knees. Those with sacral level involvement have variable plantar-flexion strength. They may present with either rocker bottom or cavus feet, with clawing of their toes.

Osteopenia frequently accompanies paralysis, and the ambulatory status and neurosegmental level of involvement are strongly correlated with decreased bone mineral density (Shook and Lubicky, 1996; Wright, 2001). As a consequence, these children may present with fractures of the insensate lower extremities. Often, there is no clear-cut trauma. There may be a significant local inflammatory reaction, which may be confused with an infection. Patients may even present with fever and increased white blood cell counts, as well as increased inflammatory parameters. Crepitation may be found only in displaced injuries; this is the least common scenario. Plain films may elucidate the diagnosis, but this must be initially suspected. In a child with MMC who presents with fever, the two most frequent differential diagnoses are urinary tract infections and pathological fracture.

REFERENCES

Boone D, Parsons D, Lachman SM, et al (1985). Spina bifida occulta: lesion or anomaly? Clin Radiol 36:159–161.

Bowman RM, McLone DG, Dias LS, et al (2001). Twenty-year outcome for nonselectively treated children with myelomeningocele. In Sarwark JF, Lubicky JP (eds): *Caring for the Child with Spina Bifida*. Shriners Hospitals for Children Symposium. Rosemont, IL: AAOS, pp. 455–461.

Carman DL, Browne RH, Birch JG (1990). Measurement of scoliosis and kyphosis radiographs. Intraobserver and interobserver variation. J Bone Joint Surg. 72(A):328.

Carstens C, Koch H, Brocai DR, et al (1991). Development of pathological lumbar kyphosis in myelomeningocele. J Bone Joint Surg 78(B):945.

Christofersen MR, Brooks AL (1985). Excision and wire fixation of rigid myelomeningocele kyphosis. J Pediatr Orthop 5:691, 696.

Cobb J (1948). Outline for the study of scoliosis. Instructional Course Lectures 5:261.

Locke MD, Dias LS, Sarwark JF (2001). The relationship between infrapelvic obliquity and scoliosis. In Sarwark JF, Lubicky JP (eds): *Caring for the Child with Spina Bifida.* Shriners Hospitals for Children Symposium. Rosemont, IL: AAOS, pp. 105–115.

Martin J, Kumar SJ, Guille JT, et al (1994). Congenital kyphosis in myelomeningocele: results following operative and nonoperative treatment. J Pediatr Orthop 14:323–328.

Morrisy RT, Goldsmith GS, Hall EC, et al (1990). Measurement of the Cobb angle on radiographs of patients who have scoliosis. Evaluation of intrinsic error. J Bone Joint Surg 72(A):320.

Risser JC (1958). The iliac apophysis: an invaluable sign in the management of scoliosis. Clin Orthop 11:111.

Sharrard WJ (1967). Paralytic deformity in the lower limb. J Bone Joint Surg 49(B):731–747.

Shook JE, Lubicky JP (1996). Paralytic scoliosis. In: Bridwell KH, DeWald RI (eds.): *The Textbook of Spinal Surgery,* 2nd ed. Philadelphia: JB Lippincot, pp. 837–880.

Swank M, Dias L (1992). Myelomeningocele: a review of the orthopaedic aspects of 206 patients treated from birth with no selection criteria. Dev Med Child Neurol 34:1047–1052.

Wright JG (2001). Neurosegmental level and functional status. Sarwark JF, Lubicky JP (eds): *Caring for the Child with Spina Bifida.* Shriners Hospital for Children Symposium. Rosemont, IL: AAOS, pp. 67–78.

6

Classification of Neural Tube Defects

CYNTHIA A. MOORE

The human neural tube develops and closes during the third and fourth weeks after conception and is normally completed by 28 days postconception (Sadler, 1998) (Fig. 6.1*A,B*). Malformations known as *neural tube defects* occur when the normal closure process fails. Several clinical types of neural tube defects are recognized, anencephaly and spina bifida being the most common; however, the basis for the variation among the recognized types is poorly understood. In this chapter, the major types of neural tube defects—anencephaly, craniorachischisis, spina bifida, encephalocele, and iniencephaly—will be defined and the classification issues surrounding each will be discussed.

IMPORTANCE OF CLASSIFICATION OF NEURAL TUBE DEFECTS

Neural tube defects are classified for clinical, research, and public health activities. In clinical practice, the differentiation of the various types of neural tube defect is important for several reasons. The outcome can vary considerably both among and within defect groups. Infants with anencephaly are stillborn or die shortly after birth (Baird and Sadovnick, 1984). In a recent population-based study in the United States, over 90% of individuals with spina bifida in a 1989–1994 birth cohort survived to age 1 year, with higher mortality occurring in those with high versus low lesions (Wong and Paulozzi, 2001). Across populations, survival of individuals with spina bifida differs, but a large majority of survivors have some degree of disability (Bowman et al., 2001; Hunt and Oakeshott, 2003). The geographical variability in survival might reflect actual differences in severity of the lesion, but more likely is a result of social and economic factors such as availability and use of treatment and selective termination of affected pregnancies after prenatal diagnosis (Kalucy et al., 1994; Shehu et al., 2000; Oneko et al., 2002; Olde Scholtenhuis et al., 2003). The likelihood of identifying a known etiology in an affected infant also varies by type of neural tube defect. For example, in clinical series, encephaloceles are more frequently associated with single-gene and chromosomal syndromes than are other types (Hunter, 1993). Finally, the presence of additional structural birth defects varies among the types of neural tube defects, with lumbosacral spina bifida being least likely to occur with other anomalies (Seller and Kalousek, 1986; Hall et al., 1988). Both factors, known etiology and additional birth defects, will influence the prognosis and family counseling about future reproductive risks (Holmes et al., 1976).

Research activities also rely on accurate and consistent classification of affected individuals. The birth prevalence of the rarer types of neural tube defects is an important consideration related to study power in prospective studies such as clinical trials. In family-based studies, recognition of form fruste variants as well as classic presentations is important in correctly identifying affected individuals for linkage and association studies (Stevenson and DeLoache, 1988). Population-based epidemiological studies struggle to find the correct balance between combining types of defects to increase the power to detect an association and stratifying by type of defect to find the risk associated with each particular defect (Khoury et al., 1992b). Finally, public health surveillance and prevention activities often have lumped together neural tube defects in determining birth prevalence and making recommendations for decreasing the risk of these defects. Recent studies of birth prevalence trends have shown differences between anencephaly and spina bifida in the magnitude of the decline in rates after fortification of cereal grains with folic acid (Honein et al., 2001; Williams et al.,

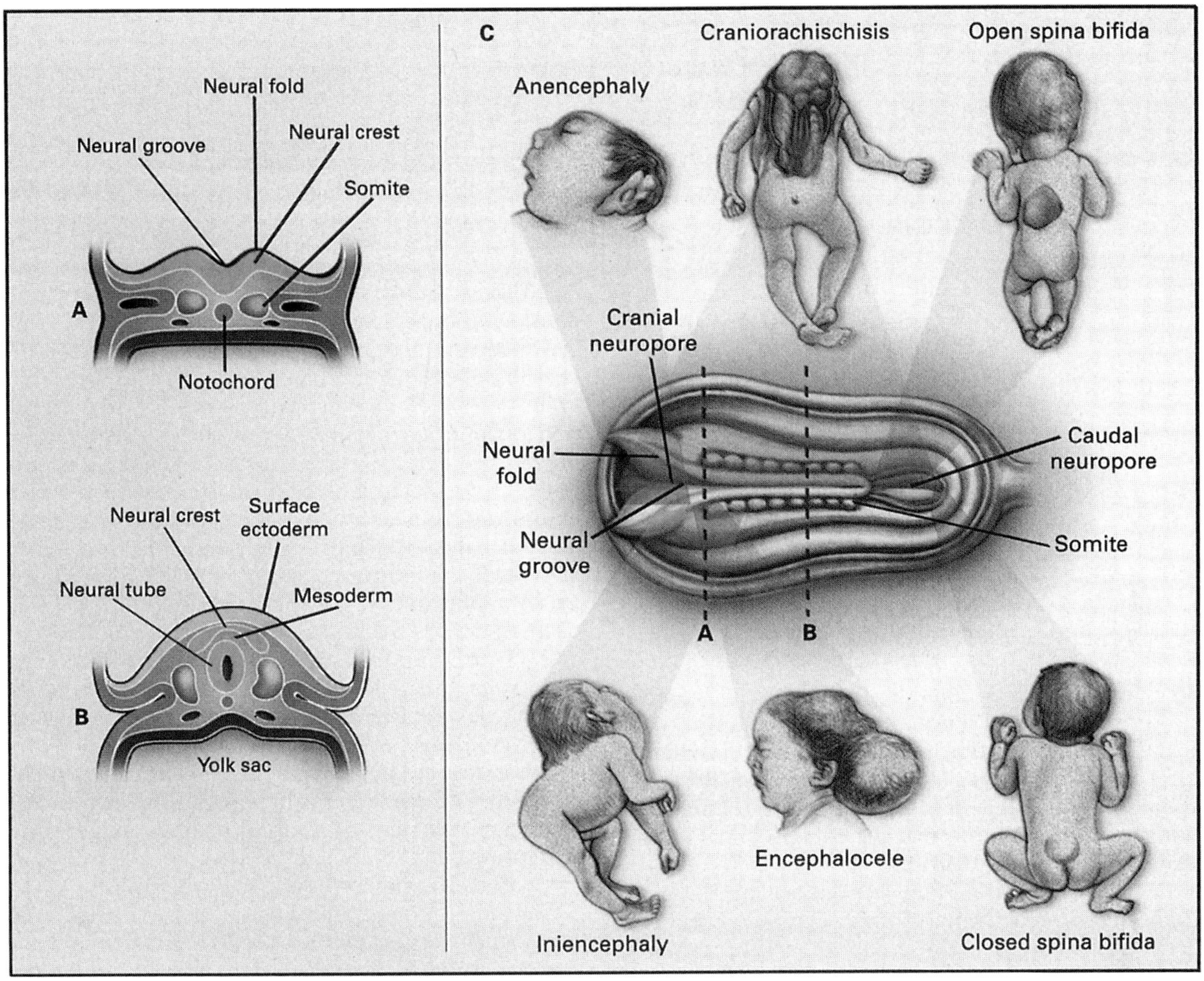

FIGURE 6.1. Features of neural tube development and neural tube defects. Panel A shows a cross section of the cranial end of the embryo at approximately 3 weeks after conception, revealing the neural fold in the process of closing, overlying the notochord. The neural folds are the rising margins of the neural tube, topped by the neural crest, and demarcating the neural groove centrally. Panel B shows a cross section of the middle portion of the embryo after the neural tube has closed. The neural tube, which will ultimately develop into the spinal cord, is not covered by surface ectoderm (later, the skin). The intervening mesoderm will form the bony spine. The notochord is regressing. Panel C shows the development and clinical features of the main types of neural tube defects. The diagram in the center is a dorsal view of a developing embryo showing a neural tube that is fused in the center but still open at the cranial and caudal ends. The dotted lines marked A and B refer to the cross sections shown in Panels A and B. Shaded bars point to the region of the neural tube relevant to each defect. The different types of neural tube defects are described further in the text. *Source:* Reprinted from Botto et al. (1999).

2002). However, data are currently not sufficient to determine if these observed differences accurately represent changes in incidence and whether the differences will vary among populations.

CLINICAL TYPES OF NEURAL TUBE DEFECTS

The distribution of neural tube defect types appears to vary in different populations and can also vary by the birth prevalence of these defects (Botto et al., 1999). In most instances, if not detected prenatally, neural tube defects are recognized at birth; however, inconsistent nomenclature has complicated the documentation and investigation of this group of defects (Borman and Cryer, 1990). Even medical professionals such as pathologists have shown marked variation in the identification of types of neural tube defects in a study by Dolk and Sellar (1993).

The most common classification schema for neural tube defects includes anencephaly, spina bifida, and encephalocele. A more complete classification includes two neural tube defects that are considered to be rarer in most populations, craniorachischisis and iniencephaly

(Fig. 6.1C). Various studies have included other defects in the neural tube defect spectrum, most commonly spina bifida occulta and other conditions broadly described as occult spinal dysraphism (such as spina lipomas and tight filum terminale) (Lorber and Levick, 1967; Carter et al., 1976; Sattar et al., 1996). Unfortunately, the term *spina bifida occulta* is also used for a defect in posterior arches, usually at the fifth lumbar or first sacral vertebral level, that is common (10%–30%) in the general population (Boone et al., 1985; Northrup and Volcik, 2000). The report of families in which the presence of multiple vertebral anomalies (Wynne-Davies, 1975), isolated hydrocephalus (Journel et al., 1989), and cutis aplasia (Stevenson and DeLoache, 1988; Drolet et al., 1995) was related to a higher occurrence of neural tube defects has raised the possibility of a relation between these defects and neural tube defects.

Anencephaly

Anencephaly results from a failure of fusion of the cranial portion of the neural tube, with resultant absence of all or part of the brain, neurocranium, and skin. The cerebral hemispheres are usually absent; the brainstem and portions of the midbrain are usually present. The pituitary gland is hypoplastic or absent, and the cranial base is abnormal. At term, variable amounts of membrane-covered tissue known as *cerebrovasculosa* or *angiomatous stroma* protrude through the bony defect. Studies of the *area cerebrovasculosa* have identified glial tissue, ependyma, and abnormally vascular choroid plexus covered with squamous epithelium (Bell and Green, 1982). Additional craniofacial defects such as exophthalmos and low-set ears are common. Small numbers of infants with anencephaly or craniorachischisis and a holoprosencephalic facial appearance have also been reported (Lemire et al., 1981; Siebert et al., 1981).

A defect similar to anencephaly, exencephaly (brain located outside the skull), is well documented in mice and has been postulated to be a precursor event to anencephaly in humans. Several reports of transformation from exencephaly to anencephaly in human fetuses visualized by ultrasonography provide support for this hypothesis (Wilkins-Haug and Freedman, 1991; Timor-Tritsch et al., 1996). Recently, Matsumoto and collegues (2002) studied mouse embryos in an exo utero development system and described two modes of tissue reduction, based on an imbalance between neural tissue and vascular growth, that led to an anencephalic phenotype in embryos that were initially exencephalic.

Two types of anencephaly are generally described, holoanencephaly and meroanencephaly, although the descriptive terms for these lesions have varied considerably over the years (Lemire and Siebert, 1990). In holoanencephaly the bony defect extends through the level of the foramen magnum, while the defect in meroanencephaly is smaller (Fig. 6.2). In the prospective Collaborative Perinatal Project, 11 (35%) of 31 infants with anencephaly were classified as having meroanencephaly (Melnick and Myrianthopoulos, 1987). Although meroanencephaly is characterized as a "milder" form of anencephaly, a prospective study of affected fetuses and infants demonstrated that there is little or no residual brain tissue in this form of anencephaly (Melnick and Myrianthopoulos, 1987). Because information on the type of anencephaly is not routinely collected for birth defects

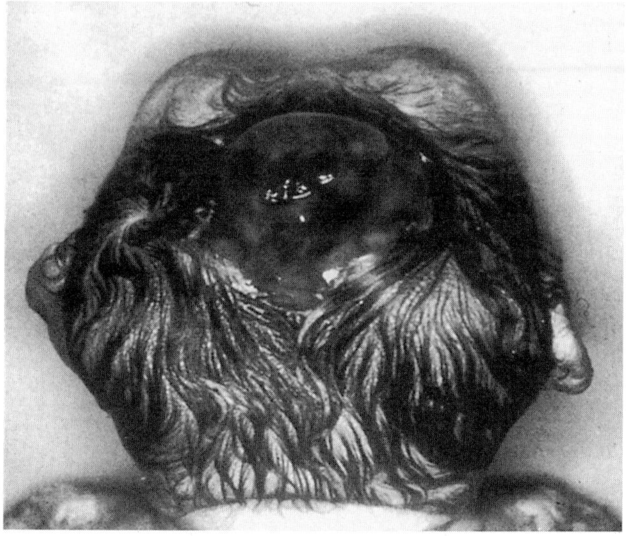

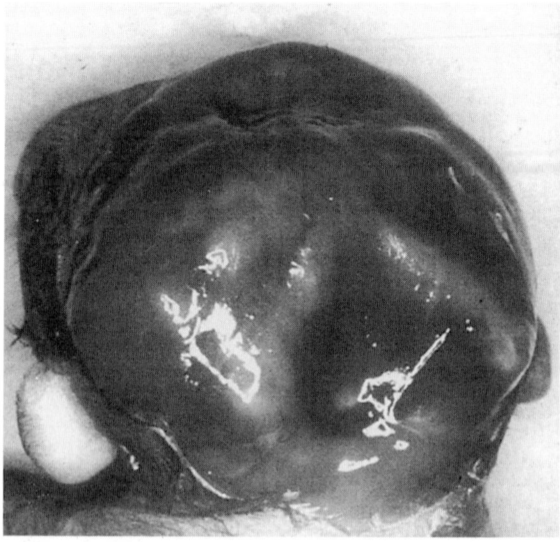

FIGURE 6.2. Clinical types of anencephaly. Posterior view of an infant with meroanencephaly (top) and holoanencephaly (bottom). *Source:* Courtesy of the Collaborative Birth Defects Surveillance Project–China, National Center for Maternal and Infant Health, Peking University.

surveillance or analytic studies, little is known about the potential demographic difference between holoanencephaly and meroanencephaly, although one study did find a difference in sex ratio (Seller, 1987).

A term that is occasionally used for anencephaly and its subtypes is *acrania*. Unfortunately, use of this term can lead to misclassification because it is sometimes used to describe acalvaria, a condition in which only the neurocranium is absent and is believed to be unrelated to neural tube defects (Harris et al., 1993). Infants with acephaly-acardia, a condition in which one twin is hypoperfused, resulting in maldevelopment of the upper half of the body (Van Allen et al., 1983), are often reported by medical professionals as having anencephaly. Because true anencephaly is also increased in twinning, careful review of such reports is needed to discriminate between the two unrelated conditions. Finally, infants with a disrupted cranium due to amniotic bands often receive the diagnosis of anencephaly, which is an incorrect use of the term. Infants with amniotic band disruption sequence often can be recognized either by the asymmetric or distorted appearance of the cranial defect or by the presence of additional anomalies such as constriction lesions or unusual facial clefts. Occasional adherence of the fetal membranes or placenta to the exposed tissue in true anencephaly can also complicate the differential process. If external examination is not sufficient to discriminate between the two conditions, characteristics of the cranial base and spine determined on autopsy or radiographs might be used to differentiate anencephaly from amniotic band disruption according to findings in two studies (Keeling and Kjaer, 1994; Kjaer et al., 1994).

Spina Bifida

The term *spina bifida* is used by both health-care professionals and the lay public to describe a group of defects that occurs when there is failure of fusion of the caudal portion of the neural tube and concomitant schisis of the posterior elements of the vertebrae. Meningomyeloocele is the most common type of spina bifida, reportedly accounting for about 90% of all spina bifida (Hunter, 1993); however, it is likely that this estimation is biased toward surgical series of patients. This lesion, most commonly located in the lumbosacral region, is characterized by a central neural placode that is covered by a sac-like membrane containing cerebrospinal fluid, hence the outdated term *spina bifida cystica*. The placode is elevated by fluid in the ventral subarachnoid space (Tortori-Donati et al., 2000). A similar lesion and a more rare form of spina bifida known as *myeloschisis* or *myelocele* lacks a membranous sac, and the open neural tissue lies at the bottom of the spinal canal (McComb, 1997). Warkany (1971) postulated that myeloschisis is a precursor to meningomyelocele that develops its cystic nature after epithelialization of the lesion. Rarely, a meningomyelocele or myeloschisis can affect only one half of a split cord; this condition is known as *hemimeningomeylocele* or *hemimyeloschisis* (McComb, 1997; Tortori-Donati et al., 2000). Arnold Chiari type II malformation (a condition in which the cerebellar portion of the brain protrudes into the spinal canal) with resultant hydrocephalus is commonly associated with meningomyelocele. A recent study reported that 81% of affected individuals required ventricular shunting (Rintoul et al., 2002).

A meningocele consists of herniated meninges through a spine defect and does not contain the spinal cord, although some neural elements such as nerve roots can be present (McComb, 1997; Tortori-Donati et al., 2000). In contrast to meningomyelocele and myeloschisis, meningoceles are usually covered by normal skin. For this reason, meningocele is often classified with other skin-covered lesions rather than with meningomyelocele or myeloschisis.

Other lesions of the spinal cord that are usually classified with neural tube defects are myelocystocele and lipomyelomeningocele and their variants. Myelocystocele, also called *syringocele*, results from dilation of the normally vestigial central canal or hydromyelia and subsequent herniation of the dilated structure through a bony defect. Although myelocystoceles can occur anywhere on the spine, in most instances the lesion occurs in the sacral region (terminal *myelocystocele*), where it may be associated with other caudal malformations such as persistent cloaca (Lemire et al., 2003). A ventral variant of myelocystocele is anterior meningocele, which can be a component of the Currarino triad (anorectal malformation, sacral bony abnormality, and presacral mass) (Lee et al., 1997). Lipomeningomyelocele, lipomeningocele, and other lipomatous malformations of the caudal cord are composed of varying amounts of fatty tissue attached to the spinal cord or filum terminale (McComb, 1997). Frequently these lipomatous defects are included with other caudal developmental lesions, such as split-cord malformation and tight filum terminale, under the nonspecific labels of *closed* or *occult spinal dysraphism*, especially in the neurosurgical or neuroradiological literature. It is uncertain which of these caudal lesions, if any, should be categorized as a neural tube defect. Certainly, the pathogenetic mechanism(s) likely differ both among the various caudal lesions and between these defects and those associated with failure of primary closure of the neural tube.

Cephaloceles

Cephaloceles are pedunculated or sessile cystic cranial lesions containing either herniated meninges and portions of the brain (encephalocele or meningoencephalocele) or meninges without brain (cranial meningocele) through a defect in the skull. The malformation is usually midline and is more likely to affect the occipital area; however, there are population differences, such as the high rate of frontoethmoidal encephaloceles in Southeast Asia (Richards, 1992). Cephaloceles can vary greatly in size and form and are usually covered with skin. Commonly, areas of skin breakdown and necrosis are present. Atretic forms of cephaloceles are usually located in the parietal area. On examination they resemble areas of cutis aplasia or are small nodular lesions consisting of fibrous tissue and dura with occasional identification of neural tissue such as glial rests (Yokota et al., 1988). Cephaloceles containing tissue from the brain and spinal cord are called encephalomyeloceles. Although a mesodermal origin has been postulated for cephaloceles, the frequent accompanying brain malformations indicate a more global developmental problem of the rostral neural tube rather than a simple herniation in most instances (Hunter, 1993).

Several classification schemas in addition to the pathological type exist for cephaloceles, and all of these are based on the location of the lesion. Broad categories such as frontal, parietal, occipital, and sphenoidal are used for most registries or epidemiological studies. In the neurosurgical literature, a distinction between anterior and posterior cephaloceles is made because of the implications for treatment and prognosis. McComb (1997) further subdivides the posterior cephaloceles based on their relation to the torcula (infratorcular and supratorcular). Anterior cephaloceles are divided into frontal, sincipital (visible), and basal (not visible). Sincipital cephaloceles occur at the fronto-midface junction, while basal cephaloceles occur within the ethmoid and sphenoid bones. The location of the various subtypes of both sincipital and basal cephaloceles is reflected by their name (e.g., *nasofrontal* and *transethmoidal*). Disruption of facial structures commonly occurs with sincipital lesions. As with anencephaly, amniotic band disruption sequence as an etiology for cephaloceles must be considered and should be suspected for any lesion that does not appear to follow known anatomical patterns.

Craniorachischisis

Anencephaly with a contiguous spina bifida is known as *craniorachischisis*. Caudal extension of anencephaly is common, occurring in 16 (80%) of 20 infants with holoanencephaly in the Collaborative Perinatal Project (Melnick and Myrianthopoulos, 1987); however, the term *craniorachischisis* is most commonly used to describe infants with significant extension of the rachischisis. The latter lesion is rare but has been reported to be more prevalent in areas with high rates of neural tube defects, such as the United Kingdom and northern China (Dolk et al., 1991; Moore et al., 1997). A subset of infants with extensive craniorachischisis will have spinal retroflexion (Fig. 6.3) and exhibit a body habitus that is very similar to that of iniencephaly, which is described in the following paragraph.

Iniencephaly

Iniencephaly is a complex neural tube defect characterized by a closed cranium, enlarged foramen magnum, and marked retroflexion of the cervical spine resulting in an upward-directed gaze and absent neck (Fig. 6.4). Infants with iniencephaly can have accompanying encephalocele or posterior spina bifida. In some literature, the term *apertus* is used if an encephalocele is present, and the term *clausus* is used in the absence of other neural tube defects. For many years, a debate has existed concerning the relation between iniencephaly and craniorachischisis with spinal retroflexion (Coffey, 1965; Lemire et al., 1972). Lemire and colleagues (1972) described an anterior spina bifida in two of two fetuses with iniencephaly and one of eight fetuses with craniorachischisis with spinal retroflexion. Blackburn and collegues (1995) examined 14 fetuses with either iniencephaly or craniorachischisis with spinal retroflexion (number of each not specified) and reported an extensive duplication of the cervical spine in those with iniencephaly that was not seen in those with craniorachischisis with spinal retroflexion. In addition, a difference in the position of craniospinal articulation (anterior in iniencephaly, posterior in craniorachischisis with spinal retroflexion) was reported. Despite similar demographic and clinical characteristics in the two conditions (e.g., female predominance, frequent additional anomalies, and increased prevalence in areas with high birth rates of infants with neural tube defects), the distinct dissimilarities in the cranial pathology suggest different timing if not different mechanisms.

CLASSIFICATION OF NEURAL TUBE DEFECTS

In an attempt to construct more homogeneous groups for analytic studies of risk factors, various classification schemas for neural tube defects have been used, including classification by type of defect, location of the lesion, and open/closed status. Lemire (1988) put forth a classification schema for neural tube defects based on location, mechanism, and timing. Both McComb (1997) and Tortori-Donati and colleagues (2000) proposed a classification schema for spinal dysraphism that segregates spina bifida by the presence or absence of a skin covering that can either be normal or have various stigmata, such as hemangiomas, hairy patches, or hyperpigmentation.

Ideally, for complete classification of a neural tube defect and the ability to further stratify as needed for subanalyses, the following information is needed: anatomical type of lesion, including other central nervous system

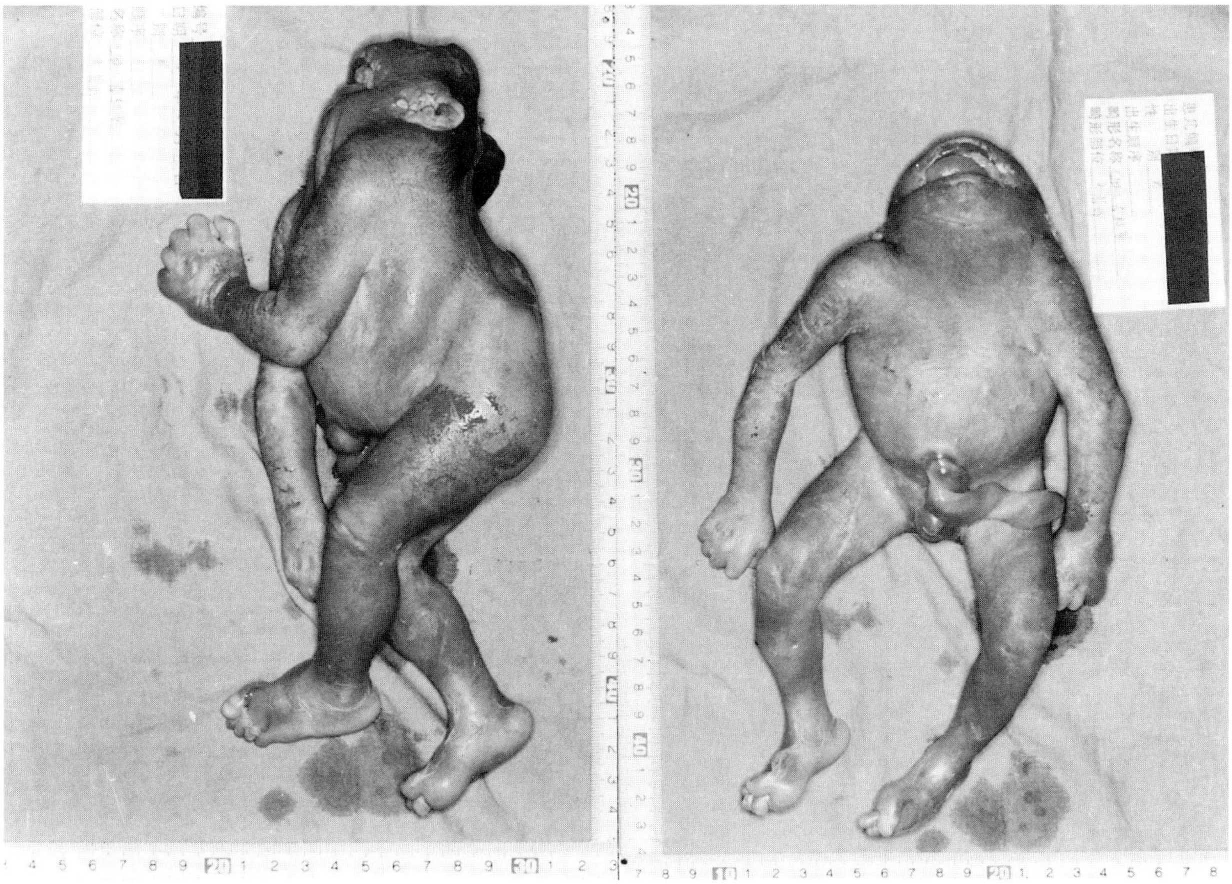

FIGURE 6.3. Infant with craniorachischisis with spinal retroflexion. Lateral and anterior views of an infant with craniorachischisis and spinal retroflexion. Note the similarity of the body habitus to iniencephaly (Fig. 6.4).

Source: Courtesy of the Collaborative Birth Defects Surveillance Project–China, National Center for Maternal and Infant Health, Peking University. Reprinted from Moore et al. (1997).

defects (confirmed by neuroimaging, surgery, or autopsy); location of the lesion (confirmed by radiographs or neuroimaging); and open/closed status. In addition, information on other associated congenital defects is necessary to classify the infant with a neural tube defect (Rasmussen et al., 2003).

Classification Based on Anatomical Type

The most obvious method of classification of neural tube defects is by type of lesion; however, lack of information or small sample size can lead to lumping of all neural tube defects. Some data sources (like vital records) that can be used to assess trends limit separation of neural tube defects into the categories of anencephaly and spina bifida and provide little or no additional information on defect subtypes or etiological factors. Even with a large study size and adequate information, dividing some types of neural tube defects into subgroups might result in small analytic groups that lead to imprecise risk estimates (Khoury et al., 1992b). Data sources such as hospital discharge data are usually limited to codes assigned according to the International Classification of Diseases, 9th Revision, Clinical Modification (ICD-9-CM) (U.S. Department of Heath and Human Services, 1980). The ICD codes are anatomically based, and the ability to uniquely and specifically code congenital defects is limited (Rasmussen and Moore, 2001). The result of these classification challenges is that the majority of information we have concerning neural tube defects risk factors is based on limited stratification, if any.

Classification Based on Location of Lesion

The location of the neural tube defect is another characteristic that can be used for classification. At a basic level, neural tube defects can be divided into cranial and spinal neural tube defects, but this is not a usual method because of concerns about comparability of defects like anencephaly and encephalocele.

Epidemiologic studies of encephaloceles have included the location of the lesion. Different rates of encephaloce-

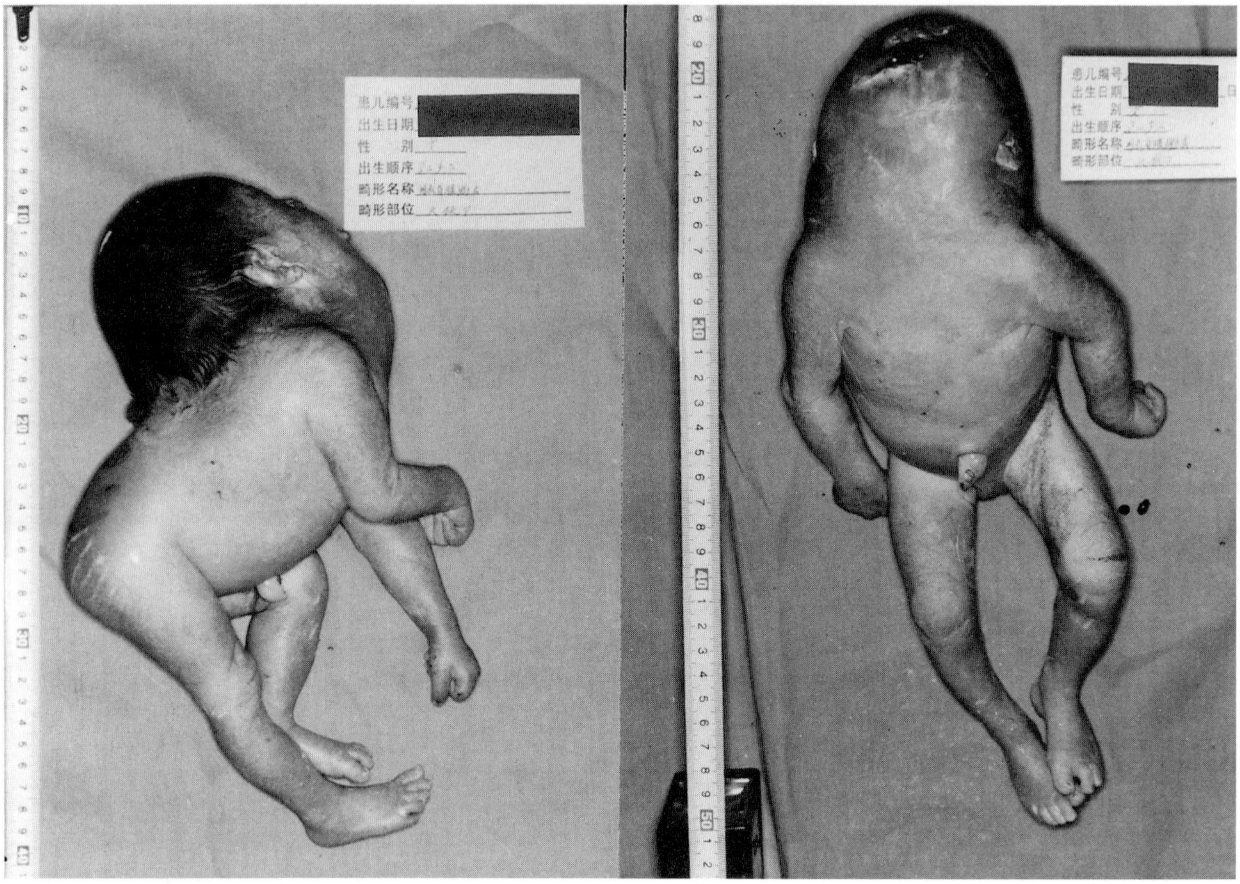

FIGURE 6.4. Infant with iniencephaly. Lateral and anterior views of an infant with iniencephaly. Note the closed cranium and retroflexed head. The infant also has thoracolumbar spina bifida. *Source:* Courtesy of the Collaborative Birth Defects Surveillance Project–China, National Center for Maternal and Infant Health, Peking University. Reprinted from Moore et al. (1997).

les in populations have been documented, such as the previously mentioned high rate of frontal encephaloceles in the Asian population (Richards, 1992).

The anatomical location of the lesion has been studied extensively for spina bifida, with the highest level of the lesion used for classification. In the majority of studies, the lesion is classified as high or low, with the 11th and 12th thoracic vertebrae being the most frequent points of division (Toriello and Higgins, 1985). Using this method, differences between the two groups have been shown in regard to demographics (Khoury et al., 1982; Park et al., 1992; Kallen et al., 1994; Shaw et al., 1994), risk factors (Blatter et al., 1997; Shaw et al., 1997; Volcik et al., 2003), recurrence risk (Hall et al., 1988; Park et al., 1992; Hunter et al., 1996), additional malformations (Toriello and Higgins, 1985), and survival (Wong and Paulozzi, 2001). The rationale for the division into high and low spina bifida has been a proposed embryological difference in the formation of the spinal cord in these regions, that is, neurulation (primary neurulation) versus canalization (secondary neurulation). However, there remains disagreement about the location of the junction between these two processes. Work by Müller and O'Rahilly (1986) indicates that the division is at the level of the future second sacral vertebra, while a more recent study places it lower, at the fifth sacral vertebra, suggesting that all spina bifida develops from defects of neurulation (Haque et al., 2001). Regardless of the exact division point, it is evident that variation previously found in multiple studies of high versus low lesions is unlikely to be related to the process (i.e., neurulation versus canalization). Another concern in these studies is that differences might exist between the clinical and radiographical assessment of the level of the lesion, and the method of establishing the level likely varies among and within studies. Hunter and colleagues (1996) documented that the level of the lesion varied between the two sources in approximately one-third of individuals studied, and the variation was not consistently in one direction.

A more comprehensive approach to classifying by location was set forth by Van Allen et al. (1993) and was based on a proposed multisite model of neural tube closure based on patterns observed in the mouse (Golden and Chernoff, 1993, 1995; Van Allen et al., 1993). In this model five closure sites were proposed, with various types of neural tube defects resulting from nonclosure at those sites. Several studies used the sites to classify neural tube defects (Seller, 1995; Martinez-Frias et al., 1996). A recent study of human embryos from the Carnegie Collection indicated that humans have only two sites of *fusion* (a term preferred to *closure*) (O'Rahilly and Muller, 2002). It has been postulated that there could be different closure or fusion mechanisms in the five areas without separate initiation sites (Sadler, 1998).

Classification Based on Open/Closed Status

Neural tube defects can also be classified as open or closed, depending on whether the skin over the lesion is intact. The term *spina bifida aperta* has been used for open lesions but has fallen into disuse. Defects without a covering or with only a membranous covering have been postulated to represent defects that happen during closure of the neural tube (primary neurulation) during embryonic stages 8–12 (days 17–30 postovulation). In contrast, those with a skin covering are thought to represent postneurulation events occurring at stage 13 or later. The relevant factor is the timing of the event (Lemire, 1988). The timing distinction becomes somewhat less clear when open and closed defects coincide in the same infant; however, one could postulate that whatever factor resulted in the defect in neurulation also affected another region of the neural tube, resulting in abnormal postclosure development. Information about open or closed status is not available from every data source, and the terms are often used incorrectly in the clinical setting (i.e., a membrane-covered lesion designated as *closed* if not *leaking*).

CLASSIFICATION OF THE INFANT WITH A NEURAL TUBE DEFECT

Although accurate classification of the neural tube defect is a principal consideration for studies, classification of the infant with the neural tube defect is also important. The etiological heterogeneity of neural tube defects, and of birth defects in general, is well recognized (Khoury et al., 1982; Seller and Kalousek, 1986; Blatter et al., 1997); however, this heterogeneity is one of several complicating factors in epidemiologic studies of potential risk factors (Khoury et al., 1992b). Schemas for the use of embryological and pathogenetic knowledge to construct more homogeneous analytic groups have been proposed (Rasmussen et al., 2003). Most commonly, infants are first separated by whether there is a known etiology, such as a single-gene, chromosomal, or teratogen-induced disorder (i.e., a syndrome). The remaining infants are then grouped based on the presence of additional major defects. These additional defects can be related to the defect of interest or there can be no apparent relation. Infants who have a neural tube defect alone or with related defects are classified into the category *isolated,* while those with additional unrelated defects are classified in the category *multiple.* Studies using this classification system have found differences in demographic characteristics and risk factors (Khoury et al., 1982); however, since the proportion of infants classified as multiple could be modest (i.e., 10%–30%), statistical power considerations arise (Khoury et al., 1992b).

Determining whether one defect is related to another can be challenging, and for neural tube defects the associated defects vary by type (Seller and Kalousek, 1986; Hall et al., 1988). Some associations are well known (e.g., spina bifida and clubfoot) (Frischhut et al., 2000), and the pathogenetic mechanism is evident. Other associations are less well documented (e.g., anencephaly and long arms), and the pathogenetic mechanism is unknown (Lemire and Siebert, 1990). Generally, defects that are found in the same organ system, in this instance the central nervous system, are considered to be related to the defect whether the pathogenetic mechanism is known (e.g., hydrocephalus) or unknown (e.g., agenesis of the corpus callosum) (Kawamura et al., 2002). For defects that occur together less often but have a proposed pathogenetic mechanism, such as mechanical induction (e.g., cleft palate and anencephaly; spinal retroflexion and omphalocele) (Seller and Kalousek, 1986), the classification decision can be based on the frequency and consistency of the finding (Rasmussen et al., 2003). However, without consistent methods of case ascertainment and defect classification, assessing the validity of reported defect associations can be difficult (David and Nixon, 1976; Seller and Kalousek, 1986; Melnick and Myrianthopoulos, 1987; Lemire and Siebert, 1990).

In summary, classification of neural tube defects for clinical, research, or public health activities can be challenging. Given the inconsistent nomenclature, comparison between published studies is difficult, and assumptions that defects are the same based on similar defect labels must often be made. For example, in a comparison of types of neural tube defects in a high-prevalence area of China (Moore et al., 1997) with those in a high-prevalence area of the United Kingdom (Dolk et al., 1991), the authors assumed that anencephaly with spina bifida equated to craniorachischisis; anencephaly with iniencephaly equated to craniorachischsis with spinal retroflexion; and iniencephaly without anencephaly equated to iniencephaly. Inferences from this comparison (e.g., rarer types of neural tube defects are a greater proportion of the total in high-prevalence areas) could be incorrect because of misclassification. In addition to problems with descriptive studies, the judgment that factors increase or decrease the risk for congenital defects is often based, in part, on the consistency of findings in well-designed analytic studies (Khoury et al., 1992a). Misclassification is one factor that can impede these comparisons as well as bias individual studies (Rothman and Greenland, 1998). In the clinical and public health settings, translating knowledge obtained through research into intervention and prevention strategies is also impeded by the same issues surrounding classification. A universally accepted nomenclature and classification system is needed to begin to address the inconsistencies and facilitate our ability to interpret findings correctly.

REFERENCES

Baird PA, Sadovnick AD (1984). Survival in infants with anencephaly. Clin Pediatr (Phila) 23:268–271.

Bell JE, Green RJ (1982). Studies on the area cerebrovasculosa of anencephalic fetuses. J Pathol 137:315–328.

Blackburn W, Maertens P, Cooley NR, Barr M (1995). Studies of the cranioskeletal anomalies associated with iniencephaly. Proc Greenwood Genet Ctr 14:87.

Blatter BM, Lafeber AB, Peters PW, Roeleveld N, Verbeek AL, Gabreels FJ (1997). Heterogeneity of spina bifida. Teratology 55:224–230.

Boone D, Parsons D, Lachmann SM, Sherwood T (1985). Spina bifida occulta: lesion or anomaly? Clin Radiol 36:159–161.

Borman B, Cryer C (1990). Fallacies of international and national comparisons of disease occurrence in the epidemiology of neural tube defects. Teratology 42:405–412.

Botto LD, Moore CA, Khoury MJ, Erickson JD (1999). Neural-tube defects. N Engl J Med 341:1509–1519.

Bowman RM, McLone DG, Grant JA, Tomita T, Ito JA (2001). Spina bifida outcome: a 25-year prospective. Pediatr Neurosurg 34:114–120.

Carter CO, Evans KA, Till K (1976). Spinal dysraphism: genetic relation to neural tube malformations. J Med Genet 13:343–350.

Coffey VP (1965). Anencephaly or iniencephaly? J Irish Med Assoc 56:96.

David TJ, Nixon A (1976). Congenital malformations associated with anencephaly and iniencephaly. J Med Genet 13:263–265.

Dolk H, De Wals P, Gillerot Y, Lechat MF, Ayme S, Cornel M, Cuschieri A, et al (1991). Heterogeneity of neural tube defects in Europe: the significance of site of defect and presence of other major anomalies in relation to geographic differences in prevalence. Teratology 44:547–559.

Dolk H, Seller MJ (1993). Neural tube defects: a survey of lesion descriptions made by different European pathologists. J Med Genet 30:942–946.

Drolet B, Prendiville J, Golden J, Enjolras O, Esterly NB (1995). "Membranous aplasia cutis" with hair collars. Congenital absence of skin or neuroectodermal defect? Arch Dermatol 131:1427–1431.

Frischhut B, Stockl B, Landauer F, Krismer M, Menardi G (2000). Foot deformities in adolescents and young adults with spina bifida. J Pediatr Orthop B 9:161–169.

Golden JA, Chernoff GF (1993). Intermittent pattern of neural tube closure in two strains of mice. Teratology 47:73–80.

Golden JA, Chernoff GF (1995). Multiple sites of anterior neural tube closure in humans: evidence from anterior neural tube defects (anencephaly). Pediatrics 95:506–510.

Hall JG, Friedman JM, Kenna BA, Popkin J, Jawanda M, Arnold W (1988). Clinical, genetic, and epidemiological factors in neural tube defects. Am J Hum Genet 43:827–837.

Haque M, Ohata K, Takami T, Soares SB Jr, Aree SN, Hakuba A, Hara M (2001). Development of lumbosacral spina bifida: three-dimensional computer graphic study of human embryos at Carnegie stage twelve. Pediatr Neurosurg 35:247–252.

Harris CP, Townsend JJ, Carey JC (1993). Acalvaria: a unique congenital anomaly. Am J Med Genet 46:694–699.

Holmes LB, Driscoll SG, Atkins L (1976). Etiologic heterogeneity of neural-tube defects. N Engl J Med 294:365–369.

Honein MA, Paulozzi LJ, Mathews TJ, Erickson JD, Wong LY (2001). Impact of folic acid fortification of the U.S. food supply on the occurrence of neural tube defects. JAMA 285:2981–2986.

Hunt GM, Oakeshott P (2003). Outcome in people with open spina bifida at age 35: prospective community based cohort study. Br Med J 326:1365–1366.

Hunter AG, Cleveland RH, Blickman JG, Holmes LB (1996). A study of level of lesion, associated malformations and sib occurrence risks in spina bifida. Teratology 54:213–218.

Hunter AGW (1993). Brain and spinal cord. In Stevenson RE, Hall JG, Goodman RM (eds): *Human Malformations and Related Anomalies,* Vol. 2. New York: Oxford University Press, pp. 109–137.

Journel H, Parent P, Roussey M, LeMarec B (1989). "Isolated" hydrocephalus in families of spina bifida and anencephaly: a coincidence? Neuropediatrics 20:220–222.

Kallen B, Cocchi G, Knudsen LB, Castilla EE, Robert E, Daltveit AK, Lancaster PL, et al (1994). International study of sex ratio and twinning of neural tube defects. Teratology 50:322–331.

Kalucy M, Bower C, Stanley F, Burton P (1994). Survival of infants with neural tube defects in Western Australia 1966–1990. Paediatr Perinatal Epidemiol 8:334–351.

Kawamura T, Nishio S, Morioka T, Fukui K (2002). Callosal anomalies in patients with spinal dysraphism: correlation of clinical and neuroimaging features with hemispheric abnormalities. Neurol Res 24:463–467.

Keeling JW, Kjaer I (1994). Diagnostic distinction between anencephaly and amnion rupture sequence based on skeletal analysis. J Med Genet 31:823–829.

Khoury MJ, Erickson JD, James LM (1982). Etiologic heterogeneity of neural tube defects: clues from epidemiology. Am J Epidemiol 115:538–548.

Khoury MJ, James LM, Flanders WD, Erickson JD (1992a). Interpretation of recurring weak associations obtained from epidemiologic studies of suspected human teratogens. Teratology 46:69–77.

Khoury MJ, Moore CA, James LM, Cordero JF (1992b). The interaction between dysmorphology and epidemiology: methodologic issues of lumping and splitting. Teratology 45:133–138.

Kjaer I, Keeling JW, Graem N (1994). Cranial base and vertebral column in human anencephalic fetuses. J Craniofac Genet Dev Biol 14:235–244.

Lee SC, Chun YS, Jung SE, Park KW, Kim WK (1997). Currarino triad: anorectal malformation, sacral bony abnormality, and presacral mass—a review of 11 cases. J Pediatr Surg 32:58–61.

Lemire RJ (1988). Neural tube defects. JAMA 259:558–562.

Lemire RJ, Beckwith JB, Shepard TH (1972). Iniencephaly and anencephaly with spinal retroflexion. A comparative study of eight human specimens. Teratology 6:27–36.

Lemire RJ, Cohen MM Jr, Beckwith JB, Kokich VG, Siebert JR (1981). The facial features of holoprosencephaly in anencephalic human specimens. I. Historical review and associated malformations. Teratology 23:297–303.

Lemire RJ, Pendergrass TW, Beckwith JB, Ellenbogen RG (2003). Tumors and malformations of the caudal spinal axis. Pediatr Neurosurg 38:174–180.

Lemire RJ, Siebert JR (1990). Anencephaly: its spectrum and relationship to neural tube defects. J Craniofac Genet Dev Biol 10:163–174.

Lorber J, Levick K (1967). Spina bifida cystica. Incidence of spina bifida occulta in parents and in controls. Arch Dis Child 42:171–173.

Martinez-Frias ML, Urioste M, Bermejo E, Sanchis A, Rodriguez-Pinilla E (1996). Epidemiological analysis of multi-site closure failure of neural tube in humans. Am J Med Genet 66:64–68.

Matsumoto A, Hatta T, Moriyama K, Otani H (2002). Sequential observations of exencephaly and subsequent morphological changes by mouse exo utero development system: analysis of the mechanism of transformation from exencephaly to anencephaly. Anat Embryol (Berl) 205:7–18.

McComb JG (1997). Spinal and cranial neural tube defects. Semin Pediatr Neurol 4:156–166.

Melnick M, Myrianthopoulos NC (1987). Studies in neural tube defects. II. Pathologic findings in a prospectively collected series of anencephalics. Am J Med Genet 26:797–810.

Moore CA, Li S, Li Z, Hong SX, Gu HQ, Berry RJ, Mulinare J, et al (1997). Elevated rates of severe neural tube defects in a high-prevalence area in northern China. Am J Med Genet 73:113–118.

Muller F, O'Rahilly R (1986). Somitic-vertebral correlation and vertebral levels in the human embryo. Am J Anat 177:3–19.

Northrup H, Volcik KA (2000). Spina bifida and other neural tube defects. Curr Probl Pediatr 30:313–332.

Olde Scholtenhuis MA, Cohen-Overbeek TE, Offringa M, Barth PG, Stoutenbeek P, Gooskens RH, Wladimiroff JW, Bilardo CM (2003). Audit of prenatal and postnatal diagnosis of isolated open spina bifida in three university hospitals in The Netherlands. Ultrasound Obstet Gynecol 21:48–52.

Oneko M, Lyamuya S, Mhando S (2002). Outcome of hydrocephalus and spina bifida surgery in a referral hospital without neurosurgical services in Tanzania. Eur J Pediatr Surg 12(Suppl 1):S39–41.

O'Rahilly R, Muller F (2002). The two sites of fusion of the neural folds and the two neuropores in the human embryo. Teratology 65:162–170.

Park CH, Stewart W, Khoury MJ, Mulinare J (1992). Is there etiologic heterogeneity between upper and lower neural tube defects? Am J Epidemiol 136:1493–1501.

Rasmussen SA, Moore CA (2001). Effective coding in birth defects surveillance. Teratology 64(Suppl 1):S3–7.

Rasmussen SA, Olney RS, Holmes LB, Lin AE, Keppler-Noreuil KM, Moore CA (2003). Guidelines for case classification for the National Birth Defects Prevention Study. Birth Defects Res Part A Clin Mol Teratol 67:193–201.

Richards CG (1992). Frontoethmoidal meningoencephalocele: a common and severe congenital abnormality in South East Asia. Arch Dis Child 67:717–719.

Rintoul NE, Sutton LN, Hubbard AM, Cohen B, Melchionni J, Pasquariello PS, Adzick NS (2002). A new look at myelomeningoceles: functional level, vertebral level, shunting, and the implications for fetal intervention. Pediatrics 109:409–413.

Rothman KJ, Greenland S (1998). *Modern Epidemiology.* Philadelphia: Lippincott-Raven.

Sadler TW (1998). Mechanisms of neural tube closure and defects. Ment Retard Dev Disabil Res Rev 4:247–253.

Sattar MT, Bannister CM, Turnbull IW (1996). Occult spinal dysraphism—the common combination of lesions and the clinical manifestations in 50 patients. Eur J Pediatr Surg 6(Suppl 1):10–14.

Seller MJ (1987). Neural tube defects and sex ratios. Am J Med Genet 26:699–707.

Seller MJ (1995). Multi-site neural tube closure in humans and maternal folate supplementation. Am J Med Genet 58:222–224.

Seller MJ, Kalousek DK (1986). Neural tube defects: heterogeneity and homogeneity. Am J Med Genet (Suppl 2):77–87.

Shaw GM, Jensvold NG, Wasserman CR, Lammer EJ (1994). Epidemiologic characteristics of phenotypically distinct neural tube defects among 0.7 million California births, 1983–1987. Teratology 49:143–149.

Shaw GM, Todoroff K, Lammer EJ (1997). NTD phenotypes in infants and fetuses whose mothers used multivitamins containing folic acid in early pregnancy compared to those who did not. Am J Med Genet 70:330–331.

Shehu BB, Ameh EA, Ismail NJ (2000). Spina bifida cystica: selective management in Zaria, Nigeria. Ann Trop Paediatr 20:239–242.

Siebert JR, Kokich VG, Beckwith JB, Cohen MM Jr, Lemire RJ (1981). The facial features of holoprosencephaly in anencephalic human specimens. II. Craniofacial anatomy. Teratology 23:305–315.

Stevenson RE, DeLoache WR (1988). Aplasia cutis congenita of the scalp. Proc Greenwood Genet Ctr 7:14–18.

Timor-Tritsch IE, Greenebaum E, Monteagudo A, Baxi L (1996). Exencephaly-anencephaly sequence: proof by ultrasound imaging and amniotic fluid cytology. J Matern Fetal Med 5:182–185.

Toriello HV, Higgins JV (1985). Possible causal heterogeneity in spina bifida cystica. Am J Med Genet 21:13–20.

Tortori-Donati P, Rossi A, Cama A (2000). Spinal dysraphism: a review of neuroradiological features with embryological correlations and proposal for a new classification. Neuroradiology 42:471–491.

U.S. Department of Heath and Human Services PHS, Health Care Financing Administration (1980). *ICD-9-CM: The International Classification of Diseases, 9th revision, Clinical Modification.* Vol. PHS 80-1260. Washington, DC: Government Printing Office.

Van Allen MI, Kalousek DK, Chernoff GF, Juriloff D, Harris M, McGillivray BC, Yong SL, et al (1993). Evidence for multi-site closure of the neural tube in humans. Am J Med Genet 47:723–743.

Van Allen MI, Smith DW, Shepard TH (1983). Twin reversed arterial perfusion (TRAP) sequence: a study of 14 twin pregnancies with acardius. Semin Perinatol 7:285–293.

Volcik KA, Shaw GM, Lammer EJ, Zhu H, Finnell RH (2003). Evaluation of infant methylenetetrahydrofolate reductase genotype, maternal vitamin use, and risk of high versus low level spina bifida defects. Birth Defects Res Part A Clin Mol Teratol 67:154–157.

Warkany J (1971). *Spina Bifida. Congenital Malformations. Notes and Comments.* Chicago: Year Book Medical, pp. 272–291.

Wilkins-Haug L, Freedman W (1991). Progression of exencephaly to anencephaly in the human fetus—an ultrasound perspective. Prenat Diagn 11:227–233.

Williams LJ, Mai CT, Edmonds LD, Shaw GM, Kirby RS, Hobbs CA, Sever LE, et al (2002). Prevalence of spina bifida and anencephaly during the transition to mandatory folic acid fortification in the United States. Teratology 66:33–39.

Wong LY, Paulozzi LJ (2001). Survival of infants with spina bifida: a population study, 1979–94. Paediatr Perinatal Epidemiol 15:374–378.

Wynne-Davies R (1975). Congenital vertebral anomalies: aetiology and relationship to spina bifida cystica. J Med Genet 12:280–288.

Yokota A, Kajiwara H, Kohchi M, Fuwa I, Wada H (1988). Parietal cephalocele: clinical importance of its atretic form and associated malformations. J Neurosurg 69:545–551.

7

Syndromes with Neural Tube Defects

LAURIE H. SEAVER
ROGER E. STEVENSON

The preponderance of all neural tube defects (NTDs) are isolated malformations of the central nervous system (CNS) and its protective encasements. Some common associated anomalies are considered secondary to the NTD, such as hydrocephalus, Arnold-Chiari malformation, and clubfoot. Only about one in five NTDs will have a co-occurring defect of non-CNS structures that is not considered a typical secondary defect. Certain of these associated structural anomalies coexist with NTDs as components of recognizable malformation syndromes of genetic or environmental etiology. Other anomalies, not typically considered secondary, may indeed be related to the NTD due to disturbance of neural crest migration or spatial limitations placed on developing tissues. Beyond these two major categories of associated defects, small numbers of other structural anomalies that lack current explanation are also found. Studies of NTDs and associated anomalies are instructive in understanding embryonic development, identifying the causes of birth defects, determining recurrence risks, and guiding expectations for the efficacy of preventive strategies.

FREQUENCY OF ASSOCIATED ANOMALIES

Overall, nonisolated cases comprise 15%–25% of most unselected series of NTDs (Table 7.1). These numbers exclude the common secondary defects (lower limb deformation, spinal curvature or vertebral anomalies, Arnold-Chiari II anomaly, and hydrocephaly). The frequency of associated anomalies appears to be related in part to the type and level of NTD and in part to the severity of the dysraphic defects (Toriello and Higgins, 1985; Hall et al., 1988; Hunter et al., 1996; Kallen et al., 1998; Stevenson et al., 2000; Seaver et al., 2002). As a generalization, the more severely dysraphic NTDs are more likely to have associated anomalies. Craniorachischisis and encephalocele have the highest rates of associated anomalies, anencephaly and high spina bifida intermediate rates, and spina bifida the lowest (Table 7.1).

The frequency of associated anomalies tends to be greater in autopsy series, perhaps reflecting selection of more complex malformations for postmortem examination (Lemire et al., 1978; Seller and Kalousek, 1986; Melnick and Myrianthopoulos, 1987). Likewise, spina bifida clinics, which deal with patients who survive, tend to report associated anomalies less frequently (Toriello and Higgins, 1985; Hunter et al., 1996). An impression that in geographic regions with a low overall NTD prevalence the defects are more commonly accompanied by non-CNS anomalies may be gained from several studies (Kallen et al., 1998; Stevenson et al., 2000). This may imply that the residual NTDs in low-prevalence regions may be weighted with syndromic cases.

Specific anomalies that occur with greatest frequency are facial clefting, cardiac defects, anotia/microtia, limb reduction defects, anophthalmia/microphthalmia, abdominal wall defects, and renal anomalies. Less common anomalies include holoprosencephaly, amniotic bands, and polydactyly (Kallen et al., 1998). In a series of 564 NTDs ascertained over 10 years in South Carolina, there were 98 (17%) cases with multiple anomalies. Of those 98 cases, 51 (52%) were recognized as having a specific underlying diagnosis (Seaver et al., 2002) (Table 7.2). Recurrence risk in these cases is based on the primary diagnosis. In those cases without a specific diagnosis, the most common associated malformations were facial clefting; heart, genitourinary, and limb defects; diaphragmatic

TABLE 7.1. *Frequency of Associated Structural Anomalies with Various Types of Neural Tube Defects*

	Anencephaly	Craniorachischisis	Upper Spina Bifida	Lower Spina Bifida	Encephalocele	All
Kallen et al. (1998)*						
$n = 2955$ infants	25%	—	35%	20%	43%	23%
$n = 734$ fetuses	26%	—	—	—	49%	25%
Seaver et al. (2002)†						
$n = 559$ infants and fetuses	11%	41%	11.6%	9.4%	33%	17%
Hall et al. (1988)‡						
$n = 512$ infants	15%	62%	19.5%	6.7%	30%	14%

*Series from French (1976–1994), Swedish (1973–1993), and California Birth Defects Registries (1983–1992).
† Series from South Carolina Surveillance Registry (1982–2002).
‡ Series from British Columbia (1958–1984).

hernia; and holoprosencephaly (Table 7.3). In some cases, including both isolated and nonisolated NTDs, a specific diagnosis cannot be made, but a recognized contributing factor may be identified, such as maternal diabetes or other teratogenic exposure or complications of twinning. Study of the frequency and types of associated defects contributes to our understanding of the potential pathogenetic mechanisms underlying NTDs with associated anomalies.

PATHOGENETIC MECHANISMS OF NTDS WITH OTHER ANOMALIES

Secondary Defects

A number of anomalies, including clubfoot or other deformation of the lower limbs, hydrocephaly, Arnold Chiari II anomaly, and spinal curvature, have been widely accepted as secondary structural abnormalities that may accompany NTDs. Observations by several investigators suggest that a much wider range of other structural anomalies that co-occur with NTDs may also represent secondary defects (Seller and Kalousek, 1986; Seaver et al., 2002). Two observations support this suggestion.

TABLE 7.2. *Diagnoses in 98 Neural Tube Defects with Additional Anomalies in South Carolina, 1992–2002*

Chromosome abnormality	17
Amniotic band disruption sequence	15
Meckel syndrome	9
Omphalocele-exstrophy of bladder-imperforate anus-spinal defect	4
Oculo-auriculo-vertebral syndrome (Goldenhar)	1
Other	5
	51

First, shortening of the trunk and cervical retroflexion accompany cranial and upper spinal NTDs and impose space limitation on the abdomen and thorax. Anomalies that may result from the lack of pleural and peritoneal space include abdominal wall defects (principally omphalocele), diaphragmatic hernia, Meckel diverticulum, and possibly cardiac defects. The second major mechanism is through the disturbance of cranial neural crest migration that accompanies cranial NTDs. Disturbance of neural crest migration plausibly interferes with formation of the face and cardiovascular structures, resulting in facial clefting and cardiac defects.

Twinning and Amniotic Bands

Regarding two phenomena commonly associated with NTDs, twinning and amniotic bands, there is controversy over whether the NTD is the primary developmental anomaly or a secondary anomaly. Twins, or other multiple pregnancies, co-occur with NTDs more commonly than any specific structural anomaly (Leck, 1974; Schinzel et al., 1979; Khoury et al., 1982; Windham et al.,

TABLE 7.3. *Additional Malformations Present in 47 South Carolina Neural Tube Defect (1992–2002) Cases Not Recognized as a Specific Diagnosis**

Facial cleft	13 (27.6%)
Heart defect	11 (23.4%)
Genitourinary defect	8 (17.0%)
Holoprosencephaly spectrum	7 (14.9%)
Diaphragmatic hernia	7 (14.9%)
Limb defect	6 (12.8%)
Omphalocele/ventral wall defect	6 (12.8%)
Other	5

*Cases may have more than one malformation in addition to the neural tube defect.

1982; Seaver et al., 2002). Schinzel et al. (1979) interpret this association to indicate that the etiology of monozygous twinning also underlies the NTD. The increased NTD rate in twins occurs more commonly among same-sex twins, and anencephaly is the usual defect (Hay and Wehrung, 1970; James, 1976; Schinzel et al., 1979). Neural tube defects are also one of the most common malformations in conjoined twins (Edmonds and Layde, 1982). Among twin pregnancies, only 5% are concordant for NTDs. Among 564 consecutive infants/fetuses (1992–2002) in the South Carolina NTD Project, 20 twin sets or multiple pregnancies occurred (3.5%), making it the most common associated diagnosis or contributing factor overall to both isolated and nonisolated NTDs. In only one (5%) of these pregnancies was there concordance for an NTD: twin males with thoracic spina bifida. Fertility drugs were used in two pregnancies, and in vitro fertilization was involved in another two pregnancies. Zygosity was determined by ultrasound examination of membranes and/or postnatal placental examination; there were eight monozygous and four dizygous pregnancies, with eight pregnancies of unknown zygosity. Remarkably, seven of the eight monozygous pregnancies were monochorionic-monoamniotic, which typically occurs in only 1%–2% of monozygous gestations. These data support multiple gestation, especially monozygosity, as a common association or contributing factor to NTDs and also suggest that late division of the zygote leading to monoamniotic gestation may be especially important (Seaver et al., 2003).

The association of amniotic bands and NTDs constitutes a second special circumstance. Evidence of amniotic bands is found in about 1% of NTDs. Bizarre anomalies of the CNS, such as fusion of the brain to the placenta and lobation of the CNS, are seen in association with other evidence of early amnion rupture or amniotic bands (Higginbottom et al., 1979). Alternative interpretations of this association have been put forth. One theory proposes that the NTD (usually anencephaly) is the primary developmental defect and that the raw CNS defect adheres to the placenta or fetal membranes, leading to amnion rupture or amniotic bands. The second theory identifies amnion rupture or band formation as the primary defect, with the CNS becoming entrapped secondarily.

Schisis Association and the Midline Developmental Field Concept

Although most co-occurring anomalies may represent pleiotropy or secondary phenomena, two other hypotheses have emerged as prominent among the attempts to explain the co-occurrence of associated structural anomalies with NTDs. Both focus on the excessive number of midline anomalies among the associated defects. The first, termed the *schisis association,* was set forth by Czeizel (1981). The concept derives from the observation that certain of the anomalies more commonly found in association with NTDs may be considered defects of closure. These include cleft lip with or without cleft palate, cardiac defects, omphalocele, and diaphragmatic hernia. The second hypothesis, the *midline developmental field concept,* suggests a particular common vulnerability of structures in the midline (Opitz and Gilbert, 1982). Hence, the insult that causes anomalous development of the neural tube defect would, at the same time, jeopardize proper formation of other structures in the midline. There exists no evidence to support either of these theories relative to NTDs and associated defects. The litany of defects called in support of the theories are in fact just as easily explained as secondary defects caused by mechanical or other pressures on development and say nothing about (*1*) their vulnerability because of their midline location or (*2*) the similarity of the causative mechanisms to that of NTDs.

COMMON DIAGNOSES AND SYNDROMES ASSOCIATED WITH NTDS

Common diagnoses contributing to NTDs are discussed in the following section. The reader is referred to Chapter 16 for further details and a more comprehensive listing of syndromes that have been associated with NTDs.

Anencephaly and Spina Bifida

Chromosome Anomalies. Numerical aneuploidies and chromosomal rearrangements have been identified in both apparently isolated NTDs and those associated with other anomalies (Hume et al., 1996; Kennedy et al., 1998) and are the most commonly found causes for spina bifida or anencephaly with other anomalies (Hunter, 1993; Kallen et al., 1998; Melvin et al., 2000; Stevenson et al., 2000). Trisomy 18 (Fig. 7.1), trisomy 13, and triploidy are the most common chromosomal conditions associated with anencephaly and spina bifida (Smith, 1969; Hodes et al., 1978; Coerdt et al., 1997). In one series of prenatally identified NTDs, aneuploidy was detected in 10 of 145 (7%) cases, with trisomy 18 found in 7 of the 10 cases (Hume et al., 1996). Although a less common cause of NTDs, the segmental aneuploidies, deletions or duplications of smaller chromosome segments, are potentially quite important in delineating smaller regions of the human genome in which to concentrate efforts to identify genes that contribute to NTDs (Melvin et al., 2000). Depending on the size of the duplication or deletion, chromosome abnormalities can be identified on routine or high-resolution analyses, although some, such as 22q11 deletions, may require fluorescence in situ hybridization (FISH). Such unbalanced

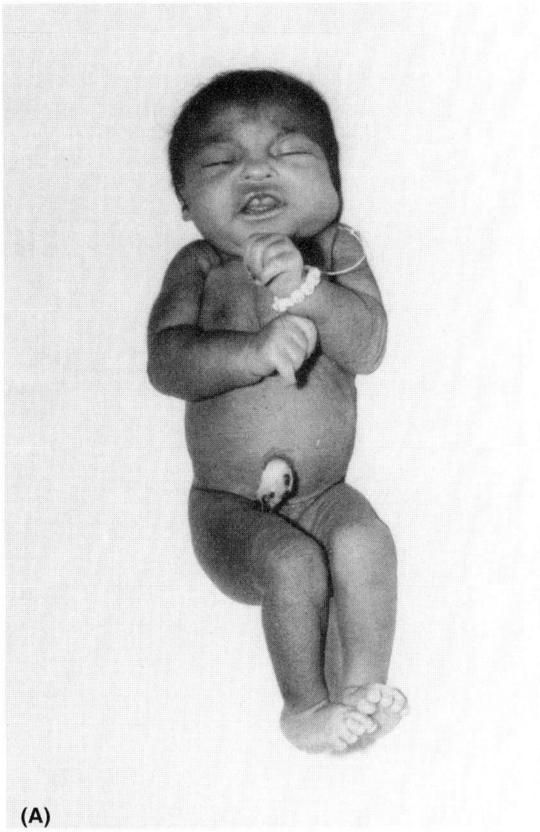

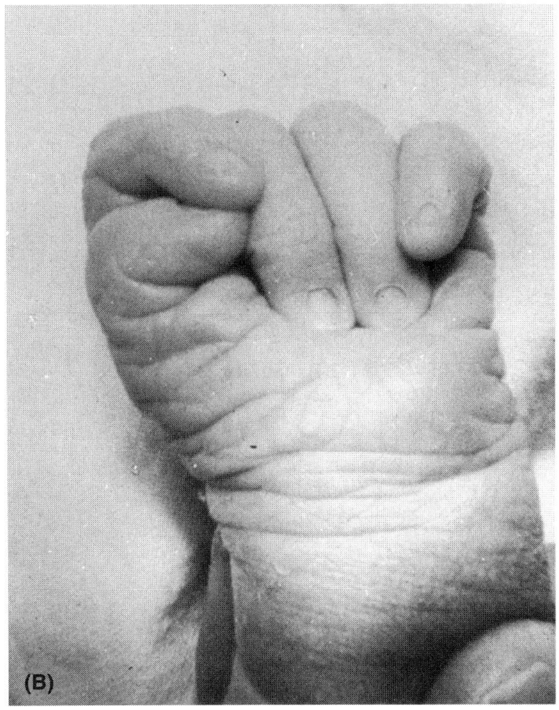

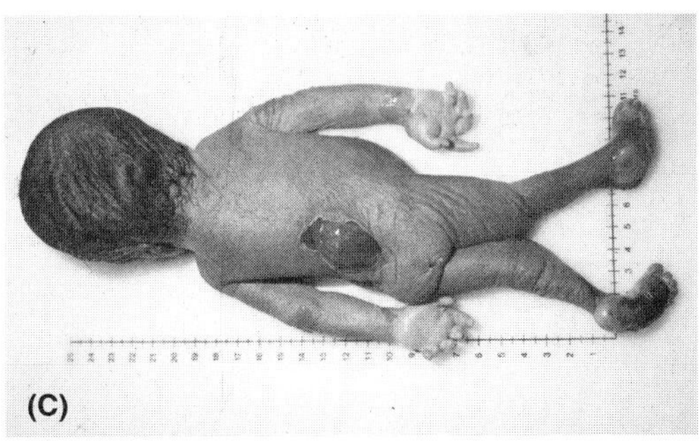

FIGURE 7.1. Trisomy 18, one of the more common chromosome aberrations associated with neural tube defects. (*A*) General appearance of infant with trisomy 18. (*B*) Typical hand appearance with overlapping digits. (*C*) Thoracolumbar spina bifida.

karyotypes in an affected case should also prompt the study of parental chromosomes, as identification of a balanced translocation carrier parent will be important in predicting the recurrence risk. Chromosome abnormalities that have been reported to be associated with anencephaly and spina bifida are shown in Table 7.4.

Amniotic Band Disruption Sequence. The amniotic band disruption sequence is a sporadic defect of unknown cause. Craniofacial defects and limb defects are typical (Jones et al., 1974; Higginbottom et al., 1979). Other cases may also involve ventral or lateral body wall defects (Miller et al., 1981). Several pathogenetic mechanisms have been proposed. The hypothesis set forth by Streeter (1930) is defective development of the amniotic cavity and germ disc in the earliest weeks of gestation. Alternative mechanisms include rupture of the early amniotic cavity, as proposed by Torpin (1968), and fetal vascular disruption, as hypothesized by Hunter and Carpenter (1986). Regardless of the primary event, the fetus becomes entangled in strands of amniotic membrane, which can often be identified at birth. The craniofacial defects and NTDs are often bizarre and atypical. The NTDs associated with amniotic bands can be difficult to classify due to their disruptive nature. There may be almost complete absence of the cranium, and these cases are often classified as anencephaly. However, CNS tissue may be present outside of the cranial vault, in which case the defect may be classified as single or multiple encephaloceles. Often there are accompanying atypical facial clefts that do not follow the usual lines of facial cleavage. Associated limb defects include amputations,

TABLE 7.4. *Chromosome Abnormalities Associated with Neural Tube Defects*

Anencephaly/Spina Bifida
Trisomy 18
Triploidy
Trisomy 13
Tetraploidy
Trisomy 9
Chromosome 1q deletion (q21q23–q25) (q42q43-qter)
Chromosome 2p duplication (p24)
Chromosome 3q duplication
Chromosome 7q deletion (q36-qter)
Chromosome 11q duplication
Chromosome 12q duplication
Chromosome 13q deletion
Chromosome 14q del (q22q23)
Chromosome 20p duplication
Isochromosome 18p
Chromosome 22q deletion (q11)
Encephalocele
Trisomy 18
Trisomy 20, mosaic
Chromosome 1q deletion (q42q43-qter) (q32q42)
Chromosome 2p duplication
Chromosome 2q deletion (q24.3)
Chromosome 3q deletion (q27-qter)
Chromosome 4q deletion (q21q22)
Chromosome 6q duplication
Chromosome 11q duplication
Chromosome 13q deletion (q21-qter) (q32)
Chromosome 15q duplication

transverse terminal limb reduction defects, distal hypoplasia, ring constrictions, and pseudosyndactyly (Jones et al., 1974). Some associated defects may also be secondary to oligohydramnios or fetal constraint, as the fetus is sometimes "tethered" to the placenta (Fig. 7.2). While the diagnosis of amniotic band disruption sequence as a cause of NTDs is usually apparent on examination, it is not always apparent on fetal ultrasound images, confirming the importance of careful postnatal examination. In addition, there are some cases where an NTD is considered to be a primary defect, and amniotic band defects are secondary (Keeling and Kjaer, 1994) (Fig. 7.3).

Limb-body wall complex is a related pattern of malformation, although controversy exists in regard to the role of amniotic bands in the pathogenesis of this disorder (Van Allen et al., 1987; Russo et al., 1993). Russo et al. distinguish between cases with craniofacial disruption with identifiable bands and/or adhesion and other cases without craniofacial involvement, but with primarily urogenital anomalies, imperforate anus, lower limb

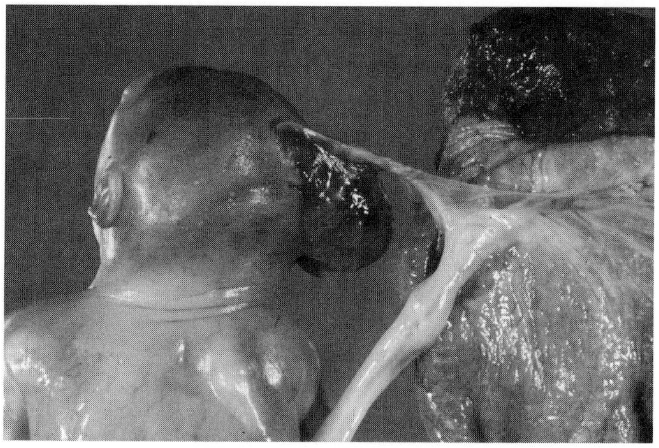

FIGURE 7.2. Encephalocele associated with amniotic bands. The fetus also had multiple limb reduction defects.

defects, very short umbilical cord, and frequently associated meningocele. Other authors refer to this latter condition as *short umbilical cord syndrome* (Blackburn and Cooley, 1993).

Meckel Syndrome. Also called *Meckel-Gruber syndrome,* this is a lethal genetic condition that includes polycystic kidneys, postaxial (ulnar) polydactyly, and CNS defects, usually microcephaly and encephalocele. Less commonly, anencephaly, hydrocephaly, or other structural abnormalities of the brain may occur. Other features can include facial clefting, cysts in the liver and pancreas, cardiac and genital defects, and clubfoot (Salonen and Paavola, 1998). Inheritance is autosomal recessive (Hsia et al., 1971), with a corresponding 25%, or one in four, risk of recurrence in siblings.

Omphalocele-Exstrophy-Imperforate Anus-Spine defects (OEIS Complex). This midline abdominal wall defect occurs sporadically. The omphalocele is located above the opening in the lower abdominal wall in which the internal surface of the bladder is visible (exstrophy). The small bowel and colon have separate openings into

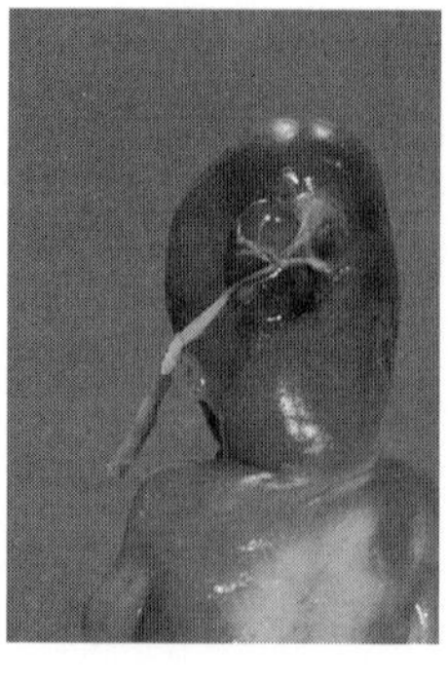

FIGURE 7.3. Occipital encephalocele associated with a single amniotic band. No other defects were present.

the bladder, and the anus is absent or imperforate. There is often an accompanying defect of the lumbosacral spine with hemivertebrae and/or a meningocele. The pelvic bones are widely separated, and the external genitalia are absent or ambiguous. Renal defects are also associated (Carey et al., 1978). The etiology of the OEIS complex is unknown. Surgical repair has been successful in some cases (Hurwitz et al., 1987).

Diabetic Embryopathy. Major malformations among infants of insulin-dependent diabetic mothers are increased approximately eightfold, based on a large population-based case-control study (Becerra et al., 1990). The relative risk of major CNS defects is 15.5, and open NTDs are the most common CNS defects. Other common features of diabetic embryopathy include heart, genitourinary, vertebral, and rib defects. Levels of hemoglobin A_{1c} in early pregnancy, as a measure of diabetic control, are positively related to the risk of birth defects (Greene et al., 1989). The basis for the teratogenesis of maternal diabetes mellitus is unknown and is probably multifactorial (Reece et al., 1996).

Valproic Acid Embryopathy. The association of maternal valproic acid use and spina bifida was first reported in 1982 (Bjerkedal et al., 1982; Robert and Guibaud, 1982), and the fetal valproate syndrome was further described in 1984 (DiLiberti et al., 1984). The facial features include epicanthal folds, flat nasal bridge, small upturned nose, long philtrum, and thin upper lip (DiLiberti et al., 1984). Preaxial (radial) limb reduction defects have also been reported (Sharony et al., 1993). The risk of associated spina bifida has been estimated at 1%–2%, although it can be as high as 5% at high valproate exposure (Bjerkedal et al., 1982, Omtzigt et al., 1992). The spinal lesions are usually low, lumbosacral, or sacral.

Syndromes Associated with Encephalocele

Chromosome Abnormalities. Encephaloceles occur less commonly than spina bifida and anencephaly in the common chromosome anomalies such as trisomies 13 and 18 but have been reported. In one study of 26 prenatally diagnosed encephaloceles, 18 were karyotyped and only one was abnormal (trisomy 18) (Budorick et al., 1995). Smaller deletions and duplications have also been associated with encephaloceles (Hunter, 1993; Melvin et al., 2000). As with other NTDs, this knowledge may lead to the identification of genes that contribute to encephalocele in those regions. Chromosome anomalies reported to be associated with encephalocele are shown in Table 7.4.

Meckel Syndrome. Occipital encephalocele is the most common CNS defect associated with Meckel syndrome (Mecke and Passarge, 1971; Sugiura et al., 1996) (Fig. 7.4). It is the most frequent single-gene disorder associated with NTDs (Simpson et al., 1991; Stevenson et al., 2000). See the above discussion on anencephaly and spina bifida for further details. A variety of occipital encephaloceles associated with Meckel syndrome are shown in Figure 7.4.

Walker-Warburg Syndrome. This condition is considered part of a spectrum of muscle-eye-brain syndromes that also includes muscle-eye-brain disease and Fukuyama congenital muscular dystrophy (Cormand et al., 2001). Walker-Warburg syndrome has variously been termed *Warburg syndrome, HARD±E syndrome* (hydrocephalus, agyria, retinal dysplasia, encephalocele), and *cobblestone lissencephaly*. Severe CNS anomalies in Walker-Warburg syndrome include microcephaly, lissencephaly, white matter dysmyelination, hydrocephalus, midbrain and cerebellar hypoplasia, Dandy Walker malformation, and occipital encephaloceles (Walker, 1942; Williams et al., 1984; Dobyns et al., 1989). Eye anomalies include microphthalmia, Peters anomaly, cataract, glaucoma, colobomata, retinal dysplasia with nonattachment or detachment, and optic nerve hypoplasia (Pagon et al., 1983; Dobyns et al., 1989). Inheritance is autosomal recessive, with a 25% recurrence risk in siblings.

Von Voss-Cherstvoy Syndrome. This autosomal recessive condition is also referred to as *DK-phocomelia*. Associated defects include occipital meningocele or encephalocele, cleft palate, phocomelia or radial defects, thrombocytopenia, and urogenital anomalies (Cherstvoy et al., 1980). Although affected siblings and consanguinity in some cases suggest autosomal recessive inheritance (Bird et al., 1994; Gilpin, 2000), one case is reported with mosaicism for deletion of chromosome 13q12 (Bamforth and Lin, 1997). The recurrence risk could be as high as 25%.

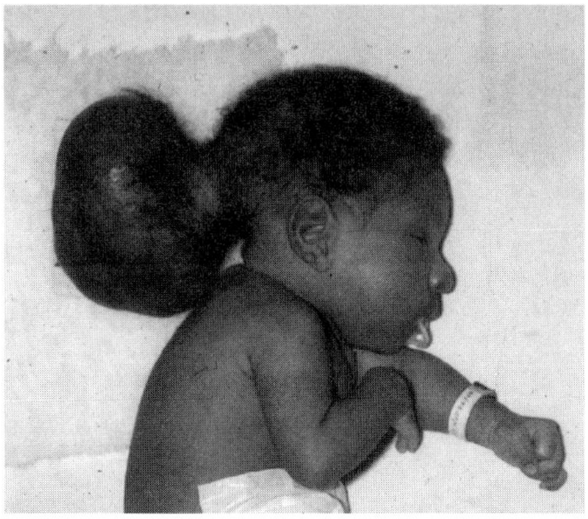

FIGURE 7.4. Large occipital encephalocele in an infant with Meckel syndrome (encephalocele, postaxial polydactyly, cystic kidneys).

Knobloch Syndrome. Knobloch syndrome is an autosomal recessive condition that includes occipital encephalocele or scalp defect and severe myopia with vitreoretinal degeneration (Knobloch and Layer, 1971; Seaver et al, 1993). Other defects are occasionally reported, and intelligence can be normal (Knobloch and Layer, 1971; Seaver et al., 1993; Wilson et al., 1998). The recurrence risk for siblings is 25%.

Warfarin Embryopathy. In a review of fetal outcomes in warfarin exposed pregnancies, 2/24 cases with suspected warfarin embryopathy had parieto-occipital or occipital encephalocele. The most common features of warfarin embryopathy include severe nasal hypoplasia and stippled calcification of epiphyses. The critical period of exposure was 6–9 weeks' gestation (Hall et al., 1980).

Frontonasal Malformation. This sporadic pattern of malformation includes extreme hypertelorism, broad nasal root, broad or absent nasal tip, and anterior cranium bifidum with herniation of cranial contents (anterior encephalocele). The terms *frontonasal dysplasia* and *median cleft face syndrome* are also used to refer to this condition (DeMyer, 1967; Sedano et al., 1970). The CNS and facial features are sometimes associated with other defects of the eyes, ears, and limbs (Toriello et al., 1986, 1995). The probability of mental retardation is increased with the severity of the facial defects and the presence of other anomalies (DeMyer, 1967). Several cases of frontonasal malformation have been associated with chromosome abnormalities (Stevens and Qumsiyeh, 1995; Stratton and Payne, 1997; Kirkpatrick and Pauli, 1998). The etiology in most cases is unknown.

SUMMARY

The minority of NTDs are associated with additional malformations. It is important, however, to recognize those cases with a specific underlying diagnosis for accurate recurrence risk counseling, prenatal diagnosis, epidemiological studies, and prevention strategies. Associated malformations have been reported in most organ systems. Study of these more complicated, or syndromic, NTDs has contributed to the identification of genetic loci, specific genes, and potential pathogenetic mechanisms that contribute to the overall burden of NTDs.

REFERENCES

Bamforth JS, Lin CC (1997). DK phocomelia phenotype (von Voss-Cherstvoy syndrome) caused by somatic mosaicism for del (13q). Am J Med Genet 73:408–411.

Becerra JE, Khoury MJ, Cordero JF, Erickson JD (1990). Diabetes mellitus during pregnancy and the risks for specific birth defects: a population-based case-control study. Pediatrics 85:1–9.

Bird LM, Newbury RO, Ruiz-Velasco R, Jones MC (1994). Recurrence of diaphragmatic agenesis associated with multiple midline defects: evidence of an autosomal gene regulating the midline. Am J Med Genet 53:33–38.

Bjerkedal T, Czeizel A, Goujard J, Kallen B, Mastroiacova P, Nevin N, Oakley G Jr, et al (1982). Valproic acid and spina bifida. Lancet 2:1096.

Blackburn W, Cooley NR Jr (1993). The umbilical cord. In Stevenson RE, Hall JG, Goodman RG (eds): *Human Malformations and Related Anomalies,* Vol. II. New York: Oxford University Press, pp. 1098–1099.

Budorick NE, Pretorius DH, McGahan JP, Grafe MR, James HE, Slivka J (1995). Cephalocele detection in utero: sonographic and clinical features. Ultrasound Obstet Gynecol 5:77–85.

Carey JC, Greenbaum B, Hall BD (1978). The OEIS complex (omphalocele, exstrophy, imperforate anus, spinal defects). Birth Defects Orig Art Ser 14(6B):253–263.

Cherstvoy E, Lazjuk G, Lurie I, Ostrovskaya T, Shved I (1980). Syndrome of multiple congenital malformations including phocomelia, thrombocytopenia, encephalocele and urogenital abnormalities (letter). Lancet 2:485.

Coerdt W, Miller K, Holzgreve W, Rauskolb R, Schwinger E, Rehder H (1997). Neural tube defects in chromosomally normal and abnormal human embryos. Ultrasound Obstet Gynecol 10:410–415.

Cormand B, Pihko H, Bayes M, Valanne L, et al (2001). Clinical and genetic distinction between Walker-Warburg syndrome and muscle-eye-brain disease. Neurology 56:1059–1069.

Czeizel A (1981). Schisis-association. Am J Med Genet 10:25–35.

DeMyer W (1967). The median cleft face syndrome. Differential diagnosis of cranium bifidum occultum, hypertelorism, and medial cleft nose, lip and palate. Neurology 17:961–971.

DiLiberti JH, Farndon PA, Dennis NR, Curry CJR (1984). The fetal valproate syndrome. Am J Med Genet 19:473–481.

Dobyns WB, Pagon RA, Armstrong D, Curry CJR, Greenberg F, Grix A, Holmes L, et al (1989). Diagnostic criteria for Walker-Warburg syndrome. Am J Med Genet 32:195–210.

Edmonds LD, Layde PM (1982). Conjoined twins in the United States. Teratology 25:301–308.

Gilpin NSN (2000). von Voss-Cherstvoy syndrome: a second family with affected siblings. Am J Hum Genet 67(Suppl 2):121.

Greene MF, Hare JW, Cloherty JP, Benacerraf BR, Soeldner JS (1989). First-trimester hemoglobin A1 and risk for major malformation and spontaneous abortion in diabetic pregnancy. Teratology 39:225–231.

Hall JG, Friedman JM, Kenna BA, Popkin J, Jawanda M, Arnold W (1988). Clinical, genetic, and epidemiological factors in neural tube defects. Am J Hum Genet 43:827–837.

Hall JG, Pauli RM, Wilson KM (1980). Maternal and fetal sequelae of anticoagulation during pregnancy. Am J Med 68:122–140.

Hay S, Wehrung DA (1970). Congenital malformations in twins. Am J Hum Genet 22:662–678.

Higginbottom MC, Jones KL, Hall BD, Smith DW (1979). The amniotic band disruption complex: timing of amniotic rupture and variable spectra of consequent defects. J Pediatr 95:544–549.

Hodes ME, Cole J, Palmer CG, Reed T (1978). Clinical experience with trisomies 18 and 13. Am J Med Genet 15:48–60.

Hsia YE, Bratu M, Herbordt A (1971). Genetics of the Meckel syndrome (dysencephalia splanchnocystica. Pediatrics 48:237–247.

Hume RF Jr, Drugan A, Reichler A, Lampinen J, Martin LS, Johnson MP, Evans MI (1996). Aneuploidy among prenatally detected neural tube defects. Am J Med Genet 61:171–173.

Hunter AGW (1993). Brain and spinal cord. In Stevenson RE, Hall JG, Goodman RM (eds): *Human Malformations and Related Anomalies,* Vol. II. New York: Oxford University Press, pp. 116–118.

Hunter AGW, Carpenter BF (1986). Implication of malformations not due to amniotic bands in the amniotic band sequence. Am J Med Genet 24:691–700.

Hunter AGW, Cleveland RH, Blickman JG, Holmes LB (1996). A study of level of lesion, association malformations and sib occurrence risks in spina bifida. Teratology 54:213–218.

Hurwitz RS, Manzoni GA, Ransley PG, Stephens FD (1987). Cloacal exstrophy: a report of 34 cases. J Urol 138(Pt 2):1060–1064.

James WH (1976). Twinning and anencephaly. Ann Hum Biol 3:401–409.

Jones KL, Smith DW, Hall BD, Hall JG, Ebbin AJ, Massoud H, Golbus MS (1974). A pattern of craniofacial and limb defects secondary to aberrant tissue bands. J Pediatr 84:90–95.

Kallen B, Robert E, Harris J (1998). Associated malformations in infants and fetuses with upper or lower neural tube defects. Teratology 57:56–63.

Keeling JW, Kjaer I (1994). Diagnostic distinction between anencephaly and amnion rupture sequence based on skeletal analysis. J Med Genet 31:823–829.

Kennedy D, Chitayat D, Winsor EJ, Silver M, Toi A (1998). Prenatally diagnosed neural tube defects: ultrasound, chromosome, and autopsy or postnatal findings in 212 cases. Am J Med Genet 77:317–321.

Khoury MJ, Erickson JD, James LM (1982). Etiologic heterogeneity of neural tube defects. II. Clues from family studies. Am J Hum Genet 34:980–987.

Kirkpatrick SJ, Pauli RM (1998). Frontonasal malformation and deletion of 22q11. Am J Med Genet 75:443–444.

Knobloch WH, Layer JM (1971). Retinal detachment and encephalocele. J Pediatr Ophthalmol 8:181–184.

Leck I (1974). Neural-tube defects and twinning. Lancet 1:178.

Lemire RJ, Beckwith JB, Warkany MD (1978). *Anencephaly.* New York: Raven Press.

Mecke S, Passarge E (1971). Encephalocele, polycystic kidneys, and polydactyly as an autosomal recessive trait simulating certain other disorders: the Meckel syndrome. Ann Genet 14:97–103.

Melnick M, Myrianthopoulos NC (1987). Studies in neural tube defects II. Pathologic findings in a prospectively collected series of anencephalics. Am J Med Genet 26:797–810.

Melvin EC, George TM, Worley G, Franklin A, Mackey J, Viles K, Shah N, et al (2000). Genetic studies in neural tube defects. Pediatr Neurosurg 32:1–9.

Miller ME, Graham JM, Higginbottom MC, Smith DW (1981). Compression-related defects from early amnion rupture: evidence for mechanical teratogenesis. J Pediatr 98:292–297.

Omtzigt JG, Los FJ, Grobbee DE, Pijpers L, Jahoda MG, Brandenburg H, Stewart PA, et al (1992). The risk of spina bifida aperta after first-trimester exposure to valproate in a prenatal cohort. Neurology 42(Suppl 5):119–125.

Opitz JM, Gilbert EF (1982). Editorial comment: CNS anomalies and the midline as a "developmental field." Am J Med Genet 12:443–455.

Pagon RA, Clarren SK, Milam DF Jr, Hendrickson AE (1983). Autosomal recessive eye and brain anomalies: Warburg syndrome. J Pediatr 102:542–546.

Reece EA, Homko CJ, Wu YK (1996). Multifactorial basis of the syndrome of diabetic embryopathy. Teratology 54:171–182.

Robert E, Guibaud P (1982). Maternal valproic acid and congenital neural tube defects. Lancet 2:937.

Russo R, D'Armiento M, Angrisani P, Vecchione R (1993). Limb body wall complex: a critical review and a nosological proposal. Am J Med Genet 47:893–900.

Salonen R, Paavola P (1998). Meckel syndrome. J Med Genet 35:497–501.

Schinzel AAGL, Smith DW, Miller JR (1979). Monozygotic twinning and structural defects. J Pediatr 95:921–930.

Seaver LH, Joffe L, Spark RP, Smith BL, Hoyme HE (1993). Congenital scalp defects and vitreoretinal degeneration: redefining the Knobloch syndrome. Am J Med Genet 46:203–208.

Seaver LH, Stevenson RE, Collins JS, Dean JH (2003). Multiple gestation and neural tube defects: data from ten years of the South Carolina Neural Tube Defect Surveillance and Prevention Project. Paper presented at the third biennial Neural Tube Defects Conference, Seabrook Island, South Carolina, September 27–30, 2003.

Seaver LH, Stevenson RE, Dean J (2002). Neural tube defects with associated anomalies: recognized and unrecognized patterns of malformation. Paper presented at the second biennial Neural Tube Defects Conference, Seabrook Island, South Carolina, May 4–7, 2002.

Sedano HO, Cohen MM Jr, Jirasek, J, Gorlin RJ (1970). Frontonasal dysplasia. J Pediatr 76:906–913.

Seller MJ, Kalousek DK (1986). Neural tube defects: heterogeneity and homogeneity. Am J Med Genet (Suppl 2):77–87.

Sharony R, Garber A, Viskochil D, Schreck R, Platt LD, Ward R, Buehler BA, et al (1993). Preaxial ray reduction defects as part of valproic acid embryofetopathy. Prenat Diagn 13:909–918.

Simpson JL, Mills J, Rhoads GG, Cunningham GC, Conley MR, Hoffman HJ (1991). Genetic heterogeneity in neural tube defects. Ann Genet 34:279–286.

Smith DW (1969). The 18 trisomy and the 13 trisomy syndromes. Birth Defect Orig Art Ser 5(5):67–71.

Stevens CA, Qumsiyeh MB (1995). Syndromal frontonasal dysostosis in a child with a complex translocation involving chromosomes 3, 7, and 11. Am J Med Genet 55:494–497.

Stevenson RE, Allen WP, Pai GS, Best R, Seaver LH, Dean J, Thompson S (2000). Decline in prevalence of neural tube defects in a high-risk region of the United States. Pediatrics 106:677–683.

Stratton RF, Payne RM (1997). Frontonasal malformation with tetralogy of Fallot associated with a submicroscopic deletion of 22q11. Am J Med Genet 69:287–289.

Streeter GL (1930). Focal deficiencies in fetal tissues and their relation to intrauterine amputation. Contrib Embryol Carnegie Inst 22:1–44.

Sugiura Y, Suzuki Y, Kobayashi M (1996). The Meckel syndrome: report of two Japanese sibs and a review of the literature. Am J Med Genet 67:312–314.

Toriello HV, Higgins JV (1985). Possible causal heterogeneity in spina bifida cystica. Am J Med Genet 21:13–20.

Toriello HV, Higgins JV, Mann R (1995). Oculoauriculofrontonasal syndrome: report of another case and review of differential diagnosis. Clin Dysmorphol 4:338–346.

Toriello HV, Radecki LL, Sharda J, Looyenga D, Mann R (1986). Frontonasal "dysplasia," cerebral anomalies, and polydactyly: report of a new syndrome and discussion from a developmental field perspective. Am J Med Genet 25(Suppl 2):89–96.

Torpin R (1968). *Fetal Malformations Caused by Amnion Rupture during Gestation.* Springfield, IL: Charles C. Thomas.

Van Allen MI, Curry C, Gallagher L (1987). Limb body wall complex: I. Pathogenesis. Am J Med Genet 28:529–548.

Walker AE (1942). Lissencephaly. Arch Neurol Psychiatry 48:13–29.

Williams R, Swisher CN, Jennings M, Ambler M, Caviness VS Jr (1984). Cerebro-ocular dysgenesis (Walker-Warburg syndrome): neuropathologic and etiologic analysis. Neurology 34:1531–1541.

Wilson C, Aftimos L, Pereira A, McKay R (1998). Report of two sibs with Knobloch syndrome (encephalocele and vitreoretinal degeneration) and other anomalies. Am J Med Genet 78:286–290.

Windham GC, Bjerkedal T, Sever LE (1982). The association of twinning and neural tube defects: studies in Los Angeles, California, and Norway. Acta Genet Med Gemellol 31:165–172.

8

The Tethered Cord Syndrome

CARY R. TEMPLIN
JOHN F. SARWARK

Tethering of the spinal cord is a clinical syndrome manifested by neurological deterioration and/or scoliosis as a result of sustained longitudinal traction on the axis of the spinal cord. The tethering of the spinal cord may be primary (tight filum terminale, fatty filum) or secondary (adhesions). Tethered cord in children with myelomeningocele is a secondary type of tethering that is the result of scarring in and around the neonatal closure of the myelomeningocele, most commonly at the last intact laminar arch.

Symptomatic secondary retethering or tethered cord syndrome following primary myelomeningocele repair occurs in 11% to 32% children during their growth years; however, it can present primarily in adults (Barson, 1970; Bowman et al., 2001; McLone, 1992; Peterson, 1992; Colak et al., 1998; Tamaki et al., 1988; Ohe et al., 2000). Although the conus medullaris is frequently found to be low-lying in children with a myelomeningocele, and may even appear adherent to the dorsal dura in a majority of cases, tethering is significant only when it is associated with clinical signs and symptoms of neurological deterioration as well as progression of scoliotic deformity (Oi et al., 1990; Banta, 1991; Mazur and Menelaus, 1991; Rekate, 1991; McEnery et al., 1992). Signs and symptoms of neurological deterioration or loss include change in the motor or sensory level in the lower extremities, spasticity of the lower extremities, rapid progression of scoliosis, back and leg pain, change in bladder tone, and/or incontinence on intermittent catheterization (McLone et al., 1990–91; Rekate, 1991).

The pathophysiology of tethered cord is not fully understood. A metabolic impairment of the cord has been noted in one study (Yamada et al., 1981) that correlated electrophysiological spinal cord dysfunction in an animal model spinal cord while under continuous traction. Another animal model study demonstrated elevation in the levels of metabolites that are indicative of ischemic injury in response to sustained tension on the cord. The presence of these metabolites coincided with decreased amplitudes and increased latency of somatosensory and motor evoked potentials (Kocak et al., 1997). Other authors have also noted that traction on the cord increases the potential for damage from extrinsic compression in the already metabolically compromised cord (Fujita and Yamamoto, 1989).

Tethered cord syndrome in children with myelomeningocele is caused by scarring or adhesive arachnoiditis around the neural placode or distal spinal cord and its subsequent adherence to the overlying dura or subcutaneous layers and skin (Reigel, 1983; Venes and Stevens, 1983; Tamaki et al., 1988; Moufarrij et al., 1989; Rekate, 1991). Whether the initial neonatal closure technique reduces clinical tethering is still controversial. Some neurosurgeons advocate pia-arachnoid repair, while others prefer a neural placode open technique (McLone and Naidich, 1985). The practice of implanting membranes such as Gore-Tex and silastic as protective barriers from adhesion has been introduced in both animal and human studies (Inoue et al., 1994; Zide et al., 1995; Aliredjo et al., 1999; Ohe et al., 2000). Although implants such as these have been shown in some instances to inhibit adhesions, concern about cerebrospinal fluid leakage, arachnoiditis, and chronic infection has limited this practice. One study has indicated that no graft material was effective in reducing tethering (Colak et al., 1998). Given the anatomical arrangement of the intraspinal compartment (placode) at infancy, often described as a shallow dish, retethering may be very difficult to avoid (Rekate, 1991).

CONTROVERSIES REGARDING EVALUATION AND SURGICAL MANAGEMENT

Debate continues as to the significance of symptomatic tethered spinal cord in children with a myelomeningocele and the approaches, if any, to it (Banta, 1991). It is widely accepted that the surgical release of a secondary retethered spinal cord in children with myelomeningocele is of benefit for symptomatic children whose magnetic resonance imaging (MRI) findings are consistent with the clinical findings of a tethered spinal cord. Numerous studies have confirmed the benefit of tethered cord release in the symptomatic patient (Garceau, 1953; Herman et al., 1993; Chaseling et al., 1985; McLone and Naidich, 1986; Tamaki et al., 1988; Mayfield, 1991; Peterson, 1992; Sarwark et al., 1996). Proponents of accepting neurological decline over time as a natural history for children have differing opinions from proponents of intervening to preserve function when neurological decline is observed. Phuong et al. (2002) demonstrated that in myelomeningocele patients symptomatic for tethered cord syndrome who were treated conservatively with observation, there was a significantly increased need for additional orthopedic and urological procedures. They showed that the rate of progression of the tethered cord symptoms was 27.5%, 40%, and 60% over 1, 2, and 5 years, respectively. By contrast, Archibeck et al. (1997) revealed that patients who underwent tethered cord release, especially those with myelomeningocele, frequently required operative revision of the index repair. They also showed that the incidence of subsequent orthopedic procedures in this population was elevated as well. It appears reasonable that whichever choice is made, the goal should be to preserve the patient's maximum independence of function.

Diagnosis

These differing philosophies result in a controversy involving the selection of children for surgical detethering. With the estimate that 11%–32% of all children with myelomeningocele ultimately develop symptomatic tethering of the spinal cord with any and all of the clinical manifestations described earlier, selection of appropriate candidates for detethering becomes critical (Tamaki et al., 1988; Oi et al., 1990; Rekate, 1991; McEnery et al., 1992; McLone, 1992; Peterson, 1992; Colak et al., 1998; Ohe et al., 2000; Bowman et al., 2001). Children who will benefit from surgical detethering must be carefully identified.

Some of the clinical manifestations of symptomatic tethered cord syndrome may be caused by or may mimic concurrent conditions (Hall et al., 1976, Park et al., 1985). This further increases the complexity of clinical decision making and surgical selection. For example, while the contribution of tethered cord syndrome to developmental scoliosis in myelomeningocele patients is well referenced in the literature (McLone et al., 1990–91; Herman et al., 1993; Reigel et al., 1994; Filler et al., 1995), progressive scoliosis in these patients may be caused by multiple other factors. These factors include bony anomalies or congenital vertebral defects; asymmetric anatomical or motor level of the lesion leading to imbalance and causing scoliosis (Mayfield, 1991); hydromyelia; or shunt malfunction with resultant hydrocephalus (Hall et al., 1979; Hughes and Dias, 1988; Weiner et al., 1988; McLone and Naidich, 1989; Rekate, 1991). Shunt malfunction, with or without hydromyelia, is extremely common in these children. A recent study showed that 86% of those with myelomeningocele required some form of shunting, and of those patients, 95% required at least one revision (Bowman et al., 2001). Given this frequency, the differentiation between a shunt malfunction and a tethered cord becomes quite difficult. Additionally, rapid growth during a rapid growth phase may be associated with curve progression and may further hinder accurate diagnosis.

Children with thoracic-level or high-lumbar-level paralysis may commonly have a neurologically based developmental scoliosis that is dependent on the anatomical and neurological levels of the lesion. This acquired scoliosis by age 15 years occurs in nearly all thoracic-level patients (Kendall et al., 1971; Banta et al., 1976; Moe et al., 1978), 23%–70% of low-lumbar-level patients (Mackel and Lindseth, 1975; Shurtleff, 1976; Moe et al., 1978), and less than 10% of sacral-level patients (Shurtleff, 1976; Moe et al., 1978). In children with higher motor-level lesions, it would be difficult to state with confidence that scoliosis is due exclusively to tethered cord alone.

Urological findings, in addition to spasticity and progression of scoliosis, contribute to the diagnosis of tethered cord syndrome. Changes in urodynamic studies, as well aspects of the history and physical examination such as urinary frequency, incontinence, urgency, or infection, may be early clues to the development of a tethered cord (Palmer et al., 1998; Kaplan, 2002). Initially, renal and bladder ultrasound examinations are performed every 3 months for the first year, then every 6 months for 5 to 7 years (Kaplan, 2002). Given the subtle changes in function and the benefit of early diagnosis, yearly urological and urodynamic evaluations may be important in evaluating these patients (Spindel et al., 1987; Palmer et al., 1998). Urodynamic testing is indicated with any change in orthopedic function or continence level, with an increase in urological infections, or with changes in the appearance of the kidneys on ultrasound scans (Kaplan, 2002). In patients with serial urodynamic studies providing evidence of nerve injury to the external sphincter, those treated with early intervention had a 59% improvement in symptoms (Bauer, 2000).

Outcome

Improvement and/or Stabilization of Scoliosis. Reigel and associates (1994) reviewed the clinical and functional status of a large group of patients with tethered cord and surgical release, nearly 90% of whom had myelomeningocele or meningocele. In those with scoliosis, the condition stabilized in 71% and continued to progress in 29%, supporting the strategy of surgical release of the cord in symptomatic patients (Reigel, 1983). In general, most cases demonstrate stabilization or improvement of scoliosis in the first year after surgical release. Further analysis of results demonstrates that in preoperative scoliotic curves of 45° or less, a larger number of children show stabilization or improvement in the first year (82% in one study). Tethered cord release may be of benefit in allowing the child to delay corrective spinal fusion or avoid it altogether (Sarwark et al., 1996). Some scoliotic curves will ultimately progress in any case, but the child benefits greatly from additional years of growth, so that surgical stabilization by fusion and instrumentation is more timely and does not result in major loss of sitting height (Schafer and Dias, 1983).

Symptomatic Retethering. Symptomatic retethering after secondary release is seen in an additional 13%–25% of patients. One report identified this 1 to 9 years after tethered cord release (Filler et al., 1995). This incidence is similar to that of pathological adhesion of the spinal cord after primary closure for myelomeningocele (Barson, 1970; Tamaki et al., 1988; McLone, 1992; Peterson, 1992; Bowman et al., 2001). It is reasonable to state that there is an inherent risk of adhesions following any closure or exploration for the tethered cord in this group of patients. The implantation of protective barriers around the neural placode at the time of index closure or at the time of secondary detethering has been discussed (Inoue et al., 1994; Aliredjo et al., 1999; Ohe et al., 2000). Despite the reported success of this technique in preventing adhesions of the neural elements to surrounding tissues, this practice has been avoided because of concerns about drainage, infection, and arachnoiditis (McLone, Personal Communication). Some patients with complex scarring may not benefit from any type of surgery. Patients undergoing surgical release of adhesions seem to maintain a constant risk of recurrence over time. Nonetheless, Banta (1991) found that tethered cord release is indicated in children with symptomatic secondary retethering of the cord with myelomeningocele.

Scoliosis Management. Children with progressive scoliosis without neurological deterioration are treated with orthoses and/or surgery. The surgical procedure most commonly performed is anterior spinal release and fusion coupled with posterior spinal fusion, usually in the same anesthetic session. In progressive scoliotic deformity without evidence of neurological deterioration, prophylactic detethering of the cord before or at the time of spinal fusion is not indicated in most instances. In cases in which neurological deterioration is present at the same time as progressive, severe scoliosis, tethered cord release may be performed 6 weeks or more before corrective spinal fusion or, in cases of established and severe scoliosis, on the same day as the staged procedures.

Based on our understanding of the pathophysiology of the tethered cord, it is reasonable to infer that detethering at an early stage will lead to a better result with respect to reversal of scoliosis, resolution of spasticity, improved urological function, and preserved motor strength. Most patients who experience a decline in motor function preoperatively stabilize after detethering (Reigel, 1983; Schmidt and Yngve, 1988). Data support the belief that release is indicated in those with symptomatic secondary retethering of the cord (Banta, 1991).

ROLE OF IMAGING IN TETHERED CORD SYNDROME

Magnetic Resonance Imaging Evaluation

The purpose of an MRI evaluation in the symptomatic child with myelomeningocele is to identify the morphology of the proposed site of surgery and to identify other possible sites of pathology prior to tethered cord release. Ultrasound can be used, particularly in the infant, to evaluate the spine for adhesions and other abnormalities, with results comparable to those of MRI. Proponents of this modality state that it is cheaper and does not require sedation (Gerscovich et al., 1999). Despite this, MRI remains the test of choice, probably because of its soft tissue detail and ease of interpretation in contrast to ultrasound. It is generally accepted that MRI is a reliable way to confirm the site of cord tethering and define the environment of the neural elements (Brunberg et al., 1988; Peterson, 1992; Westcott et al., 1992; Ohe et al., 2000). All clinically symptomatic patients who were found to have a cord or conus that abutted the dorsal dura on MRI demonstrated a tethered cord at surgery. Interestingly, in some patients with tethering, the cord follows a ventral route at the thoracolumbar junction. Patients with this finding had more severe lower extremity weakness (Saita et al., 1998).

Johnson and Levy (1995) studied neurologically symptomatic children with phase MRI. They showed that those patients who demonstrated only slightly or moderately decreased cord motion remained stable with observation or had better outcomes after surgical detethering. Those with severe limitation of motion did not improve following detethering. Magnetic resonance imaging provides valuable information regarding scarring around the cord and decreasing cord motion; however, it is important to note that the diagnosis of tethered cord syndrome must be based on signs and symptoms of neurological loss, with MRI findings serving as an adjunct to this diagnosis. The MRI findings alone do not indicate a tethered cord.

EFFECTS OF SURGICAL DETETHERING IN THE SYMPTOMATIC CHILD

As noted earlier, tethered cord release for symptomatic secondary retethering and myelomeningocele is generally beneficial in properly selected patients.

Potential Neurological Complications

Because of the nature of this procedure, there is inherent risk of injury to motor and sensory roots. Damage to these roots may be neurologically catastrophic and must be avoided. Neurophysiological monitoring is effective in differentiating the thickened filum terminale from the lumbosacral nerve roots and should be used in tethered cord release (Von Koch et al., 2002).

Effects of Detethering

In an effort to clearly analyze the effect of surgical detethering, a study group of strictly defined, symptomatic, highly functioning children with only secondary tethering was evaluated (Sarwark et al., 1996). Only patients who had been functioning at the L3 motor level or better (community ambulation) were included. Patients with other concomitant neurological problems were excluded, as were those who had moderate to severe associated hydromyelia, shunt malfunction requiring recent shunt revision, central nervous system complications other than hydromyelia (infection, cerebral palsy), posterior rhizotomy performed at the time of release, inaccurate records of their spinal cord imaging studies, or incomplete clinical data concerning their course prior to the time of tethered cord release (Sarwark et al., 1996).

The average age at the time of tethered cord release in this group was 7 years, with the range of ages from 1 year, 1 month to 14 years, 5 months. The neurological level was either low lumbar motor level (L4–L5) or sacral motor level.

Thirty-three cases were ultimately analyzed in this study for clinical presentations and postoperative (detethering) results. Clinical findings evaluated in this study included new or rapidly progressive scoliosis in patients with no primary vertebral anomalies, deterioration of motor function, spasticity (frequently seen in the hamstring muscles, ankle dorsiflexors/evertors), and back pain at the site of closure.

Scoliosis

In the aforementioned study, 60% of the patients presented with new-onset or recently progressing scoliosis in the absence of primary vertebral abnormality (congenital scoliosis). The majority were curves of 45° or less. Forty-nine percent of the patients presented with lower extremity spasticity. Forty-two percent demonstrated a decrease in muscle/motor function, and 9% presented with low back pain of recent onset at the site of closure. The majority of patients presented with more than one clinical finding.

In most cases, the scoliosis either improved (by more than 10°) or was stable in the first year following tethered cord release. The best results in terms of scoliosis improvement were seen in patients with a scoliotic curve of 45° or less preoperatively. The worst results were cases in which the curvature was greater than 45° prior to the release.

Spasticity

With respect to spasticity (improved, not improved, or worsened based on serial examinations), 44% of the patients improved following tethered cord release, 56% showed no clear improvement, and none worsened. With respect to improvement in motor function, 79% of the patients showed some improvement postoperatively, 21% showed no clear improvement, and none deteriorated. All of the patients who reported back pain prior to surgery experienced resolution of the pain. Four of 33 patients developed symptomatic retethering requiring another surgical release.

Pierz and associates (2000) also studied the effects of detethering on scoliosis in persons with myelomeningocele and had similar results. They found that 86% of curves greater than 40° at presentation progressed to require fusion. Another interesting finding was that 100% of thoracic-level patients went on to require spinal fusion. Those with curves less than 40° had greater potential for improvement following tethered cord release.

Conclusion

These studies support the position that in the correctly selected patient, release of the tethered cord is beneficial to maintaining function and therefore is indicated. Our continued goal should be to provide maximum independence of function to our patients with myelomeningocele.

REFERENCES

Aliredjo RP, deVries J, Menovsky T, Grotenhuis JA, Merx J (1999). The use of Gore-Tex membrane for adhesion prevention in tethered spinal cord surgery: technical case reports. Neurosurgery 44(3):674–677.

Archibeck MJ, Smith JT, Carroll KL, Davitt JS, Stevens PM (1997). Surgical release of tethered spinal cord: survivorship analysis and orthopedic outcome. J Pediatr Ortho 17(6):773–776.

Banta JV (1991). The tethered cord in myelomeningocele: should it be untethered? Dev Med Child Neurol 33:173–176.

Banta JV, Whiteman S, Dyck PM, Hartleip DL, Gilbert D (1976). Fifteen years review of myelodysplasia. J Bone Joint Surg 58A:726.

Barson AJ (1970). The vertebral level of termination of the spinal cord during normal and abnormal development. J Anat 106:489–497.

Bauer SB (2000). The argument for early assessment and treatment of infants with spina bifida. Dialogues Pediatr Urol 23:2–30.

Bowman RM, McClone DG, Grant JA, Tomita T, Ito JA (2001). Spina bifida outcome: a twenty-five year prospective. Pediatr Neurosurg 34(3):114–120.

Brunberg JA, Latchaw RE, Kanal E, Burk L, Albright L (1988). Magnetic resonance imaging of spinal dysraphism. Radiol Clin North Am 26:181–204.

Chaseling RW, Johnston IH, Besser M (1985). Meningocele and the tethered cord syndrome. Child Nerv Syst 1:105–108.

Colak A, Pollack IF, Albright AL (1998). Recurrent tethering: a common long-term problem after lipomyelomeningocele repair. Pediatr Neurosurg 29(4):184–190.

Filler AG, Britton JA, Uttley D, Marsh HT (1995). Adult post repair myelomeningocoele and tethered cord syndrome: good surgical outcome after abrupt neurological decline. Br J Neurosurg 9(5):659–666.

Fujita Y, Yamamoto H (1989). An experimental study on spinal cord traction effect. Spine 14:698–705.

Garceau GJ (1953). The filum terminale syndrome. J Bone Joint Surg 35A:711–716.

Gerscovich EO, Maslen L, Cronan MS, Poirier V, Anderson MW, McDonald C, Boggan JE, Ivanovic M (1999). Spinal sonography and magnetic resonance imaging in patients with repaired myelomeningocele: comparison of modalities. J Ultrasound Med 18(9):655–664.

Hall PV, Lindseth R, Campbell R, Kalsbeck J (1976). Myelodysplasia and developmental scoliosis: a manifestation of syringomyelia. Spine 1:49–55.

Hall PV, Lindseth R, Campbell R, Kalsbeck J, Desousa A (1979). Scoliosis and hydrocephalus in myelocele patients, the effects of ventricular shunting. J Neurosurg 50:174–178.

Herman JM, McLone D, Storrs B, Dauser R (1993). Analysis of 153 patients with myelomeningocele or spinal lipoma reoperated upon for a tethered cord. Pediatr Neurosurg 19:243–249.

Hughes WA, Dias LS (1988). Scoliosis in myelomeningocele. The role of tethered cord and hydromyelia. Dev Med Child Neurol Suppl 57:26.

Inoue HK, Kobayashi S, Ohbayashi K, Kohga H, Nakamura M (1994). Treatment and prevention of tethered and retethered spinal cord using a Gore-Tex surgical membrane. J Neurosurg 80(4):689–693.

Johnson DL, Levy LM (1995). Predicting outcome in the tethered cord syndrome: a study of cord motion. Pediatr Neurosurg 22(3):115–119.

Kaplan WE (2002). Surgical urologic management of children with spina bifida. In Sarwark JF, Lubicky JP, (eds): *Caring for the Child with Spina Bifida.* Rosemont, IL: AAOS, pp. 551–560.

Kendall HO, Kendall PK, Wadsworth GE (1971). *Muscles, Testing and Function,* 2nd ed. Baltimore: Williams & Wilkins.

Kocak A, Kilic A, Nurlu G, Konan A, Kilinc K, Cirak B, Colak A (1997). A new model for tethered cord syndrome: a biochemical, electrophysical, and electron microscopic study. Pediatr Neurosurg 26(3):120–126.

Mackel JL, Lindseth RE (1975). Scoliosis in myelodysplasia. J Bone Joint Surg 57A:1031.

Mayfield JK (1991). Comprehensive orthopaedic management in myelomeningocele. In Rekate HL (ed): *Comprehensive Management of Spina Bifida.* Boston: CRC Press, pp. 113–164.

Mazur JM, Menelaus MB (1991). Neurologic status of spina bifida patients and the orthopaedic surgeon. Clin Orthop Relat Res 264:54–64.

McEnery G, Borzyskowski M, Cox TCS, Neville, BGR (1992). The spinal cord in neurologically stable spina bifida: a clinical and MRI study. Dev Med Child Neurol 34:342–347.

McLone DG (1992). Continuing concepts in management of children with spina bifida. Pediatr Neurosurg 18(5–6):254–256.

McLone DG, Herman JM, Gabrieli AP, Dias L (1990–1991). Tethered cord as a cause of scoliosis in children with myelomeningocele. Pediatr Neurosurg 16(1):8–13.

McLone DG, Naidich TP (1985). Spinal dysraphism: experimental and clinical. In Holtzman RN, Stein BM (eds): *The Tethered Spinal Cord.* New York: Thiem-Stratton, pp. 14–28.

McLone D, Naidich T (1986). Laser resection of fifty spinal lipomas. Neurosurgery 18:611–615.

McLone D, Naidich T (1989). The tethered spinal cord. In McLaurin RL, Schut L, Venes JL, Epstein F (eds): *Pediatric Neurosurgery,* 2nd ed. Philadelphia, WB Saunders, pp. 71–97.

Moe JH, Winter RB, Bradford DL, Lonstein JE (1978). *Scoliosis and Other Spinal Deformities.* Philadelphia: WB Saunders.

Moufarrij NA, Palmer JM, Hahn JF, Weinstein MA (1989). Correlation between magnetic resonance imaging and surgical findings in the tethered spinal cord. Neurosurgery 25:341–346.

Ohe N, Futamura A, Kawada R, Minatsu H, Kohmura H, Hayashi K, Miwa K, Sakai N (2000). Secondary tethered cord syndrome in spinal dysraphism. Child Nerv Syst 16(7):457–461.

Oi S, Yamada H, Matsumoto S (1990). Tethered cord syndrome versus low-placed conus medullaris in an overdistended spinal cord following initial repair for myelodysplasia. Child Nerv Syst 6:264–269.

Palmer LS, Richards I, Kaplan WE (1998). Subclinical changes in bladder function in children presenting with nonurologic symptoms of the tethered cord syndrome. J Urol 159:231–234.

Park TS, Cail WS, Maggio WM, Mitchell DC (1985). Progressive spasticity and scoliosis in children with myelomeningocele: radiological investigation and surgical treatment. J Neurosurg 62:367–375.

Peterson MC (1992). Tethered cord syndrome in myelodysplasia: correlation between level of lesion and height at time of presentation. Dev Med Child Neurol 34:604–610.

Phuong LK, Schoeberl KA, Raffel C (2002). Natural history of tethered cord in patients with myelomeningocele. Neurosurgery 50(5):989–993.

Pierz K, Banta J, Thomson J, Gahm N, Hartford J (2000). The effect of tethered cord release on scoliosis in myelomeningocele. J Pediatr Orthop 20(3):362–365.

Reigel DH (1983). Tethered spinal cord. In Humphreys RP (ed): *Concepts in Pediatric Neurosurgery,* Vol. 40 Basel: Karger, pp. 142–64.

Reigel DH, Tchernoukha K, Bazmi B, Kortyna R, Rotenstein D (1994). Change in spinal curvature following release of tethered spinal cord associated with spina bifida. Pediatr Neurosurg 20(1):30–42.

Rekate HL (1991). Neurosurgical management of the child with spina bifida. In Rekate HL (ed): *Comprehensive Management of Spina Bifida.* Boston: CRC Press, pp. 93–112.

Saita K, Nakamura K, Takeshita K, Kawaguchi H, Kurokawa T (1998). Tethered cord syndrome: ventral displacement of the spinal cord at the thoracolumbar junction in magnetic resonance imaging. Eur J Radiol 27(3):254–257.

Sarwark JF, Weber DT, Gabrieli AP, McLone DG, Dias L (1996). Tethered cord syndrome in low motor level children with myelomeningocele. J Pediatr Neurosurg 25(6):295–301.

Schafer MF, Dias LS (1983). *Myelomeningocele: Orthopaedic Treatment.* Baltimore: Williams & Wilkins.

Schmidt F, Yngve D (1988). Tethered cord release: risks and benefits. Dev Med Child Neurol Suppl 57:27.

Shurtleff DB (1976). Myelodysplasia: the natural history of kyphosis and scoliosis. Dev Med Child Neurol Suppl 18(37):126.

Spindel MR, Bauer SB, Dyro FM, et al (1987). The changing neurological lesion in myelodysplasia. JAMA 258:1630.

Tamaki N, Shirataki K, Kojima N, Shouse Y, Matsumoto S (1988). Tethered cord syndrome of delayed onset following repair of myelomeningocele. J Neurosurg 69:393–398.

Venes JL, Stevens EA (1983). Surgical pathology in tethered cord secondary to myelomeningocele repair. In Humphreys RP (ed): *Concepts in Pediatric Neurosurgery,* Vol. 4. Basel: Karger, pp. 165–185.

Von Koch CS, Quinones-Hinojosa A, Gulati M, Lyon R, Peacock WJ, Yingling CD (2002). Clinical outcome in children undergoing tethered cord release utilizing intra-operative neurophysiological monitoring. Pediatr Neurosurg 37(2):81–86.

Weiner LS, Burke SW, Root L (1988). The use of MRI in myelodysplasia. Dev Med Child Neurol Suppl 57:27.

Westcott MA, Dynes MC, Remer EM, Donaldson JS, Dias LS (1992). Congenital and acquired orthopedic abnormalities in patients with myelomeningocele. Radiographics 12(6):1155–1173.

Yamada S, Zinke DE, Sanders D (1981). Pathophysiology of tethered cord syndrome. J Neurosurg 54:494–503.

Zide B, Constantini S, Epstein FJ (1995). Prevention of recurrent tethered spinal cord. Pediatr Neurosurg 22(2):111–114.

9

Prenatal Screening and Diagnosis of Neural Tube Defects

GLENN J. GARDENER
CHARLES H. RODECK

Neural tube defects are a spectrum of serious malformations of the cranium, spine, and nervous system. The spectrum includes anencephaly, spina bifida, cephalocele, and iniencephaly. Anencephaly and spina bifida, the two most common are important contributors to perinatal mortality and morbidity. Anencephaly is a lethal condition, and infants with spina bifida who survive are likely to have severe, lifelong disabilities (Date et al., 1993; Botto et al., 1999).

Antenatal screening and diagnosis of neural tube defects involves the application of biochemical and/or ultrasound techniques during pregnancy. Antenatal screening identifies pregnancies at risk for the condition so that diagnostic tests can be applied. Ultrasound scanning can be used as both a screening and a diagnostic test for the prenatal detection of neural tube defects. The introduction of maternal serum and ultrasound screening programs over the past 25 years has contributed to a significant reduction in the birth incidence of neural tube defects (Cragan et al., 1995). This chapter describes the development of screening and diagnostic tests used for the prenatal detection of neural tube defects and their current application. With interest developing in fetal therapy for spina bifida, the emergence of novel methods of imaging including three-dimensional ultrasound and fetal magnetic resonance imaging is also discussed.

PRENATAL BIOCHEMICAL SCREENING AND DIAGNOSIS OF NEURAL TUBE DEFECTS

Alpha fetoprotein (AFP) is a glycoprotein that is structurally and functionally similar to albumin. Fetal AFP is sequentially produced by the fetal yolk sac, the gastrointestinal tract, and the liver, reaching peak concentrations in the fetal serum at the end of the first trimester. Fetal serum concentrations of AFP decline exponentially from 14 to 32 weeks' gestation due to both an expanding intravascular compartment and decreased fetal synthesis. Alpha fetoprotein is secreted by the fetal kidney into urine and then excreted into the amniotic fluid. Alpha fetoprotein levels in amniotic fluid show a rise and fall with gestation similar to the levels of AFP in fetal serum. In addition, AFP can pass into the amniotic fluid as a transudate across the membrane and blood vessel surfaces that are exposed in open neural tube defects. Alpha fetoprotein reaches the maternal circulation by a combination of transplacental and transamniotic diffusion, and this forms the pathophysiological basis of the maternal serum screening test for open neural tube defects Maternal serum AFP (MSAFP) concentrations are much lower than the AFP concentrations found in amniotic fluid. In contrast to fetal serum and amniotic fluid levels, the MSAFP level peaks between 28 and 32 weeks' gestation and then slowly declines (Habib, 1977; Lemire, 1988; Haddow, 1990; Bock, 1992).

A specific role for AFP in pregnancy has not yet been established. Various functions for AFP have been postulated, including a role as an intravascular transport protein, to help maintain oncotic pressure, or as an immunosuppressant to prevent a maternal antibody response to paternally derived fetal antigens. Pregnancies without fetal tissues (e.g., hydatidiform moles) may have very low levels of AFP. Pregnancies with an AFP deficiency have also been reported without apparent adverse effects (Filly et al., 1993; Mizejewski, 2003, 2004).

In 1972, Brock and Sutcliffe first reported the association between raised amniotic fluid AFP levels and open neural tube defects. Reports soon followed suggesting a similar association with MSAFP (Wald et al., 1974). In a multicenter study involving more than 18,000 pregnancies across 19 centers, the UK Collaborative AFP Study Group demonstrated the scientific basis for antenatal screening for open neural tube defects by the measurement of MSAFP (Wald et al., 1977). Population screening programs for open neural tube defects using MSAFP then followed in England and the United States. The success of biochemical screening programs in the detection of fetuses with open neural tube defects has been clearly demonstrated, even in regions with lower NTD prevalence (Burton et al., 1983; Cowan et al., 1989; Milunsky et al., 1989).

The distinction between open and closed neural tube defects is an important one from the point of view of antenatal biochemical screening. Closed neural tube defects are covered by skin or a thick membrane that generally does not allow the transfer of AFP into the amniotic fluid. The vast majority of fetuses with anencephaly and approximately 85% of those with spina bifida have open lesions, and it is these pregnancies that will demonstrate increased levels of AFP in both amniotic fluid and maternal serum.

A multitude of congenital abnormalities and disease states have been ascribed to both high and low levels of AFP in recent years. Table 9.1 lists many of the conditions that have been reported to be associated with abnormal AFP levels in pregnancy (Seppala et al., 1976; Wald et al., 1977; Monteagudo and Timor-Tritsch, 1996; Mizejewski, 2003).

TABLE 9.1. *Conditions Associated with Abnormal Alpha Fetoprotein Levels During Pregnancy*

Increased AFP Levels
Open neural tube defects
Ventral wall defects—omphalocele, gastroschisis
Multiple gestation
Sacrococcygeal teratoma
Placental tumors—chorioangioma
Pentalogy of Cantrell
Congenital nephrosis (Finnish type)
Congenital skin defects—epidermolysis bullosa, congenital icthyosis
Amnion rupture sequence
Fetal bowel obstruction
Diaphragmatic hernia
Congenital cystic adenomatoid malformation of the lung
Fetal-maternal hemorrhage
Maternal liver disease
Maternal systemic lupus erythematosus
Maternal germ cell tumor
Rh immunization/hydrops fetalis
Placental abruption
Placenta accreta
Decreased AFP Levels
Insulin-dependent diabetes
Spontaneous abortion
Fetal demise
Trisomies 13, 18, and 21
Molar pregnancy
Fetal growth restriction
Polyhydramnios
Preeclampsia
Thyroid disease

Maternal serum AFP values are usually expressed as a multiple of the median (MoM) at the relevant gestational age. The MoM is simply the observed value divided by the expected value. An advantage of using the median is that, unlike the mean, it is not influenced by outlying values. The MoM values are easy to derive and allow for interlaboratory variation and comparison. Most centers use a cutoff of more than 2.0–2.5 MoM as an abnormal result. The threshold chosen depends on the balance between the detection rate and the false-positive rate. The distributions of MSAFP levels in pregnancies with open neural tube defects and those seen in unaffected pregnancies has the greatest difference at 16–18 weeks' gestation. Although MSAFP screening is most accurate when performed between 16 and 18 weeks' gestation, it can be performed between 15 and 22 weeks (Wald, 2000).

The discriminating power of a test is expressed in terms of the detection rate (the proportion of affected individuals with a positive result) and the false-positive rate (the proportion of unaffected individuals with a positive result). Maternal serum AFP values are a continuous variable, and as such, the detection rate and the false-positive rate vary and are determined by the cutoff level chosen. Moving the cutoff level to reduce the false-positive rate will automatically reduce the detection rate, and moving the cutoff level to increase the detection rate will increase the false-positive rate (Fig. 9.1).

The performance of MSAFP screening improves when the gestation is based on ultrasound measurement of the biparietal diameter (BPD) rather than dating from the last normal menstrual period (LNMP). This is due to both increased precision in estimating gestational age by ultrasound imaging and the advantageous error that fetuses with spina bifida generally have smaller BPDs, leading to MoM values that are higher than those obtained when dated by the LNMP (Wald et al., 1980b).

Using a MSAFP cutoff of greater than 2.5 MoM, the UK Collaborative AFP Study Group detected 79% of open spina bifida and 88% of anencephaly, with a false-positive rate of 3.3% (Wald et al., 1977). Improvements in assay precision and correction of AFP levels for

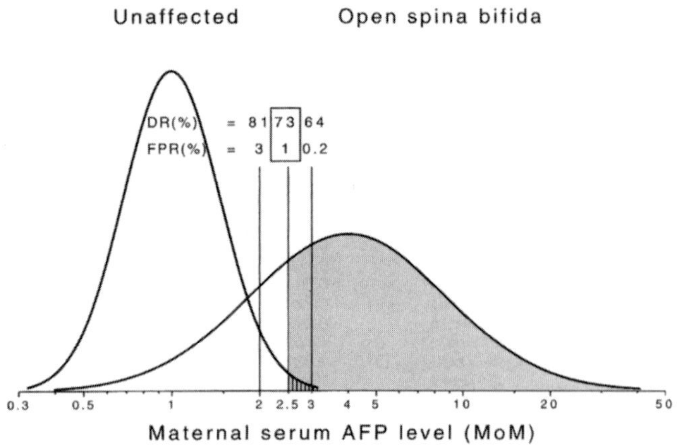

FIGURE 9.1. Distribution of maternal serum alpha-fetoprotein levels in pregnancies with and without open spina bifida at 17 weeks' gestation. Three different MoM cutoffs are shown (2.0, 2.5, and 3.0) with their corresponding detection rates (DR) and false-positive rates (FPR). MoM, multiple of the median.
Source: Wald N and Leck I (2000). *Antenatal and Neonatal Screening*, 2nd edition, with permission.

maternal weight have increased the screening performance. Using an AFP cutoff level of 2.5 MoM or greater, the detection rate for open spina bifida at 17 weeks' gestation according to dates is 73%, with a false-positive rate of 1% when the AFP values are corrected for maternal weight (Fig. 9.1). In addition to gestational age and maternal weight, other variables may influence the distribution pattern of MSAFP values, including insulin-dependent diabetes, multiple pregnancy, and ethnic group. Correction for these factors can further improve the screening performance of MSAFP (Wald, 2000).

When a MSAFP level is found to be elevated, further evaluation is required. The availability and quality of ultrasound services may determine the next action to take. A first elevated test may be repeated because as many as 30% of moderately elevated MSAFP results will be below the threshold level on subsequent testing without increasing the risk of false-negative neural tube defect diagnoses (Wald et al., 1977). In addition, a direct correlation has been reported between the degree of MSAFP elevation and the incidence of fetal anomalies (Reichler et al., 1994). An initial ultrasound assessment can sometimes explain the raised MSAFP immediately by correctly dating the pregnancy, diagnosing a multiple gestation, or identifying a neural tube defect, ventral wall defect, or other anomaly. If the initial ultrasound examination does not provide an explanation for the raised MSAFP, a comprehensive level 2 or level 3 fetal ultrasound examination should be performed.

The decision to then perform amniotic fluid biochemical tests using AFP and/or acetylcholinesterase (AChE) depends on the availability and standard of the ultrasound service and the quality of the images obtained (Sepulveda et al., 1995). The main disadvantage of amniotic fluid testing is the risk of fetal loss related to amniocentesis, widely quoted to be between 0.5 and 1% (Tabor et al., 1986; Wilson, 2000; Alfirevic et al., 2003). Traditionally, amniocentesis for the biochemical diagnosis of neural tube defects was performed before detailed fetal assessment, but with improvements in ultrasound resolution and detection of neural tube defects, invasive assessment to measure amniotic fluid AChE and AFP should be now considered complementary for those cases where the ultrasound findings are inconclusive. One advantage of amniocentesis is that amniotic fluid can also be obtained for chromosomal analysis.

Acetylcholinesterase is derived from neural tissue and is not normally present in amniotic fluid. The AChE test is performed by either gel electrophoresis or immunoassay (Bonham et al., 1987; Rasmussen Loft et al., 1990). The Second Report of the Collaborative Acetylcholinesterase Study showed that amniotic fluid AChE measurement was a better diagnostic test for open neural tube defects than amniotic fluid AFP. The detection rate for open spina bifida using amniotic fluid AChE was 99%, with a false-positive rate of 0.34%, compared with amniotic fluid AFP rates of 90% and 0.46%, respectively. Blood contamination of amniotic fluid is an important cause of false-positive results using amniotic fluid AFP and to a lesser extent AChE (Wald et al., 1989, 2000). The Second Report concluded that an effective policy was to perform an AChE test on samples with amniotic fluid AFP levels greater than 2.0 MoM. The expected open spina bifida detection rate with this policy would be 96% for a false-positive rate of 0.14% (Wald et al., 1989).

Maternal serum AFP screening for neural tube defects may be unnecessary in a population already routinely screened by second trimester ultrasound. Where access to ultrasound screening is limited, MSAFP screening is an effective way of selecting women for targeted ultrasound diagnosis or amniotic fluid biochemical diagnosis. Many centers have abandoned MSAFP screening without firm evidence that ultrasound screening for neural tube defects is at least as reliable. Maternal serum AFP measurement, however, is likely to continue in areas that utilize second trimester biochemical screening for Down syndrome, for which AFP is also a marker (Chan et al., 1995; Wald, 2000).

PRENATAL ULTRASOUND SCREENING AND DIAGNOSIS OF NEURAL TUBE DEFECTS

Antenatal ultrasound scanning can diagnose neural tube defects directly, and as such is used as both a screening test and a diagnostic test. By calculating the gestational age based on measurement of the BPD, ultrasound also improves the performance of MSAFP screening (Wald et al., 1982). The performance of ultrasound in the detection of neural tube defects is dependent on the skill of the operator, the quality of the ultrasound machine, and whether it is used to screen a low-risk population or to target a high-risk population. Prenatal ultrasound detection of neural tube defects initially relied on direct visualization of signs that provided high rates of detection for anencephaly but poor rates for spina bifida. The discovery of indirect cranial and intracranial signs of spina bifida and improvements in ultrasound resolution have increased the detection rates to more than 90% in experienced hands (Nadel et al., 1990; Watson et al., 1991; Sepulveda et al., 1995).

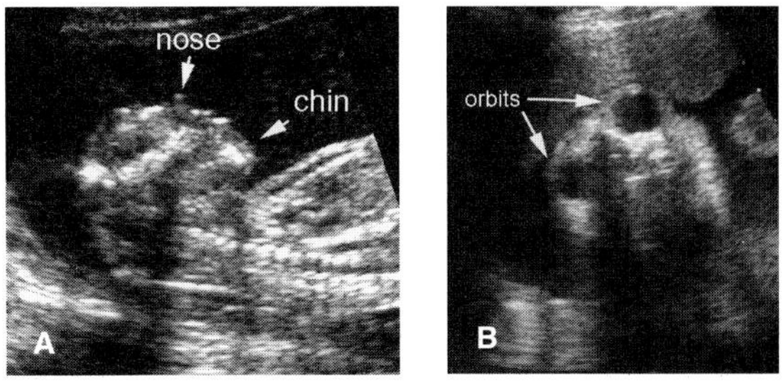

FIGURE 9.2. Second trimester ultrasound images of a fetus with anencephaly. (*a*) Midline sagittal view through the fetal head and thorax showing the facial profile and absence of the calvarium and cerebral hemispheres. (*b*) Coronal view of the fetal face with the orbits visible but nothing above them creating the appearance of frog's eyes.

Acrania/Anencephaly

A synonym for *acrania/anencephaly* is *exencephaly/anencephaly sequence.* Acrania/anencephaly refers to partial or complete absence of the cranial vault and the brain. Cerebral hemispheres and midbrain structures are usually completely absent, leaving remnants of the forebrain and a generally well-formed medulla. In exencephaly, the brain is present but is not covered by the vault of the skull and is therefore exposed to the amniotic fluid. There is now increasing evidence to support the theory that exencephaly is the precursor to anencephaly, with the exposed brain in exencephaly disintegrating secondary to exposure to the amniotic fluid, thus giving rise to the exencephaly/anencephaly sequence (Wilkins-Haug and Freedman, 1991; Timor-Tritsch et al., 1996).

Anencephaly was the first fetal malformation to be detected prenatally using transabdominal ultrasonography (Campbell et al., 1972). In the second and third trimesters, the sonographic diagnosis of anencephaly is based on the symmetrical partial or total absence of the cranial vault above the orbits and varying degrees of disintegration of the cerebral hemispheres (Hidalgo et al., 1982). In a coronal view, facial features can be seen, with the orbits clearly visible and with nothing above them. The prominent, bulging eyes give the anencephalic fetus a typical ultrasound appearance designated "frog's eyes" (Fig. 9.2*a*). In a sagittal view, the face can be identified with normal lips and chin, but the absence of the calvarium above the orbital ridge is clearly seen (Fig. 9.2*b*). Polyhydramnios, which complicates up to 50% of pregnancies with anencephalic fetuses, is often a feature in the second half of the pregnancy (Salamanca et al., 1992).

Late first trimester diagnosis of anencephaly relies upon absence of the cranial vault, which begins to ossify at 10 weeks' gestation (Johnson et al., 1997b; Green and Hobbins, 1988). Unlike the appearances of anencephaly in the second trimester, the cerebral hemispheres may be intact, giving rise to the "Mickey Mouse" sign (Fig. 9.3*a,b*) (Chatzipapas et al., 1999). Diagnosis of exencephaly has been reported at less than 10 weeks' gestation by transvaginal ultrasound on the basis of abnormal cranial pole features (Becker et al., 2000).

Anencephaly is uniformly lethal, with 75% of fetuses dying in utero and the majority of those born alive dying in the first week of life (Baird and Sadovnick, 1984; Pomerance et al., 1989).

Iniencephaly

Iniencephaly is a rare neural tube defect consisting of an occipital bone defect, fixed retroflexion of the head with lordosis of the cervicothoracic spine, and varying degrees of open spinal defects (Sahid et al., 2000). Prenatal sonographic diagnosis of iniencephaly is based on detection of the above features. Two types have been described, iniencephalus apertus with an occipital cephalocele and iniencephalus clausus without an associated occipital cephalocele (Hrgovic et al., 1989).

Other intracranial and extracranial anomalies that may occur in association with iniencephaly include hydrocephalus, holoprosencephaly, posterior fossa defects, diaphragmatic hernia, urinary tract anomalies, cleft lip and palate, omphalocele, and talipes (David and Nixon, 1976; Morocz et al., 1986; Dogan et al., 1996).

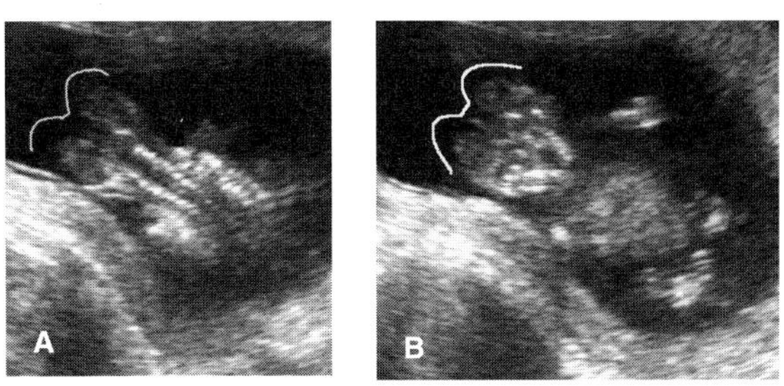

FIGURE 9.3. Fetus with exencephaly in the first trimester showing the "Mickey-mouse" sign. (*a*) Coronal view showing the posterior aspect of the fetal head and thorax. The bony calvarium is absent and the cerebral hemispheres are exposed to the amniotic fluid. (*b*) Coronal view showing the anterior aspect of the fetal head and thorax with acrania and exposed cerebral hemispheres.

Cephalocele

Cephalocele is defined as a herniation of intracranial contents through a bony defect in the skull. Herniation of the meninges alone is termed a *meningocele,* and if any brain parenchyma exits the cranium via a bony defect, it is called an *encephalocele.* When the cerebellum is herniated as part of the cephalocele, it is called the *Chiari type III deformity.* Cephaloceles are subdivided into occipital, frontal, temporal, and parietal types according to the location of the bony defect on the fetal head. The occurrence of the different types reflects geographic variation. In Europe and North America the majority of cephaloceles are occipital, while in Southeast Asia frontal cephaloceles are more common (Chervanak et al., 1984; David and Proudman, 1989; Richards, 1992).

Cephaloceles usually occur as isolated lesions but may occur as part of a chromosomal or genetic syndrome (Nyberg et al., 1990; Wininger and Donnefeld, 1994). Chromosomal abnormalities associated with cephaloceles include trisomies 13, 14, 15, and 18, partial trisomy 6q, monosomy X, triploidy, mosaic trisomy 20, deletion (13q),(2)(q21–q24), and duplications (6)(q21-qter), (7)(pter-q11), and (8)(q23-qter) (Monteagudo and Timor-Tritsch, 1996; Hall and Solehdin, 1998). Among the most common genetic syndromes found with a cephalocele is the Meckel-Gruber syndrome. This is a lethal autosomal recessive condition that also consistently features bilateral enlarged cystic kidneys and postaxial polydactyly (Nyberg et al., 1990).

Cephaloceles may also result from a disruption in the formation of the fetal skull due to amniotic bands or amnion rupture. Cephaloceles due to amniotic bands tend to have irregular surfaces and asymmetric placement (Chervanak et al., 1984).

The sonographic appearance of cephaloceles is diverse and varies according to the site and size of the bony defect and its herniated contents. A meningocele appears as a purely cystic mass, with herniation of the meninges and containing cerebrospinal fluid only (Fig. 9.4*a*). The diagnosis of encephalocele is suggested when the contents of the sac appear solid or mixed solid/cystic, depending on the volume of brain parenchyma within the lesion (Fig. 9.4*b*). The bony defect within the calvarium is usually visible and can vary in size. The cephalocele sac may also vary in size from a few millimeters to a size exceeding that of the normal fetal head. Microcephaly may be a feature if the cephalocele is large. With an encephalocele, distortion of the remaining intracranial contents can occur, producing secondary abnormalities such as ventriculomegaly.

In the absence of identification of a skull defect, the main differential diagnoses include cystic hygroma, cervical myelomeningocele, hemangioma, teratoma, or epidermal cyst of the skull. In view of the association with aneuploidy and other genetic syndromes, a detailed examination of the fetus is required and karyotyping should be offered. Positive prognostic signs include the absence of brain tissue from the sac and an anterior location (Brown and Sheridan-Pereira, 1992).

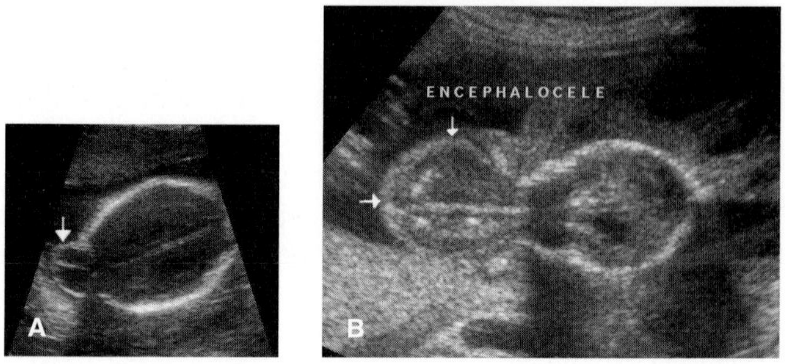

FIGURE 9.4. Ultrasound images of two occipital cephaloceles. (*a*) Transverse section through the fetal head showing an occipital meningocele. The meninges are protruding through a bony defect and after delivery, the sac was confirmed to contain cerebral spinal fluid only. (*b*) Transverse section through the fetal head showing an occipital encephalocele protruding through a bony defect in the calvarium.

Spina Bifida

Spina bifida results from nonfusion of the vertebral arch surrounding the spinal cord and is associated with exposure or protrusion of the spinal contents through the bony defect. In spina bifida occulta, one or more vertebral arches have not closed and there is no externally visible lesion. In contrast, spina bifida aperta or open spina bifida has an externally visible defect consisting of a neural plaque and/or a dorsally protruding sac. If the sac contains only dura, arachnoid, and cerebrospinal fluid, it is a meningocele. If the sac also contains neural tissue, it is a myelomeningocele (synonomous with *meningomyelocele*). Approximately 10% of spina bifida cystica lesions are meningoceles, and the remainder are myelomeningoceles. The majority of open spina bifida lesions occur in the thoracolumbar area and may extend to involve the sacrum. Approximately 10% occur in the thoracic region, and 5% are cervically located (Osborn, 1994; Hahn, 1995).

Prior to the mid-1980s, the prenatal diagnosis of open spina bifida by ultrasound relied upon the identification of a vertebral defect, with detection rates ranging from 33% to 80% (Roberts et al., 1983; Birnbacher et al., 2002). The introduction of indirect cranial and cerebellar signs of open spina bifida in 1986 and continuous improvements in ultrasound quality have steadily increased the diagnostic sensitivity of ultrasound to more than 90% (Nicolaides et al., 1986; Peralta et al., 2003).

Diagnosis of open spina bifida in the first trimester is more difficult and has been originally reported based on visualization of the vertebrae and overlying skin (Braithwaite et al., 1996). Craniocerebral signs associated with open spina bifida in the late first trimester have also been reported, but their reliability in early diagnosis has not been validated (Bernard et al., 1997; Blaas et al., 2000; Buisson et al., 2002).

The fetal spine can be examined in the sagittal, axial, and coronal planes from late in the first trimester on. The recognition of spinal defects requires a systematic examination of each neural arch from the cervical to the sacral region. On transverse section, the open spine has a U shape (Fig. 9.5*b*). However, it is the cleft in the soft tissues that is recognized more easily than the bony defect itself such that closed lesions are relatively rarely detected in utero. On a coronal section, the affected bony segment shows a divergent configuration that replaces the typical parallel lines of the normal vertebral arches. In the presence of a meningocele or myelomeningocele, the defect, overlying skin, and tissues may be seen as a cystic extension from the posterior aspect of the spine (Fig. 9.5*a*). In the sagittal plane, the defect, overlying skin, and tissues may be seen. The presence of neural tissue within the sac indicates the presence of a myelomeningocele. Sonography may have some difficulty in distinguishing reliably between a meningocele and a myelomeningocele (Monteagudo and Timor-Tritsch, 1996).

There are several cranial and intracranial features associated with spina bifida. In the second trimester, fetuses with open spina bifida tend to have a disproportionately small BPD for the gestational age (Wald et al., 1980b) Varying degrees of ventriculomegaly occur in almost all fetuses by the third trimester but only in about 70% of those in the second trimester (Fig. 9.6*b*). In 1986, Nicolaides and co-workers reported the "lemon" and "banana" signs, which have been a significant aid to the prenatal sonographic diagnosis of spina bifida (Fig. 9.6*a,b*). The lemon sign refers to a loss of the convex outward shape of the frontal bones with mild flattening. It is present in virtually all fetuses with spina bifida between 16 and 24 weeks' gestation, but is a less reliable marker after 24 weeks' gestation, when it is present in only 30%–50% of cases (Fig. 9.3) (Penso et al., 1987; Nyberg et al., 1988; Thiagarajah et al., 1990). In the majority of cases of spina bifida, the cerebellum is either not detectable sonographically or has a banana-shaped appearance (Fig. 9.6*a*). Downward displacement of the cerebellum into the foramen magnum, causing the Arnold Chiari type II malformation, occurs in almost all cases of open spina bifida. With the inferior displacement of the medulla and fourth ventricle into the upper cervical canal, the cerebellum becomes compressed and is flattened at the level of the vermis. This abnormal shape may be seen from 14 weeks on (Blumenfeld et al., 1993). Cerebellar abnormalities are present in more than 90% of fetuses with open spina bifida irrespective of the age of gestation. The cerebellar abnormality seen most commonly before 24 weeks' gestation is the banana sign, whereas in later pregnancy the cerebellum is more often absent (Van den Hof et al., 1990). While false-positive cerebellar signs are rare, the lemon sign is found in as many as 1%–2% of normal fetuses (Pilu and Hobbins, 2002).

Recognition of the lemon and banana signs has considerably enhanced prenatal sonographic diagnosis and screening for spina bifida in both low- and high-risk populations (Wald, 2000). Examination of the low lumbar sacral region of the spine can sometimes be difficult in the second trimester due to the fetal position and/or maternal obesity, and lesions in this area may be missed. The fetal head is usually more readily visualized, and identification of the cranial and intracranial signs associated with spina bifida should prompt a detailed sonographic examination of the spine (Chitty, 1995).

Following the identification of spina bifida, detailed examination of the fetus should be performed to look for other signs that may indicate an associated chromosomal or genetic syndrome. In addition, ultrasound can be used to find evidence of neurological damage such as talipes or a dilated renal tract. Karyotyping should be offered when

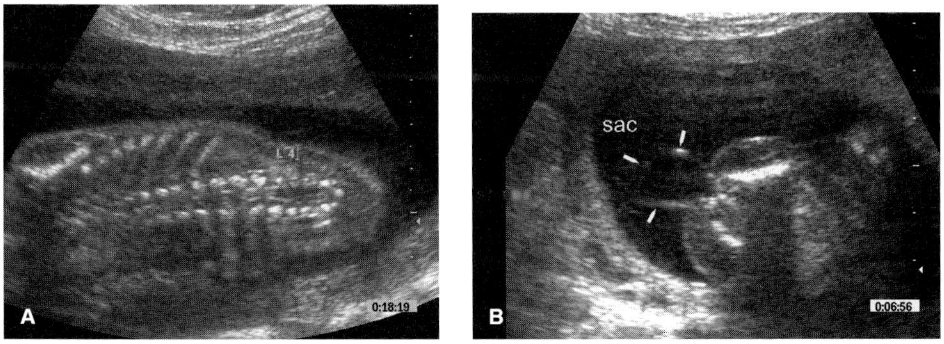

FIGURE 9.5. Ultrasound images of a fetus with a lumbar open spina bifida. (*a*) Coronal view of the fetal spine showing splaying of lumbosacral vertebrae. (*b*) Transverse section through the fetal pelvis showing the dorsally protruding sac and U-shaped vertebral body.

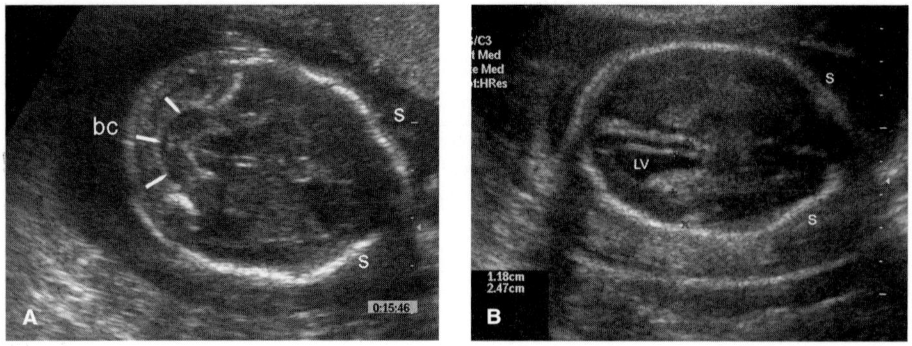

FIGURE 9.6. Cranial and intracranial ultrasound signs seen in association with open spina bifida. (*a*) Transverse section of the fetal head at the level of the cavum septum pellucidum (csp) anteriorly and cerebellum posteriorly showing scalloped frontal bones (s) creating the lemon sign and the curved cerebellum (bc) demonstrating the banana sign. (*b*) Transverse section of the fetal head at the level of the lateral ventricles showing a lemon-shaped head and dilatation of the lateral cerebral ventricles.

other abnormalities are detected or other risk factors such as older maternal age are present. In an analysis of 200 fetuses with neural tube defects, 6.5% had chromosomal abnormalities. However, the absence of associated sonographic abnormalities was not necessarily predictive of a normal karyotype, with 2.4% of fetuses in this category having a chromosomal abnormality. Conversely, 72% of fetuses with additional findings on ultrasound had normal chromosomes. When classified according to the site of the neural tube defect, 2.3% of anencephalics, 7.1% of encephaloceles, and 10.2% of myelomeningoceles had an abnormal karyotype (Kennedy et al., 1998).

The prognostic value of prenatal sonographic features of open spina bifida has not been established but is likely to gain importance as fetal surgery is investigated. Postnatally determined lesion levels have correlated with functional status and survival, and limited data has suggested that prenatal sonographic determination of lesion level is useful in predicting the ambulatory potential of fetuses with open spina bifida (Hunt and Poulton, 1995; Biggio et al., 2001). The following landmarks may be helpful in assessing the level of involvement. In the second trimester, the last sacral ossification center is S4 and in the third trimester it is S5. T12 can be localized by identifying the last ribs; alternatively, the site of the lesion can be estimated by counting upward from the tip of the sacrum. Kollias et al. (1992) reported an accurate sonographic estimation of the level of the spinal defect to within one spinal segment in 79% of the 28 cases reviewed. In general, the prognosis is worse the higher and larger the lesion and in the presence of associated abnormalities. Normal fetal lower limb movements and an intact urinary tract appear to have little prognostic value (Lorber, 1971).

THREE-DIMENSIONAL ULTRASOUND

Three-dimensional (3-D) ultrasound has potential advantages over two-dimensional (2-D) ultrasound for imaging of the fetal spine and vertebral column. This is due to the ability of 3-D ultrasound to present the fetal spine as a continuous structure rather than as independent 2-D views (Johnson et al., 1997a). In addition, 3-D volume data sets of fetal spinal anatomy can be stored and manipulated for further analysis at a later date.

Translating the 3-D potential for improved visualization over current 2-D techniques into practical benefits for the diagnosis and management of neural tube defects, however, is yet to be established. Predicting the level of the spinal defect with 3-D ultrasound at least appears to correlate well with the 2-D technique (Lee et al., 2002). In addition, 3-D ultrasound imaging of a neural tube defect may be helpful in describing the anomaly when counseling parents. While it is likely that 3-D ultrasound will become a complementary imaging modality for the assessment of neural tube defects, further studies are required to examine the diagnostic accuracy, efficiency, and cost-effectiveness of this technology.

FETAL MAGNETIC RESONANCE IMAGING

As interest in fetal surgery for open spina bifida has increased, so has the need for more detailed information from imaging of the fetal brain and spine. While ultrasound continues to be the first-line modality of choice for fetal assessment, magnetic resonance imaging (MRI) may provide additional information in some specific areas. Evaluation of the fetal central nervous system by ultrasound can sometimes be limited by technical factors such as maternal obesity and fetal ossification, both of which can obscure visualization. Magnetic resonance imaging allows for direct and multiplanar views of fetal intracranial anatomy, which can improve visualization of the posterior fossa in cases of Chiari II malformation and to help demonstrate extremely low open spinal defects (Mangels et al., 2000; Levine, 2002). Serial fetal MRI has been used to demonstrate improvement in hindbrain herniation following fetal surgery for spina bifida (Sutton et al., 1999). Additional information may also be gained with MRI evaluation of cephaloceles, which may be important for counseling and preparation prior to delivery (Levine, 2002; Breysem et al., 2003).

The progress made in the detection of fetuses with neural tube defects has been a public health success. The initial MSAFP screening studies developed in England in the 1970s have become a model for other population screening programs used worldwide. Invasive procedures using biochemical tests to detect neural tube defects have now largely been replaced by high-resolution ultrasound. Ultrasound technology combined with improved knowledge of the disorder has progressed to enable the possibility of direct diagnostic ultrasound for both the screening and diagnosis of neural tube defects. The future holds the hope of even better and more accurate diagnostic ability with the further development of 3-D and four-dimensional ultrasound and the use of additional modalities such as MRI.

REFERENCES

Alfirevic Z, Sundberg K, Brigham S (2003). Amniocentesis and chorionic villus sampling for prenatal diagnosis. Cochrane Database Syst Rev 3:CD003252.

Baird PA, Sadovnick AD (1984). Survival in infants with anencephaly. Clin Pediatr (Phila) 23:268–271.

Becker R, Mende B, Stiemer B, Entezami M (2000). Sonographic markers of exencephaly at 9 $^{+3}$ weeks of gestation. Ultrasound Obstet Gynecol 16:582–584.

Bernard JP, Suarez B, Rambaud C, Muller F, Ville Y (1997). Prenatal diagnosis of neural tube defect before 12 weeks' gestation: direct and indirect ultrasonographic semeiology. Ultrasound Obstet Gynecol 10:406–409.

Biggio JR Jr, Owen J, Wenstrom KD, Oakes WJ (2001). Can prenatal ultrasound findings predict ambulatory status in fetuses with open spina bifida? Am J Obstet Gynecol 185:1016–1020.

Birnbacher R, Messerschmidt AM, Pollak AP (2002). Diagnosis and prevention of neural tube defects. Curr Opin Urol 12:461–464.

Blaas HG, Eik-Nes SH, Isaksen CV (2000). The detection of spina bifida before 10 gestational weeks using two- and three-dimensional ultrasound. Ultrasound Obstet Gynecol 16:25–29.

Blumenfeld Z, Siegler E, Bronshtein M (1993). The early diagnosis of neural tube defects. Prenat Diagn 13:863–871.

Bock JL (1992). Current issues in maternal serum alpha-fetoprotein screening. Am J Clin Pathol 97:541–554.

Bonham JR, Dale G, Atack JR (1987). Neural tube defect–specific acetylcholinesterase: its properties and quantitation in the detection of anencephaly and spina bifida. Clin Chim Acta 70:69–77.

Botto LD, Moore CA, Khoury MJ, Erickson JD (1999). Neural-tube defects. N Engl J Med 41:1509–1519.

Braithwaite JM, Armstrong MA, Economides DL (1996). Assessment of fetal anatomy at 12 to 13 weeks of gestation by transabdominal and transvaginal sonography. Br J Obstet Gynaecol 103:82–85.

Breysem L, Bosmans H, Dymarkowski S, Schoubroeck DV, Witters I, Deprest J, Demaerel P, et al (2003). The value of fast MR imaging as an adjunct to ultrasound in prenatal diagnosis. Eur Radiol. Published online DOI 10.1007/s00330-002-1811-6.

Brock DJH, Sutcliffe RG (1972). Alpha-fetoprotein in the antenatal diagnosis of anencephaly and spina bifida. Lancet 2:197–199.

Brown MS, Sheridan-Pereira M (1992). Outlook for the child with a cephalocele. Pediatrics 90:914–919.

Buisson O, De Keersmaecker B, Senat MV, Bernard JP, Moscoso G, Ville Y (2002). Sonographic diagnosis of spina bifida at 12 weeks: heading towards indirect signs. Ultrasound Obstet Gynecol 19:290–292.

Burton BK, Sowers SG, Nelson LH (1983). Maternal serum alpha-fetoprotein screening in North Carolina: experience with more than twelve thousand pregnancies. Am J Obstet Gynecol 146:439–444.

Campbell S, Johnstone FD, Holt EM, May P (1972). Anencephaly: early ultrasonic diagnosis and active management. Lancet 2:1226–1227.

Chan A, Robertson EF, Haan EA, Ranieri E, Keane RJ (1995). The sensitivity of ultrasound and serum alpha-fetoprotein in population-based antenatal screening for neural tube defects. South Australia 1986–1991. Br J Obstet Gynaecol 102:370–376.

Chatzipapas IK, Whitlow BJ, Economides DL (1999). The "Mickey Mouse" sign and the diagnosis of anencephaly in early pregnancy. Ultrasound Obstet Gynecol 13:196–199.

Chervenak FA, Isaacson G, Mahoney MJ, Berkowitz RL, Tortora M, Hobbins JC (1984). Diagnosis and management of fetal cephalocele. Obstet Gynecol 64:86–91.

Chitty LS (1995). Ultrasound screening for fetal abnormalities [see comments]. Prenat Diagn 15:1241–1257.

Cowan LS, Phelps-Sandall B, Hanson FW, Peterson AG, Tennant FR (1989). A prenatal diagnostic center's first-year experience with the California alpha-fetoprotein screening program. Am J Obstet Gynecol 160:1496–1503.

Cragan JD, Roberts HE, Edmonds LD, Khoury MJ, Kirby RS, Shaw GM, Velie EM, et al (1995). Surveillance for anencephaly and spina bifida and the impact of prenatal diagnosis—United States, 1985–1994. Morb Mortal Wkly Rep 44:1–13.

Date I, Yagyu Y, Asari S, Ohmoto T (1993). Long-term outcome in surgically treated spina bifida cystica. Surg Neurol 40:471–475.

David DJ, Proudman TW (1989). Cephaloceles: classification, pathology, and management. World J Surg 13:349–357.

David TJ, Nixon A (1976). Congenital malformations associated with anencephaly and iniencephaly. J Med Genet 13:263–265.

Dogan MM, Ekici E, Yapar EG, Soysal ME, Soysal SK, Gokmen O (1996). Iniencephaly: sonographic–pathologic correlation of 19 cases. J Perinat Med 24:501–511.

Filly RA, Callen PW, Goldstein RB (1993). Alpha-fetoprotein screening programs: what every obstetric sonologist should know. Radiology 188:1–9

Green JJ, Hobbins JC (1988). Abdominal ultrasound examination of the first-trimester fetus. Am J Obstet Gynecol 159:165–175.

Habib ZA (1977). Maternal serum alpha-fetoprotein: its value in antenatal diagnosis of genetic disease and obstetrical-gynaecological care. Acta Obstet Gynecol Scand (Suppl 61):1–92.

Haddow JE (1990). Prenatal screening for open neural tube defects, Down's syndrome, and other major fetal disorders. Semin Perinatol 14:488–503.

Haddow JE, Kloza EM, Knight GJ, Smith DE (1981). Relation between maternal weight and serum alpha-fetoprotein concentration during the second trimester. Clin Chem 27:133–134.

Hahn YS (1995). Open myelomeningocele. Neurosurg Clin North Am 6:231–241.

Hall JG, Solehdin F (1998). Genetics of neural tube defects. Ment Retard Dev Disabil Res Rev 4:269–281

Hidalgo H, Bowie J, Rosenberg ER, Ram PC, Ford K, Lipsit E (1982). Review. In utero sonographic diagnosis of fetal cerebral anomalies. Am J Roentgenol 139:143–148.

Hrgovic Z, Pantiz HG, Kurjak A, Jurkovic D (1989). Contribution to the recognition of iniencephaly on the basis of a new case. J Perinat Med 17:375–379.

Hunt G, Poulton A (1995). Open spina bifida: a complete cohort reviewed 25 years after closure. Dev Med Child Neurol 37:19–29.

Johnson DD, Pretorius DH, Riccabona M, Budorick NE, Nelson TR (1997a). Three-dimensional ultrasound of the fetal spine. Obstet Gynecol 89:434–438.

Johnson SP, Sebire NJ, Snijders RJ, Tunkel S, Nicolaides KH (1997b). Ultrasound screening for anencephaly at 10–14 weeks of gestation. Ultrasound Obstet Gynecol 9:14–16.

Kennedy D, Chitayat D, Winsor EJ, Silver M, Toi A (1998). Prenatally diagnosed neural tube defects: ultrasound, chromosome, and autopsy or postnatal findings in 212 cases. Am J Med Genet 77:317–321.

Kollias SS, Goldstein RB, Cogen PH, Filly RA (1992). Prenatally detected myelomeningoceles: sonographic accuracy in estimation of the spinal level. Radiology 185:109–112.

Lee W, Chaiworapongsa T, Romero R, Williams R, McNie B, Johnson A, Treadwell M, et al (2002). A diagnostic approach for the evaluation of spina bifida by three-dimensional ultrasonography. J Ultrasound Med 21:619–626.

Lemire RJ (1988). Neural tube defects. JAMA 259:558–562.

Levine D (2002). MR imaging of fetal central nervous system abnormalities. Brain Cogn 50:432–448.

Lorber J (1971). Results of treatment of myelomeningocele. An analysis of 524 unselected cases, with special reference to possible selection for treatment. Dev Med Child Neurol 13:279–303.

Mangels KJ, Tulipan N, Tsao LY, Alarcon J, Bruner JP (2000). Fetal MRI in the evaluation of intrauterine myelomeningocele. Pediatr Neurosurg 32:124–131.

Milunsky A, Jick SS, Bruell CL, MacLaughlin DS, Tsung YK, Jick H, Rothman KJ, et al (1989). Predictive values, relative risks, and overall benefits of high and low maternal serum alpha-fetoprotein screening in singleton pregnancies: new epidemiologic data. Am J Obstet Gynecol 161:291–297.

Mizejewski GJ (2003). Levels of alpha-fetoprotein during pregnancy and early infancy in normal and disease states. Obstet Gynecol Surv 58:804–826.

Mizejewski GJ (2004). Biological roles of alpha-fetoprotein during pregnancy and perinatal development. Exp Biol Med 229:439–463

Monteagudo A, Timor-Tritsch IE (1996). Fetal neurosonography of congenital brain anomalies. In Timor-Tritsch IE, Monteagudo A, Cohen HL (eds): *Ultrasonography of the Prenatal and Neonatal Brain.* Stamford, CT: Appleton and Lange, pp. 148–219.

Morocz I, Szeifert GT, Molnar P, Toth Z, Csecsei K, Papp Z (1986). Prenatal diagnosis and pathoanatomy of iniencephaly. Clin Genet 30:81–86.

Nadel AS, Green JK, Holmes LB, Frigoletto FD Jr, Benacerraf BR (1990). Absence of need for amniocentesis in patients with elevated levels of maternal serum alpha-fetoprotein and normal ultrasonographic examinations. N Engl J Med 323:557–561.

Nicolaides KH, Campbell S, Gabbe SG, Guidetti R (1986). Ultrasound screening for spina bifida: cranial and cerebellar signs. Lancet 2:72–74.

Nyberg DA, Hallesy D, Mahony BS, Hirsch JH, Luthy DA, Hickok D (1990). Meckel-Gruber syndrome. Importance of prenatal diagnosis. J Ultrasound Med 9:691–696.

Nyberg DA, Mack LA, Hirsch J, Mahony BS (1988). Abnormalities of fetal cranial contour in sonographic detection of spina bifida: evaluation of the "lemon" sign. Radiology 167:387–392.

Osborn AG (1994). *Diagnostic Neuroradiology: Normal Anatomy and Congenital Anomalies of the Spine and Spinal Cord.* St Louis: Mosby-Year Book, pp. 799–807.

Penso C, Redline RW, Benacerraf BR (1987). A sonographic sign which predicts which fetuses with hydrocephalus have an associated neural tube defect. J Ultrasound Med 6:307–311.

Peralta CF, Bunduki V, Plese JP, Figueiredo EG, Miguelez J, Zugaib M (2003). Association between prenatal sonographic findings and post-natal outcomes in 30 cases of isolated spina bifida aperta. Prenat Diagn 23:311–314.

Pilu G, Hobbins JC (2002). Sonography of fetal cerebrospinal anomalies. Prenat Diagn 22:321–330.

Pomerance JJ, Morrison A, Williams RL, Schifrin BS (1989). Anencephalic infants: life expectancy and organ donation. J Perinatol 9:33–37.

Rasmussen Loft AG, Nanchahal K, Cuckle HS, Wald NJ, Hulten M, Leedham P, Norgaard-Pedersen B (1990). Amniotic fluid acetylcholinesterase in the prenatal diagnosis of open neural tube defects and abdominal wall defects: a comparison of gel electrophoresis and a monoclonal antibody immunoassay. Prenat Diagn 10:449–459.

Reichler A, Hume RF Jr, Drugan A, Bardicef M, Isada NB, Johnson MP, Evans MI (1994).

Risk of anomalies as a function of level of elevated maternal serum alpha-fetoprotein. Am J Obstet Gynecol 171:1052–1055.

Richards CG (1992). Frontoethmoidal meningoencephalocele: a common and severe congenital abnormality in South East Asia. Arch Dis Child 67:717–719.

Roberts CJ, Evans KT, Hibbard BM, Laurence KM, Roberts EE, Robertson IB (1983). Diagnostic effectiveness of ultrasound in detection of neural tube defects. The South Wales experience of 2509 scans (1977–1982) in high-risk mothers. Lancet 2:1068–1069.

Sahid S, Sepulveda W, Dezerega V, Gutierrez J, Rodriguez L, Corral E (2000). Iniencephaly: prenatal diagnosis and management. Prenat Diagn 20:202–205.

Salamanca A, Gonzalez-Gomez F, Padilla MC, Sabatel RM, Camara M, Cuadros JL (1992). Prenatal ultrasound semiography of anencephaly: sonographic–pathological correlations. Ultrasound Obstet Gynecol 2:95–100.

Seppala M, Rapola J, Huttunen NP, Aula P, Karjalainen O, Ruoslahti E (1976). Congenital nephrotic syndrome: prenatal diagnosis and genetic counselling by estimation of aminotic-fluid and maternal serum alpha-fetoprotein. Lancet 2:123–125.

Sepulveda W, Donaldson A, Johnson RD, Davies G, Fisk NM (1995). Are routine alpha-fetoprotein and acetylcholinesterase determinations still necessary at second-trimester amniocentesis? Impact of high-resolution ultrasonography. Obstet Gynecol 85:107–112.

Sutton LN, Adzick NS, Bilaniuk LT, Johnson MP, Crombleholme TM, Flake AW (1999). Improvement in hindbrain herniation demonstrated by serial fetal magnetic resonance imaging following fetal surgery for myelomeningocele. JAMA 282:1826–1831.

Tabor A, Philip J, Madsen M, Bang J, Obel EB, Norgaard-Pedersen B (1986). Randomised controlled trial of genetic amniocentesis in 4606 low-risk women. Lancet 1:1287–1293.

Thiagarajah S, Henke J, Hogge WA, Abbitt PL, Breeden N, Ferguson JE (1990). Early diagnosis of spina bifida: the value of cranial ultrasound markers. Obstet Gynecol 76:54–57.

Timor-Tritsch IE, Greenebaum E, Monteagudo A, Baxi L (1996). Exencephaly-anencephaly sequence: proof by ultrasound imaging and amniotic fluid cytology. J Matern Fetal Med 5:182–185.

Van den Hof MC, Nicolaides KH, Campbell J, Campbell S (1990). Evaluation of the lemon and banana signs in one hundred thirty fetuses with open spina bifida. Am J Obstet Gynecol 162:322–327.

Wald N (2000). Neural tube defects. In Wald N, Leck I (eds): *Antenatal and Neonatal Screening,* 2nd ed. Oxford: Oxford University Press, pp. 61–84.

Wald NJ, Brock DJH, Bonnar J (1974). Prenatal diagnosis of spina bifida and anencephaly by maternal serum alpha-fetoprotein measurement. A controlled study. Lancet 1:765–767.

Wald NJ, Cuckle HS, Barlow RD, Smith AD, Stirrat GM, Turnbull AC, Bobrow M, et al (1980a). Early antenatal diagnosis of exomphalos. Lancet 1:1368–1369.

Wald N, Cuckle H, Boreham J, Stirrat G (1980b). Small biparietal diameter of fetuses with spina bifida: implications for antenatal screening. Br J Obstet Gynaecol 87:219–221.

Wald N, Cuckle H, Boreham J, Turnbull AC (1982). Effect of estimating gestational age by ultrasound cephalometry on the specificity of alpha-fetoprotein screening for open neural-tube defects. Br J Obstet Gynaecol 89:1050–1053.

Wald NJ, Cuckle H, Brock JH, Peto R, Polani PE, Woodford FP (1977). Maternal serum-alpha-fetoprotein measurement in antenatal screening for anencephaly and spina bifida in early pregnancy. Report of U.K. collaborative study on alpha-fetoprotein in relation to neural-tube defects. Lancet 1:1323–1332.

Wald N, Cuckle H, Nanchahal K (1989). Amniotic fluid acetylcholinesterase measurement in the prenatal diagnosis of open neural tube defects. Second report of the Collaborative Acetylcholinesterase Study. Prenat Diagn 9:813–829.

Wald NJ, Hackshaw AK, Cuckle HS (2000). Maternal serum alphafetoprotein screening for open neural tube defects: revised statistical parameters. BJOG 107:296–298.

Watson WJ, Chescheir NC, Katz VL, Seeds JW (1991). The role of ultrasound in evaluation of patients with elevated maternal serum alpha-fetoprotein: a review. Obstet Gynecol 78:123–128.

Wilkins-Haug L, Freedman W (1991). Progression of exencephaly to anencephaly in the human fetus—an ultrasound perspective. Prenat Diagn 11:227–233.

Wilson RD (2000). Amniocentesis and chorionic villus sampling. Curr Opin Obstet Gynecol 12:81–86.

Wininger SJ, Donnenfeld AE (1994). Syndromes identified in fetuses with prenatally diagnosed cephaloceles. Prenat Diagn 14:839–843.

III

Epidemiology of Neural Tube Defects

10

Methodological Issues in the Study of Neural Tube Defects

RUSSELL S. KIRBY

The design and conduct of epidemiologic investigations into the etiology of neural tube defects (NTDs) requires attention to several methodological issues. While some of these issues are common to perinatal research, others are more specific to the epidemiology of birth defects in general and NTDs in particular. In this chapter, we begin by examining some methodological issues associated with assessment of the occurrence of NTDs, followed by a discussion of methodological issues specific to the study of NTDs using the major epidemiologic study designs.

ASSESSING THE OCCURRENCE OF NEURAL TUBE DEFECTS

Completeness of Case Ascertainment

An issue common to all epidemiologic studies of NTDs is the completeness of case ascertainment. This involves several distinct yet overlapping aspects, including the choice of case definition and the methods of clinical/diagnostic evaluation, the types of data sources used, and case ascertainment methods.

What cases should be included in an epidemiologic analysis, and how should they be identified or diagnosed? All cases classified as NTDs should be rigorously evaluated using established clinical criteria. Some administrative data sources contain diagnosis codes created for administrative purposes that may not reflect an accurate assessment of the case. Of special concern is the location of the lesion on the spine; the International Classification of Diseases, Version 9, Clinical Modification (ICD-9-CM) codes do not differentiate between high and low lesions, nor do they identify the size or complexity of the lesion. If the data are acquired from a hospital labor and delivery database or vital statistics, they most likely include only live birth or possibly fetal death events. Cases terminated antenatally, through induced or spontaneous abortion, will be lost. For many birth defects this is not a major issue, but several recent European and North American studies have examined the rate of prenatal diagnosis for NTDs overall, or specific to anencephaly and spina bifida, and found it to be considerable. Stoll et al. (2001, 2002) found that the prenatal diagnosis rate for anencephaly was 96.4% with a pregnancy termination rate of 73.2%; for spina bifida the rates were 68.6% and 40.7%, respectively. Two recent American studies found 74% of NTDs diagnosed antenatally, with 48% terminated in Hawaii during 1986–97 (Forrester and Merz, 2000), and 36% of all pregnancies affected by NTDs found in Utah were terminated during 1990–2000 (Feldkamp et al., 2002). In examining trends over time, researchers must consider secular changes in beliefs and attitudes concerning prenatal diagnosis and elective termination of pregnancies, improvements in diagnostic technologies and incorporation of these procedures into routine obstetrical care, differences in population genetics, diet, government policies concerning fortification of food supplies with folic acid, and a host of environmental factors. In a recent study, Morris and Wald (1999) estimated that the 96% decline in the prevalence of NTDs in England and Wales from 1970 to 1997 could be apportioned, with 40% due to prenatal diagnosis and termination and 56% due to the secular decline in incidence. Cross-national or subnational comparisons may be invalid if the studies are based on registries or case-ascertainment approaches that use different methods for identifying cases diagnosed prenatally or terminated electively. Williams et al.

(2002) illustrated this point in examining recent trends in anencephaly and spina bifida across a large number of American state-level surveillance programs. If access to prenatal diagnosis or pregnancy termination services is associated with socioeconomic status, or if decisions about pregnancy termination vary across ethnic or cultural groups, NTD studies based only on liveborn infants may bias observed associations between NTDs and maternal sociodemographic characteristics. More problematic are undetected cases of spontaneous abortion during the first trimester, which might involve NTDs. These cases are not amenable to identification through birth defects surveillance strategies, but could perhaps be tracked in a cohort of women actively seeking pregnancy in a controlled clinical setting.

A second aspect of completeness of case ascertainment involves the types of data sources used for case identification and/or ascertainment. Although the vast majority, perhaps all cases, of NTDs should be diagnosable at delivery, by no means are all cases reported in commonly used administrative health data sources. Watkins et al. (1996) estimated the sensitivity and predictive positive value of birth certificates for identifying anencephaly at 86% and for spina bidifa at 40%, but these data concern liveborn infants only. Greb et al. (1987) examined the reliability and validity of fetal death records in an era prior to routine antenatal diagnosis and found anencephaly correctly reported in only two of three cases (sensitivity of 67%), with a predictive value positive of only 50%. Hospital discharge summaries fare somewhat better (Hexter et al., 1990; Calle and Khoury, 1991), but researchers should remember that neither vital statistics nor hospital discharge databases capture diagnoses made in outpatient settings or at pregnancy termination, and also that hospital discharges do not include separate records describing fetal demise. Although the newborn discharge is a separate reporting event, maternity discharge summaries in cases of stillbirth contain limited data concerning the condition of the fetus or its cause of death. Cases can also be identified through pediatric surgery databases, neonatal intensive care unit databases, clinical genetics centers (both prenatal and pediatric), spinal cord injury registries, and spina bifida clinics and treatment centers.

The value of a multisource approach to case ascertainment of birth defects, including NTDs, cannot be overstated. Case ascertainment methods have been classified in a hierarchy from active case-finding (trained abstracters review medical source documents on site), to passive-aggressive (cases are reported directly to the registry, with quality assurance and regular review of related data sources), to passive-compliant (the registry accepts whatever records it receives, with minimal follow-up or record review), to impassive case-finding (no reports are filed for the purpose of identifying cases, and the registry consists of "cases" identified through record linkage across a variety of administrative and public health program databases). Ideally, the case ascertainment methodology should be active or at least passive-aggressive. Case-finding based on impassive methods, although multisource, is likely to underidentify NTDs systematically. These case ascertainment strategies are defined and compared across the American state birth defects registries as of the late 1990s (Kirby, 2000).

Validity of Case Coding and Classification

Coding and classification methods are another methodological issue affecting all types of study designs for the epidemiology of NTDs. In the United States, birth defects are commonly coded using the ICD-9-CM in hospital discharge and billing claims records, while most birth defects surveillance programs use a modification of the British Paediatric Association classification for birth defects, which is based on the ICD-9-CM with a sixth digit for additional diagnostic detail (BPA-CDC). Death certificates use a less detailed version of the ICD; since 1999 in the United States the ICD-10 has been used, while from 1979 to 1998 the ICD-9 was used. Hoyert (2003) shows the effect of changes in ICD versions on overall rates of birth defect mortality since the 1950s and on mortality for specific types of birth defects in the conversion from ICD-9 to ICD-10. Care must be taken in comparing data from different countries or registries to ensure that coding methods are compatible.

Three conditions are commonly considered to be NTDs: anencephaly, spina bifida, and encephalocele. In addition to the diagnostic heterogeneity surrounding the classification of cases of anencephaly, classification practices can affect the enumeration of spina bifida co-occurring with anencephaly. By convention, anencephaly is reported as all cases of isolated anencephaly (ICD-9-CM 740.0 with no other NTD) or of anencephaly with spina bifida (ICD-9-CM 740.0 with 741.0 or 741.9), while spina bifida counts do not include the cases of anencephaly with spina bifida. This concern may be more apparent than real. In the New York State Congenital Malformations Registry for the period 1983–2000, a total of 390 cases of anencephaly, 1645 cases of spina bifida, and 11 of both were identified. Failure to count the 11 cases as cases of spina bifida results in a decrease of less than 1% in the total number of cases of spina bifida. Also from New York State, for a western region where even more rigorous surveillance of NTDs was conducted for 1990–2002, a total of 89 cases of anencephaly, 126 cases of spina bifida, and 3 of both were identified; again, excluding the cases of both from the spina bifida total affects the total by less than 3% (C. Druschel, personal communications, September 4 and 5, 2003).

There are additional concerns regarding the classification of encephalocele. This condition is coded outside the ICD-9-CM rubric for NTDs (740–741) as an "other congenital anomaly of the central nervous system" (742.0), but it is frequently grouped together with anencephaly and spina bifida for reporting purposes (Mulinare and Erickson, 1997; Siffel et al., 2003). Emerging evidence from secular trends indicates that the prevalence of encephalocele has not declined similarly to spina bifida, suggesting that encephalocele may not be as responsive to folic acid supplementation or fortification (Stevenson et al., 2000). Researchers should evaluate the question of whether encephalocele is a birth defect structurally and etiologically distinct from anencephaly and spina bifida and whether it should not be included in their epidemiologic case definitions for neural tube defects.

Researchers should also consider whether to analyze all NTDs as a group or to conduct their analyses across strata, defined by condition, location of the lesion on the spine (Park et al., 1992), or whether the NTD occurs in isolation or with birth defects affecting other organ systems. Infants or fetuses with complex patterns of birth defects in addition to an NTD may have genetic disorders or syndromes, or could perhaps present new observations that help to identify previously unknown teratogens. Some researchers prefer to separate cases into "isolated" and "multiple" categories to gain additional insights into the roles of risk factors and gene–environment interactions (Khoury et al., 1992, 1994a; Rasmussen et al., 2003). Cases of NTDs may be nonsyndromic as opposed to syndromic in nature or origin. In conducting an epidemiologic study, sufficient clinically descriptive data should be available to classify cases of NTDs into these two categories so that each can be analyzed separately.

Assessment of Maternal Exposures

Another methodological issue in the design of epidemiologic studies of NTDs is the assessment of maternal exposures before and during pregnancy (Gray and Becker, 2000). It is difficult to collect samples for measurement of biomarkers retrospectively, although some substances have half-lives that remain detectable after a pregnancy. When researchers rely on maternal recall, selective bias may result. Prospective data collection methods based on biomonitoring are preferred, and associations identified in retrospective studies should be confirmed with cohort studies where maternal exposures are adequately measured.

Incidence or Prevalence?

Epidemiologists will probably debate the issue of whether NTDs statistics represent incidence or prevalence, and rates or ratios, as long as epidemiologists conduct research and NTDs continue to occur. Researchers making cross-national and even state-to-state comparisons must be wary of differences in the calculation of statistics (Borman and Cryer, 1990) and carefully consider the meaning of their rates and measures. Most birth defects epidemiologists prefer to report population-based statistics as birth prevalence measures, but the term *incidence* is in common usage. Often denominators are incompletely specified and not all cases are included in the numerator. When statistics are compared across jurisdictions, differences in the measurement of both numerator and denominator can lead to erroneous conclusions.

Summary

The implications of these issues for the design, analysis, and interpretation of epidemiologic studies of NTDs vary with the study design and the research hypothesis. In the next section, we review the characteristics of the most commonly uses methodological approaches in epidemiologic research and consider the strengths, limitations, and informativeness of each major study design for the study of the descriptive epidemiology, risk factors, and etiology of NTDs.

EPIDEMIOLOGIC STUDY DESIGNS: IMPLICATIONS FOR EPIDEMIOLOGIC RESEARCH ON THE ETIOLOGY AND RISK FACTORS FOR NEURAL TUBE DEFECTS

Epidemiologic research employs both observational and analytical approaches, and most epidemiologic study designs can be found in the research literature on the epidemiology of NTDs. A useful introduction to general design and analytical issues in epidemiologic and clinical research can be found in Hulley et al. (2001). Here we briefly describe each study design, provide some examples involving NTD research, and discuss relevant methodological concerns and problems.

Cross-Sectional and Descriptive Studies

Most descriptive studies of NTDs are derived from population-based surveillance programs or case series. Examples include analyses of trends over time, comparisons across categories of maternal characteristics (maternal age, race/ethnicity, plurality, recurrence of NTDs), and analyses of regional or small area variation in the prevalence of NTDs. Frequently, population-based descriptive studies use cross-sectional study designs (in which events that occur during a specified time interval are analyzed, with exposure and outcome data collected simultaneously). The limitations of cross-sectional study designs are valid for analyses of the descriptive epidemiology of NTDs: the antecedent–consequent relationship between exposure and outcome cannot be determined; bias may be present in the forms of recall bias, selection bias, and survival bias; and direct estimates of risk cannot be made. However, the cross-sectional study is often a useful first step in examining demographic patterns, trends, and prevalence patterns.

A brief comparison of two recent cross-sectional studies of trends in the prevalence of anencephaly and spina bifida in the United States may be instructive. Both Honein et al. (2001) and Williams et al. (2002) examined the effect of folic acid fortification on the population-based prevalence of these conditions, the former study using primarily birth certificate data and the latter study relying on data from population-based birth defects surveillance programs. Both studies were designed to monitor the influence of a regulatory change in fortification of the food supply on the prevalence of NTDs, but while the vital statistics study contains national data, its focus on birth events limits its ability to fully calibrate the changes in prevalence of anencephaly and spina bifida.

Case-Control Studies

Case-control studies compare the incidence of risk factors between subjects representative of a disease or health condition (cases) and control subjects representative of the reference population from which the cases are drawn. The basic methods and epidemiologic issues in conducting case-control studies are described in Schlesselman (1982) and Breslow and Day (1980), with supporting details concerning various methodological issues throughout the peer-reviewed epidemiologic literature. Generally, case-control studies of NTDs rely on birth defects surveillance data linked to related databases for the initial identification of cases (e.g., Thompson et al., 2003), although some studies are based on data from a single clinic or hospital source or from hospital-based registries (Werler et al., 1999). The National Birth Defects Prevention Study is a large multistate case-control study that should support testing of a wide range of hypotheses concerning demographic, behavioral, environmental, and genetic risk factors and their association with NTDs and many other birth defects (Yoon et al., 2001; Rasmussen et al., 2003). Case-control studies often involve retrospective data collection, interviews, and collection of biological and occasionally environmental samples. Examples of recent case-control studies concerning risk factors associated with NTDs include a study of the role of vitamin B_{12} (Suarez et al., 2003), studies of the role of paternal occupation (Brender et al., 2002; Shaw et al., 2002), and environmental exposures (e.g., Marshall et al., 1997). Comparatively few studies thus far have examined gene–gene interaction in the etiology of NTDs (e.g., de Franchis et al., 2002); this will be an exciting area for future research.

Case-control studies are a very common epidemiologic study design because they are relatively inexpensive and provide a flexible methodology to test multiple hypotheses. However, the inherently retrospective approach limits the generalizability of study findings, and biomarkers and environmental samples contemporaneous with actual exposures are generally unavailable. Researchers must also take steps to prevent differential reporting bias between parents of cases and controls, and to take care that controls are selected in a manner that ensures that they are drawn from a population with the same opportunity for exposure to putative risk factors as are the cases (Swan et al., 1992; Khoury et al., 1994b). Case-control study designs cannot directly estimate relative risks because they are not based on measures of incidence, and care must be taken to control for recall bias. While care must be taken not to overinterpret the results of case-control studies of risk factors for NTDs, these studies can provide important insights that can be tested further with more definitive research designs.

Two variations on the case-control study design have recently been proposed for birth defects epidemiology. Case-crossover and case-time-control designs (Hernandez-Diaz et al., 2003) may be useful for NTD research. The case-crossover design includes only cases, observed in an at-risk period (case window) and one or more control windows, with exposure frequencies compared between the two windows and with odds ratios calculated on matched subjects. The case-time-control design uses both cases and controls, each measured over the case window and control window. Neither of these designs has been widely used to date, but when used with care they may yield some insights into the role of embryologically sensitive exposures. While the potential of these approaches for studies of NTDs remains to be demonstrated, the narrow time window for exposures during the preconception period and the first weeks of embryonic development appears to be suitable for these study designs.

Cohort and Longitudinal Studies

Cohort studies involve the formation of groups of study participants who are followed prospectively for a specified time interval or until the occurrence of a health event or outcome (Breslow and Day, 1987). In perinatal epidemiology, a classic example is the National Collaborative Perinatal Project (NCPP), in which approximately 60,000 pregnancies were enrolled from 1959 to 1965, with prospective documentation of the pregnancy, neonatal and infant outcomes, and follow-up of the children at ages 7 and 8 (Hardy, 2003; Melnick and Myrianthopoulos, 1987; Myrianthopoulos and Melnick, 1987).

Cohort study designs can model the effect of an exposure on health outcomes. For studies of the etiology of NTDs, it is imperative that study subjects be identified during the preconceptional period, and followed through conception and antenatally to the pregnancy outcome. Cohort studies focusing solely on NTDs are unusual; more commonly, perinatal cohorts are formed to study the broad range of perinatal outcomes.

Randomized Trials and Intervention Studies

Randomized controlled clinical trials are experiments in which study subjects who meet inclusion criteria and provide informed consent are randomized to two or more experimental treatment and control groups. These trials have rarely been conducted to study the effects of treatments on the prevalence of birth defects. However, we do have two classic examples, both involving the use of folic acid supplementation to reduce the birth prevalence of NTDs (MRC, 1991; Czeizel and Dudas, 1992).

Randomized controlled clinical trials examine very specific hypotheses with specific outcomes and require blinding, extensive interaction with study participants including multiple visits, documentation, and follow-up. A similar study design, the community intervention trial, can sometimes be conducted without the need for randomization. An important example, also involving the use of folic acid supplements to reduce the prevalence of NTDs, is the China birth defects study (Berry et al., 1999; Berry and Li, 2002).

Emerging Issues

In using any of these study designs, researchers should consider the potential for gene–gene and gene–environment interactions (Sever, 1995; Botto and Mastroiacovo, 1998) and place their studies in the proper context (Khoury and Dorman, 1998). Many epidemiologic studies are designed to test a primary environmental hypothesis and overlook potential genetic factors, while genetic epidemiologic studies often fail to incorporate data concerning known demographic or environmental risk factors. As with many chronic diseases and perinatal outcomes, when all the pieces of the puzzle of determinants of NTDs are known, the answer is likely to be a combination of these factors.

SUMMARY

In this chapter, we reviewed a series of common methodological issues in the classification and measurement of NTDs, and examined their impact on the design, conduct, and interpretation of the most common epidemiologic study designs for the analysis of these defects. There is no substitute for well-designed scientific methods for this research. However, our studies are only as good as the underlying data sources for cross-sectional and case-control studies, and only as strong as our foresight and diligence in the design and conduct of prospective analyses, including longitudinal or cohort studies, and randomized controlled clinical trials and intervention trials.

REFERENCES

Berry RJ, Li Z (2002). Folic acid alone prevents neural tube defects: evidence from the China study. Epidemiology 13:114–116.

Berry RJ, Li Z, Erickson JD, Li S, Moore CA, Wang H, Mulinare J, Zhao P, Wong LY, Gindler J, Hong SX, Correa A (1999). Prevention of neural-tube defects with folic acid in China. China-U.S. Collaborative Project for Neural Tube Defect Prevention. N Engl J Med 341:1485–1490.

Borman B, Cryer C (1990). Fallacies of international and national comparisons of disease occurrence in the epidemiology of neural tube defects. Teratology 42(4):405–412.

Botto LD, Mastroiacovo P (1998). Exploring gene-gene interactions in the etiology of neural tube defects. Clin Genet 53:456–459.

Brender J, Suarez L, Hendricks K, Baetz RA, Larsen R (2002). Parental occupation and neural tube defect–affected pregnancies among Mexican Americans. J Occup Environ Med 44:650–656.

Breslow NE, Day NE (1980). *Statistical Methods in Cancer Research*, Vol. I. *The Analysis of Case-Control Studies*. Lyon, France: International Agency for Research on Cancer.

Breslow NE, Day NE (1987). *Statistical Methods in Cancer Research*, Vol. II. *The Design and Analysis of Cohort Studies*. Lyon, France: International Agency for Research on Cancer.

Calle EE, Khoury MJ (1991). Completeness of the discharge diagnoses as a measure of birth defects recorded in the hospital medical record. Am J Epidemiol 134:69–77.

Czeizel AE, Dudas I (1992). Prevention of the first occurrence of neural-tube defects by periconceptional vitamin supplementation. N Engl J Med 327:1832–1835.

deFranchis R, Botto LD, Sebastio G, Ricci R, Iolascon A, Capra V, Andria G, Mastroiacovo P (2002). Spina bifida and folate-related genes: a study of gene-gene interactions. Genet Med 4:126–130.

Feldkamp M, Friedrichs M, Carey JC (2002). Decreasing prevalence of neural tube defects in Utah, 1985–2000. Teratology 66 (Suppl 1):S23–S28.

Forrester MB, Merz RD (2000). Prenatal diagnosis and elective termination of neural tube defects in Hawaii, 1986–1997. Fetal Diagn Ther 15:146–151.

Gray RH, Becker S (2000). Selected topics in the epidemiology of reproductive outcomes. Epidemiol Rev 22:71–5.

Greb AE, Pauli RM, Kirby RS (1987). Accuracy of fetal death reports: comparison with data from an independent stillbirth assessment program. Am J Public Health 77:1202–1206.

Hardy JB (2003). The Collaborative Perinatal Project: lessons and legacy. Ann Epidemiol 13:303–311.

Hernández-Díaz S, Hernán MA, Meyer K, Werler MM, Mitchell AA (2003). Case-crossover and case-time-control designs in birth defects epidemiology. Am J Epidemiol 158:385–391.

Hexter AC, Harris JA, Roeper P, Croen LA, Krueger P, Gant D (1990). Evaluation of the hospital discharge diagnoses index and the birth certificate as sources of information on birth defects. Public Health Rep 105:296–307.

Honein MA, Paulozzi LJ, Mathews TJ, Erickson JD, Wong LY (2001). Impact of folic acid fortification of the U.S. food supply on the occurrence of neural tube defects. JAMA 285:2981–2986.

Hoyert DL (2003). Mortality associated with birth defects: influence of successive disease classification revisions. Birth Defects Res (Pt A) 67:651–655.

Hulley SB, Cummings SR, Browner WS, Grady D, Hearst N, Newman TB (2001). *Designing Clinical Research,* 2nd ed. Philadelphia: Lippincott Williams & Wilkins.

Khoury MJ, Botto L, Mastroiacovo P, Skaerven R, Castilla EE, Erickson JD (1994a). Monitoring for multiple congenital anomalies: an international perspective. Epidemiol Rev 16:335–350.

Khoury MJ, Dorman JS (1998). The Human Genome Epidemiology Network. Am J Epidemiol 148:1–3.

Khoury MJ, James LM, Erickson JD (1994b). On the use of affected controls to address recall bias in case-control studies of birth defects. Teratology 49:273–281.

Khoury MJ, Moore CA, James LM, Cordero JF (1992). The interaction between dsymorphology and epidemiology: methodologic issues of lumping and splitting. Teratology 45:133–138.

Kirby RS (2000). Analytical resources for assessment of clinical genetics services in public health: current status and future prospects. Teratology 61:9–16.

Marshall EG, Gensburg LJ, Deres SA, Geary NS, Cayo MR (1997). Maternal residential exposure to hazardous wastes and risk of central nervous system and musculoskeletal birth defects. Arch Environ Health 52:416–425.

Melnick M, Myrianthopoulos NC (1987). Studies in neural tube defects. II. Pathologic findings in a prospectively collected series of anencephalics. Am J Med Genet 26:797–810.

Morris JK, Wald NJ (1999). Quantifying the decline in the birth prevalence of neural tube defects in England and Wales. J Med Screen 6:182–185.

MRC Vitamin Study Research Group (1991). Prevention of neural tube defects: results of the Medical Research Council Vitamin Study. Lancet 338:131–137.

Mulinare J, Erickson JD (1997). Prevention of neural tube defects. Teratology 56:17–18.

Myrianthopoulos NC, Melnick M (1987). Studies in neural tube defects. I. Epidemiologic and etiologic aspects. Am J Med Genet 26:783–796.

Park CH, Stewart W, Khoury MJ, Mulinare J (1992). Is there etiologic heterogeneity between upper and lower neural tube defects? Am J Epidemiol 136:1493–1501.

Rasmussen SA, Olney RS, Holmes LB, Lin AE, Keppler-Noreuil KM, Moore CA and the National Birth Defects Prevention Study (2003). Guidelines for case classification for the National Birth Defects Prevention Study. Birth Defects Res (Pt A) 67:193–201.

Schlesselman JJ (1982). *Case-Control Studies: Design, Conduct, Analysis.* New York: Oxford University Press.

Sever LE (1995). Looking for causes of neural tube defects: where does the environment fit in? Environ Health Perspect 103 (Suppl 6):165–171.

Shaw GM, Nelson V, Olshan AF (2002). Paternal occupational group and risk of offspring with neural tube defects. Paediatr Perinatal Epidemiol 16:328–333.

Siffel C, Wong LC, Olney RS, Correa A (2003). Survival of infants diagnosed with encephalocele in Atlanta, 1979–1998. Paediatr Perinatal Epidemiol 17:40–48.

Stevenson RE, Allen WP, Pai GS, Best R, Seaver LH, Dean J, Thompson S (2000). Decline in prevalence of neural tube defects in a high-risk region of the United States. Pediatrics 106:677–683.

Stoll C, Alembik Y, Dott B, Roth MP (2002). Impact of prenatal diagnosis on livebirth prevalence of children with congenital anomalies. Ann Genet 45:115–121.

Stoll C, Tenconi R, Clementi M, and the Euroscan Study Group (2001). Detection of congenital anomalies by fetal ultrasonographic examination across Europe. Commun Genet 4:225–232.

Suarez L, Hendricks K, Felkner M, Gunter E (2003). Maternal serum B_{12} levels and risk for neural tube defects in a Texas-Mexico border population. Ann Epidemiol 13:81–88.

Swan SH, Shaw GM, Schulman J (1992). Reporting and selection bias in case-control studies of congenital malformations. Epidemiology 3:356–363.

Thompson SJ, Torres ME, Stevenson RE, Dean JH, Best RG (2003). Periconceptional multivitamin folic acid use, dietary folate, total folate and risk of neural tube defects in South Carolina. Ann Epidemiol 13:412–418.

Watkins ML, Edmonds L, McClearn A, Mullins L, Mulinare J, Khoury M (1996). The surveillance of birth defects: the usefulness of the revised U.S. standard birth certificate. Am J Public Health 86:731–734.

Werler MM, Hayes C, Louik C, Shapiro S, Mitchell AA (1999). Multivitamin supplementation and risk of birth defects. Am J Epidemiol 150:675–682.

Williams LJ, Mai CT, Edmonds LD, Shaw GM, Kirby RS, Hobbs CA, Sever LE, Miller LA, Meaney FJ, Levitt M (2002). Prevalence of spina bifida and anencephaly during the transition to mandatory folic acid fortification in the United States. Teratology 66:33–39.

Yoon PW, Rasmussen SA, Lynberg MC, Moore CA, Anderka M, Carmichael SL, Costa P, Druschel C, Hobbs CA, Romitti PA, Langlois PH, Edmonds LD (2001). The National Birth Defects Prevention Study. Public Health Rep 116:32–40.

11

Birth Defects Surveillance Systems and Neural Tube Defects

LOWELL E. SEVER

Birth defects surveillance programs, particularly in Europe and the United States, developed following the recognition of the teratogenicity of thalidomide. The argument was that if there had been a routine way of monitoring the occurrence of birth defects, the introduction of a drug or any other environmental agent that caused abnormal development would have been recognized earlier than through the observations of alert practitioners. Acceptance of this premise continues; the introduction of the Birth Defects Prevention Act of 1998 included the justification that the presence of a birth defects surveillance program in Texas would have alerted the medical community to an "epidemic" of anencephaly in the Lower Rio Grande Valley earlier than occurred through the observations of an alert nurse. Supposedly, had there been an earlier recognition of the epidemic, something could have been done to stop it. While the logic of this premise holds, birth defects surveillance programs have yet to be the first to identify a new teratogen, and investigations of birth defect clusters identified through surveillance have yet to establish a responsible agent. Indeed, it has been argued (Khoury and Holtzman, 1987) that surveillance systems are inefficient in detecting even powerful teratogens and that the alert clinician is still a more important early warning system than a surveillance system. Clearly, there must be other reasons for conducting birth defects surveillance; there are.

During the past decade, recognition of multiple reasons to conduct birth defects surveillance has grown. It is useful to begin with the definition of public health or epidemiologic surveillance established by the United States Centers for Disease Control and Prevention (CDC). As "the Nation's public health agency," the CDC plays key roles in the practice of public health in the United States and in other parts of the world. The CDC (1988) defines public health surveillance as

> [t]he ongoing, systematic collection, analysis, and interpretation of health data essential to the planning, implementation and evaluation of public health practice, closely integrated with the timely dissemination of these data to those who need to know. The final link of the surveillance chain is the application of these data to prevention and control. A surveillance system includes a functional capacity for data collection, analysis, and dissemination linked to public health programs.

This chapter addresses issues of neural tube defects (NTDs) from the perspective of public health surveillance. We begin with a brief consideration of epidemiologic aspects of expressing measures of disease occurrence. The design of birth defects surveillance programs will be discussed briefly, along with the general functions programs fulfill and how data are used. Case definition and methods used to ascertain (identify) cases will be considered in some detail, followed by a brief discussion of measures of occurrence for birth defects that grow out of the ascertainment of cases and the population defined to be at risk. The chapter closes with a consideration of applications of these measures and the role of surveillance in prevention and the evaluation of prevention interventions.

TERMINOLOGY ON MEASURES OF OCCURRENCE

There is considerable confusion in the terminology surrounding presentation of data on the occurrence of birth defects. In epidemiology two basic measures, incidence and prevalence, are used to describe the frequency of disease. The simplest definition of incidence is that it is the "number of new cases of a disease that occur during specified period of time in a population at risk of developing the disease" (Gordis, 2000). Sometimes incidence is expressed as a rate that brings in a time dimension for being at risk. Prevalence, on the other hand, is defined as the "number of affected persons present in the population at a specific time divided by the number of persons in the population at that time" (Gordis, 2000). While there are a number of nuances with respect to these terms, which provide fodder for students and practitioners of epidemiology, most simply put, incidence can be expressed in the form of a rate, whereas prevalence is a proportion. Thus, although it is not uncommon to see the use of the term *prevalence rate* (EUROCAT, 2002) or reference to prevalence as *rates* (National Birth Defects Prevention Network, 2002), technically these are not rates but proportions. This chapter uses the term *prevalence* to represent the frequency of occurrence of NTDs in a population. For reasons that have been discussed extensively elsewhere, it is not correct to refer to the *incidence* of most congenital malformations, since neither the number of new cases occurring nor the population at risk is known (Sever, 1983a, 1983b).

DESIGN OF BIRTH DEFECT SURVEILLANCE PROGRAMS

As noted, surveillance for birth defects, including NTDs, can be carried out for many purposes. It is essential that the objectives of a surveillance program be established as one of the initial steps in planning, since different objectives may lead to different system requirements. Common objectives include monitoring trends in occurrence; identifying potential "clusters"; identifying children in need of special health-care and educational services; evaluating the population-based results of primary prevention and prenatal screening programs; and ascertaining cases for epidemiologic studies, particularly for case-control studies searching for etiologic agents. For any of these objectives, it is essential to define what the population at risk—the population of interest—is, what constitutes a case, how the cases will be ascertained, and what information will be obtained about them.

Since most surveillance systems fulfill many functions, the system must be designed with the most demanding requirements in mind. For example, if the system is established only to identify children with special health-care needs, then the population of interest would include only live births and identifiers would be necessary. If the system is developed to track prevalence, then ideally it would identify cases occurring among live births, fetal deaths, and prenatally diagnosed cases, since, as discussed subsequently, increasing availability of prenatal diagnosis and pregnancy termination can have a dramatic effect on prevalence based solely on births. On the other hand, personal identifiers are not crucial if the interest is only in prevalence and changes in it. If one of the major objectives is to identify clusters, then precise information regarding the mother's residence is important, and ideally, residence early in gestation and not just residence at the time of birth.

COMPARING DISEASE OCCURRENCE

Borman and Cryer (1990) present a very illuminating discussion of "Fallacies of International Comparisons of Disease Occurrence in the Epidemiology of Neural Tube Defects." They address the following points: definition of NTDs, incidence and prevalence, late fetal deaths, secular trends, and ascertainment. With the exception of secular trends, all of these topics are of relevance to routine NTD surveillances.

In a more recent consideration of sources of variability among surveillance systems in birth defects prevalence, Hobbs and colleagues (2001) discuss the potential impact of seven factors on the prevalence of defects included in the 2000 Congenital Malformations Surveillance Report from the National Birth Defects Prevention Network (NBDPN) (National Birth Defects Prevention Network, 2000). They refer to the surveillance methods used both by EUROCAT and by the state birth defects surveillance programs contributing to the NBDPN report and note that there may be defect-specific differences in impact. The potential sources of variability are:

- Case ascertainment methods
- Case ascertainment sources
- Case inclusion criteria
- Inclusion of elective terminations and stillbirths
- Age limit at time of diagnosis
- Methods of diagnosis confirmation
- Diagnostic precision

The first four of these clearly are relevant to surveillance for NTDs, while the last three may be of less importance.

In birth defects surveillance programs in the United States, approaches to case ascertainment traditionally have been grouped into two general categories: passive and active (Lynberg and Edmonds, 1992). Passive surveillance is based on submission of reports of cases from data sources to the surveillance system. This may include vital records or reporting of case information by staff from hospitals, clinics, or other sources. The key feature of passive systems is that the actual case ascertainment is not done by surveillance program staff; some passive programs do have staff carry out case verification. Active surveillance, as the name implies, is based on identification of cases by trained surveillance program staff who actively seek cases in hospitals, clinics, or other sources through systematic review of medical records, specialty clinic logs, discharge indices, and so on. The key difference between passive and active surveillance is who has direct responsibility for case ascertainment (identification): nonprogram versus program staff.

DEFINING CASES OF NEURAL TUBE DEFECTS

An important component of surveillance is to provide data on rates of occurrence in ways that are comparable across time and space. This is essential when one wants to make comparisons of the prevalence of NTDs among pregnancies in one population with the prevalence in another. Populations can be defined as pregnancies among one ethnic group versus another, one geographic location versus another, or one time period versus another. Two things are essential for comparability: the cases (outcomes) are defined similarly, and the cases are ascertained (identified) using similar methods and from comparable populations.

In any epidemiologic study, including a surveillance study, it is important to establish what the outcomes being studied include and how they are defined. This is in addition to defining the population from which the cases come and how they are ascertained. Therefore, there are two key aspects of case definition: what specific malformations are eligible for inclusion and the population from which these eligible cases come. For example, usually individual malformations are coded using a standard classification system such as the International Classification of Diseases (ICD). Based on the ICD Revision 9 Clinical Modification (ICD-9-CM), the broad category "neural tube defects" includes defects with the codes 740 (anencephalus and similar anomalies), 741 (spina bifida, excluding spina bifida occulta), and 742.0 (encephalocele) (International Classification of Diseases, 1998). Note that the three-digit rubrics for ancencephalus and spina bifida subsume all fourth-digit classifications. For anencephalus and similar anomalies, this includes anencephalus, craniorachischisis, and ininecephaly; for spina bifida, it includes spina bifida with hydrocephalus and spina bifida without mention of hydrocephalus. Importantly, the three-digit rubric that includes encephalocele is "other congenital anomalies of the central nervous system." Only one defect in this category, encephalocele (742.0), is an NTD. Other central nervous system malformations are included in this three-digit rubric, two of which (microcephalus, 742.1, and congenital hydrocephalus, 742.3) are relatively common specific abnormalities.

Because of its increased specificity, many surveillance programs are using the British Paediatric Association (BPA) coding system (British Paediatric Association, 1979). As an example, these are definitions used by EUROCAT in their 1991 surveillance report (EUROCAT Working Group, 1991).

> Neural Tube defects include anencephaly (BPA codes: 7400, 7401), encephalocele (BPA code: 7420), spina bifida (BPA code: 741), and iniencephaly (BPA code: 7402). Cases were subdivided into mutually exclusive categories as follows: 1) anencephaly with or without spina bifida including cra-niorachischisis, 2) spina bifida excluding spina bifida occulta and cases associated with anencephaly, encephalocele or iniencephaly, 3) encephalocele excluding cases associated with anencephaly or iniencephaly and 4) iniencephaly excluding cases associated with anencephaly.

In conducting surveillance and reporting prevalence, it is preferable to provide information on the defects individually, that is, to report anencephalus, spina bifida, and encephalocele separately. This way, comparison can be made between the individual defects or NTDs as a group. Often in the older literature there is reference to "central nervous system malformations" as a category, leading to problems in making comparisons to more recent data.

SOURCES OF CASES

The second definitional point was in reference to the population at risk and methods of case ascertainment. Since in many populations cases of anencephalus and spina bifida commonly are diagnosed prenatally, it is essential to be clear about whether these cases are included if the pregnancy is terminated. In addition, defects observed among spontaneous abortions may be included as cases. In both of these instances, the contribution of these cases to the numerator is much more significant than the contribution that either terminated pregnancies or observed spontaneous abortions would make to the denominator used for prevalence.

One should be able to look at the reported prevalence and know precisely what defects are included and the populations from which they came. Data from the surveillance programs participating in EUROCAT (e.g., EUROCAT Working Group, 1997) and the International Clearinghouse for Birth Defects Monitoring Systems (e.g., International Clearinghouse for Birth Defects Monitoring Systems, 2002) are presented in a way that allows determination of the sources of case ascertainment. For EUROCAT, prevalence for each registry is shown for live births plus fetal deaths plus induced abortions, live births plus fetal deaths, and live births. For those registries that do not ascertain terminated cases, the first two prevalences will be identical.

The terminology used by the International Clearinghouse is slightly different. Their annual report (International Clearinghouse for Birth Defects Monitoring Systems, 2002) provides the number of cases of birth defects by each of three pregnancy outcomes: live births, stillbirths, and terminations of pregnancy for birth defects. These data are presented by individual monitoring programs, and prevalence is provided for live births and stillbirths combined and for live births and stillbirths plus terminations of pregnancy. Since in some countries termination of pregnancy for birth defects is not permitted, this allows comparisons to be made among prevalences based on comparable source populations. The report notes, appropriately:

> It is unwise to compare rates of a birth defect among programmes, as there are important differences in the methodology of registration, in defining live births, stillbirths and abortions, including birth defects observed in pregnancy terminations, and last but not least, in defining every single birth defect.

With respect to the United States, in the congenital malformations surveillance report from the NBDPN, state-specific NTD rates (reported as "rates" but really proportions—prevalence) are presented in both tabular and graphic form (National Birth Defects Prevention Network, 2002). In the graphical presentations, the states are organized by three groupings of the pregnancy outcomes on which prevalence was based:

- Live births/stillbirths/spontaneous abortion/elective terminations
- Live births/stillbirths/spontaneous abortion
- Live births only

It is worth noting that there has been extensive discussion in the past regarding the use of the terms *fetal deaths* and *stillbirths* with respect to the reporting of birth defect occurrence, specifically NTDs (Hook 1982, 1983; Sever 1983a, 1983b). The term *fetal death* is preferable, following the suggestions of Gaudino et al. (1994): "Since 1950, the term fetal death has been used in preference to other terms to reflect the adoption of the WHO's recommended definition and to end confusion between the terms stillbirth, abortion, and miscarriage."

USING SURVEILLANCE DATA

Epidemiologic Applications

Common epidemiologic applications of surveillance include monitoring prevalence (EUROCAT Working Group, 1997; Lowry et al., 2000; National Birth Defects Prevention Network, 2002), identifying clusters (Harris and Wynne, 1994; Sever, 1994; Williams et al., 2002a), and serving as a source of cases for etiologic studies (Yoon et al., 2001). Such uses are commonly known and understood, and programs may place different emphases on which ones they carry out. For example, the California Birth Defects Monitoring Program is perhaps best known for the high quality of the etiologic studies that have grown out of their surveillance activities (e.g., Shaw et al., 2002). Similarly, the Metropolitan Atlanta Congenital Defects Program (MACDP) has made important contributions to our understanding of birth defects causes and prevention, such as a case-control study of the role of folic acid in reducing the risk of occurrence of NTDs (Mulinare et al., 1988).

Surveillance to Evaluate the Impact of Folic Acid Education and Fortification

Clearly, one of the most exciting and public health–relevant aspects of the epidemiologic history of NTDs is the recognition of the role of folic acid in reducing the risk. This topic is considered extensively in Chapters 15 and 29. Discussed here are surveillance activities undertaken to evaluate the changes in prevalence at birth during the period in the United States when there was a transition to mandatory folic acid fortification of cereal grains (Honein et al., 2001; Williams et al., 2002b). Reed and Meaney (1988) suggested that surveillance activities can be grouped into three categories: "1) epidemiological, 2) preventative (sic)/planning, and 3) social/educational." The surveillance for NTDs reported by Williams et al. (2002b) actually supports all three of these activities.

Following the introduction of folic acid fortification of cereal grains in the United States, there was interest in attempting to document the impact of this public health intervention on NTD occurrence. The question was addressed by review of birth certificate data by Honein et al. (2001), who compared the birth prevalence of anencephaly and spina bifida before and after fortification. The prevalences of both defects decreased from the prefortification, to the optional, to the mandatory fortification periods; differences between the two defects were observed. The authors note the problems of basing their assessment of the effectiveness of folic acid on NTD occurrence only on cases reported on certificates of live births, given the extensive literature on the impact of prenatal diagnosis on prevalence at birth (e.g., EUROCAT Working Group, 1991; Limb and Holmes, 1994; Cragan et al., 1995; Velie and Shaw, 1996; Ethan and Canfield, 2002). For example, it is not safe to assume that the ratio of terminated to nonterminated cases remains fairly constant from year to year.

To overcome some of the limitations of the Honein et al. (2001) study, the NBDPN, in collaboration with the CDC, undertook an NTD rapid ascertainment surveillance project. The methods and results of the project have been published (Williams et al., 2002a). State-based birth defects surveillance programs were eligible to participate if they could:

- Ascertain NTD cases from sources other than birth certificates.
- Submit date from January 1995 through December 1999 for counts of pregnancies affected by either spina bifida or anencephaly.
- Provide annual prevalences of spina bifida and anencephaly for 1995 and 1996.
- Report data from 1997 to 1999 by quarter of birth, using expected dates of delivery for pregnancy terminations and fetal deaths.

A total of 24 state programs participated in the project. While these states used both active and passive methods of case ascertainment and multiple sources of information, all were able to supply timely data. Of particular importance for this discussion, nine of the programs ascertained prenatally diagnosed NTD cases. The goal of the study was to compare the prevalences of spina bifida and anencephaly by year and quarter for the periods during optional folic acid fortification (1997 through the third quarter of 1998) and mandatory fortification (fourth quarter of 1998 through 1999) with the prevalences before fortification. The results of this study are presented in Figures 11.1 to 11.3. It should be noted that not only are there are important differences in terms of the changes in the rates of spina bifida and anencephaly, but also that the magnitude of these differences is influenced strongly by the inclusion of prenatally ascertained (electively terminated) cases. When the data were stratified by prenatal ascertainment, there was no significant decline in anencephaly prevalence among those programs that did not include prenatally ascertained cases. The declining trend for spina bifida was similar between programs with and without prenatal ascertainment, consistent with earlier suggestions that prenatal diagnosis and subsequent termination of pregnancy occur less frequently in pregnancies affected by spina bifida (Cragan et al., 1995).

These two studies in the United States, and others that have used surveillance data to evaluate the impact of folic acid on the occurrence of NTDs, provide two important lessons: first, the necessity of including prenatally diagnosed cases when measuring trends, and, second, the fact that there may be etiological differences between anencephaly and spina bifida, leading to differences in the effectiveness of folic acid in their prevention.

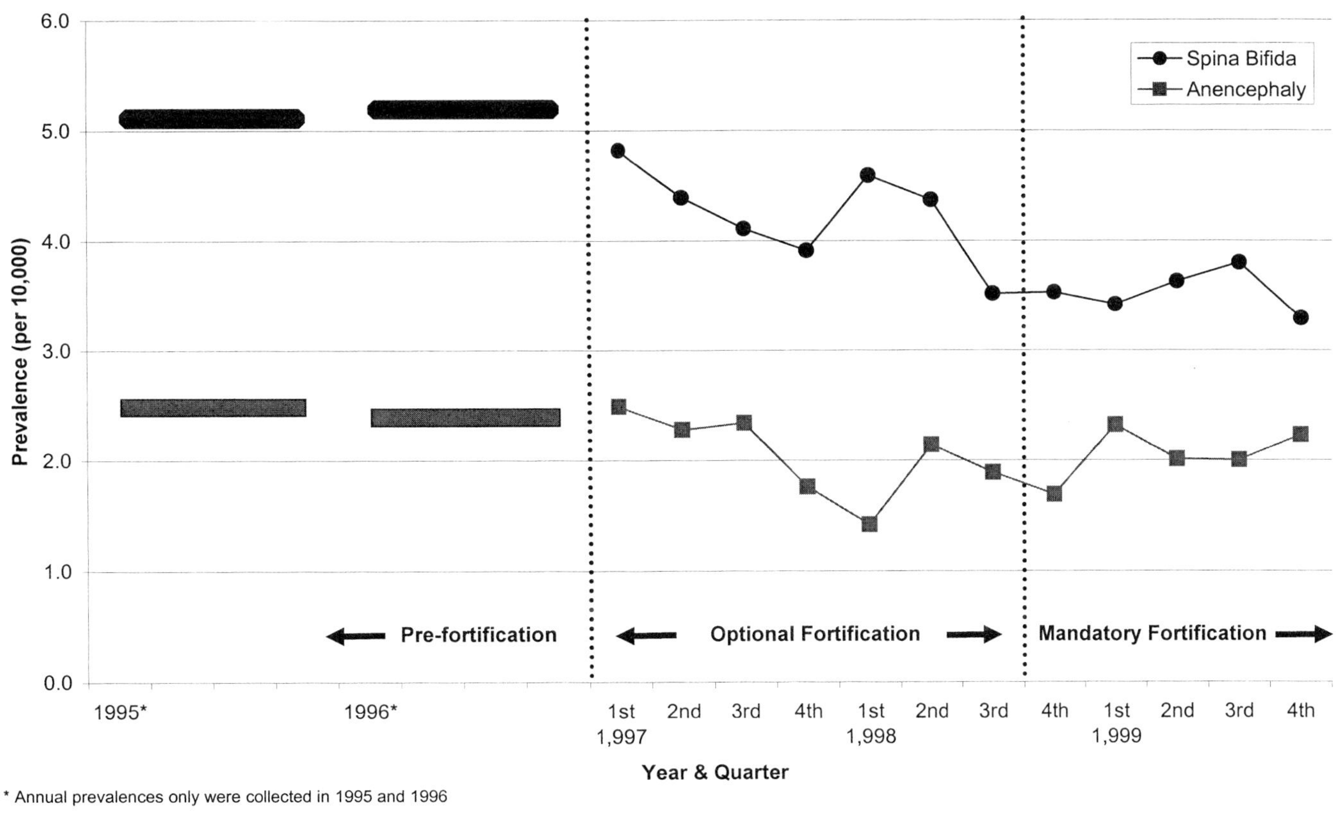

FIGURE 11.1. Prevalences of spina bifida and anencephaly by year and quarter of birth for 24 surveillance programs (1995–1999). *Source:* Williams et al. (2002b).

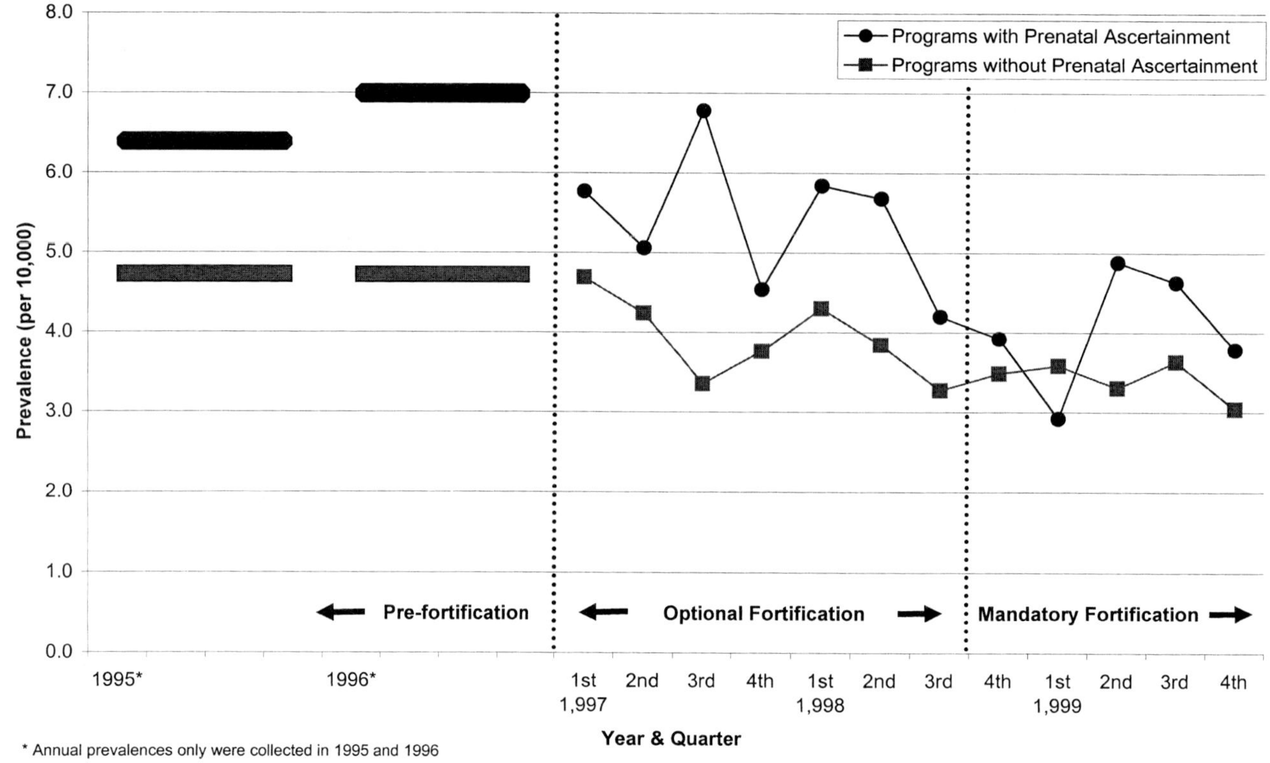

FIGURE 11.2. Prevalence of spina bifida for programs with prenatal ascertainment (9) and programs without prenatal ascertainment (13). *Source:* Williams et al. (2002b).

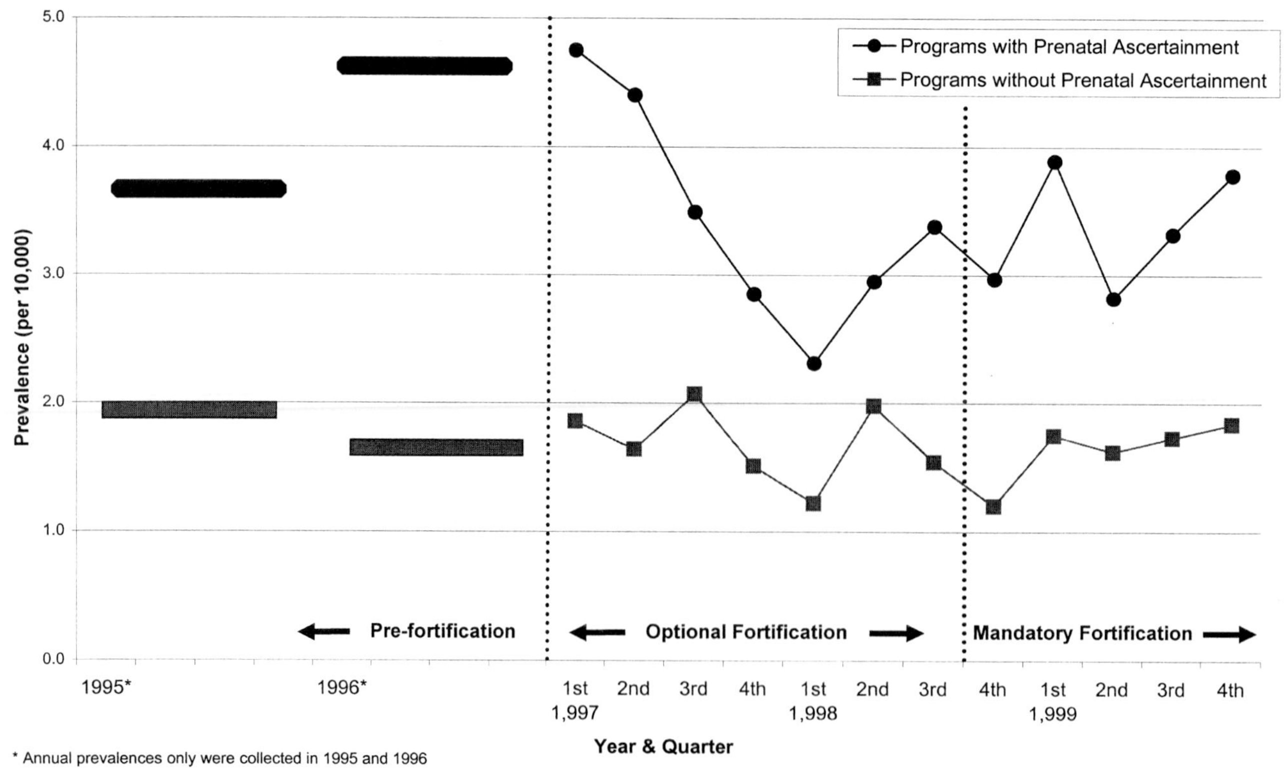

FIGURE 11.3. Prevalence of anencephaly for programs with prenatal ascertainment (9) and programs without prenatal ascertainment (13). *Source:* Williams et al. (2002b).

Surveillance to Target Prevention Interventions

A third example of the use of surveillance with respect to folic acid and NTDs is a project conducted by the Texas Department of Health and funded by the CDC. The Texas Neural Tube Defect Project (TNTDP) was a program of NTD surveillance and risk-reduction activities in the 14 Texas counties that border Mexico (Hendricks et al., 2000). This project was initiated following the recognition of a cluster of cases of anencephaly in Brownsville (Cameron County), Texas, in 1990–1991 (Hendricks et al., 1999). This cluster received widespread attention and played an important role in gathering support in the United States for the Birth Defects Prevention Act of 1998 (Pew Environmental Health Commission, 1999). This project shows the application of surveillance to a specific birth defects prevention problem and a subsequent public health intervention.

As noted earlier, there is clear and convincing evidence that increasing women's intake of folic acid reduces their risk of having a baby with an NTD. The protective role of folic acid was first demonstrated by reducing the recurrence risk of women who had had an affected pregnancy (Smithells et al., 1983; MRC, 1991). The argument put forward with respect to the cluster of anencephaly in Brownsville was that although the cause of the cluster was unknown, there was evidence that the use of folic acid during the preconception period reduces the risk. Therefore, it was important to adopt a multipronged approach to the cluster that included conducting studies to search for the etiology and increasing women's intake of folic acid. The latter included two major components: a community education and vitamin distribution program and a recurrence prevention program. The recurrence prevention program is the focus of the discussion here.

Multiple sources, including hospitals, midwives, and genetic and prenatal diagnostic centers, participated in prospective case finding for the TNTDP. The primary objective of the TNTDP was to prevent NTD recurrence among the women identified through this surveillance activity. The women were contacted and, after giving informed consent, were enrolled in a program that included NTD risk reduction counseling and education and were provided with folic acid supplements. The preliminary results of this study suggested that the use of active NTD surveillance in a high-risk population, coupled with an appropriate intervention—in this case provision of folic acid—can significantly reduce the risk of NTD recurrence (Hendricks et al., 2000).

As a final example of the application and use of surveillance for NTDs for prevention interventions, activities carried out in the State of South Carolina are considered (Stevenson et al., 2000). With support from the CDC, a program was designed (*1*) to conduct surveillance for NTDs in this state, an area where prevalence had traditionally been high, and (*2*) to prevent NTD occurrence and recurrence through the periconceptional use of folic acid. Recurrence was prevented through individual genetic counseling of women who had had an affected pregnancy, and occurrence was reduced through a campaign aimed at developing public awareness of the benefits of preconceptional folic acid use. The program was highly successful, as there were no recurrences among 113 subsequent pregnancies to women who had had a previous pregnancy affected by an isolated NTD. In addition, the prevalence of NTDs among births in this high-risk region declined coincident with the increased use of periconceptional folic acid supplements among women of reproductive age (Stevenson et al., 2000).

Two aspects of the South Carolina project are particularly informative relative to points made earlier about case ascertainment methods and differences in the effects of folic acid supplementation on anencephaly and spina bifida. First, the authors note that "prenatal diagnosis through ultrasonography, MSAFP [maternal serum alpha fetoprotein] screening and amniocentesis may influence NTD surveillance substantially" (Stevenson et al., 2000). They reported that 44% of the cases from the years 1992–1998 were diagnosed prenatally, with the pregnancies terminated prior to the end of the 20th week of gestation. As they stated, failure to include these prenatally diagnosed and terminated cases in surveillance will result in inaccurate lower rates of NTDs. Second, there were marked differences in the reduction in the prevalence of spina bifida compared with anencephaly. As is illustrated clearly in their Figure 1, the reduction in the prevalence of NTDs over the period 1992–1998 can be attributed primarily to a reduction in the prevalence of spina bifida (Stevenson et al., 2000).

CONCLUSIONS

As mentioned above, in a paper published over 15 years ago, Borman and Cryer (1990) discussed the "Fallacies of International and National Comparisons of Disease Occurrence in the Epidemiology of Neural Tube Defects." As noted, many of their comments are particularly relevant to surveillance for NTDs, since key surveillance activities relate to comparisons, either between populations or within a population over time. The following factors they discussed have been considered in the context of this chapter:

- Definition of NTDs
- Incidence and prevalence
- Late fetal deaths
- Ascertainment

In their conclusions, Borman and Cryer (1990) note that "the nonuniformity in the duration and diligence of case ascertainment and the definition of the denominator remain principle problems in evaluating the epidemiology of NTDs." It is hoped that some of the suggestions made in this chapter can contribute to increasing uniformity in surveillance methods, allowing continual improvement in understanding the distribution and determinants of these important birth defects.

REFERENCES

Borman B, Cryer C (1990). Fallacies of international and national comparisons of disease occurrence in the epidemiology of neural tube defects. Teratology 42:405–412.

British Paediatric Association (1979). *Classification of Diseases*. London: British Paediatric Association.

Centers for Disease Control (1988). *CDC Surveillance Update, January 1988*. Atlanta: CDC.

Cragan JD, Roberts HE, Edmonds LD, Muin JK, Kirby RS, Shaw GM, Merz RD, et al (1995). Surveillance for anencephaly and spina bifida and the impact of pre-natal diagnosis—United States, 1985–1994. MMWR CDC Surveill Summ 44:1–13.

Ethen MK, Canfield MA (2002). Impact of including elective pregnancy terminations before 20 weeks gestation on birth defect rates. Teratology 66:S32–S35.

EUROCAT Working Group (1991). Prevalence of neural tube defects in 20 regions of Europe and the impact of prenatal diagnosis 1980–1986. J Epidemiol Commun Health 45:52–58

EUROCAT Working Group (1997). *Report 7: 15 Years of Surveillance of Congenital Anomalies in Europe, 1980–1994*. Brussels: Scientific Institute of Public Health—Louis Pasteur.

EUROCAT Working Group (2002). *Report 8: Surveillance of Congenital Anomalies in Europe, 1980–1999*. Newtownabbey, Northern Ireland: EUROCAT Central Registry, University of Ulster.

Gaudino JA, Hoyert DL, MacDorman MF, Gazmararian JA, Adams MM, Kiely JL (1994). Fetal deaths. In Wilcox LS, Marks JS (eds): *From Data to Action: CDC's Public Health Surveillance for Women, Infants, and Children*. Atlanta: U.S. Department of Health and Human Services, pp. 163–178.

Gordis L (2000). *Epidemiology*, 2nd ed. Philadelphia: WB Saunders.

Harris JA, Wynne JW (1994). Birth defects clusters: evaluating community reports. Health Environ Dig 7:1–3.

Hendricks KA, Larsen R, Suarez L (2000). Neural tube defect surveillance and folic acid intervention: Texas–Mexico border, 1993–1998. MMWR 49(1):1–4.

Hendricks KA, Simpson JS, Larson RD (1999). Neural tube defects along the Texas–Mexico border, 1993–1995. Am J Epidemiol 149:1119–1127.

Hobbs CA, Hopkins SE, Simmons CJ (2001). Sources of variability in birth defects prevalence rates. Teratology 64:S8–S13.

Honein MA, Paulozzi LJ, Mathews TJ, Erickson JD, Wong LC (2001). Impact of folic acid fortification of the U.S. food supply on the occurrence of neural tube defects. JAMA 285:2981–2236.

Hook EB (1982). Incidence and prevalence as measures of the frequency of birth defects. Am J Epidemiol 116:743–747.

Hook EB (1983). Problems in interpretation of reported birth prevalence rates of neural tube defects. Teratology 27:125–126.

International Classification of Diseases (1998). *International Classification of Diseases, 9th Revision, Clinical Modification*. Washington, DC: National Center for Health Statistics and the Health Care Financing Agency.

International Clearinghouse for Birth Defects Monitoring Systems (2002). *Annual Report 2002, with Data for 2000*. Rome: International Centre for Birth Defects.

Khoury MJ, Holtzman NA (1987). On the ability of birth defects monitoring to detect new teratogens. Am J Epidemiol 126:136–143.

Limb CJ, Holmes LB (1994). Anencephaly: changes in prenatal detection and birth status, 1972 through 1990. Am J Obstet Gynecol 170:1333–1338.

Lowry B, Castilla EE, Mastroiacovo P, Ciffel C, eds. (2000). *International Clearinghouse for Birth Defects Monitoring Systems Annual Report 2000*. Rome: International Center for Birth Defects.

Lynberg MC, Edmonds LD (1992). Surveillance of birth defects. In Halperin W, Baker E (eds): *Public Health Surveillance*. New York: Van Nostrand Reinhold, pp 157–177.

MRC Vitamin Study Research Group (1991). Prevention of neural tube defects: results of the Medical Research Council Vitamin Study. Lancet 338:131–137.

Mulinare J, Cordero JF, Erickson JD, Berry RJ (1988). Periconceptional use of multivitamins and the occurrence of neural tube defects. JAMA 260:3141–3145.

National Birth Defects Prevention Network (NBDPN) (2000). Birth defects surveillance data from selected states, 1989–1996. Teratology 61:86–158.

National Birth Defects Prevention Network (NBDPN) (2002). Birth defects surveillance data from selected states, 1995–1999. Teratology 66:S129–S211.

Pew Environmental Health Commission (1999). *Healthy from the Start: Why America Needs a Better System to Track and Understand Birth Defects and the Environment*. Baltimore: Pew Environmental Health Commission.

Reed T, Meaney FJ (1988). Birth defects registries: a survey of state programs. Indiana Med 81:232–237.

Sever LE (1983a). Fetal deaths, stillbirths, and the prevalence of neural tube defects. Teratology 27:127–128.

Sever LE (1983b). Re: Incidence and prevalence as measures of the frequency of birth defects. Am J Epidemiol 118:608–609.

Sever LE (1994). The conundrum of birth defects clusters. Health Environ Dig 7:4–6.

Shaw GM, Nelson V, Carmichael SL, Lammer EJ, Finnell RH, Rosenquist TH (2002). Maternal periconceptional vitamins: interactions with selected factors and congenital anomalies? Epidemiology 13:625–630.

Smithells RW, Seller MJ, Harris R, Fielding DW, Schorah CJ, Nevin NC, Sheppard S, et al (1983). Further experience of vitamin supplementation for prevention of neural tube defect recurrences. Lancet 1:1027–1031.

Stevenson RE, Allen WP, Pai GS, Best R, Seaver LH, Dean J, Thompson S (2000). Decline in prevalence of neural tube defects in a high-risk region of the United States. Pediatrics 106:677–683.

Velie EM, Shaw GM (1996). Impact of prenatal diagnosis and elective termination on prevalence and risk estimates of neural tube defects in California, 1989–1991. Am J Epidemiol 144:473–479.

Williams LJ, Honein MA, Rasmussen SJ (2002a). Methods for a public health response to birth defects clusters. Teratology 66:S50–S58.

Williams LJ, Mai CT, Edmonds LD, Shaw GM, Kirby RS, Hobbs, CA, Sever LE, et al (2002b). Prevalence of spina bifida and anencephaly during the transition to mandatory folic acid fortification in the United States. Teratology 66:33–39.

Yoon PA, Rasmussen SA, Lynberg MC, Moore CA, Anderka M, Carmichael SL, Costa P, Druschel C, Hobbs CA, et al (2001). The National Birth Defects Prevention Study. Public Health Rep 116:32–40.

12

An International Perspective on Anencephaly and Spina Bifida: Prevalences by the Turn of the Century

ROLV T. LIE

Neural tube defects are dramatic birth defects that probably have occurred since ancient times around the world (Elwood et al., 1992; Smith, 2001). Excavations of ancient skeletons with neural tube defects have been found in South and North America and in Africa. A mummy from Egypt has a verified spina bifida. There are texts from Babylonia that possibly describe neural tube defects, and ancient texts from India, Greece, and Rome discuss the occurrence of birth defects in different contexts.

How prevalent neural tube defects were is, of course, impossible to assess. Since 1970, prevalence estimation has become an increasingly important part of public health. Recent changes in prevention strategies for neural tube defects may, however, completely alter their epidemiology. This chapter gives an update of the most recent prevalence estimates from around the world.

DEFINITION OF THE CONDITIONS

Neural tube defects are a series of different types of defects with the common feature that the closure of the neural tube is incomplete or that there has been some form of damage to the neural tube. Relatively distinct but still broad categories of neural tube defects are anencephaly, encephalocele, and spina bifida. Smaller subtypes may also be defined. Anencephaly and spina bifida are the most common categories. Anencephaly probably results from nonclosure of the upper part of the neural tube, resulting in an open cranium. Spina bifida similarly is a result of nonclosure of the lower parts of the neural tube, again affecting the formation of the spine. The categories may be overlapping, but cases with both anencephaly and spina bifida are by some conventions supposed to be classified as anencephaly.

Children with anencephaly or spina bifida have increased susceptibility to a spectrum of other types of birth defects. Cases with accompanying defects and cases with known syndromes are often classified as separate categories. A distinction can also be made between whether the neural tube is open or closed. Given the great heterogeneity of neural tube defects, it may be difficult to know what in practice is included in the categories of anencephaly and spina bifida in a specific study.

Most reports on the occurrence of neural tube defects provide numbers separately for anencephaly and spina bifida. Spina bifida may usually be assumed to be synonymous with meningomyelocele. There are also studies that deal only with one of the two categories. It is therefore natural to attempt to describe the epidemiology of the two categories separately in an overview of the epidemiology of neural tube defects.

DEFINITION OF PREVALENCE

Neural tube defects are serious defects with a very high mortality. All cases of anencephaly and about half of the ascertained cases of spina bifida die around the time of birth. Because of this high mortality, it is essential for a description of the occurrence of these defects to state what explicit criteria are used for inclusion of a case (Borman and Cryer, 1990). Neural tube defects occur within the first month of a pregnancy. Since a significant number of affected fetuses probably are aborted spontaneously before they are recognized, perhaps even before the pregnancy is recognized, it is unrealistic to attempt to estimate the total occurrence, or incidence, of these defects. The occurrence is therefore best measured as a prevalence of affected fetuses at a certain age, for example at 16 weeks of gestation. This, of course, requires that all pregnancies in a population with a gestational age of at least 16 weeks are identified and counted, and that all cases among those pregnancies also are diagnosed and counted. If the prevalence is restricted to later stages of the pregnancy or even to live births, the prevalence will drop because of the lethality of these defects and, more recently, elective termination of affected pregnancies.

In most Western populations, as well as in developing countries, prenatal diagnosis combined with induced abortion are used specifically to reduce the prevalence of affected fetuses in the population of term births. Any rigid prevalence at ages beyond the gestational age at which induced abortion based on prenatal diagnoses is used may greatly underestimate the natural prevalence of the birth defects. This has become a key problem for epidemiologic estimation of prevalences of anencephaly and spina bifida. Any study of prevalences since 1980 is potentially affected by these problems. Even in developing countries, antenatal care with ultrasound is becoming more common (Kunzel et al., 1996; Bussmann et al., 2001), but the effects on prevalences of birth defects is largely unknown.

Studies from the 1990s show that most cases of anencephaly and more than half of the cases of spina bifida may be detected prenatally and electively aborted (Boyd et al., 1998). In 1990, half of the anencephaly cases and one-third of the spina bifida cases were elective terminations of pregnancies after a prenatal diagnosis in California (Velie and Shaw, 1996). Studies show that elimination of cases that are aborted would estimate very low prevalences (Alembiek et al., 1997; Ethen and Canfield, 2002). Estimation of a residual of non-aborted cases could make clinical sense but would have limited value in epidemiology.

One way to compensate for the epidemiologic problems of selective abortion of cases is to add aborted cases to the number of cases ascertained at birth (beyond a certain gestational age) and then calculate the total proportion of cases (using all births beyond a certain gestational age plus all aborted cases as the denominator) to estimate the natural prevalence. It is, however, difficult to reconstruct natural prevalences from such quasi-prevalences, since the number of electively aborted cases that would have been spontaneously aborted or stillborn by a certain gestational age is unknown. Still, a prevalence defined by all cases among births beyond a certain gestational age plus all cases among induced abortions based on a prenatal diagnosis may be the best measure for epidemiologic purposes. Such prevalences have been systematically collected by registries involved in The International Clearinghouse for Birth Defects Monitoring Systems (ICBDMS, www.icbd.org) since the mid-1990s (Rosano et al., 1999; ICBDMS, 2002). Registries in Australia and China, for example, also calculate quasi-prevalences of birth defects by counting all pregnancies at 20 weeks' gestation plus all elective terminations after prenatal diagnosis (Bower et al., 2001; Li et al., 2003).

Since systematic efforts to include cases from induced abortions have started quite recently, an epidemiologic overview of prevalences around the world should focus on data that include aborted cases. Prevalences of neural tube defects that do not include such data may perhaps be used only to assess the impact of prenatal screening for neural tube defects. They may have very little value in assessing the natural prevalences, for example in studies of effects of primary prevention measures like supplementation of folic acid (Borman and Cryer, 1990; Yen et al., 1992, Birnbacher et al., 2002).

ASCERTAINMENT

Even if inclusion criteria in a prevalence study or a registry are well defined, finding and registering all cases of neural tube defects is a notoriously difficult enterprise. One would expect that no case of a neural tube defect would go unrecognized by the health-care personnel involved, and that is probably true. In reality, however, there are always failures in compliance with obligations to record and report cases. The reasons could be many, for example that in the exceptionally dramatic circumstances surrounding the rare event of a neural tube defect, reporting appeared to be less important or perhaps everybody involved thought it was somebody else's responsibility to report. Even when reporting is compulsory by law and there are staff designated for the work, underreporting still occurs. Therefore, any single registration system must work extremely hard to maintain a high degree of ascertainment of cases.

Since no system of reporting can be trusted to be complete, several epidemiologists have argued that reliable estimation of a prevalence requires that multiple more or less independent sources of ascertainment be used. One example would be two or more different registries operating in the same population. Such multiple sources of ascertainment increase the chances of finding any particular case when the data are combined. In addition, these sources would shed light on each other's tendency to underreport cases.

Epidemiologists have also recommended more formal methods of using multiple sources of ascertainment to estimate the prevalence of neural tube defects. Hook et al. (1980) suggested the use of capture-recapture methods for data on spina bifida prevalence in New York. The same data were recently reanalyzed by Farrington (2002) using a refined methodology. Several other groups interested in assessing the degree of underreporting of neural tube defects by a particular source have also used capture-recapture or similar double-sampling methods (Hey et al., 1994; Lie et al., 1994; Honein and Paulozzi, 1999, Bower et al., 2001). The weakness of formal capture-recapture analyses is that usually little is known about dependencies between the different sources of ascertainment. The important lesson from all those exercises, however, is that no single source is complete and that prevalence studies should assess their degree of underascertainment.

PURPOSES OF PREVALENCE ESTIMATION

Prevalence studies and registries of neural tube defects around the world may have different purposes. The most common purpose is epidemiologic surveillance of birth defects, particularly for preparedness to detect new potent teratogens that may cause new epidemics of birth defects. Registries like those involved in ICBDMS have this as their main objective. One important new surveillance purpose of great public health importance is to monitor any effects on prevalences of neural tube defects of folic acid supplementation programs around the world.

Registries that have surveillance as their main purpose may know that they have an incomplete ascertainment of neural tube defects, but may still be more concerned that their ascertainment is constant and provided by a stable and sustainable system of reporting (Hey et al., 1994; Lie et al., 1994). Prevalences from such registries may have less value as a basis for making comparisons between countries than for comparing estimates over time within the country. Still, these registry data may represent the best data available.

A series of studies have addressed the impact of prenatal screening programs on the prevalence of neural tube defects (Velie and Shawn, 1996; Alembiek et al., 1997; Ethen and Canfield, 2002). A study designed to estimate a live-birth prevalence to assess the public health challenge represented by cases that need future care may be irrelevant for an international comparison of natural prevalences.

A study based on a series of births at one or a couple of large hospitals may aim at estimating the prevalence in the population surrounding the hospitals. If the hospitals are referral hospitals, there will always be uncertainties about whether the prevalence estimates are too high, because cases from a larger population than the births at the hospitals are included, or whether the prevalences are too low because prenatally diagnosed cases or cases delivered preterm are not delivered at the hospitals. In developing countries, such studies may still be important and the problems involved are smaller than for a hospital-based study in a developed country.

If a prevalence study is performed to provide documentation of rumors of a particularly high prevalence in a local population, the study may be better described as a cluster report than a prevalence study. Some of the studies included in this overview are documentations of particularly high prevalences in smaller areas (Mocan et al., 1992; Verma et al., 1991).

Precise estimation of a well-defined prevalence from a large population is therefore one of the most challenging tasks in epidemiology. Running a good case-control study or a cohort study may in many ways be simpler. All the complications and limitations mentioned above need to be taken into account when prevalence estimates of neural tube defects from different parts of the world, collected in different ways and under very different circumstances, are compared. Variation in methodology may often be a much more likely explanation of differences between populations than environmental teratogens or genetics.

FOCUS ON RECENT PREVALENCES

Because modern prenatal diagnostics and folate supplementation programs have created a completely new situation, this overview will focus on prevalence reports from the 1990s. Prevalences will, if possible, be kept separate for the first and second halves of the decade. Inclusion of terminated cases became routine for several registries involved in the ICBDMS collaboration in the mid-1990s. Unfortunately, these changes in reporting policies coincided with the introduction of folic acid prevention programs and may make it more difficult to separate effects of a changed ascertainment from changes due to prevention. Still, it makes sense to focus on recent prevalences from the 1990s and separate the first from the second half of the period. It is, however, important to recognize that the current overview is purely descriptive, and is not a formal analysis of the effects of prenatal diagnostics and folic acid prevention programs on prevalences.

Another reason to focus this overview on prevalences from the 1990s is that prevalence reports from around the world up to 1990 were extensively reviewed by Elwood and colleagues (1992). The current review may therefore also be viewed as an update of and a supplement to that historic review. Identification of prevalence reports is based on searches of Medline and review of reports from ICBDMS and EUROCAT, a collaboration of European birth defects registries. Another source of prevalence information is the WHO World Atlas of Birth Defects (WHO, 2003).

The overview is organized alphabetically by geographical continent and by countries within continents. Tables 12.1 and 12.2 provide prevalences of anencephaly

TABLE 12.1. *Reported Prevalences of Anencephaly in the Period 1991–2000 for Different Geographic Areas*

	1991–1995		1996–2000				
Geographical Region	Total Births	Prevalence (per 10,000)	Total Births	Prevalence (per 10,000)	Source Type*	Prevalence Type†	Reference
Africa							
Ghana	19,094	8.4			H	LS	Anyebuno et al. (1993)
Nigeria	5,977	3.3‡			H	LS	Airede (1992)
South Africa	222,614	0.8	123,879	2.2	H	L	ICBDMS (1994–97, 1999, 2001–2)
Cape Town	516,252	7.8‡			P	LST	Buccimazza et al. (1994)
North America							
Canada			1,062,296	1.2	P	LS	ICBDMS (1998–2001)
Alberta	38,784	1.8	187,359	2.8	P	LST (97–)	ICBDMS (1997–2002)
Br. Columbia			40,775	1.5	P	LS	ICBDMS (2002)
Quebec	21,254	4.7			P	LST	De Wals et al. (1999)
Jamaica	54,200	2.6			P	LS	Coard et al. (1990)
Mexico	288,684	16.0	181,013	13.5	H	LS	ICBDMS (1993–2002)
USA	17,712,087	1.4	17,641,571	1.1	P	LS	Mathews et al (2002)
USA	24,726,932	1.4	4,381,901	1.0	P	LS	Honein et al. (2001)
USA	915,199	1.2			H	LS	ICBDMS (1993–95)
USA (1995–96) vs. (1998–99)	3,127,161	2.4	2,406,427	2.1	P	LST	Williams et al. (2002)
Atlanta	196,813	2.0	227,847	2.7	P	LST	ICBDMS (1993–2002)
California	568,282	2.0			P	LS	ICBDMS (1994, 1997)
California	1,618,279	4.8			P	LST	Feuchtbaum et al. (1999)
Vietnamese	45,453	2.2			P	LS	Shaw et al. (2002)
Non-Hispanic white	1,257,853	1.5			P	LS	Shaw et al. (2002)
Hawaii	~250,000	3.6			P	LST	Forrester and Merz, (2000)
South Carolina	278,122	4.2			P	LST	Stevenson et al. (2000)
Texas (Tex–Mex border)	135,221	6.4			P	LST	Hendricks et al. (1999)
Arkansas	108,519	3.7			P	LST	Cragan et al. (1995)
California	708,129	4.0			P	LST	Cragan et al. (1995)
Atlanta	77,022	4.8			P	LST	Cragan et al. (1995)
Hawaii	148,092	3.0			P	LST	Cragan et al. (1995)
Iowa	234,113	3.5			P	LST	Cragan et al. (1995)
South Carolina	16,641	6.0			P	LST	Cragan et al. (1995)
South America							
South America	952,372	7.5	766,460	7.2	H	LS	ICBDMS (1993–2002)
Venezuela	32,331	7.5			H	LST	Moreno-Fuenmajor et al. (1996)
Asia							
China			2,281,616	5.0	H	LS	Dai et al. (2002)
China			1,242,752	5.0	H	LS	ICBDMS (1999–2002)
Beijing			549,574	3.2	P	LS	ICBDMS (1999–2002)
Sichuan	113,822	4.2			H	LS	ICBDMS (1993, 1994)
India, Punjab	10,000	36			H	LS	Verma et al. (1991)
Uttar Pradesh	9,405	21.3			H	LS	Agarwal et al. (1991)
Israel	78,764	0.6	101,249	0.6	H	LST (95–)	ICBDMS (1993–2002)
Jews			181,307	5.3	P	LST	Zlotogora et al. (2002)
Non-Jews			80,895	8.8	P	LST	Zlotogora et al. (2002)
Palestinians	26,934	24.1			H	LST	Dudin (1997)
Japan	554,477	3.5	482,195	1.7	H	LS	ICBDMS (1993–2002)
Tokyo	27,573	6.5‡			H	LS	ICBDMS (1991–93)
Oman	242,764	6.9			P	LS	Rajab et al. (1998)
Singapore, Chinese	19,955	4.5			H	LS	Ho (1991)

TABLE 12.1. *Reported Prevalences of Anencephaly in the Period 1991–2000 for Different Geographic Areas (Continued)*

	1991–1995		1996–2000				
Geographical Region	Total Births	Prevalence (per 10,000)	Total Births	Prevalence (per 10,000)	Source Type*	Prevalence Type†	Reference
Singapore, Malay	8,303	8.4			H	LS	Ho (1991)
South Korea	1,202,835	3.4			P	M	Jung et al. (1999)
Turkey, Ankara	9,160	10.9			H	L(S)T	Himmetoglu et al. (1996)
Ankara	20,677	11.6			H	LS	Tunchbilek et al. (1999)
Izmir	82,720	15.0			H	LS	Posaci et al. (1992)
Eastern Black Sea Region	7,624	36.7			H	LS	Mocan et al. (1992)
Elazig	5,240	38.2			H	LS	Guvenc et al. (1993)
United Arab Emirates			38,052	5.5	H	LS	ICBDMS (1998–2002)
Europe							
Croatia	~17,500	1.7	~16,000	1.3	P	LST	Loncarek et al. (2001)
Czech Republic	577,964	1.1	453,465	3.1	P	LST	ICBDMS (1993–2002)
Denmark	135,742	0.7			P	LS	ICBDMS (1995, 1996)
England/Wales	3,388,435	1.4	3,168,907	2.8	P	LST	ICBDMS (1993–2002)
North England	190,627	7.7			P	LST	Rankin et al. (2000)
Finland	326,669	0.3	292,234	3.1	P	LST (96–)	ICBDMS (1993–2002)
France, Central East Region	513,514	0.9	521,168	1.5	P	LST	CBDMS (1993–2002)
Paris	202,740	2.4	191,800	5.4	P	LST	ICBDMS (1993–2002)
Strassbourg	66,792	4.3	68,136	3.8	P	LST	ICBDMS (1993–2002)
Northeast Region	94,500	5.8			P	LST	Alembik et al. (1997)
Germany, Saxony-Anhalt			18,799	1.6	P	LST	ICBDMS (2002)
Hungary	595,926	0.7	497,741	1.4	P	LST	ICBDMS (1993–2002)
Ireland, Dublin			97,627	3.3	P	LS	ICBDMS (1998–2002)
Dublin	~20,000	4.4			P	LS	McDonell et al. (1999)
Italy	189,655	0.6			H	LS	ICBDMS (1993–1996)
Emilia-Romagna	126,923	1.3	123,541	1.9	P	LST	ICBDMS (1993–2002)
Campania	87,188	3.2	246,252	3.0	H	LST	ICBDMS (1996–2002)
Toscana			102,610	2.5	P	LST	ICBDMS (1999–2002)
Northeast			274,197	2.1	H	LST	ICBDMS (1998–2002)
Sicily			70,073	1.3	H	LST	ICBDMS (2002)
Malta			8,611	3.5	P	LS	ICBDMS (2001–2)
Netherlands, Northern	77,106	2.1	98,999	2.9	P	LST	ICBDMS (1993–2002)
Norway	303,092	3.2	299,153	3.4	P	LST	ICBDMS (1993–2002)
Russia, Moscow			45,092	4.0	P	LST	ICBDMS (2002)
Scotland	~67,000	5.2			P	LST	Davis and Young, (1991)
Glasgow	142,882	13.7			P	LST	Omran et al. (1992)
Spain	430,098	1.0	499,650	0.4	H	LS	ICBDMS (1993–2002)
Sweden	247,271	0.4	179,308	3.1	P	LST (99–)	ICBDMS (1993– 94, 2001–2)
Ukraine			26,025	8.8	P	LST	ICBDMS (2002)
Oceania							
Australia	1,109,159	2.6	757,724	4.4	P	LST (95–)	ICBDMS (1993–2002)
Victoria			~60,000	7.9	P	LST	Owen et al. (2000)
Western Australia	~120,000	8.0	~120,000	6.0	P	LST	Bower et al. (2002)
New Zealand	293,819	0.7	286,412	0.5	P	L	ICBDMS (1993–2002)

*Source types: H, hospital-based; P, population-based.

†Prevalence type: L, including live births; M, medical insurance data; S, including stillbirths; T, including terminations after prenatal diagnoses (period indicated).

‡Data from before 1991.

TABLE 12.2. *Reported Prevalences of Spina Bifida in the Period 1991–2000 for Different Geographic Areas*

Geographical Region	1991–1995 Total Births	1991–1995 Prevalence (per 10,000)	1996–2000 Total Births	1996–2000 Prevalence (per 10,000)	Source Type*	Prevalence Type†	Reference
Africa							
Ghana	19,094	3.1			H	LS	Anyebuno et al. (1993)
Nigeria	5,977	4.8‡			H	LS	Airede (1992)
South Africa	222,614	4.4	123,879	5.8	H	L	ICBDMS (1994–1997, 1999, 2001–2)
Cape Town	516,252	3.2‡			P	LST	Buccimazza et al. (1994)
North America							
Canada			1,062,296	4.7	P	LS	ICBDMS (1998–2001)
Alberta	38,784	6.5	187,359	3.7	P	LST (97–)	ICBDMS (1997–2002)
Br. Columbia			40,775	2.5	P	LS	ICBDMS (2002)
Quebec	21,254	4.7			P	LST	De Wals et al. (1999)
Mexico	288,684	15.8	181,013	14.4	H	LS	ICBDMS (1993–2002)
USA	17,712,087	2.5	17,641,571	2.3	P	LS	Mathews et al. (2002)
USA	24,726,932	2.5	4,381,901	2.0	P	LS	Honein et al. (2001) w. erratum
USA	915,199	4.2			H	LS	ICBDMS (1993–95)
USA (1995–96) vs. (1998–99)	3,127,161	5.2	2,406,427	3.5	P	LST	Williams et al. (2002)
USA	7,244,380	4.6‡			P	L(S)	Lary and Edmonds (1996)
Atlanta	196,813	3.0	227,847	3.1	P	LST	ICBDMS (1993–2002)
California	568,282	3.5			P	LS	ICBDMS (1994, 1997)
California	1,618,279	4.0			P	LST	Feuchtbaum et al. (1999)
Vietnamese	45,453	1.8			P	LS	Shaw et al. (2002)
Non-Hispanic white	1,257,853	3.5			P	LS	Shaw et al. (2002)
Hawaii	~250,000	4.5			P	LST	Forrester and Merz (2000)
South Carolina	278,122	5.2			P	LST	Stevenson et al. (2000)
Texas	135,221	7.1			P	LST	Hendricks et al. (1999)
Arkansas	108,519	6.6			P	LST	Cragan et al. (1995)
California	708,129	5.0			P	LST	Cragan et al. (1995)
Atlanta	77,022	5.1			P	LST	Cragan et al. (1995)
Hawaii	148,092	4.1			P	LST	Cragan et al. (1995)
Iowa	234,113	5.5			P	LST	Cragan et al. (1995)
South Carolina	16,641	9.6			P	LST	Cragan et al. (1995)
South America							
South America	952,372	7.9	766,460	10.4	H	LS	ICBDMS (1993–2002)
Asia							
China			2,281,616	6.3	H	LS	Dai et al. (2002)
China			1,242,752	7.5	H	LS	ICBDMS (1999–2002)
Beijing			549,574	2.9	P	LS	ICBDMS (1999–2002)
Sichuan	113,822	1.8			H	LS	ICBDMS (1993, 1994)
India, Punjab	10,000	1.0‡			H	LS	Verma et al. (1991)
Uttar Pradesh	9,405	21.3‡			H	LS	Agarwal et al. (1991)
Israel	78,764	2.4	101,249	2.6	H	LST (95–)	ICBDMS (1993–2002)
Jews			181,307	4.6	P	LST	Zlotogora et al. (2002)
Non-Jews			80,895	10.3	P	LST	Zlotogora et al. (2002)
Palestinians	26,934	22.3			H	LST	Dudin (1997)
Japan	554,477	3.6	482,195	3.8	H	LS	ICBDMS (1993–2002)
Tokyo	27,573	4.0‡			H	LS	ICBDMS (1991–93)
Oman	242,764	4.5			P	LS	Rajab et al. (1998)
South Korea	1,202,835	2.8			P	M	Jung et al. (1999)

TABLE 12.2. *Reported Prevalences of Spina Bifida in the Period 1991–2000 for Different Geographic Areas (Continued)*

	1991–1995		1996–2000				
Geographical Region	Total Births	Prevalence (per 10,000)	Total Births	Prevalence (per 10,000)	Source Type*	Prevalence Type†	Reference
Turkey, Ankara	9,160	14.2			H	L(S)T	Himmetogulu et al. (1996)
Ankara	20,677	14.0			H	LS	Tunchbilek et al. (1999)
Izmir	82,720	7.4‡			H	LS	Posaci et al. (1992)
United Arab Emirates			38,052	5.8	H	LS	ICBDMS (1998–2002)
Europe							
Czechoslovakia	577,964	2.2	453,465	4.2	P	LST	ICBDMS (1993–2002)
Denmark	135,742	2.7			P	LS	ICBDMS (1995, 1996)
England/Wales	3,388,435	1.7	3,168,907	2.9	P	LST	ICBDMS (1993–2002)
North England	190,627	7.8			P	LST	Rankin et al. (2000)
Finland	326,669	2.4	292,234	4.7	P	LST (96–)	ICBDMS (1993–2002)
France, Central East	513,514	3.0	521,168	3.6	P	LST	ICBDMS (1993–2002)
Paris	202,740	3.1	191,800	5.2	P	LST	ICBDMS (1993–2002)
Strassbourg	66,792	3.7	68,136	7.3	P	LST	ICBDMS (1993–2002)
Northeast Region	94,500	4.7			P	LST	Alembik et al. (1997)
Germany, Saxony-Anhalt			18,799	8.0	P	LST	ICBDMS (2002)
Hungary	595,926	1.8	497,741	3.0	P	LST	ICBDMS (1993–2002)
Ireland, Dublin			97,627	5.0	P	LS	ICBDMS (1998–2002)
Dublin	~20,000	5.5			P	LS	McDonell et al. (1999)
Italy	189,655	4.2			H	LS	ICBDMS (1993–1996)
Emilia-Romagna	126,923	3.9	123,541	3.6	P	LST	ICBDMS (1993–2002)
Campania	87,188	3.8	246,252	3.3	H	LST	ICBDMS (1996–2002)
Toscana			102,610	3.4	P	LST	ICBDMS (1999–2002)
Northeast			274,197	3.3	H	LST	ICBDMS (1998–2002)
Sicily			70,073	2.4	H	LST	ICBDMS (2002)
Malta			8,611	5.8	P	LS	ICBDMS (2001–2)
Netherlands, Northern	77,106	4.3	98,999	5.4	P	LST	ICBDMS (1993–2002)
Norway	303,092	4.9	299,153	5.5	P	LST	ICBDMS (1993–2002)
Russia, Moscow			45,092	7.1	P	LST	ICBDMS (2002)
Scotland	~67,000	5.8‡			P	LST	Davis and Young, (1991)
Glasgow	142,882	16.4‡			P	LST	Omran et al. (1992)
Spain	430,098	3.1	499,650	2.1	H	LS	ICBDMS (1993–2002)
Sweden	247,271	4.9	179,308	5.1	P	LST (99–)	ICBDMS (1993–94, 2001–2)
Ukraine			26,025	9.6	P	LST	ICBDMS (2002)
Oceania							
Australia	1,109,159	4.7	757,724	5.2	P	LST (95–)	ICBDMS (1993–2002)
Victoria			~60,000	8.8	P	LST	Owen et al. (2000)
Western Australia	~120,000	10.0	~120,000	6.0	P	LST	Bower et al. (2002)
New Zealand	293,819	4.0	286,412	3.1	P	L	ICBDMS (1993–2002)

*Source types: H, hospital-based; P, population-based.
†Prevalence type: L, including live births; M, medical insurance data; S, including stillbirths; T, including terminations after prenatal diagnoses (period indicated).
‡Data from before 1991.

and spina bifida per 10,000 babies. Total number of births or pregnancies (the denominator of the prevalence) is also provided for each study to give an impression of the precision of the estimate and facilitate calculation of confidence intervals. Denominators range from a couple of thousand to more than 20 million.

OVERVIEW OF PREVALENCES

Figures 12.1 and 12.2 present maps of total prevalences by country for anencephaly and spina bifida. For each country, a weighted average was calculated using all available data from that country. There are several problems

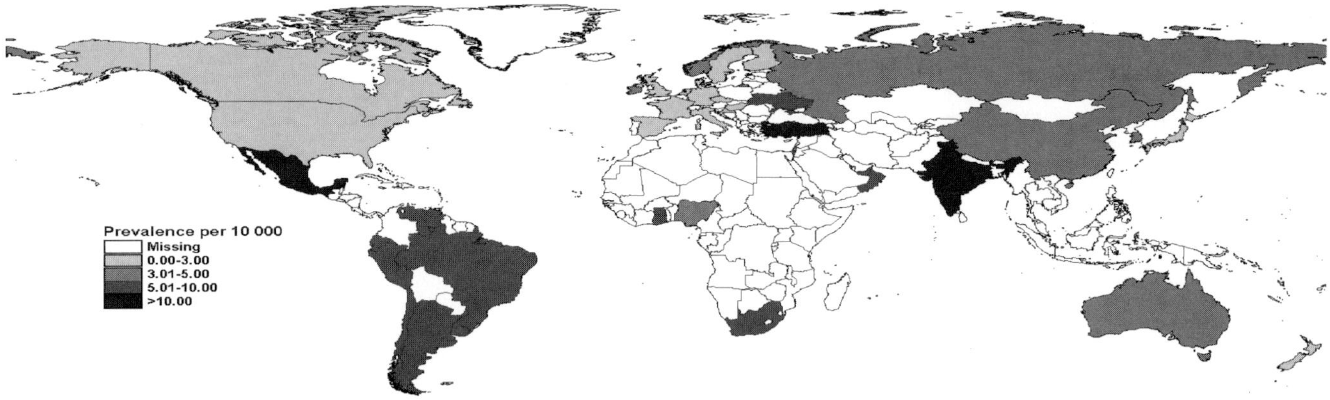

FIGURE 12.1. Average prevalence of anencephaly by country based on reports from the 1990s. Some countries are represented only by data from a smaller region.

with this presentation. One is that the average could be calculated from a very heterogeneous set of high and low prevalences from different studies in a country. Another problem is that a prevalence from only one region or city could represent a whole country. Inspection of the maps should therefore be taken as a very crude guide to global geographic variation.

Africa

There was limited information about prevalences of neural tube defects in the period 1990 to 2000 in the continent of Africa. Data on both anencephaly and spina bifida are, however, available for South Africa and for Ghana and Nigeria in West Africa.

Data for South Africa came from a surveillance system based on 9 to 15 hospitals across the country and covering up to 50,000 births per year (5% of the population) (ICBDMS, 1996, 2002). Ascertainment was based on reports from obstetric and pediatric units of the hospitals and on live births. The prevalence of anencephaly was 0.8 per 10,000 in 1991–1995 and 2.2 in 1996–2000. These prevalences are low and probably related to an ascertainment based only on live births. A population-based study in the Cape Town area showed a prevalence of 7.8 per 10,000 for the years 1990–1992 (Table 12.1) (Buccimazza et al., 1994). Ascertainment was based on review of clinical records including records of stillbirths and prenatal diagnoses. The high prevalence may be explained partly by a higher proportion of white children (50% of cases) and a threefold risk among these children.

The prevalence of spina bifida in South Africa was estimated at 4.4 and 5.8 per 10,000 for the two periods, respectively, from the ICBDMS registry (ICBDMS, 1993–2002), while an estimate for Cape Town was 3.2 per 10,000 for the first period (Buccimazza et al., 1994).

A hospital-based study from Ghana estimated a higher prevalence of anencephaly of 8.4 per 10,000 for 1991–1992 (Anyebuno et al., 1993). Ascertainment includes stillbirths. The study estimated a prevalence of 3.1 per 10,000 for spina bifida.

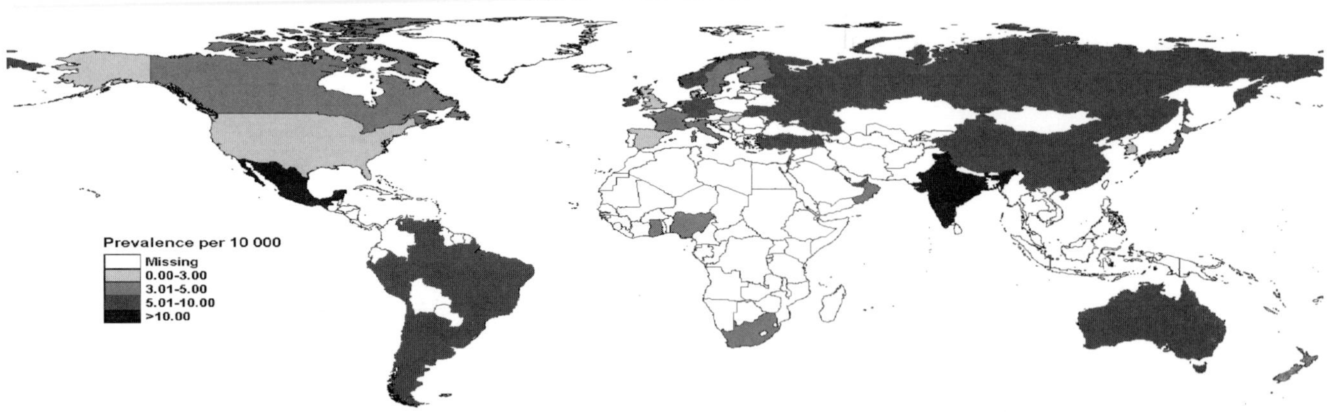

FIGURE 12.2. Average prevalence of spina bifida by country based on reports from the 1990s. Some countries are represented only by data from a smaller region.

Another slightly older hospital-based study from Nigeria estimated a prevalence of anencephaly of 3.3 per 10,000 (data for 1988–1990) (Airede, 1992). This study estimated a prevalence of 4.8 per 10,000 for spina bifida.

These recent studies seem to indicate that the prevalence of anencephaly could be high in some black African populations. The numbers still fall in the lower range of older prevalences from Africa, varying from 4.0 to 17.5 (Elwood et al., 1992). The prevalence of spina bifida was much more consistent and within a range of 3.1 to 5.8 per 10,000.

North America

Data on neural tube defects from Canada were mainly available from ICBDMS registries. Estimated prevalences of anencephaly were not very high, 1.2 per 10,000 in the second period from national data, 1.8 per 10,000 in the first, and 2.8 in the second period in Alberta and 1.5 per 10,000 in British Columbia. These Canadian registries cover both liveborn and stillborn babies. The Alberta registry also covers terminations from 1997, which probably explains the higher prevalence in the second period (ICBDMS, 1993–2002). A population-based study from Quebec included both stillbirths and terminations (De Wals et al., 1999). The study estimated a slightly higher prevalence of 3.3 per 10,000 for 1992.

Prevalence of spina bifida in Canada was 4.7 per 10,000 in the second half of the 1990s for the national registry and 6.5 and 3.7 per 10,000 in each half of the 1990s in the Alberta registry (ICBDMS, 1993–2002). In Quebec the prevalence was 4.7 per 10,000 in the first half and in British Columbia 2.5 in the second half of the 1990s.

There is little recent information about prevalences on the Caribbean isles. A small study based on stillbirths and neonatal deaths in Jamaica estimated a prevalence of 2.6 per 10,000 for anencephaly just prior to the 1990s (Coard et al., 1990).

Mexico has been recognized as a high-prevalence area for neural tube defects. Data from ICBDMS (1993–2002) show that the prevalence of anencephaly was 16 per 10,000 in the first period and 13.5 in the second. This registry is based on a series of hospitals and covers livebirths and stillbirths. The prevalence of spina bifida was also high, 15.8 and 14.4 per 10,000 for the two periods.

The interest in neural tube defects was particularly high in the United States in the 1990s. The recommendation was first given in 1992 that all fertile women should use folic acid supplementation. In 1996 fortification of food products was started specifically to prevent neural tube defects. A series of studies provide estimates of prevalences and discuss possible effects of the prevention program.

National data from the United States based on birth certificate data estimated relatively low prevalences of anencephaly. Mathews et al. (2002) showed a drop from 1.4 to 1.1 per 10,000 from the first to the second period. Similar data, with a drop from 1.4 to 1.0, were shown by Honein et al. (2001). Data from ICBDMS showed a prevalence of 1.2 per 10,000 in the first period (1991–1993) for the United States, based on a registry of discharge diagnoses from 1200 hospitals (ICBDMS, 1993–1995).

In a study of 24 population-based registries in the United States, some counting and some not counting terminations, Williams et al. (2002) estimated a prevalence of anencephaly of 2.4 per 10,000 for 1995–1996 prior to fortification and 2.1 for 1998–1999, also consistent with a decline.

A couple of local surveillance systems provide similar prevalences for anencephaly. A prevalence estimate for Atlanta, Georgia, increased from 2.0 to 2.7 per 10,000 from the first to the second period (ICBDMS, 1993–2002). An estimate for California was 2.0 for the first period (ICBDMS, 1994, 1997). A study also using population-based data from California showed that the prevalence was higher among people of Vietnamese origin (2.2 per 10,000) than among non-Hispanic whites (1.5 per 10,000) in the first period (Shaw et al., 2002).

A study from Utah that included stillbirths and terminations showed a falling trend in the prevalence of anencephaly from 1985 to 2000 graphically (Feldkamp et al., 2002, Fig. 2). By visual inspection, anencephaly prevalences were estimated at around 3 per 10,000 for the first period and 2 per 10,000 for the second period.

There are several studies of anencephaly prevalences from U.S. states in the first period that have made a special effort to include prenatal diagnoses. A study from California estimated a prevalence of 4.8 per 10,000 for anencephaly for the period 1990–1994 (Feuchtbaum et al., 1999), a study from Hawaii found a prevalence of 3.6 for the period 1986–1997 (Forrester and Merz, 2000), and another study from South Carolina a prevalence of 4.2 for the period 1992–1998 (Stevenson et al., 2000). Based on previous reports that the Texas–Mexico border area had particularly high prevalences, Hendricks (1999) estimated a prevalence of 6.4 per 10,000 in this area. A study from the first period (Cragan et al., 1995) estimated a prevalence of 3.7 per 10,000 for Arkansas, 4.0 for California, 4.8 for Atlanta, Georgia, 3.0 for Hawaii, 3.5 for Iowa, and 6.0 for South Carolina. The study showed that overall, around half of the cases of anencephaly were terminated after a prenatal diagnosis in this period, and that the impact of prenatal diagnoses on prevalence estimates was great and varied among the states.

The national data from the United States estimated slightly higher prevalences for spina bifida than for anencephaly. Mathews et al. (2002) estimated a prevalence of 2.5 per 10,000 for spina bifida in the first half of the 1990s and 2.3 in the second. The similar data from Honein et al. (2001) estimated 2.5 and 2.0 for the two periods. The ICBDMS data from 1200 hospitals provide a higher prevalence of 4.2 per 10,000 in the first period (1991–1993) for the United States (ICBDMS, 1993–1995). Williams' study (2002), covering most of the United States, estimated an even higher prevalence of spina bifida of 5.2 per 10,000 for 1995–1996 prior to folic acid fortification, but with a drop to 3.5 for 1998–1999.

Prevalence estimates provided by the registry in Atlanta, Georgia, were 3.0 for the first period and 3.1 per 10,000 for the second period (ICBDMS 1993–2002). For California the estimate was 3.5 for the first period (ICBDMS, 1994, 1997). A lower prevalence among people of Vietnamese origin than among non-Hispanic whites in California has also been estimated (1.8 vs. 3.5 per 10,000) in the first period (Shaw et al., 2002).

Studies of prevalences that also include prenatal diagnoses generally estimate higher prevalences for spina bifida than for anencephaly. The study from Utah including both stillbirths and terminations also showed a falling trend in the prevalence of spina bifida from 1985 to 2000 (Feldkamp et al., 2002, Fig. 2) graphically. By visual inspection, anencephaly prevalences were estimated at around 5 per 10,000 for the first period and 3.5 per 10,000 for the second period. In California, the prevalence was 4.0 per 10,000 for the period 1990–1994 (Feuchtbaum et al., 1999), and the studies from Hawaii (Forrester and Merz, 2000) and South Carolina (Stevenson et al., 2000) estimated prevalences of 4.5 and 5.2 per 10,000. The suspected high prevalence on the Texas–Mexico border (Hendricks et al., 1999) was estimated at 7.1 per 10,000. Cragan et al. (1995) estimated a prevalence of 6.6 per 10,000 for Arkansas, 5.0 for California, 5.1 for Atlanta, Georgia, 4.1 for Hawaii, 5.5 for Iowa, and 9.6 for South Carolina. The authors showed that one-fifth of spina bifida cases were terminated after a prenatal diagnosis in the first half of the 1990s and that the impact of prenatal diagnoses on the birth prevalence varied among the states even for spina bifida.

South America

A large registry that covers most of South America has reported prevalences of anencephaly for more than 30 years. The system is based on hospitals and covers livebirths and stillbirths (ICBDMS, 1993–2002). Prevalences of anencephaly in this system have been quite stable and were 7.5 per 10,000 in 1991–1995 and 7.2 per 10,000 in 1996–2000. A study based on data from Venezuela estimated a prevalence of 7.5 for the first period, similar to the overall prevalence for South America (Moreno-Fuenmajor et al., 1996).

Data from the South America registry estimated a prevalence of spina bifida of 7.9 per 10,000 for the first half of the 1990s and 10.4 for the second half.

Asia

Prevalences of neural tube defects show great variation across the huge continent of Asia. Even within regions there are probably great differences. Previous reports, for example from Punjab in India, have estimated very high prevalences (Elwood et al., 1992). A paper on the effect of folic acid supplementation in China shows a very high baseline risk of 65 per 10,000 for all neural tube defects combined in the northern province of Hebei and a baseline risk of 8 per 10,000 in the southern provinces of Zhejiang and Jiangsu (Berry et al., 1999). Specific data for anencephaly are, however, not provided for these provinces.

Other data on anencephaly from China are quite consistent. Dai et al. (2002) estimated a prevalence of 5.0 per 10,000 for the second period. The data are from the hospital-based Chinese Birth Defects Monitoring Network covering 31 provinces. A population-based registry in Beijing estimated a prevalence of 3.2 (ICBDMS, 1999–2002). Data from Sichuan showed a prevalence of 4.2 per 10,000 for the first period (ICBDMS, 1993–1994), while data from an extension of the database to 31 provinces showed a prevalence of 5.0, similar to the data of Dai et al. (2002), for the second period (ICBDMS, 1999–2002).

Dai et al. (2002) estimated a prevalence of 6.3 per 10,000 for spina bifida in China in the second period. The population-based registry in Beijing estimated a prevalence of 2.9 for the second period (ICBDMS, 1999–2002). Sichuan data estimated a prevalence of only 1.8 per 10,000 for the first period (ICBDMS, 1993–1994), while the extended data for 31 provinces for the second period gave a prevalence of 7.5 (ICBDMS, 1999–2002), again similar to the data of Dai et al. (2002).

Two hospital-based studies from India showed prevalences of anencephaly of 36 per 10,000 in Punjab (Verma et al., 1991) and 21.3 per 10,000 in Lucknow, Uttar Pradesh (Agarwal et al., 1991) just before the 1990s. Another report of an extremely high prevalence of a slightly larger category of central nervous system defects of 118 per 10,000 just prior to the 1990s in Uttar Pradesh was given by Kulkarni and Kurian (1990). A high degree of consanguinity was suggested as an explanation. An extensive review of older prevalences in India was given in Elwood et al. 1992). Several of these are among the highest reported prevalences of anencephaly in the world, for example those from Punjab of around .5%.

While the study by Verma et al. (1991) estimated a low prevalence of spina bifida in Punjab (1.0 per 10,000), Agarwal et al.'s (1991) study reported a high prevalence of 21.3 per 10,000 from Uttar Pradesh.

National data from Israel (three hospitals) showed very low prevalences of anencephaly, 0.6 per 10,000 for both periods (ICBDMS, 1993–2002). The ascertainment should include livebirths, stillbirths, and terminations since 1995. A study overlapping with the first half of the 1990s (1986–1993), however, estimated a prevalence of 24.1 per 10,000 for Palestinians in Israel (Dudin, 1997). Data from a new registry of neural tube defects designed to monitor effects of folic acid supplementation policies and using data from all units diagnosing neural tube defects in Israel estimated a prevalence of 5.3 per 10,000 among Jews and 8.8 among non-Jews in the second half of the 1990s (1999–2000) (Zlotogora et al., 2002).

The prevalence of spina bifida in Israel was estimated at 2.4 per 10,000 for the first period and 2.6 for the second period (ICBDMS, 1993–2002). The study from the period 1986–1993, however, estimated a much higher prevalence of 22.3 per 10,000 for Palestinians in Israel (Dudin, 1997). Data from the new registry of neural tube defects in Israel estimated a prevalence of 4.6 per 10,000 among Jews and 10.3 among non-Jews in the second half of the 1990s (Zlotogora et al., 2002).

A birth defects registry in Japan provided data throughout the whole decade (IDBDMS, 1993–2002). The registry was based on 330 hospitals and covered livebirths and stillbirths. In the first half of the 1990s the prevalence of anencephaly was estimated at 3.5 per 10,000 and in the second, 1.7 (ICBDMS, 1993–2002). A smaller system operating in Tokyo up to 1991 estimated a prevalence of 6.5 per 10,000 for the period 1989–1991 (ICBDMS, 1991–1993).

The national data for Japan showed a prevalence of 3.6 per 10,000 in the first period and 3.8 in the second period. The Tokyo registry estimated a lower prevalence of 1.5 per 10,000 for the first period.

A study from South Korea used national medical insurance data to estimate the prevalence of birth defects for the years 1993 and 1994 (Jung et al., 1999). The prevalence of anencephaly was estimated at 3.4 per 10,000 and the prevalence of spina bifida at 2.8 per 10,000.

By retrospective review of medical records, Rajab et al. (1998) estimated prevalences of neural tube defects for the period 1992–1995 in Oman. The prevalence of anencephaly was 6.9 per 10,000. This study also noted consanguinity as a possible explanation for the relatively high prevalence. The prevalence of spina bifida was 4.5 per 10,000.

For Singapore, the prevalence of anencephaly was estimated separately for the Chinese and Malayan populations just prior to the 1990s (Ho, 1991). The study was hospital-based and estimated a prevalence of 4.5 per 10,000 for Chinese births and 8.4 for Malay births. Surprisingly, only one case of spina bifida was found in the study of 31,000 births.

There are several recent reports of fairly high prevalences of neural tube defects from Turkey. A report of a particularly high prevalence just prior to the 1990s, perhaps related to the radioactive fallout from the Chernobyl nuclear power plant accident in 1986, was given by Mocan et al. (1992). They reported a prevalence of anencephaly of 36.7 per 10,000 for the eastern Black Sea region of Turkey. Another small study (Guvenc, 1993) reported a similar prevalence of anencephaly of 38.2 for the period 1984–1990 for Elazig in central east Turkey, with a particularly high prevalence in 1988. From Izmir in west Turkey, particularly high prevalences of neural tube defects were also reported just after the Chernobyl accident (Posaci et al., 1992). The prevalence of anencephaly was estimated at 15 per 10,000 for the period 1980–1990. All three studies from Turkey were hospital-based.

Two hospital-based studies from Ankara (Himmetoglu et al., 1996; Tunchbilek et al., 1999) estimated quite high and similar prevalences of anencephaly for the first half of the 1990s. Himmetogulu et al. found a prevalence of 10.9 per 10,000 and Tunckbilek a prevalence of 11.6.

The prevalence of spina bifida in Izmir in west Turkey was estimated at 7.4 per 10,000 just before the 1990s (Posaci et al., 1992). From Ankara, high estimates of 14.2 and 14.0 are reported by the two studies from the 1990s (Himmetogulu 1996, Tunchbilek 1999).

The United Arab Emirates has contributed data to the ICBDMS since 1996. The registry is based on three large hospitals and covers livebirths and stillbirths. For the second half of the 1990s, the prevalence of anencephaly was estimated at 5.5 per 10,000 (ICBDMS, 1998–2002). The prevalence of spina bifida was 5.8 per 10,000.

Europe

A surveillance network in Western Europe (EUROCAT) has systematically provided prevalence data for birth defects for European countries since 1980 (EUROCAT, 2002). Most EUROCAT registries, however, also provide data to ICBDMS. Although most references to European data here are based on ICBDMS reports, these data are also available from EUROCAT reports and from the EUROCAT Web site (www.eurocat.ulster.ac.uk). We will not distinguish between registries in the ICBDMS that are and are not members of EUROCAT.

A population-based registry in the Czech Republic has provided data for the whole decade of the 1990s. The registry covers both livebirths and stillbirths as well as terminations, and estimated a prevalence of anencephaly of 1.1 per 10,000 for the first half of the decade and 3.1 for the second (ICBDMS, 1993–2002). The prevalence of spina bifida was 2.2 per 10,000 for the first half of the decade and 4.2 for the second half.

The prevalence of anencephaly has been estimated for both halves of the decade for the region of Rijeka in Croatia (Loncarek et al., 2001). The study included terminations. Estimates were, however, still low, 1.7 and 1.3 per 10,000 for the two periods.

Denmark provided data for 1992 and 1993 to ICBDMS (ICBDMS, 1994, 1995) based on a national medical birth registry and a registry of birth defects. The estimated prevalence of anencephaly for the 2 years was, however, as low as 0.7 per 10,000. For spina bifida the prevalence was 2.7 per 10,000.

Data for England and Wales are available from a national registry collecting diagnoses from several sources. Since 1994 the registry has included reports on terminations. The prevalence of anencephaly was estimated at 1.4 per 10,000 for the first half of the decade and 2.8 for the second half (ICBDMS, 1993–2002). A study from the North of England, also including terminations (Rankin et al., 2000), estimated a similar prevalence of anencephaly of 7.9 per 10,000 for 1991–1996.

The prevalence of spina bifida in England and Wales was 1.7 per 10,000 in the first period and 2.9 in the second period from the national registry (ICBDMS, 1993–2002). As for anencephaly, the increase is probably due to inclusion of terminations from 1994. However, the study from the North of England (Rankin et al., 2000) estimated a prevalence of spina bifida of 7.8 per 10,000 for 1991–1996.

Another country where terminations have been included in the ascertainment recently (since 1996) is Finland (ICBDMS, 1993–2002). This effected an increase in the estimated prevalence of anencephaly from the first to the second half of the 1990s from 0.3 to 3.1 per 10,000. A smaller increase was seen for the spina bifida prevalence, from 2.4 to 4.7 per 10,000.

France has several regional registries that report prevalences of anencephaly and include terminations. A registry in the North east region (around Strassbourg) reported prevalences of 4.3 per 10,000 for the first half of the 1990s and 3.8 for the second half (ICBDMS, 1993–2002). A separate study estimated a slightly higher prevalence (5.8 per 10,000) for the same region for the first period (Alembik et al., 1997). A registry in the Central East Region has included terminations since 1994. Estimates of the prevalence of anencephaly were 0.9 and 1.5 per 10,000 for the first and second halves of the decade (ICBDMS, 1993–2002). Paris has a separate registry that also has reported terminations since 1994. This registry estimated a prevalence of anencephaly of 2.4 for the first half of the decade, but with a more complete ascertainment of terminations in the second half, the prevalence increased to 5.4 per 10,000 (ICBDMS, 1993–2002).

The estimated prevalence of spina bifida in different regions of France showed less variation. In the Northeast Region the prevalence was 3.7 per 10,000 for the first period and 7.3 for the second (ICBDMS, 1993–2002). The prevalence was, however, slightly higher in the first period according to the separate study by Alembik et al. (1997) (4.7 per 10,000). Again, these differences may partly be caused by different coverage of terminations. The registry in the Central East Region (including terminations since 1994) estimated a prevalence of spina bifida of 3.0 and 3.6 per 10,000 for the first and second halves of the decade (ICBDMS, 1993–2002). In Paris the prevalence was estimated at 3.1 for the first half of the decade, but again, with a more complete ascertainment of terminations in the second half, the prevalence was increased to 5.2 per 10,000 (ICBDMS, 1993–2002).

A small population-based registry in Germany, for Saxony-Anhalt, that includes stillbirths and terminations reported data for 2000 (ICBDMS, 2002). The prevalence of anencephaly was still as low as 1.6 per 10,000. However, the prevalence of spina bifida was 8.0 per 10,000.

A national registry of birth defects in Hungary has provided data to ICBDMS for three decades. The registry includes stillbirths and terminations, but still estimated a prevalence of only 0.7 per 10,000 in the first half and 1.4 in the second half of the 1990s for anencephaly (ICBDMS, 1993–2002). The estimated prevalence of spina bifida was also relatively low, but increased from 1.8 to 3.0 per 10,000.

Ireland has provided data for counties surrounding Dublin to ICBDMS since 1996 (ICBDMS, 1998–2002). Stillbirths are included, and abortion is illegal. The registry estimated a prevalence of 3.3 per 10,000 for the second half of the 1990s. A study also from Dublin (McDonell et al., 1999) estimated a prevalence of anencephaly of 4.4 per 10,000 in 1994. This study also showed a fourfold reduction in Dublin since 1980.

Irish data on spina bifida showed a prevalence of 5.0 per 10,000 for Dublin for the last part of the 1990s (ICBDMS, 1998–2002). A consistent number of 5.5 per 10,000 was published for 1994 (McDonell et al., 1999) by a study that showed a downward trend since 1980 for spina bifida.

The data on prevalences from Italy has changed, according to ICBDMS reports from the first to the second half of the 1990s, in that several local registries have replaced a centralized registry (ICBDMS, 1993–2002). This registry was based on many hospitals throughout Italy and covered livebirths and stillbirths. For the first period, the centralized registry reported a prevalence of anencephaly of 0.6 per 10,000 (Table 12.1). All the local registries in Italy are hospital-based except those in Emilia-Romagna and Tuscany, which are population-based. All these registries collected information on terminations in the second half of the 1990s. Sicily, however, started in

2000. In Emilia-Romagna the prevalence of anencephaly was estimated at 1.3 per 10,000 in 1991–1995 and 1.9 in 1996–2002 (Table 12.1). In Campania, the prevalences were 3.2 and 3.0, respectively, for the two periods. Tuscany estimated a prevalence of anencephaly of 2.5 per 10,000 for the second half of the 1990s, and, for the same period, the northeast of Italy and Sicily estimated prevalences of 2.1 and 1.3 per 10,000, respectively.

The prevalence of spina bifida in Italy was estimated for the first period by the centralized registry at 3.9 per 10,000. Similar prevalences were reported from the separate regional registries. In Emilia-Romagna the prevalence of spina bifida was 3.9 per 10,000 in 1991–1995 and 3.6 in 1996–2000. In Campania the prevalence was 3.8 in the first period and 3.3 in the second. For the second period the prevalence was 3.4 in Tuscany, 3.3 in the northeast of Italy, and 2.4 per 10,000 in Sicily.

A registry covering the small population of Malta reported a prevalence of anencephaly of 3.5 per 10,000 for 1999 and 2000 (ICBDMS, 2001, 2002). The reports do not include any terminations. For spina bifida the prevalence was 5.8 per 10,000.

Parts of the northern Netherlands have been covered by a population-based registry for the whole period. The registration is voluntary, based on informed consent, and also covers terminations (ICBDMS, 1993–2002). The prevalence of anencephaly was estimated at 2.1 per 10,000 for the first half of the 1990s and 2.9 for the second. For spina bifida the prevalences were 4.3 and 5.4 per 10,000 for the two periods.

In Norway, a population-based registry has reported data including terminations for the whole decade (ICBDMS, 1993–2002). The estimated prevalence of anencephaly was quite stable at 3.2 per 10,000 for the first half and 3.4 for the second half of the decade. The prevalence of spina bifida was 4.9 in the first period and 5.5 in the second. These prevalences are similar to the recent figures from Finland.

The region of Moscow in Russia started reporting birth defects to ICBDMS in 2000. Terminations are included. For 2000 the prevalence of anencephaly was estimated at 4.0 per 10,000, and that of spina bifida was 7.1 per 10,000 (ICBDMS, 2002).

Two studies performed just prior to the 1990s estimated prevalences in Scotland (Davis and Young, 1991; Omran et al., 1992). Omran et al. describe a falling prevalence of anencephaly in Glasgow over three decades and estimate a prevalence of 13.7 per 10,000 in the 1980s. The study included terminations. Davis et al. estimated a prevalence of anencephaly of 5.2 per 10,000 in 1988 for all of Scotland and also showed a falling trend prior to 1988. The data from Glasgow showed a high prevalence of spina bifida of 16.4 per 10,000 in the 1980s (Omran et al., 1992), while the data for Scotland estimated a prevalence of 5.8 also in the 1980s (Davis and Young, 1991). Whether prevalences are still high for populations with a Celtic background is not clear.

A registry in Spain has reported prevalences to ICBDMS for decades. The registry is hospital-based and covers stillbirths but not terminations (ICBDMS, 1993–2002). Prevalences of anencephaly estimated from the registry data were 1.0 per 10,000 for the first half of the 1990s and 0.4 for the second half. For spina bifida, the prevalences were 3.2 and 2.1 per 10,000, respectively, for the two periods.

Sweden reported birth defects to ICBDMS up to 1992 from a population-based registry with multiple sources of ascertainment (ICBDMS, 1993–94). Since 1999, Sweden has again reported, and the reports now cover terminations as well (ICBDMS, 2001–2002). The prevalence of anencephaly increased from 0.4 per 10,000 in 1991–1992 to 3.1 in 1999–2000, very close to recent prevalences for Norway and Finland. For spina bifida, prevalences of 4.9 and 5.1 for the first and second periods are similar to recent numbers from Norway and Finland.

In 2000 a registry in Ukraine, covering the regions of Rivne and Volyn, also started reporting data to ICBDMS. The registry covers terminations of pregnancies based on prenatal diagnoses. A prevalence of anencephaly of 8.8 per 10,000 was estimated for 2000. A high prevalence of spina bifida, 9.6 per 10,000, was also estimated.

Oceania

Data up to 1998 from a registry covering most of Australia are available from ICBDMS reports (ICBDMS, 1993–2001). Reports from multiple sources also included terminations of pregnancies. The registry estimated a prevalence of anencephaly of 2.6 per 10,000 for the first half of the 1990s and 4.4 for the second half. Slightly higher prevalences were, however, reported from Victoria (Owen et al., 2000) and Western Australia (Bower et al., 2002). For Victoria a prevalence of 7.9 per 10,000 for 1997 may be derived from a graphical presentation. Also from graphical presentations, prevalences of around 8 per 10,000 and 6 per 10,000 may be estimated for the first and the second halves of the 1990s for Western Australia.

Australian data on spina bifida estimate a prevalence of 4.7 and 5.2 per 10,000 for the two periods (ICBDMS, 1993–2001), quite similar to other prevalences from primarily Caucasian populations. Other studies, however, indicate slightly higher prevalences of 8.8 per 10,000 in 1997 in Victoria (Owen et al., 2000), as well as 10 per 10,000 for the first half of the 1990s and 6 per 10,000 for the second half in Western Australia (Bower et al., 2002).

A population-based registry in New Zealand covers live births prospectively and is updated with stillbirths retrospectively (ICBDMS, 1993–2002). No terminations are included. The registry estimated very low prevalences of anencephaly of 0.7 per 10,000 in the first half of the 1990s and 0.5 in the second half. The prevalence of spina bifida was 4.0 per 10,000 in the first period and 3.1 per 10,000 in the second period.

CONCLUDING REMARKS

The overall prevalence of anencephaly for all studies combined was 2.2 per 10,000 for the period 1991–1995 and 2.1 for the period 1996–2000. If we restrict our analysis to studies that provide data for both halves of the 1990s, the total prevalence increased from 1.6 to 1.9 per 10,000. These total prevalences, however, make little sense because of the great variation among prevalences. The range was 100-fold in the first period (38.2 per 10,000 in Turkey vs. 0.3 in Finland) and 30-fold in the second period (13.5 per 10,000 in Mexico vs. 0.4 in Spain).

For spina bifida, the total prevalence was 3.1 per 10,000 for all studies combined for the period 1991–1995 and 3.4 for the period 1996–2000. By restricting the analysis to studies that provide data for both periods, the prevalences were 2.9 and 3.1 per 10,000. For spina bifida the variation among studies was smaller but still substantial. The range was 15-fold (from 22.3 per 10,000 among Palestinians in Israel to 1.5 in Tokyo) in 1991–1995 and 6-fold (14.4 per 10,000 in Mexico to 2.3 in the United States) for the period 1996–2000.

As expected, the total prevalence varied, depending on whether registration was hospital-based or population-based, but only when the prevalence calculation did not include terminations. For anencephaly the average prevalence was similar for population-based and hospital-based studies that included terminations (2.8 vs.3.0 per 10,000). For studies that did not include terminations, however, the average prevalence was much higher for hospital-based than for population-based studies (4.8 vs. 1.4 per 10,000). This pattern was similar for spina bifida. The average prevalence was similar for hospital-based and population-based studies when terminations were included (3.9 vs. 3.8 per 10,000). When terminations were not included, the prevalence was much higher for hospital-based studies (6.4 vs. 2.7 per 10,000).

Underlying this pattern is, of course, also specific geographic variation. The high prevalence of hospital-based studies that did not include terminations included prevalences from high-risk areas like India, Mexico, South America, and Turkey. One could speculate, however, that low prevalences (in the 1990s) in areas with population-based data but no data on terminations could be due to problems of ascertainment. Terminations are likely to occur in several of those populations. It is also interesting to observe that studies that include terminations show the same average prevalence, regardless of whether the data were hospital- or population-based.

It seems clear, however, that ascertainment is an important source of variation in prevalence estimates across the world for anencephaly. One might question whether prevalences below the total average of 2 per 10,000 can be trusted or have sufficient credibility to serve any useful purpose. Even surveillance over time of such prevalences may have limited value since they may be greatly influenced by changes in reporting. It is therefore hard to use the available data to identify true low-prevalence populations of anencephaly.

Very high prevalence estimates, however, particularly consistent ones like those from areas in China, India, Mexico, and the Middle East, probably identify populations with a higher prevalence.

Prevalences appear to show falling trends in historic high-risk areas like the British Isles and North America. This also underscores the importance of regular updates of local prevalences.

The fact that introduction of folic acid prevention programs coincides with the change in the epidemiology of neural tube defects caused by new and widely used methods of early diagnosis and termination of affected pregnancies makes it more difficult to evaluate historically the effect of the prevention programs. Many surveillance programs have problems establishing relevant baseline prevalences from before the 1990s simply because the data had a different basis. As expected, these problems appear to be smaller for spina bifida than for anencephaly. The problems do, however, also influence studies of spina bifida.

Similar to the problem of any prevalence study of finding all eligible cases, this overview must be assumed to have had problems of ascertaining all prevalence studies from around the world. It is likely that some studies that were published as master theses, as reports, or even as scientific papers and should have been represented here were missed. One effect could be an underrepresentation of developing countries in the tables and maps.

This overview of prevalences of anencephaly and spina bifida has focused especially on prevalence reports from the 1990s. Particular emphasis has been placed on the reliability of estimates. The purpose has not been to provide a basis for a formal analysis of the effects of prenatal diagnosis or folic acid supplementation programs. Still, the overview could be helpful for studies with specific knowledge about ongoing programs.

REFERENCES

Agarwal SS, Singh U, Singh PS, Singh SS, Das V, Sharma A, Mehra P, Chandravati, Malik GK, Misra PK (1991). Prevalence and spectrum of congenital malformations in a prospective study at a teaching hospital. Indian J Med Res 94:413–419.

Airede KI (1992). Neural tube defects in the middle belt of Nigeria. J Trop Pediatr 38:27–30.

Alembik Y, Dott B, Roth MP, Stoll C (1997). Prevalence of neural tube defects in northeastern France, 1979–1994. Impact of prenatal diagnosis. Ann Genet 40:69–71.

Anyebuno M, Amofa G, Peprah S, Affram A (1993). Neural tube defects at Korle Bu Teaching Hospital, Accra, Ghana. East Afr Med J 70:572–574.

Berry RJ, Li Z, Erickson JD, Li S, Moore CA, Wang H, et al (1999). Prevention of neural-tube defects with folic acid in China. China-U.S. Collaborative Project for Neural Tube Defect Prevention. N Engl J Med 341:1485–1490.

Birnbacher R, Messerschmidt AM, Pollak AP (2002). Diagnosis and prevention of neural tube defects. Curr Opin Urol 12:461–464.

Borman B, Cryer C (1990). Fallacies of international and national comparisons of disease occurrence in the epidemiology of neural tube defects (review). Teratology 42:405–412.

Bower C, Ryan A, Rudy E (2001). Ascertainment of pregnancies terminated because of birth defects: effect on completeness of adding a new source of data. Teratology 63:23–25. (Erratum: Teratology 2001 63:164)

Bower C, Ryan A, Rudy E, Miller M (2002). Trends in neural tube defects in Western Australia. Aust NZ J Public Health 26:150–151.

Boyd PA, Chamberlain P, Hicks NR (1998). 6-year experience of prenatal diagnosis in an unselected population in Oxford, UK. Lancet 352:1577–1581.

Buccimazza SS, Molteno CD, Dunne TT, Viljoen DL (1994). Prevalence of neural tube defects in Cape Town, South Africa. Teratology 50:194–199.

Bussmann H, Koen E, Arhin-Tenkorang D, Munyadzwe G, Troeger J (2001). Feasibility of an ultrasound service on district health care level in Botswana. Trop Med Int Health 6:1023–1031.

Coard K, Escoffery C, Golding J, Ashley D (1990). Incidence of anencephaly in Jamaica. Teratology 41:173–176.

Cragan JD, Roberts HE, Edmonds LD, Khoury MJ, Kirby RS, Shaw GM, Velie EM, Merz RD, Forrester MB, Williamson RA, et al (1995). Surveillance for anencephaly and spina bifida and the impact of prenatal diagnosis—United States, 1985–1994. MMWR CDC Surveill Summ 44:1–13.

Dai L, Zhu J, Zhou G, Wang Y, Wu Y, Miao L, Liang J (2002). Dynamic monitoring of neural tube defects in China during 1996 to 2000. Zhonghua Yu Fang Yi Xue Za Zhi 36:402–405. (In Chinese)

Davis CF, Young DG (1991). The changing incidence of neural tube defects in Scotland. J Pediatr Surg 26:516–518.

De Wals P, Trochet C, Pinsonneault L (1999). Prevalence of neural tube defects in the province of Quebec, 1992. Can J Public Health 90:237–239.

Dudin A (1997). Neural tube defect among Palestinians: a hospital-based study. Ann Trop Paediatr 17:217–222.

Elwood JM, Little J, Elwood JH (1992). *Epidemiology and Control of Neural Tube Defects*. Oxford: Oxford University Press.

Ethen MK, Canfield MA (2002). Impact of including elective pregnancy terminations before 20 weeks gestation on birth defect rates. Teratology 66(Suppl):S32–S35.

EUROCAT Report 8: Surveillance of Congenital Anomalies in Europe 1980–1999 (2002). Ulster: EUROCAT, University of Ulster.

Farrington CP (2002). Interval estimation for Poisson capture-recapture models in epidemiology. Stat Med 21:3079–3092.

Feldkamp M, Friedrichs M, Carey JC (2002). Decreasing prevalence of neural tube defects in Utah, 1985–2000. Teratology 66(Suppl):S23–S28.

Feuchtbaum LB, Currier RJ, Riggle S, Roberson M, Lorey FW, Cunningham GC (1999). Neural tube defect prevalence in California (1990–1994): eliciting patterns by type of defect and maternal race/ethnicity. Genet Test 3:265–272.

Forrester MB, Merz RD (2000). Epidemiology of neural tube defects, Hawaii, 1986–1997. Hawaii Med J 59:323–327, 341.

Guvenc H, Uslu MA, Guvenc M, Ozekici U, Kocabay K, Bektas S (1993). Changing trend of neural tube defects in eastern Turkey. J Epidemiol Community Health 47:40–41.

Hendricks KA, Simpson JS, Larsen RD (1999). Neural tube defects along the Texas–Mexico border, 1993–1995. Am J Epidemiol 149:1119–1127.

Hey K, O'Donnell M, Murphy M, Jones N, Botting B (1994). Use of local neural tube defect registers to interpret national trends. Arch Dis Child Fetal Neonatal Ed 71:F198–F202.

Himmetoglu O, Tiras MB, Gursoy R, Karabacak O, Sahin I, Onan A (1996). The incidence of congenital malformations in a Turkish population. Int J Gynaecol Obstet 55:117–121.

Ho NK (1991). Congenital malformations in Toa Payoh hospital—a 18 year experience (1972–1989). Ann Acad Med Singapore 20:183–189.

Honein MA, Paulozzi LJ (1999). Birth defects surveillance: assessing the "gold standard." Am J Public Health 89:1238–1240.

Honein MA, Paulozzi LJ, Mathews TJ, Erickson JD, Wong LY (2001). Impact of folic acid fortification of the U.S. food supply on the occurrence of neural tube defects. JAMA 285:2981–2986.

Hook EB, Albright SG, Cross PK (1980). Use of Bernoulli census and log-linear methods for estimating the prevalence of spina bifida in livebirths and the completeness of vital record reports in New York State. Am J Epidemiol 112:750–758. (Erratum: Am J Epidemiol, 1993, 137:1285)

ICBDMS (1993). *The International Centre for Birth Defects. Annual Report 1993 (with Data for 1991)—International Clearinghouse for Birth Defects Monitoring Systems.* Rome: International Centre for Birth Defects.

ICBDMS (1994). *The International Centre for Birth Defects. Annual Report 1994 (with Data for 1992)—International Clearinghouse for Birth Defects Monitoring Systems.* Rome: International Centre for Birth Defects.

ICBDMS (1995). *The International Centre for Birth Defects. Annual Report 1995 (with Data for 1993)—International Clearinghouse for Birth Defects Monitoring Systems.* Rome: International Centre for Birth Defects.

ICBDMS (1996). *The International Centre for Birth Defects. Annual Report 1996 (with Data for 1994)—International Clearinghouse for Birth Defects Monitoring Systems.* Rome: International Centre for Birth Defects.

ICBDMS (1997). *The International Centre for Birth Defects. Annual Report 1997 (with Data for 1995)—International Clearinghouse for Birth Defects Monitoring Systems.* Rome: International Centre for Birth Defects.

ICBDMS (1998). *The International Centre for Birth Defects. Annual Report 1998 (with Data for 1996)—International Clearinghouse for Birth Defects Monitoring Systems.* Rome: International Centre for Birth Defects.

ICBDMS (1999). *The International Centre for Birth Defects. Annual Report 1999 (with Data for 1997)—International Clearinghouse for Birth Defects Monitoring Systems.* Rome: International Centre for Birth Defects.

ICBDMS (2000). *The International Centre for Birth Defects. Annual Report 2000 (with Data for 1998)—International Clearinghouse for Birth Defects Monitoring Systems.* Rome: International Centre for Birth Defects.

ICBDMS (2001). *The International Centre for Birth Defects. Annual Report 2001 (with Data for 1999)—International Clearinghouse for Birth Defects Monitoring Systems.* Rome: International Centre for Birth Defects.

ICBDMS (2002). *The International Centre for Birth Defects. Annual Report 2002 (with Data for 2000)—International Clearinghouse for Birth Defects Monitoring Systems.* Rome: International Centre for Birth Defects.

Jung SC, Kim SS, Yoon KS, Lee JS (1999). Prevalence of congenital malformations and genetic diseases in Korea. J Hum Genet 44:30–34.

Kulkarni ML, Kurian M (1990). Consanguinity and its effect on fetal growth and development: a south Indian study. J Med Genet 27:348–352.

Kunzel W, Herrero J, Onwuhafua P, Staub T, Hornung C (1996). Maternal and perinatal health in Mali, Togo and Nigeria. Eur J Obstet Gynecol Reprod Biol 69:11–17.

Lary JM, Edmonds LD (1996). Prevalence of spina bifida at birth—United States, 1983–1990: a comparison of two surveillance systems. MMWR CDC Surveill Summ 45:15–26.

Li S, Moore CA, Li Z, et al (2003). A population-based birth defects surveillance system in the People's Republic of China. Ped Pediatr Epidemiol 17:287–293.

Lie RT, Heuch I, Irgens LM (1994). Maximum likelihood estimation of the proportion of congenital malformations using double registration systems. Biometrics 50:433–444.

Loncarek K, Mustac E, Frkovic A, Prodan M (2001). Prevalence of anencephaly in the region of Rijeka, Croatia. Eur J Epidemiol 17:241–244.

Mathews TJ, Honein MA, Erickson JD (2002). Spina bifida and anencephaly prevalence—United States, 1991–2001. MMWR Recomm Rep 51:9–11.

McDonnell RJ, Johnson Z, Delaney V, Dack P (1999). East Ireland 1980–1994: epidemiology of neural tube defects. J Epidemiol Community Health 53:782–788.

Mocan H, Bozkaya H, Ozbay G, Mocan MZ, Aydemir V (1992). Neural tube defects in eastern Black Sea region in 1990. Paediatr Perinat Epidemiol 6:465.

Moreno-Fuenmayor H, Valera V, Socorro-Candanoza L, Bracho A, Herrera M, Rodriguez Z, Concho E (1996). Preventive program of birth defects: incidence of anencephaly in Maracaibo, Venezuela. 1993–1996 period. Invest Clin 37:271–278. (In Spanish)

Omran M, Stone DH, McLoone P (1992). The Chief Scientist reports. Pattern of decline in prevalence of anencephaly and spina bifida in a high risk area. Health Bull 50:407–413.

Owen TJ, Halliday JL, Stone CA (2000). Neural tube defects in Victoria, Australia: potential contributing factors and public health implications. Aust NZ J Public Health 24:584–589.

Posaci C, Celiloglu M, Karabacak O (1992). The epidemiology of neural tube defects in Izmir, Turkey. Int J Gynaecol Obstet 39:135–136.

Rajab A, Vaishnav A, Freeman NV, Patton MA (1998). Neural tube defects and congenital hydrocephalus in the Sultanate of Oman. J Trop Pediatr 44:300–303.

Rankin J, Glinianaia S, Brown R, Renwick M (2000). The changing prevalence of neural tube defects: a population-based study in the north of England, 1984–96. Northern Congenital Abnormality Survey Steering Group. Paediatr Perinat Epidemiol 14:104–110.

Rosano A, Smithells D, Cacciani L, Botting B, Castilla E, Cornel M, Erickson D, Goujard J, Irgens L, Merlob P, Robert E, Siffel C, Stoll C, Sumiyoshi Y (1999). Time trends in neural tube defects prevalence in relation to preventive strategies: an international study. J Epidemiol Community Health 53:630–635.

Shaw GM, Carmichael SL, Nelson V (2002). Congenital malformations in offspring of Vietnamese women in California, 1985–97. Teratology 65:121–124.

Smith GK (2001). The history of spina bifida, hydrocephalus, paraplegia, and incontinence. Pediatr Surg Int 17:424–432.

Stevenson RE, Allen WP, Pai GS, Best R, Seaver LH, Dean J, Thompson S (2000). Decline in prevalence of neural tube defects in a high-risk region of the United States. Pediatrics 106:677–683.

Tuncbilek E, Boduroglu K, Alikasifoglu M (1999). Neural tube defects in Turkey: prevalence, distribution and risk factors. Turk J Pediatr 41:299–305.

Velie EM, Shaw GM (1996). Impact of prenatal diagnosis and elective termination on prevalence and risk estimates of neural tube defects in California, 1989–1991. Am J Epidemiol 144:473–479.

Verma M, Chhatwal J, Singh D (1991). Congenital malformations—a retrospective study of 10,000 cases. Indian J Pediatr 58:245–252.

WHO (2003). *World Atlas of Birth Defects.* Geneva: World Health Organization. Available from http://www.who.int/genomics/publications/en/

Williams LJ, Mai CT, Edmonds LD, Shaw GM, Kirby RS, Hobbs CA, Sever LE, Miller LA, Meaney FJ, Levitt M (2002). Prevalence of spina bifida and anencephaly during the transition to mandatory folic acid fortification in the United States. Teratology 66:33–39.

Yen IH, Khoury MJ, Erickson JD, James LM, Waters GD, Berry RJ (1992). The changing epidemiology of neural tube defects. United States, 1968–1989. Am J Dis Child 146:857–861.

Zlotogora J, Amitai Y, Kaluski DN, Leventhal A (2002). Surveillance of neural tube defects in Israel. Isr Med Assoc J 4:1111–1114.

13

Maternal Exposure to Selected Environmental Factors and Risk for Neural Tube Defects in the Offspring

DIEGO F. WYSZYNSKI

Among many populations, defects of neural tube closure, commonly known as *neural tube defects* (NTDs), are significant causes of infant mortality and morbidity. Neural tube defects include anencephaly, spina bifida cystica or meningomyelocele, and encephalocele. They are complex heterogeneous conditions, with multiple genes interacting with environmental factors (Seller, 1994). Although they have been studied extensively, many of their causes remain unknown (Sever, 1995). Intriguing observations about environmental factors that may play a role in the etiology of NTDs have been unveiled. For example, the protective value of increased dietary folic acid (FA) intake to 400 μg daily has been documented (Mulinare et al., 1988; Milunsky et al., 1989; Smithells et al., 1989; Wald et al., 1991; Czeizel and Dudas, 1992; Berry et al., 1999). Folic acid supplementation decreases the recurrence risk of NTDs by approximately 70% among women who have already had an affected pregnancy and shows a similar benefit in women who have not (Table 13.1). Although folate's protective effect is recognized, the mechanism by which some women develop low folate levels and presumably predispose their offspring to NTDs and other potential birth defects is still a matter of debate (see Chapter 29).

This chapter focuses on environmental causes or precursors of NTDs. It is important to realize that although there are no overwhelming data to support a role for environmental agents in the etiology of NTDs, there are data suggesting that extrinsic agents need to be evaluated further (Sever, 1995). A few selected factors have been described; some have significant evidence linking them to NTDs, while others are still mostly speculative (Table 13.2).

PREGNANCY WEIGHT

More than 45 years ago, Kalter and Warkany (1959) reviewed the literature and found an association between maternal malnutrition and increased occurrence of congenital malformations in mammals. Analyzing medical charts of 833 infants with birth defects in South Wales between 1964 and 1966, Richards (1969) found that the major anomalies were of the central nervous system, particularly anencephaly. The mothers had a higher frequency of "not balanced" and "doubtful" diets during the first trimester of pregnancy than controls. It was also noted that mothers with anencephalic babies were significantly heavier than those of controls ($p < .05$). This is consistent with the prevailing theory that vitamin deficiency is an important cause of NTDs, given that women who are underweight have lower caloric intake and women who are obese have been shown to be malnourished in spite of their high caloric intake (Hotzel, 1986; Waller et al., 1994).

Obesity is now pandemic in the United States. Most authors define obesity using the body mass index (BMI), which portrays body weight adjusted for height. Body mass index can be calculated using pounds and inches in the equation [weight in pounds/(height in inches)^2] × 703 or, using kilograms and meters [weight in kilograms/(height in meters)^2]. Obesity is then defined as BMI ≥

TABLE 13.1. *Studies of Periconceptional Folic Acid Supplementation and Risk for Recurrent Neural Tube Defects*

References	Study Type	Sample Size	Dose of Folic Acid	Results
Smithells et al. (1983)	Nonrandomized controlled	Fully supplemented, 454 Partially supplemented, 114 Unsupplemented, 543	0.36 mg	85% risk reduction
Seller and Nevin (1984)	Nonrandomized	Unsupplemented, 543 Supplemented, 421	0.36 mg	Risk reduction
Mulinare et al. (1988)	Case-control	Cases, 181 Controls, 1480	Multivitamins with folic acid	60% risk reduction
Milunsky et al. (1989)	Cohort	23,491		71% risk reduction
Wald et al. (1991)	Randomized, double-blind, controlled	1195	4.0 mg	72% risk reduction
Czeizel and Dudas (1992)	Randomized controlled	Vitamin supplement (incl. folic acid), 2420	0.8 mg	No defects with folic acid supplementation
Werler et al. (1993)	Case-control	Cases, 436 Controls, 2615		60% risk reduction
Werler et al. (1996)	Case-control	Cases, 604 Controls, 1658	Folic acid supplement	Folic acid did not decrease rates in women weighing >70 kg

Source: Adapted from Lewis et al. (1998).

TABLE 13.2. *Putative Risk Factors for Neural Tube Defects*

Putative Risk Factor	Amount of Convincing Evidence
Maternal Pregnancy weight	
Underweight	↑↑↑
Overweight	↑
Obesity (BMI ≥ 29 kg/m²)	↑↑↑↑↑
Maternal Smoking	↑↑
Maternal Illnesses	
Diabetes	↑↑↑
Hyperthermia/fever	↑↑↑↑
Antiepileptic Drugs (Valproic Acid, Carbamazepine)	↑↑↑↑↑
Dietary Factors	
Water chlorination	↑↑↑
Inositol (reduces risk)	↑↑↑↑↑
Simple sugars	↑↑↑
Iron, magnesium, niacin	↑↑↑
Maternal or Paternal Occupation	
Organic solvents	↑
Mercury	↑
Agricultural workers	↑↑
Ionizing radiation	↑
Health-care workers	↑
Other Exposures	
Socioeconomic inequalities	↑↑↑↑↑
Advanced maternal/paternal age	↑↑↑
Increased parity/birth order	↑↑↑
Prenatal maternal stress	↑↑↑
Environmental pollution	↑↑
Nitrosable drugs	↑↑

30.0 and divided into three classes: class I obesity (30.0 to 34.9), class II obesity (35.0 to 39.9), and class III obesity (≥40.0). Obesity is associated with a number of metabolic abnormalities, including impaired glucose metabolism, which is a known cause of birth defects in women with diabetes (Mills et al., 1988), and such an association is of considerable public health importance. The prevalence of obesity has steadily increased over the years among both genders, all ages, all racial/ethnic groups, all educational levels, and all smoking levels (Mokdad et al., 2003). From 1960 to 2000, the prevalence of obesity more than doubled from 13.3% to 30.9%, with most of this rise occurring in the past 20 years (Flegal et al., 2002). From 1988 to 2000, the prevalence of extreme obesity (BMI > 40.0) increased from 2.9% to 4.7%, up from 0.8% in 1960 (Flegal et al., 1998, 2002). In 1991, four states had obesity rates of 15% or higher, and none had obesity rates above 16%. By 2000, every state except Colorado had obesity rates of 15% or more, and 22 states had obesity rates of 20% or more (Mokdad et al., 2001). As the prevalence of obesity has risen in developed countries, overweight among pregnant women has become increasingly common. In the United States, the incidence of obesity among pregnant women ranges from 18.5% to 38.3%, according to the cohort studied and the cutoff point used to define overweight (Garbaciak et al., 1985; Abrams and Laros, 1986; Naeye, 1990; Taffel et al., 1993; Siega-Riz et al., 1994; Cogswell et al., 1995; Galtier-Dereure et al., 2000). In a study of 435 pregnant women seen consecutively at the Obstetric and Gynecology Department of Montpellier University Hospital (France), 74 (17.0%) had a BMI > 25 and 54 (12.6%)

had a BMI > 26 before becoming pregnant (Galtier-Dereure et al., 2000).

Naeye (1990) studied relative maternal pregravid body weight and pregnancy outcomes in 56,857 children born between 1959 and 1966 in the United States. Mothers were divided into four categories according to their BMI: thin (<20), normal (20 to 24), mildly overweight (25 to 30), and obese (>30). After confounding factors, such as age, parity, cigarette smoking, weight gain during pregnancy, presence of diabetes mellitus, and hypertensive disorder were taken into account, a positive correlation was observed between maternal pregravid weight and all congenital malformations (analyzed in aggregate). The prevalence of newborns with congenital anomalies was 4.0% among thin women, 4.5% in the normal group (compared to thin mothers: $p < .01$), 5.4% in the mildly overweight ($p < .001$), and 5.5% among obese mothers ($p < 0.001$). Naeye (1990) was unable to determine whether the increase in malformations was inherent in the metabolic milieu of increasing relative maternal body weight or if it was the result of unidentified lifestyle influences that change with maternal body weight. Other studies have since confirmed an association between obesity and increased risk of congenital anomalies (Waller et al., 1994; Shaw et al., 1996b; Watkins and Botto, 2001; Shaw et al., 2000a, 2000b; Cedergren and Källén, 2003; Honein et al., 2003; Watkins et al., 2003).

During the period called the *Dutch Hunger Winter* of 1944 to 1945, a nearly twofold increase at birth of NTDs among male offspring was observed (Susser et al., 1998). During the height of the famine, the daily ration consisted mainly of bread, potatoes, and sugar beets, yielding less than 1000 kcal (Burger et al., 1948). This tragic period provided the data for a series of randomized controlled clinical trials demonstrating that periconceptional folate supplementation in pregnant women has a significant preventive effect against NTDs. Interestingly, applying a narrower definition of starvation and analyzing the risk of death due to spina bifida as the outcome, a statistically significant effect of early prenatal malnutrition was seen only in males: relative risk (RR) of death from spina bifida in males = 2.62 (95% confidence interval [CI]: 1.14–6.01); RR of death from spina bifida in females = 0.59 (95% CI: 0.14–2.37). These findings indicate that severe periconceptional nutrient deficiency may have a greater effect on the occurrence of spina bifida in males versus females. Other potential explanations include sex-specific effects of prenatal famine on prenatal or postnatal survival rates of cases (Brown and Susser, 1997).

Richards (1969) first showed that the mean prepregnancy weight of mothers of anencephalic infants was higher than that of mothers of normal infants (Table 13.3). Waller et al. (1994) studied 99 mothers of offspring with NTDs, 337 mothers of offspring with other major birth defects, and 534 mothers of offspring without birth defects residing in California and Illinois. After adjusting for significant confounders such as age, race, education, and family income, comparison with women of normal weight (BMI = 19 to 27) showed women with BMI > 31 to be at a significantly increased risk of having an infant with an NTD. The odds ratios (ORs) were 3.0 (95% CI: 1.2–7.7) for women with BMI ≥ 38 and 1.8 (95% CI: 1.0–3.2) for women with BMI 31–37. Neither women who were underweight (BMI ≤ 18) nor those who were overweight (BMI = 28–30) had a statistically significant increased risk of having an offspring with an NTD. When analyses were done by the type of NTD, women who had a BMI ≥ 31 had an increased risk of having an infant with spina bifida (OR: 2.6, 95% CI: 1.5–4.5). When intake of the recommended daily allowance of FA was included in the statistical model, the results remained unchanged.

Shaw et al. (1996b) studied the risk of NTDs among obese California women using the Institute of Medicine's (1990) definition of obesity of BMI ≥ 29. When 538 cases and 539 nonmalformed controls were studied, an increased risk of an NTD-affected pregnancy was observed among obese women (OR: 1.9, 95% CI: 1.3–2.9), which was not attributable to lower folate intake, diabetes, diet pills, or NTD pregnancy history. A limitation of this study is that BMI was calculated from self-reported measures of height and weight. A certain amount of nondifferential misclassification is expected. Davis and Gergen (1994) and Rosner et al. (1998), however, have found high correlations between reported and measured values of weight and height among young Mexican-American mothers and suggest that the reported values can be used as continuous variables with the expectation of only small errors.

Watkins et al. (1996) studied 307 women residing in Atlanta (Georgia) who had either live or stillborn infants with anencephaly or spina bifida (case group) and 2755 women from the same area who had infants without birth defects (control group) between 1968 and 1980. Cases and controls were matched by ethnicity and hospital of birth. After adjusting for maternal age, education, smoking status, alcohol use, chronic illness, and vitamin use, the authors found that, compared with average-weight women, obese women (pregravid BMI ≥ 30) had almost twice the risk of having infants with spina bifida or anencephaly (OR: 1.9; 95% CI: 1.1–3.4). A woman's risk increased with her BMI: adjusted OR ranged from 0.6 (95% CI: 0.3–2.1) for underweight (pregravid BMI < 18.5) women to 1.9 for obese women. As in the study of Waller et al. (1994), the percentage of obese women who reported using vitamins during the periconceptional period was essentially the same as that of nonobese women (15.2% and 15.0%, respectively), suggesting that the metabolic and endocrine disturbances

TABLE 13.3. *Published Studies on Maternal Obesity and Neural Tube Defects*

Reference	Study Design	Site, Year of Birth	BMI (mg/kg^2) for Risk and Referent Group	Defect(s) Studied	Findings
Richards (1969)	Case-control	South Wales, 1964–1966	Not given	Anencephaly	Maternal weight heavier than that of controls ($p < .05$)
Haddow et al. (1981)	Cohort	U.S., years of birth not given	Not given	Anencephaly and spina bifida	No significant differences in mean maternal weight between cases and controls
Wald et al. (1991)	Cohort	United Kingdom, 1972–1980	Not given	Anencephaly and spina bifida	Median maternal weight for NTDs less than for unaffected pregnancies
Waller et al. (1994)	Case-control	U.S., 6/85–4/87 (IL) and 8/85–4/87 (CA)	BMI ≥ 31 vs. BMI = 19–27	NTDs	AOR = 1.8 (95% CI: 1.1–3.0)
				Anencephaly	AOR = 1.5 (95% CI: 0.8–3.0)
				Spina bifida	AOR = 2.6 (95% CI: 1.5–4.5)
				Encephalocele	AOR = 0.8 (95% CI: 0.2–3.7)
				Other NTDs	AOR = 4.2 (95% CI: 1.2–14.6)
Shaw et al. (1996b)	Case-control	U.S., 6/1989–5/1991	BMI > 29 vs. BMI ≤ 29	NTDs	OR = 1.9 (95% CI: 1.08–3.40)
Watkins et al. 1996	Case-control	U.S., 1968–1980	BMI > 29 vs. BMI = 19.8–26	Spina bifida or anencephaly	AOR = 1.92 (95% CI: 1.08–3.40)
Werler et al. (1996)	Case-control	U.S. and Canada, 1988–1994	BMI ≥ 29 vs. 19–23.9	NTDs	AOR = 2.0 (95% CI: 1.0–4.0)
Källén (1998)	Cohort	Sweden, 1983–1989, 1992–1993	BMI > 26 vs. BMI ≤ 26	NTDs	AOR = 1.35 (95% CI: 1.00–1.83)
Shaw et al. (2000c)	Case-control	U.S., 6/89–5/91 (study 1)	BMI ≥ 29 vs. BMI ≤ 29	NTDs (study 1)	OR† = 1.9 (95% CI: 1.3–2.9)
		U.S., 1/87–12/88 (study 2)		NTDs (study 2)	OR† = 1.8 (95% CI: 1.1–3.0)
Moore et al. (2000)	Cohort	U.S., 10/1984–6/1987	BMI ≥ 28 vs. BMI < 28	NTDs	PR*† = 2.22 (95% CI: 0.49–10.10)
				Hydrocephaly	PR*† = 3.69 (95% CI: 1.19–11.44)
Hendricks et al. (2001)	Case-control	U.S.–Mexico border, 1995–2000	BMI ≥ 30 vs. BMI < 30	NTDs	OR = 1.73 (95% CI: 1.03–2.92) AOR = 1.40 (95% CI: 0.80–2.47) OR adjusted for hyperinsulinemia only = 1.45 (95% CI: 0.84–2.51)
Watkins et al. (2003)	Case-control	Atlanta, 1993–1997	Underweight (BMI < 18.5)	All NTDS	1.1 (0.3–3.8)
				Anencephaly	1.3 (0.2–11.3)
				Spina bifida	1.6 (0.3–7.6)
				Anencephaly and spina bifida	1.5 (0.4–5.4)
				Encephalocele	—
			Overweight (BMI = 25–29.9)	All NTDS	1.4 (0.6–3.3)
				Anencephaly	1.3 (0.3–6.5)
				Spina bifida	1.5 (0.5–5.1)
				Anencephaly and spina bifida	1.5 (0.5–3.9)
				Encephalocele	1.3 (0.3–6.5)
			Obese (BMI ≥ 30)	All NTDS	1.5 (0.3–7.2)
				Anencephaly	2.7 (1.2–6.1)
				Spina bifida	2.9 (0.7–12.3)
				Anencephaly and spina bifida	3.3 (1.4–8.1)
				Encephalocele	1.0 (0.1–8.4)

*Excludes diabetic mothers.
†Calculated from extracted data.
AOR, adjusted odds ratio; NTD, neural tube defect; PR, prevalence ratio.
Source: Modified from Watkins et al. (2003).

associated with obesity may either alter folate metabolism or increase folate requirements, or both. In a follow-up study conducted between January 1993 and August 1997, Watkins et al. (2003) found that obese women were more likely than average-weight women to have an infant with spina bifida (unadjusted OR: 3.5; 95% CI: 1.2–10.3) or with anencephaly and spina bifida (OR: 3.3, 95% CI: 1.4–8.1). No significant excess risk was observed among underweight (BMI < 18.5) or overweight mothers (BMI 25–29.9). The risk estimates were higher than those previously reported, but wide CI's limit the conclusions that can be drawn from the findings. If future studies confirm these higher risk estimates, the cause might possibly be the increase over time of the average weight of women in the obese category.

Werler et al. (1996) identified 604 cases (136 with anencephaly, 407 with spina bifida, and 61 with encephalocele) and 1658 controls (fetuses or infants with other major malformations) in tertiary and birth hospitals in the greater metropolitan areas of Boston and Philadelphia, and in southeastern Ontario, between 1988 and 1994 in order to identify maternal prepregnancy weight categories as risk factors for NTDs. Prepregnancy weight was categorized as <50, 50 to 59 (the "reference"), 60 to 69, 70 to 79, 80 to 89, 90 to 99, 100 to 109, or ≥110 kg. Since height was collected as well, BMI categories were <19.0, 19.0 to 23.9 (the reference), 24.0 to 27.9, 28.0 to 31.9 and ≥32.0. Multivariate RR estimates increased from 1.9 (95% CI: 1.2–2.9) for women weighing 80 to 89 kg to 4.0 (95% CI: 1.6–9.9) for women weighing 110 kg or more (for the trend, $p < .001$). A similar increase was observed when BMI categories were analyzed: RR: 1.7 (95% CI: 0.9–3.2) for women with a BMI of 24.0 to 27.9 increased to RR: 2.8 (95% CI: 1.1–6.7) for women with a BMI ≥32. For obese women (BMI ≥ 29), the RR was 2.0 (95% CI: 1.0–4.0). The association did not appear to be mediated by folate; an approximately threefold increase in risk was estimated for the heaviest women, regardless of whether folate intake was below or above the recommended level of 400 μg/day.

Källén (1998) looked at the relationship between NTDs, maternal smoking, and BMI in 1,199,701 Swedish infants born between 1983 and 1993 with known smoking exposure in early pregnancy; 621 infants with NTDs were selected. Women with BMI > 26.0 had a higher risk of having infants with NTDs compared to women in other BMI classes (adjusted OR: 1.35, 95% CI: 1.00–1.83). For women with BMI ≥ 29, the corresponding OR was 1.29 (95% CI: 0.81–2.05).

Given the mounting evidence implicating prepregnant obesity as a risk factor for NTDs, Shaw et al. (2000c) collected data from 277 spina bifida cases and 517 nonmalformed controls to determine if phenotypic classifications of spina bifida, in combination with other factors, were associated with a BMI > 29. Women whose prepregnant BMI was >29 had an OR of 2.2 (95% CI: 1.4–3.3) for spina bifida births compared with women whose BMI was ≤ 29. An elevated risk was observed for each spina bifida subphenotype, but the magnitude of the risk varied somewhat by subphenotype: open spina bifida, OR: 2.0 (95% CI: 1.2–3.1); closed, 3.3 (1.4–7.5); isolated, 2.2 (1.4–3.4); nonisolated, 1.9 (0.9–4.2); high, 4.5 (2.1–9.6); low, 1.9 (1.2–2.9); open/isolated/high, 7.1 (2.8–18.1); and open/isolated/low, 1.8 (1.1–3.1). The finding of elevated effect estimates associated with obesity for essentially every type of spina bifida suggests a heterogeneous pathogenesis contributing to an increased risk of both abnormal neurulation and caudal dysgenesis. Similarly, associations observed for both isolated and nonisolated spina bifida suggest that at least some of the obesity-related pathogenetic processes are not unique to neural tube formation, but adversely affect the embryogenesis of other tissues as well. Further stratification showed that female infants or fetuses whose mothers had a BMI > 29 were at elevated risk compared with male infants or fetuses whose mothers had a BMI ≤ 29, particularly for the phenotypes closed (OR_{female}: 8.3, 95% CI: 2.9–23.6 vs. OR_{male}: 1.1; 95% CI: 0.5–9.0), high (OR_{female}: 6.4, 95% CI: 2.2–18.6 vs. OR_{male}: 4.9; 95% CI: 1.6–14.9), and open/isolated/high (OR_{female}: 14.2, 95% CI: 3.3–60.4 vs. OR_{male}: 3.1; 95% CI: 3.1–55.3). In general, risks were also elevated, but to a lesser extent, for female infants whose mothers did not have a BMI > 29 and for males whose mothers had a BMI >29. In a related study, Shaw et al. (2000c) looked at the relationship between maternal prepregnant BMI and height and the risk of NTDs and found an increased NTD risk with increasing maternal prepregnant BMI, controlling for height. A smaller but significant increase in risk for decreasing height after controlling for maternal BMI was also seen. The mechanism underlying the inverse association between maternal height and risk for a NTD-affected pregnancy is unknown. Some investigators have speculated that the NTD risk may be associated with disturbances in earlier developmental and growth processes of the mother herself (Emanuel and Sever, 1973). Shorter maternal height may, indeed, reflect stunting due to nutritional deprivation or other biological processes and thus may provide some indirect support for this speculation (Shaw et al., 2000c).

In response to the recurrent criticism that in many studies maternal prepregnant weight data are collected as late as several years after birth, Moore et al. (2000) prospectively evaluated the effects of maternal obesity on the risk of NTDs. Between October 1984 and June 1987, 24,559 women from more than 100 obstetrics practices who underwent early second-trimester amniocentesis or alpha-fetoprotein screening studies were invited to participate in the study. Of the 24,559 eligible women who underwent either of these studies between

1984 and 1987, data on height, prepregnancy weight, pregnancy outcome, and confounding data were analyzed for 22,951 subjects. No excess risk of NTDs in the offspring of obese women (BMI ≥ 28) without diabetes (RR: 0.90, 95% CI: 0.39–2.1) was demonstrated. Several differences between this and the previous studies might explain the disparate results: (*1*) Moore's study was prospective; therefore, most of the NTD cases in the dataset resulted in elective termination. (*2*) Seventy percent of the women in Moore's study had some college education compared to 20–50% of women in other studies. (*3*) Observation bias might be a concern in Moore's study if the physicians looked more closely for defects among the offspring of women who were obese. (*4*) The ascertainment of defects in Moore's study was confined to those observed at birth or shortly thereafter. The absence of ongoing defect surveillance in this cohort probably led to an overall underascertainment of anomalies, particularly for those defects that are more difficult to detect at birth. (*5*) In the multivariate analysis, Moore combined defects into broad categories (i.e., "all neurological") that may be etiologically dissimilar. This broad classification would most likely lead to an underestimation of the true effects of BMI on specific types of NTDs.

Shaw et al. (2001) studied 708,129 live births and fetal deaths in California in 1989–1991 and conducted interviews with mothers of 538 NTD cases (including those electively terminated, stillborn, or live-born) and with mothers of 539 nonmalformed live-born controls within an average of 5 months from the term delivery date. Respondent-reported weight gain during pregnancy was analyzed. Compared to women who gained ≥10 kg during ≥38-week gestations, an increased risk of NTD offspring was observed among women who gained <10 kg (OR: 3.2, 95% CI : 2.3–4.6). The risk was greater for anencephaly (adjusted OR: 11.8, 95% CI: 3.2–43.3) but was still elevated for spina bifida (adjusted OR: 1.7, 95% CI: 0.9–3.2). The increased risk was not attributable to maternal nonuse of a multivitamin containing FA, diabetes, NTD-pregnancy history, age, race/ethnicity, education, gravidity, alcohol use, cigarette use, prepregnant obesity, low socioeconomic status (SES), dieting, or nausea, or to lower dietary intakes of FA, zinc, energy (from fat, protein, or carbohydrates), or methionine. Gaining <10 kg during pregnancy may result from either an innate metabolic abnormality or from lifestyle factors (e.g., diet, exercise, or stress) that limit weight gain. Thus, it is possible that lowered weight gain is a reflection of other factors that the authors did not measure, though what these factors might be is unknown. Factors considered most likely to contribute to such an association, given their postulated role in the occurrence of NTDs, were in fact measured. They included maternal use of vitamins containing FA, maternal dietary intake of folate and selected other nutrients, and prepregnant obesity. However, none of these factors fully accounted for the elevated risks (Shaw et al., 2001).

Carmichael et al. (2003) examined maternal dieting behaviors and increased NTD risk among offspring in California by interview and analysis of 538 cases and 539 nonmalformed controls born between 1989 and 1991. Among reported dieting behaviors, diets to lose weight (OR: 2.1, 95% CI: 1.1, 4.1), fasting diets (OR: 5.8, 95% CI: 1.7, 20.0), and eating disorders (OR: 1.7, 95% CI: 0.8, 3.6) were associated with an increased NTD risk during the first trimester of pregnancy. Risk estimates for these behaviors during the 3 months before conception tended to be closer to 1. The fourth behavior, "other special diets," was not associated with an increased NTD risk during either period. Women also reported whether they took diet pills, laxatives, or diuretics, engaged in binge eating, induced vomiting, or exercised excessively from the first 3 months before conception through the end of pregnancy; only the intake of diuretics was associated with a substantially increased NTD risk (OR: 2.7, 95% CI: 0.7, 10.2). This study suggests that maternal dieting behaviors involving restricted food intake during the first trimester may be associated with an increased NTD risk.

MATERNAL SMOKING

Although associations between maternal smoking and decreased birth weight, miscarriage, premature delivery, and sudden infant death syndrome have been observed in many epidemiologic studies (Cnattingius, 2004), an estimated 17.3% of pregnant women in the United States aged 15–44 years smoked cigarettes during pregnancy in 2002 (Substance Abuse and Mental Health Services Administration, 2003). These associations have important implications globally, in light of the increased targeting of women by tobacco companies, both in developed and developing countries (Kaufman and Nichter, 2001). Much less attention has focused on the relationship between maternal smoking and congenital malformations in the offspring; when such studies have been done, they were generally retrospective. Most studies have indicated only a small, if any, association between maternal smoking and congenital malformations (Kelsey et al., 1978), with an estimated relative risk generally ranging from 1.1 to 1.5 (Andrews and McGarry, 1972; Seidman et al., 1990; McDonald et al., 1992). However, a positive association with maternal smoking has been found for such specific malformations as oral clefts (Ericson et al., 1979; Khoury et al., 1989; Källén, 1997a; Wyszynski et al., 1997; Wyszynski and Wu, 2002; Little et al., 2004), limb reduction defects (Czeizel et al., 1994; Källén, 1997b), and kidney malformations (Li et al., 1996; Källén, 1997c). Table 13.4 shows the results of

TABLE 13.4. *Published Studies on Maternal Smoking and Neural Tube Defects*

Study and NTD Reported	Cigarettes Smoked per Day	Odds Ratio	95% Confidence Interval
Kelsey et al. (1978)			
All NTDs (*n* = 82)	1–20	1.3	
(hydrocephalus included)	≥21	1.8	
Ericson et al. (1979)			
All NTDs (*n* = 57)	Any smoking	1.31	0.65–2.62
Evens et al. (1979)	Any smoking	1.30	0.97–1.84
Anencephaly (*n* = 132)*	1–9	0.97	0.58–1.60
	10–19	1.44	0.92–2.20
	≥20	1.73	1.00–2.87
Spina bifida (*n* = 178)	Any smoking	0.99	0.74–1.33
	1–9	0.57	0.34–0.92
	10–19	1.18	0.81–1.71
	≥20	1.49	0.94–2.30
Christianson (1980)	Any smoking	0.96	0.70–1.30
CNS (*n* = 194)	1–19	0.91	0.63–1.30
	≥20	1.02	0.67–1.50
Hemminki et al. (1983)	Smoke sporadically or regularly	0.97¶	
CNS (*n* = ?)	Smoke regularly	1.16¶	
	≥5	1.25¶	
Shiono et al. (1986)			
Anencephaly and spina bifida (*n* = 30)	Any smoking	1.1	0.5–2.4
Malloy et al. (1989)			
Anencephaly (*n* = 67)	Any smoking	0.77	0.44–1.36
Other CNS (*n* = 489)	Any smoking	1.04	0.85–1.26
Van den Eeden et al. (1990)			
Anencephaly (*n* = 34)	Any smoking	0.5	0.2–1.3
Spina bifida (*n* = 58)	Any smoking	0.6	0.3–1.2
Seidman et al. (1990)			
Spina bifida (*n* = 13)	Any smoking	1.62	0.38–5.46
Other CNS (*n* = 42)	Any smoking	0.73	0.26–1.74
Wasserman et al. (1996)			
Anencephaly (*n* = 123)	1–19	0.77	0.43–1.4
	≥20	0.80	0.26–2.3
	(Any smoking, unadjusted)	0.77	0.45–1.29
Spina bifida (*n* = 114)	1–19	0.61	0.33–1.1
	≥20	1.2	0.48–2.9
	(Any smoking, unadjusted)	0.73	0.42–1.21
Shaw et al. (1996a)			
NTDs (*n* = 538)	1–19	0.90	0.61–1.3
	≥20	0.69	0.35–1.4
	(Any smoking, unadjusted)	0.75	0.55–1.03
Källén (1998)			
Anencephaly (*n* = 16)	Any smoking	0.49	0.28–0.85
	<10	0.64	0.35–1.19
	≥20	0.22	0.07–0.67
Spina bifida (*n* = 114)	Any smoking	0.76	0.61–0.95
	<10	0.77	0.59–1.01
	≥20	0.74	0.30–2.60
Encephalocele (*n* =15)	Any smoking	1.16	0.16–2.21
	<10	1.34	0.66–2.71
	≥20	0.88	0.30–2.60
Van Rooij et al. (2002)			
Spina bifida (*n* = 39)	Any smoking, unadjusted	1.36	0.51–3.52

*p for trend <.05.
¶p > .1.
CNS, central nervous system.
Source: Modified from Källén (1998).

studies on the relationship between maternal smoking and NTDs.

The largest study to date (Shaw et al., 1996a) was negative, a finding that agreed with several published reports (Christenson, 1980; Hemminki et al., 1983; Malloy et al., 1989; Van den Eeden et al., 1990; Wasserman et al., 1996) but was not consistent with the findings of earlier studies (Kelsey et al., 1978; Ericson et al., 1979; Evans et al., 1979). Three possible factors might account for these differences. The first is response bias, or the possibility that the cases and controls understated or overstated their smoking habits. The greater amount of time that elapsed between the interviews of case mothers and the births of their children compared with the time that elapsed between the interviews of control mothers could have added to this possible bias. In general, it is impossible to say whether such bias has an effect on the results of a study. A second possible problem is that both smoking and NTDs are associated with some third factor that may be distorting the true relationship between these two factors. For example, Evans et al. (1979) reported an unadjusted association between maternal smoking and anencephaly (RR: 1.76 for smokers of >20 cigarettes per day). When the relation was examined by SES, the dose–response relation between smoking and anencephaly was not apparent in the lowest socioeconomic strata and was inconsistent in the upper strata. Both SES and ethnicity, as well as smoking, have been reported to be associated with congenital anomalies (Chung and Myrianthopoulos, 1975a; Baird, 1980; Sever and Emanuel, 1981). Consumption of FA, nutrition, maternal age, and parity are other relevant variables that need to be considered. A third potential factor is the definition of congenital anomaly. During the 24 years that elapsed between the study of Kelsey et al. (1978) and that of van Rooij et al. (2002), new syndromes have been delineated and identified, and the technological capacity to make an accurate diagnosis has greatly improved. Still, there is no recognized satisfactory classification of anomalies. Comparisons among studies can only be made in general terms since ascertainment and definition of anomalies, temporal or geographic variations in levels of cigarette constituents such as tar and nicotine, or the proportion of filtered cigarettes smoked may vary from study to study. Detailed descriptions of the challenges in assessing exposures in studies of birth defects can be found in Werler (2002) and in Chapter 10 of this book.

In addition to these methodological problems, consideration also needs to be given to the biological plausibility of an association between maternal smoking and NTDs in offspring. Smoking by pregnant women substantially raises the carboxyhemoglobin level of the blood of the fetus (Cole et al., 1972), a high induced concentration of carboxyhemoglobin in pregnant rabbits is associated with an increased frequency of congenital malformations in offspring (Astrup et al., 1972), and *N*-nitroso compounds in cigarette smoke are teratogenic in rats (Magee et al., 1976). An increase in the risk for NTDs from cigarette smoke would therefore appear to be biologically plausible, although it is unknown exactly which mechanisms are involved (Kelsey et al., 1978). Recognizing that tobacco smoke contains many different chemicals, including cadmium, nicotine, and carbon monoxide, which have been shown to be teratogenic in animals (Wasserman et al., 1996), that it induces many physiological changes, and that smokers differ from nonsmokers with regard to both lifestyle and biological characteristics (Yerushalmy, 1971) further enhances the idea that the underlying causal mechanisms are indeed complex. It is possible that maternal factors relating to self-selection of smokers, one or more chemical components of cigarette smoke, or a combination of these also is contributing to the observed associations.

In summary, an increase in the risk of giving birth to offspring with NTDs among women who smoke more than one pack of cigarettes a day during pregnancy remains plausible but by no means certain. The associations reported have not been strong, and if maternal smoking is causally related to NTDs in offspring, it is likely to account for only a modest proportion of all cases.

MATERNAL ILLNESSES

Diabetes

Maternal diabetes significantly increases the risk of congenital malformations in humans and in animal models (Pederson et al., 1964; Kucera, 1971; Chung and Myrianthopolous, 1975b; Eriksson et al., 1996; Chang and Loeken, 1999). Congenital abnormalities have replaced respiratory distress syndrome (RDS) and antepartum asphyxia as the leading cause of death in offspring of women with insulin-requiring pregestational diabetes mellitus (Greene, 1993). The incidence of major malformations is 6% to 9%, which is three- to fourfold higher than the rate observed in the general population, and accounts for 33% to 66% of perinatal deaths (Hoet and Beard, 1979; Reece and Hobbins, 1986). These malformations arise at the beginning of organogenesis, during the first 8 weeks of gestation in human embryos and during the first 7 to 10 days in mouse and rat embryos (Eriksson et al., 1996). Diabetic embryopathy can affect any developing organ system. Generally, however, the birth defects most commonly associated with maternal diabetes are caudal regression, situs inversus, kidney malformations, cardiac anomalies, and NTDs (Kucera, 1971; Mills, 1982; Martinez-Frias, 1994; Becerra et al., 1990). Fine et al. (1999) showed that excess glucose surrounding the embryo is responsible for the adverse effects of diabetic pregnancy. It is hypothesized that the exposure of the embryo to excess glucose at critical times during induction of developmental control genes can compromise subsequent morphogenetic processes (Pani et al., 2002). Other hypotheses, such as alterations of fuels or fuel-related factors essential for embryogenesis, arachidonic acid and *myo*-inositol deficiency, and excessive production of free oxygen radicals relative to the antioxidant reserve (i.e., oxidative stress) have been proposed (Reece and Hobbins, 1986). Administration of antioxidants to diabetic pregnant rodents can reduce the risk of diabetic-associated embryopathy, suggesting that oxidative stress may be involved in the cause of malformations (Viana et al., 1996; Reece and Wu, 1997; Siman and Eriksson, 1997). In humans, susceptibility to diabetic complications such as nephropathy is influenced by the genetic background, indicating that there are polymorphic genes that modify the cellular responses to hyperglycemia (Doria et al., 1995).

Milunsky et al. (1982) reported that in 24,000 pregnancies, including 411 pregnant insulin-dependent diabetic women, more than a 10-fold increase (19.5/1000) in the frequency of NTDs was observed in the offspring of these diabetic patients ($p < .000001$). Also, serum alpha-fetoprotein values were lower in diabetic than in nondiabetic women. Zacharias et al. (1984) observed a significantly increased incidence of NTDs in African-American insulin-dependent diabetic women, although the numbers in their study were small. Becerra et al. (1990) studied 4929 live and stillborn Georgian (U.S.) babies with major malformations in the first year of life. The study also included 3029 nonmalformed live babies who were frequency-matched to case babies by race, period of birth, and hospital of birth. The RR for major malformations among infants of mothers with insulin-dependent diabetes mellitus ($n = 28$) compared with infants of nondiabetic mothers was 7.9 (95% CI: 1.9–33.5), and for major central nervous system and cardiovascular system defects the RR's were 15.5 (95% CI: 3.3–73.8) and 18.0 (95% CI: 3.9–82.5), respectively. The absolute risks for major, central nervous system, and cardiovascular system malformations among infants of diabetic mothers were 18.4, 5.3, and 8.5 per 100 live births, respectively. Infants of mothers with gestational diabetes mellitus who required insulin during the third trimester of pregnancy were 20.6 (95% CI: 2.5–168.5) times more likely to have major cardiovascular system defects than infants of nondiabetic mothers. The absolute risk for infants of this group of diabetic mothers was 9.7%. No statistically significant differences were found among infants of mothers with gestational diabetes mellitus who did not require insulin during pregnancy.

Because the protective effect of multivitamin supplements against birth defects is reported to occur with supplements used regularly during the periconceptional period (defined as the 3 months before pregnancy and the first trimester of pregnancy), evaluation of the protective effect of multivitamin supplements focused on the comparison of nonusers and regular users of multivitamin supplements during the periconceptional period. Correa et al. (2003) identified Georgian (U.S.) infants born between 1968 and 1980 with nonsyndromic birth defects that were reported to be associated with diabetes ($n = 3278$) and compared them with controls without birth defects ($n = 3029$). Classification of maternal use of multivitamins was based on the mothers' responses to two questions about vitamin use during the periconceptional period. Using the answers and a definition of regular use of multivitamins as intake at least three times a week, the authors grouped the mothers into the following mutually exclusive categories: (*1*) nonusers; (*2*) periconceptional users; (*3*) other users; and (*4*) unknown or uncodable. The results showed that offspring of mothers with diabetes did not have an increased risk of spina bifida or anencephaly, although they did have an increased risk for hydrocephaly, outflow tract defects, septal defects, respiratory tract defects, pyloric stenosis, and anal atresia or stenosis. However, the increased risk seemed to be limited to offspring of mothers who had diabetes and had not taken multivitamins during the periconceptional period. Offspring of mothers who had taken multivitamins during the periconceptional period had no increased risk of birth defects, regardless of whether or not the mother had diabetes.

Hyperthermia

Hyperthermia is an abnormal elevation of body temperature. There is concern when body temperature reaches 102°F (38.9°C) or higher during pregnancy for an extended period of time. Beginning with the report of Coffey and Jessop in 1959, several clinical and epidemiologic studies have shown an increased risk for NTDs in infants exposed to maternal hyperthermia or fever-producing illness. In 1978, Miller et al. reported that 7 out of a group of 63 mothers of anencephalic infants had suffered hyperthermic interludes near the presumed time of anterior groove closure. Five had fever, with a maximum recorded temperature ranging from 38.9°C to 40.0°C, and two had possible hyperthermia following sauna bathing. Layde et al. (1980) interviewed mothers of children with NTDs as well as mothers of children with Down syndrome. They found a higher incidence of fever during the first trimester in the NTD group compared to the Down syndrome group. Shiota (1982) studied NTDs in 113 Japanese embryos and noted that maternal fever had occurred in 18% of the 50 embryos with anterior NTDs, significantly higher than the 4.9% in the matched controls. Among the 63 embryos with myeloschisis, 11.1% had a history of fever. In a larger study, Hunter (1984) interviewed 264 women who gave birth to children with NTDs between 1961 and 1981 and found that 32 (12%) reported fevers during pregnancy. Thirteen of these women reported that the fever occurred within the first 4 weeks of pregnancy; nine of them had children with anencephaly. Christo et al. (1987) studied the pregnancy history of the mothers of 30 children born with central nervous system abnormalities and found that four (13%) had significant fevers during the first trimester. Milunsky et al. (1992) conducted a large-scale prospective study that used a cohort of 23,491 women who were receiving prenatal care or having amniocentesis. Fever during the first trimester of pregnancy was associated with increased risk for NTDs; the RR, adjusted for maternal age, FA supplement use, a family history of NTDs, and exposure to other heat sources, was 1.8 (95% CI: 0.8–4.1). Lynberg et al. (1994) evaluated the risk for NTDs in infants born in Georgia (U.S.) between 1968 and 1980 whose mothers had influenza during pregnancy: a total of 385 infants with NTDs, 3647 infants with other birth defects, and 2676 infants without birth defects were included. Of the 385 mothers of NTD infants, 31 reported having a 2-day or longer episode of flu with fever from 1 month before through 3 months after conception (OR: 3.0; 95% CI: 1.9–4.7). Infants of mothers who took medications for their flu with fever had an even higher risk for NTDs (OR: 4.3, 95% CI: 2.6–7.1). When mothers of infants with birth defects other than NTDs were used as controls, an increased risk for NTDs remained for flu with fever (OR: 1.7, 95% CI 1.1–2.5). Surprisingly, there was no increased risk for NTDs among the infants of mothers who reported fever from causes other than flu.

Shaw et al. (1998) studied fetuses and live-born infants with NTDs among 708,129 births in California (includes fetal deaths) between June 1989 and May 1991. Interviews were conducted with mothers of 538 cases with NTDs and 539 controls. Women were asked if they had any febrile illnesses during their first and second trimesters and, if appropriate, the specific dates and name(s) of medication(s) taken at that time. The results revealed a statistically significant association between fever and febrile illness in the first trimester and anencephaly—OR: 2.64 (95% CI: 1.57–3.72) for fever and OR: 2.48 (95% CI: 1.31–4.69) for febrile illness—and spina bifida—OR: 1.69 (95% CI: 1.12–2.55) for fever and OR: 1.74 (95% CI: 0.94–3.20) for febrile illness. Risk estimates were not substantially altered after adjustment for maternal age, race/ethnicity, education, vitamin use, and BMI. The risk associated with maternal febrile illness in the second trimester (an irrelevant embryonic period for neural tube development because the neural tube closes approximately 28 days after conception) was not as elevated (OR: 1.10, 95% CI: 0.64–1.92), arguing against reporting bias as the alternative explanation of their findings.

Chambers et al. (1998) prospectively studied 115 women who reported fever ≥38.9°C lasting for at least 24 hours (high-fever group) and 147 women who reported fever of either <38.9°C or fever lasting for less than 24 hours (low-fever group). An additional 298 pregnant women who reported having no fever at any time during pregnancy were enrolled as a control group. Two of 34 (or 5.9%) women who had high fever during the critical period for neural tube closure carried fetuses with anencephaly compared to no anencephalic births in the low-fever group or controls, supporting the hypothesis that high maternal fever early in pregnancy is a human teratogen. Although the numbers are small, the lower bound of the confidence interval for the prevalence of anencephaly (1.0%) in the study is 10-fold the birth prevalence of all NTDs in the general population (1/1000 or 0.1%).

In an intriguing study, Shin and Shiota (1999) treated five groups of 12 ICR strain pregnant mice with different therapies: hyperthermia (exposure to 43°C for 8.5 minutes), FA (3 mg/kg/day), FA followed by hyperthermia, *myo*-inositol—which reduces the incidence of NTD in *curly tail* mice, as described below—(500 mg/kg/day), and *myo*-inositol followed by hyperthermia. When pregnant mice received hyperthermia, 23.5% of the implanted conceptuses were resorbed, indicating that they died early in the postimplantation period. Treatment of pregnant females with FA or *myo*-inositol alone produced neither teratogenic nor embryolethal effects. Among the fetuses that survived to term in the hyperthermia group, 38.6% had cranial NTDs (exencephaly and anencephaly). When pregnant mice were treated with FA and hyperthermia, the prevalence of NTDs in the fetuses was 26.6%, significantly lower than in the hyperthermia alone group ($p < .05$). When pregnant mice were treated with MI and hyperthermia, the prevalence rate of NTDs was 31.2%, not significantly different from that of the hyperthermia only group. In this study, the prevalence of NTDs in embryos treated with hyperthermia in utero was reduced by about two-thirds in the FA and hyperthermia groups. It is not clear how FA can prevent heat-induced NTD in mice; this is now under investigation in several laboratories. Seller (1994) speculated that NTDs may be produced by factors that result in decreased cell proliferation. Shin and Shiota (1999) found that brief maternal hyperthermia can cause a transient arrest of cell proliferation in neurulating mouse embryos. Although the numbers are small, this study indicates that FA may possibly ameliorate mitotic arrest of neural precursor cells in heated embryos and reduce the risk of NTD.

ANTIEPILEPTIC DRUGS

The majority of women with epilepsy bear normal, healthy children. However, women with epilepsy have an increased risk for adverse pregnancy outcomes, of which congenital malformations are the most widely reported (Yerby, 2003). Infants exposed to antiepileptic drugs (AEDs) in utero are twice as likely to develop birth defects as infants not exposed to these drugs. Hernández-Díaz et al. (2001) examined data from an ongoing case-control study of birth defects (1979–1998) in the United States and Canada, noting that among the 1242 infants with NTDs, 2.2% ($n = 27$) were exposed to folic acid antagonists (FAAs) early in pregnancy, while among the 6660 malformed controls, only 1.0% ($n = 67$) were exposed. The estimated adjusted OR for women exposed to FAAs compared with women not exposed was 2.8 (95% CI: 1.7–4.6). For NTD type, ORs were 6.4 (95% CI: 2.7–15.3) for anencephaly, 2.7 (95% CI: 1.6–4.7) for spina bifida, and 0.0 (95%: 0.0–2.5) for encephalocele (there were no exposed cases). Restriction of the analysis to infants without a family history of NTDs yielded an OR of 5.8 (95% CI: 2.5–13.7).

There is an established association between maternal use of the AED valproic acid (VPA) and the development of NTDs in offspring (see the recent review of Alsdorf and Wyszynski, 2005). During 1976 and from 1978 through September 1982, the birth defects surveillance system at the Institut Europeen des Genomutations in Lyon, France, ascertained 146 cases of spina bifida aperta. Among these cases, nine (6.2%) of the mothers had epilepsy and had taken between 400 mg and 2 g VPA daily during the first trimester (MMWR, 1982). Five of the nine patients with spina bifida were exposed to VPA monotherapy, and four were exposed to additional anticonvulsants. Twenty-one (0.32%) of the mothers of the 6616 infants in the surveillance system with other malformations had taken the drug. The OR was statistically significant (20.6, 95% CI: 8.2–47.9) for spina bifida and use of VPA during the first trimester of pregnancy compared with other structural malformations. To isolate the effect of VPA from the possible effects of seizure disorders and other drug therapy, further analysis was confined to the 71 epileptic mothers. Nine (90%) of the 10 epileptic mothers of spina bifida infants had taken VPA compared with 21 (34.4%) of the 61 mothers of infants with other defects (OR: 17.1, 95% CI: 2.8–103.7). It has been estimated that in the United States, 700–1000 pregnant women take VPA each year. Given the U.S. spina bifida rate of approximately 10 per 10,000 births and a relative risk of 20.6 (as indicated by the French data above), the estimated risk of VPA-exposed women having children with spina bifida is approximately 2%. This risk is similar to that for women who have had previous children with NTDs (anencephaly or spina bifida) (Bjerkedal et al., 1982; Lindhout and Meinardi, 1984; Omtzigt et al., 1992).

Lindhout and colleagues (1992) found an association between NTDs and infants exposed prenatally to AEDs, specifically VPA and carbamazepine (CBZ), with an anencephaly to lumbosacral spina bifida ratio of 1:33. This suggests a specific association with caudal central nervous system defects. It is still unclear how VPA initiates the molecular and biochemical events that ultimately lead to aberrant neurulation, but it may involve the disruption of normal pH within the embryonic milieu, inhibition of peroxisome proliferator receptors, and/or alteration of folate metabolism (Nau and Scott, 1986; Lampen et al., 1999; Karabiber et al., 2003). Recently, the North American Antiepileptic Drug Pregnancy Registry released its results on maternal exposure to VPA (Wyszynski et al., 2005). In their sample of 149 VPA-exposed women, 16 cases had infants with major congenital anomalies. All women took either multivitamins containing FA or FA supplements during the periconceptional period. Three cases with spina bifida were noted among the VPA-exposed women who took the daily recommended amount of FA (prevalence: 2.8%, 95% CI: 0.6–8.0%), approximately 28 times higher than in the general population.

The risk for CBZ-exposed infants presenting with an NTD ranges between 0.5% and 1% (Rosa, 1991). In a Dutch study of the offspring of epileptic women (Samren et al., 1997), two-thirds of the 34 NTD cases had been exposed in utero to VPA (RR 4.9; 95% CI: 1.6–15.0), and nearly one-fifth of the cases received CBZ (RR 4.9; 95% CI: 1.3–18.0). Morrow et al. (2004) reported data on 2967 UK pregnancies exposed to AEDs: of the 775 cases exposed to CBZ, 2 had an NTD (prevalence: 2.6/1000), while only 1 case with an NTD was found among women not exposed to any AED (prevalence: 5/1000). The evidence suggesting that maternal exposure to CBZ during the first trimester of gestation is a risk factor for NTDs is still inconclusive.

DIETARY FACTORS

Water Chlorination

In 1974, Rook demonstrated that chlorination of water containing natural organic material results in production of volatile halogenated organic compounds (Rook, 1974). Since then, many other chlorination by-products such as trihalomethanes (THMs), haloacetic acids, chlorophenols, chloral hydrate, and haloacetonitriles have been identified, most resulting from the process of chlorination but also from chloramination, chlorine dioxide disinfection, and ozonation (Tibbets, 1995; Hwang et al., 2002). Generally, the THMs are the most prevalent volatile halogenated organic compounds in chlorinated water, but there is no direct evidence of their teratogenic effect (Nieuwenhuijsen et al., 2000). Studies have suggested an increased risk of birth defects and other abnormal perinatal outcomes with exposure to disinfection by-products, but the findings are inconsistent for NTDs (see Table 13.5 for specific

TABLE 13.5. *Summary of Epidemiologic Studies on Chlorinated Disinfection By-Products and Adverse Reproductive Outcomes*

Reference	Study Details (Location, Time, Sample Size)	Cases	Exposure Assessment	Other Risk Factors Included	Main Positive Findings OR (95% CI)
Kramer et al. (1992)	Iowa 151 Towns with a single water source 1989–90 Sample population: 4028	588 (Total) 159 Low birth weight 342 Preterm delivery 187 Intrauterine growth retardation, small for gestational age	Based on maternal residential address and one municipal water survey to estimate individual THM concentrations (two or three exposure categories)	Maternal age Parity Marital status Education Smoking Prenatal care	Chloroform, no vs. medium (1–9 μg/L) vs. high (≥10 μg/L): Low birth weight Chloroform, 1 vs. 1.1 (0.7–1.6) vs. 1.3 (0.8–2.2) Intrauterine growth retardation Chloroform, 1 vs. 1.3 (0.9–1.8) vs. 1.8 (1.1–2.9) Intrauterine growth retardation Dichlorobromomethane, 1 vs. 1.2 (0.8–1.7) vs. 1.7 (0.9–2.9)
Aschengrau et al. (1993)	Massachusetts 2 Hospitals 1977–80 Sample population: 2348	1171 (Total) 1039 Major congenital malformations Urinary tract defects Respiratory tract defects 77 Stillbirths 55 Neonatal deaths	Based on maternal residential address to ascertain type of water supply, chlorination vs. chloramination, and ground water or mixed water vs. surface water	Maternal age Pregnancy history Alcohol Ethnicity Hospital payment Other water contaminants	Chlorinated vs. chloraminated: Stillbirth 2.6 (0.9 to 7.5) Neonatal deaths 1.1 (95% CI not provided) Congenital malformations Major malformations 1.5 (0.7–2.1) Respiratory defects 3.2 (1.1–9.5) Urinary tract defects 4.1 (1.2–14.1)
Bove et al. (1995)	New Jersey 75 Towns with a public water supply 1985–88 Sample population: 81,602	29,268 (Total) Live births: 1853 Low birth weight 905 Very low birth weight 4082 Small for gestational age 7167 Preterm 594 Fetal deaths All birth defects: 669 Surveillance 118 Central nervous system defects 83 Oral clefts 56 Neural tube defects 108 Major cardiac anomalies	Based on maternal residential address and municipal water surveys to estimate monthly TTHM concentrations (five or six exposure categories)	Maternal age Ethnicity Sex of baby Primipara Prenatal care Education Previous still or miscarriage Other contaminants	TTHM concentrations > 100 μg/L vs. ≤20 μg/L: Low birth weight 1.4 (50% CI 1.2–1.7) Intrauterine growth retardation or small for gestational age 1.5 (90% CI 1.2–1.9) TTHM concentrations >80 μg/L vs. ≤20 μg/L: Surveillance Register defects 1.6 (90% CI 1–2 to 2.0) CNS system defects 2.6 (90% CI: 1.5–4.3) Neural tube defects 3.0 (90% CI: 1.3–6.6) Major cardiac defects 1.8 (90% CI: 1.0–3.3) TTHM concentrations >100 μg/L vs. ≤20 μg/L: Oral cleft defects 3.2 (90% CI: 1.2–7.3)
Savitz et al. (1995)	North Carolina 6 Hospitals 1988–91 Sample population: 1003	548 (Total) 126 Spontaneous abortions 244 Preterm 178 Low birth weight	Based on maternal residential address and quarterly municipal water surveys to estimate average TTHM concentrations. Analysis of (*1*) surface vs. ground water source, (*2*) TTHM concentrations, (three exposure categories), (*3*) Consumption during pregnancy, (*4*) Water	Maternal age Ethnicity Hospital Education Marital status Poverty level Smoking Alcohol consumption	40.8–59.9 vs. 81.1–168.8 μg/L TTHM: Spontaneous abortion 1.2 (0.6–2.4) 40.8–63.3 vs. 82.8–168.8 μg/L TTHM: Low birth weight 1.3 (0.8–2.1)

			source × amount, (*5*) TTHM dose (concentration × amount)	Employment Nausea	Per 50 μg/L TTHM increment change: Spontaneous abortion 1.7 (1.1–2.7)
Kanitz et al. (1996)	Liguria, Italy 2 Hospitals 1988–89 Sample population: 676	548 Live births in exposed area 50 Preterm 141 Cesarean section 133 Neonatal jaundice 20 Low birth weight 288 Small body length 370 Small cranial circumference	Based on maternal residential address to ascertain type of water source (chlorine dioxide or hypochlorite vs. not treated)	Maternal age Education Smoking Alcohol Sex of child	Sodium hypochlorite treated (8–16 μg/L TTHMs) vs. non-treated water: Neonatal jaundice 1.1 (0.7–2.8) Low birth weight 6.0 (0.6–12.6) Small body length 2.3 (1.3–4.2) Small cranial circumference 3.5 (2.1–8.5)
Waller et al. (1998)	California 3 Regions of surface, ground, and mixed drinking water 1989–91 Sample population: 5144 pregnancies	499 Spontaneous abortions	Based on maternal residential address and quarterly municipal water surveys to estimate average TTHM and individual THM concentrations. Analysis based on (*1*) THM concentrations (3 or 10 exposure categories), and (*2*) consumption during first trimester from interviews (two exposure categories)	Maternal age Gestational age Smoking History of pregnancy loss Ethnicity Employment	High TTHM dose (≥5 glasses/day + ≥75 μg/L) vs. low dose (<5 glasses/day + <75 μg/L): Spontaneous abortion 1.8 (1.1–3.0) High BDCM dose (≥5 glasses/day + ≥18 μg/L) vs. low dose (<5 glasses/day + <18 μg/L): Spontaneous abortion 3.0 (1.4–6.6)
Gallagher et al. (1998)	Colorado 28 Census blocks in 2 water districts 1990–93 Sample population: 1244 live births	72 Low birth weight 29 Term low birth weight 68 Preterm delivery	Based on maternal residential address and municipal water surveys. Estimate of household TTHM concentration during last trimester based on hydraulic modeling (four exposure categories)	Maternal age Smoking Marital status Parity Education Employment Prenatal care	High TTHM concentration (≥61 μg/L) vs. lowest (≤20 μg/L): Low birth weight 2.1 (1.0–4.8) Term low birth weight 5.9 (2.0–17.0)
Dodds et al. (1999)	Nova Scotia, Canada 1988–95 Sample population: 49,842 births	4673 Small for gestational age 2393 Low birth weight 342 Very low birth weight 2689 Preterm delivery 77 Neural tube defects 82 Cleft defects 430 Major cardiac defects 197 Stillbirths 96 Chromosomal abnormalities	Based on maternal residential address and TTHM concentrations for public water facilities (three sampling locations) modeled with linear regression on the basis of observations by year, month, and facility (four exposure categories)	Maternal age Parity Maternal smoking Attendance at prenatal classes Neighborhood family income Sex Pregnancy and predelivery weight	0–49 μg/L vs. >100 μg/L TTHMs Stillbirth 1.66 (1.09–2.52) Chromosomal abnormalities 1.38 (0.73–2.59) Small for gestation age 1.08 (0.99–1.18) Neural tube defects 1.18 (0.67–2.10)
Klotz and Pyrch (1999)	New Jersey 1993–94 Sample population: all births, of which 112 cases and 248 controls were selected	112 Neural tube defects	Based on residential address and public water facility TTHM data, and tap water sampling for TTHMs, HANs, and HAAs (three to five exposure categories)	Sociodemographics Pregnancy and medical history Parental occupational Use of vitamins	TTHMs public monitoring data, Known residence and isolated cases <5 μg/L vs. >40 μg/L Neural tube defects 2.1 (1.1–4.0)
Magnus et al. (1999)	Norway Sample population: 141,077	2608 All birth defects 62 Neural tube defects 250 Major cardiac defects	Chlorination: yes vs. no Color: high vs. low (in chlorinated water average	Maternal age Parity	No chlorination (low color) vs. chlorination (high color) All birth defects

(*continued*)

TABLE 13.5. *Summary of Epidemiologic Studies on Chlorinated Disinfection By-Products and Adverse Reproductive Outcomes (Continued)*

Reference	Study Details (Location, Time, Sample Size)	Cases	Exposure Assessment	Other Risk Factors Included	Main Positive Findings OR (95% CI)
		91 Respiratory defects 122 Urinary defects 143 Oral clefts	TTHMs = 9.4 μg/L, average HAAs = 14.6 μ/g/L)	Geographical placement Population density Industry profile	1.14 (0.99–1.31) Urinary tract defects 1.99 (1.10–3.57) Neural tube defects 1.26 (0.61–2.62) Major cardiac defects 1.05 (0.76–1.46) Respiratory tract defects 1.07 (0.52–2.19)
Jaakkola et al. (2001)	Norway Sample population: 137,145 infants	6249 Low birth weight 5372 Small for gestational age 7886 Preterm	Chlorination and high color; chlorination and low color; no chlorination and high color vs. no chlorination and low color	Maternal age and parity, the child's place of birth in the three university clinics located in the three largest cities in Norway (yes or no), and municipal indicators of socioeconomic level such as centrality, population density, and industrial profile of the municipality where the mother lived during pregnancy	Low birth weight 0.97 (0.89–1.06) Small for gestational age 1.00 (0.91–1.10) Preterm delivery 0.91 (0.84–0.99)
Wright et al. (2003)	Massachusetts 1990 56,513 infants between 22 and 45 gestational weeks weighing more than 200 g at birth	1325 Low birth weight 5310 Small for gestational age 3173 Preterm	Maternal trihalomethane exposure was estimated from the average TTHM concentration for the town of residence. TTHM >80 μg/L vs. 0 to 60 μg/L	Diabetes, eclampsia, hydramnios, chronic hypertension, hypertension during pregnancy, incompetent cervix, lung disease, renal disease, uterine bleeding, previous preterm delivery, previous birth of an infant weighing >4000 g, gestational age	Low birth weight 1.05 (0.85–1.29) Small for gestational age 1.14 (1.02–1.26) Preterm delivery 0.90 (0.77–1.04)

BCDM, bromodiculoromethane; CNS, central nervous system; HAA, haloacetic acid; HAN, haloacetonitrile; THM, trihalomethane; TTHM, total trihalomethane.
Source: Modified from Nieuwenhuijsen et al. (2000).

studies). Discrepant results might be due to many factors: (*1*) the type of disinfection process of the mother's residential water source, (*2*) the mother's consumption of tap water, (*3*) the level of toxicants present in the water supply during the critical exposure period, and (*4*) exposure through pathways other than ingestion (inhalation; dermal contact; and uptake while showering, bathing, and swimming) (Beech et al., 1980; McKone, 1993; Levesque et al., 1994; Weisel and Jo, 1996; Lindstrom et al., 1997; Weisel et al., 1999). Several reproductive epidemiologic studies relied on crude exposure data, and some used comparisons between water source (ground vs. surface) and between water treatments (chlorinated vs. nonchlorinated) (Aschengrau et al., 1993; Kanitz et al., 1996). Other studies used routinely collected total trihalomethane (TTHM) measurements (TTHM is obtained by adding the estimated concentrations of chloroform, bromodichloromethane, chlorodibromomethane, and bromoform) to form exposure categories (Kramer et al., 1992; Bove et al., 1995; Gallagher et al., 1998; Dodds et al., 1999). More recent studies have measured individual exposure with routinely collected THM measurements combined with an attempted measure of ingestion, such as number of glasses of water drunk per day (Savitz et al., 1995; Swan et al., 1998; Klotz and Pyrch, 1999; King et al., 2004). Miscalculation of exposure as a result of crude assessment measures may lead to biased risk estimates and make interpretation of the studies more difficult (Swan and Waller, 1998).

Klotz and Pyrch (1999) carried out a population-based case-control study in New Jersey during 1993 and 1994 to examine the relation between public monitoring of THMs and estimates of THMs, haloacetonitriles (HANs), and haloacetic acids (HAAs) in tap water and their effects on NTDs. Using 112 eligible cases and 248 controls (and excluding term births weighing <2500 g as well as infants with other defects), they obtained data on demographics, pregnancy, medical history, parental occupation, ingestion of tap water, showering, bathing, and swimming patterns. The strongest association was found between public monitoring of TTHM and isolated cases of NTDs with known residency at conception (OR: 2.1 95% CI 1.1–4.0 for <5 vs. >40 μg/L). The results were not disproportionately attributable to chloroform or brominated THMs. Only a slight, but not significant, excess risk was found for HANs and HAAs and NTDs, and there was no association between showering, bathing, and swimming and NTDs. No changes were found when ingested doses were calculated and used. Dodds and King (2001) evaluated the risk of birth defects relative to exposure to specific THMs in public water supplies of Nova Scotia. For NTDs, excess risk was found only at the highest level of exposure to bromodichloromethane (≥20 μg/L) and there was no evidence of a dose–response pattern with its increasing concentration. The adjusted RR at exposure to the highest concentration of bromodichloromethane relative to exposure to concentrations less than 5 μg/L was 2.5 (95% CI: 1.2 to 5.1). The few cases in this category result in a fairly unstable point estimate, as indicated by the width of the 95% CI. There was no evidence of an association between chloroform and NTDs.

Hwang et al. (2002) grouped the risk of birth defects for 285,631 Norwegian births between 1993 and 1998 into four chlorination by-product exposure categories—high (chlorination, color ≥20 mg pt/L), medium (chlorination, color 10 to 19.9), low (chlorination, color <10), and a reference category of no chlorination and low color (color <10)—where color represented the amount of dissolved organic compounds. The authors identified 138 live births (0.08%) with NTDs, including 46 (0.03%) cases with anencephaly and 81 (0.04%) with spina bifida. Although there was no consistent association of chlorination and color with the risk of NTDs (adjusted OR for combined medium and high exposure: 1.05, 95% CI: 0.54–2.03), risk was related to color without chlorination; the adjusted OR was 2.60 (95% CI: 1.30–5.26) in the high-color category. Of the specific NTDs, the adjusted OR for spina bifida was 1.43 (95% CI: 0.58–3.48) in the medium color category and 3.11 (95% CI: 1.22–7.95) in the high-color category.

Although the available evidence suggests that the risks, if any, are small, the large number of people exposed to chlorinated water supplies means that the population attributable risk is potentially high. The inability to eliminate the possibility that other risk factors or possible biases might explain these small excess risks, coupled with the insufficient animal data to evaluate the biological mechanisms by which these agents may exert teratogenic and other birth effects, makes interpretation of such small increases in risk difficult. Moreover, many of these apparent associations have been found at TTHM concentrations well below the established maximum standards, currently 100 μg/L in the United Kingdom and the United States. Reducing concentrations of chlorination dibutyl phthalates further while still using chlorine becomes increasingly difficult. The public health benefits of chlorination in terms of microbiological safety far exceed the potential health risks, but alternatives to chlorination should be and are being explored (Nieuwenhuijsen et al., 2000).

Inositol

As previously discussed in this chapter, FA supplementation is widely used to prevent NTDs. Yet, not all cases of NTD appear to respond to FA. For example, in the randomized controlled trial sponsored by the Medical Research Council (Wald et al., 1991), 6 NTD recurrences were noted among 593 women (1%) who received full

FA supplementation compared with 21 recurrences among 602 unsupplemented pregnancies (3.5%; OR: 0.28, 95% CI: 0.09–0.73). Therefore, 28% of NTD cases were not prevented by administration of FA. Studies in mice provide evidence for FA-sensitive and FA-resistant NTD types. Neural tube defects in mice homozygous for mutations of the *Pax3, Cart1,* and *crooked tail* genes can be prevented by FA (Zhao et al., 1996; Fleming and Copp, 1998; Carter et al., 1999), whereas NTDs in the *curly tail* (*Ct;* a mouse model for human NTDs, in which 50%–60% of the offspring have spina bifida and exencephaly [van Straaten and Copp, 2001]) mutant mouse are resistant to FA (Seller, 1994). A potentially novel therapy for folate-resistant NTDs was suggested by Greene and Copp (1997), who found that treatment of pregnant female mice with *myo*-inositol, during early pregnancy can prevent the majority of NTD cases in the *ct* mouse (Cavalli and Copp, 2002). *Myo*-inositol is crucial for normal embryonic and fetal development (Greene and Copp, 1997; Beemster et al., 2002). Dietary inositol also reduces the frequency of NTDs in a diabetic rat model (Reece and Wu 1997). Cogram et al. (2002) alternatively administered D-*chiro*- or *myo*-inositol to pregnant mice. D-*chiro*-inositol consistently exhibited the more potent effect, reducing spina bifida by 73%–86% compared with the 53%–56% reduction seen with *myo*-inositol.

Cavalli and Copp (2002) reported the first use of periconceptional inositol in human pregnancy. Two unrelated healthy Italian parents of European origin (mother aged 25, father aged 30) elected to terminate two consecutive pregnancies following ultrasound findings of myelomeningocele that occurred despite administration of 4 mg FA daily, starting 3 months before conception. For their third pregnancy, the mother underwent combination treatment of 500 mg inositol and 2.5 mg FA daily, starting at least 3 months before conception and continuing through the first 60 days of pregnancy. During this pregnancy, maternal serum and amniotic fluid alpha-fetoprotein measurements were within the normal range at the 15th week of pregnancy, and ultrasound examinations at 15, 20, and 22 weeks showed normal fetal and placental growth parameters. The pregnancy progressed uneventfully, with no particular episodes of uterine contraction, and a healthy baby boy weighing 3900 g was delivered spontaneously at 40 weeks.

It has been postulated that the high glucose concentration in diabetic mothers interferes with the cellular uptake of *myo*-inositol, resulting in a tissue-specific *myo*-inositol shortage (Greene and Copp, 1997; Reece and Wu, 1997). Groenen et al. (2003) demonstrated that this lack of *myo*-inositol may result in a derangement of DNA transcription and in disturbances of migration and differentiation of neural crest cells, which are important processes in the formation of the neural tube. Between January 1991 and January 2000, amniotic fluid samples were obtained from 76 Dutch women aged 20–44. Twenty-seven women carried a fetus with a spina bifida, that is, meningo(myelo)cele, diagnosed by ultrasonography and alpha-fetoprotein level, with postpartum confirmation. The control group comprised a random sample of 49 women who underwent amniocentesis indicated for high maternal age (≥36 years). At the gestational age of 15 weeks, in contrast to the *myo*-inositol concentration, the estimated mean concentrations of glucose and zinc in amniotic fluid of women carrying fetuses with spina bifida were significantly different from those of controls. These findings partially support the study hypothesis that the transfer or metabolism of glucose and zinc is deranged in spina bifida fetuses and/or their mothers. Using the transmission disequilibrium test (described in Chapter 14 of this book), Groenen et al. (2004a) also studied the biochemical concentrations of *myo*-inositol, glucose, and zinc and polymorphisms in the *myo*-inositol transporter SLC5A11, *myo*-inositol synthase *ISYNA1,* and the zinc transporter *SLC39A4* in association with the spina bifida risk. The results suggest that the combination of maternal glucose <4.5 mmol/L and *ISYNA1* 1029A > G polymorphism protects against spina bifida offspring ($OR_{Glucose \geq 4.5 mmol/L}$: 1.27 and $OR_{Glucose<4.5 mmol/L}$: 0.35, χ^2 interaction: 4.361, $p < .05$). This, in turn, may suggest that the *ISYNA1* gene, or a tightly associated mutation, is implicated in pathways involved in neural tube development that can be modulated by glucose status.

Simple Sugars

Shaw et al. (2003) interviewed California mothers of 454 NTD cases (including fetuses and infants who were electively terminated, stillborn, or born alive) and mothers of 462 nonmalformed controls within an average of 5 months from the term delivery date to assess the effect of maternal periconceptional dietary intakes of sucrose, glucose, fructose, and foods with higher glycemic index values on the NTD-affected pregnancy risk. A 100-item food-frequency questionnaire developed by Block et al. (1986) was used to assess nutrient intake. Periconceptional intake of glucose or fructose did not substantially increase the risk of having an NTD-affected pregnancy, although elevated risks were observed for higher intake of sucrose (>46.25 g, OR: 2.34, 95% CI: 1.39–3.96) and foods with higher glycemic index values (index > 55.56 and spina bifida, OR: 2.11, 95% CI: 1.36–3.27). An elevated risk was observed for high sucrose intake irrespective of adjustment for other covariates, such as maternal FA intake. For higher glycemic index values, adjusted elevated risks were observed in women with BMI > 29 (index 53.23 to 55.56 OR: 5.74, 95% CI: 1.32–24.90; index >55.56, OR:

4.05, 95% CI: 1.04–15.73). These results indicate an elevated NTD risk associated with maternal intake of periconceptional foods with higher glycemic index values and higher sucrose content but do not indicate an elevated risk associated with higher intake of glucose and fructose.

Trace Elements and Other Nutrients

In addition to FA, other nutrients have been suggested to reduce the NTD risk, such as vitamin C (Schorah et al., 1983), zinc (Sever and Emanuel, 1973; Velie et al., 1999), and methionine (Shaw et al., 1997). Shaw et al. (1999) interviewed California mothers of 409 NTD fetal and infant cases and 420 nonmalformed controls from 1989 to 1991, obtaining information about vitamin/mineral supplement use during the 3 months before conception and in each trimester of pregnancy. A 100-item food frequency questionnaire was administered to each case and control mother. Adjusted analyses revealed a statistically significant decreased NTD risk with increased intake of lutein (OR: 0.6, 95% CI: 0.4–0.8) for women who did not use vitamin supplements periconceptionally. Reduced risks (albeit not statistically significant) were also found in this group for intake of methionine, magnesium, zinc, and thiamine. In women who used supplements, decreased NTD risks were associated with increased intake of linoleic acid, cysteine, calcium, and zinc. Increased NTD risks were associated with increased intake of oleic acid (OR: 5.8, 95% CI: 0.5–70.1). Whether or not vitamin supplements were used, although not statistically significant, reduced risks with increased intake of grains and dairy products were noted.

Groenen et al. (2004b) administered a similar food-frequency questionnaire to mothers of 106 Dutch cases with spina bifida and mothers of 181 controls between August 1999 and December 2001. The results showed that dietary intakes of iron, magnesium, niacin, fibers, plant proteins, and polysaccharides were significantly lower in case mothers compared with control mothers. The lowest intakes were associated with a two- to five-fold increased risk for spina bifida in the offspring, independent of periconceptional FA use (plant protein 20.5–28.8 g/day, OR: 5.4, 95% CI: 2.3–12.4; fiber 13.0–22.0 g/day, OR: 3.1, 95% CI: 1.5–6.8; iron 7.6–11.2 mg/day, OR: 3.5, 95% CI: 1.4–8.3; magnesium 186.7–330.3 mg/day, OR 1.9, 95% CI: 0.9–4.1; niacin 8.4–15.7 mg/day, OR 2.5, 95% CI: 1.2–5.2). By contrast, high dietary intake of mono- and disaccharides (143.0–218.7 g/day) increased the spina bifida risk 2.9-fold (95% CI: 1.4–6.3), whereas the intake of polysaccharides (142.8–184.1 g/day) was associated with a reduction in spina bifida risk (OR: 0.5, 95% CI: 0.3–1.0). Interestingly, except for iron and folate, the overall intake of all nutrients in case mothers were comparable and, in some cases, higher than that proposed by the Dutch National Food Consumption Survey and the Dutch Recommended Daily Allowances report.

MATERNAL OR PATERNAL OCCUPATION

Finnish women working in industrial occupations and construction were found to have more children with central nervous system malformations than referent mothers (OR: 1.6, $p < .05$) (Hemminki et al., 1980). No statistically significant ORs were found with respect to paternal occupation in this study. Noteworthy is the fact that differences in the risk of malformations were more pronounced by occupational group than by social class, suggesting that occupation, or related factors, play a greater role in risk determination than does social class. In a subsequent article, Hemminki et al. (1981) reported results from the same sample, adjusting for a number of confounding factors such as social class, tobacco smoking, and medication. Controlling for these factors increased the risk of central nervous system malformations for mothers employed in industry, construction, transport, and communication (OR = 2.0, $p < .001$), again suggesting that social class was not as prominent a risk factor determinant.

Because most teratogenic substances are thought to affect the child through the mother, relatively few studies have been carried out with the specific aim of investigating the relation between NTDs and paternal occupational exposure. However, paternal occupational exposure to chemicals or radiation could theoretically result in genetic damage to germ cells or in concentrations of teratogenic substances in the seminal fluid (Blatter et al., 1997). These substances might affect the child at the time of conception or later, during embryonic development (Hales et al., 1986). Also, indirect exposure of the mother could be caused by "carry-home exposure" of the father (Blatter et al., 1997). Reviewing the occupations of the fathers of children with anencephaly, as described on the birth certificates, Fedrick (1976) compared these with the occupations of all fathers in the Oxford, England, area and, although the numbers were small, found statistically significant associations for printers (RR: 6.7, $p < .001$), painters and decorators (RR: 2.5, $p < .005$), and transport and communication workers (RR: 1.7, $p < .01$), who were mainly drivers of road vehicles. McDonald et al. (1989) found an association between developmental defects and fathers working in the food and beverage and wood and textile processing industries. The observed number of NTDs was higher than expected (O/E ratio: 5/1.8), but the sample size was small. Hearey et al. (1984) investigated a cluster of anencephaly and spina bifida births with regard to a range of factors, including occupation and chemical exposure. They concluded that none of these exposures was associated with NTDs. However, this study included only 9 cases and 27 controls. A larger study did not reveal any significant association with maternal occupation either, although the case mothers had slightly more occupations where chemical exposure is likely (Ericson et al., 1988). Elwood and Elwood (1984) noted a slight but statistically significant increase in the risk for anencephaly among mother who reported working during pregnancy (RR = 1.3, $p < .01$). Brender and Suarez (1990) examined the association between parental occupation and anencephalic births among 585 cases and 1286 controls, with special attention paid to pesticide and solvent exposure. With respect to the mothers, the number of exposed cases and controls was too low to find any exposure effect. However, women working as laborers had the highest risk for anencephalic offspring when women working in professional, managerial, and technical positions were used as a reference group. As for the fathers, exposure to solvents was associated with a significantly elevated risk for anencephalic offspring (OR = 2.5, 95% CI: 1.6–4.1). Painters had a more than threefold risk, and plastic production workers had a twofold risk. Olshan et al. (1991) compared paternal occupations of 534 cases of spina bifida with 1033 referents. Increased risks were observed for fathers who were forestry and logging workers, paper workers, painters, service-station attendants, and personal service workers. Hammond and Canache (1991) observed remarkable differences in certain occupations between Venezuelan parents of children with NTDs and control parents. Thirteen percent of case mothers were hairdressers compared with 1.3% of control mothers; 8% of case mothers were farmers compared with none of the control mothers. As for fathers, 31.6% of the cases were farmers compared with 13.2% controls ($p = .01$), and 19.7% of the cases were bricklayers compared with 5.3% of controls ($p = .01$). Using telephone interviews, Schnitzer et al. (1995) obtained information on parental occupation for 176 cases of spina bifida and 2279 controls. There were moderately increased risks for vehicle manufacturers, electronic equipment operators, welders, and carpenters and woodworkers, although the latter three effect estimates were imprecise. Through job-specific telephone interviews with 122 case fathers and 411 control fathers in the Netherlands, Blatter et al. (1997) collected detailed exposure information on specific tasks, use of chemical or physical agents, frequency of exposure, and use of protective equipment. The study yielded statistically significant associations between spina bifida and low exposure to welding fumes (OR: 1.6, 95% CI: 1.0–2.6) and low exposure to ultraviolet (UV) radiation during welding (OR: 2.6, 95% CI: 1.2–5.6), and, although not statistically significantly, it suggests an association between spina bifida and moderate or high exposure to cleaning agents (OR: 2.1, 95% CI: 0.7–6.5), to moderate or high pesticide exposure (OR: 1.7, 95% CI: 0.7–4.0), and to any amount of stainless steel dust exposure (OR: 2.0, 95% CI: 0.8–5.2). No associations were identified for other paternal occupational exposures, such as organic solvents. The slightly increased risk for exposure to welding fumes was primarily caused by an increase among painters, printers, plastic and paper workers, construction workers, and agricultural workers, but not by an increase among professional welders or metal workers. The level of exposure to welding fumes in these workers was low, but less protective equipment was used by these workers than by professional welders (46% compared with 86%). The increased risk for UV radiation exposure during welding might be a proxy for the risk of exposure to welding fumes. Because UV radiation is visible to the worker, it might be less prone to subjective interpretation of the participant.

In summary, only some specific occupations were evaluated and many of these studies were small-scale. Occupations that were identified as a risk factor in two or more of these studies are painter, transport and communication worker, and farmer. Following are descriptions of individual exposure-specific or occupation-specific findings. They are included in this chapter because their results are interesting, despite the dearth of confirmatory studies.

Organic Solvents

Organic solvents are volatile liquids that belong to a structurally diverse group of chemicals having a low molecular weight and dissolve other organic such as lipids and high molecular weight compounds. Presently, they are widely used in both work and home environments. Usually, incidental exposure can take place around the house, while extensive exposure mostly occurs in the workplace. The use of organic solvents is widespread; they are used in a variety of occupations such as painting, dry cleaning, printing, and various jobs within the chemical industry. Thus, many employees are exposed extensively to organic solvents (Logman et al., 2005). Holmberg and Nurminen (1980) found that significantly more mothers of children with central nervous system defects had been exposed to organic solvents during the first trimester of pregnancy compared with control mothers. Among the 14 cases of central nervous system defects in which the mother had been exposed were 8 children with anencephaly or spina bifida (proportion: 57.1%, 95% CI: 28.9–82.3%). Logman et al. (2005) conducted a meta-analysis to assess the risks of major malformations after paternal exposure to organic solvents. They identified five studies (total of 180,242 participants) that examined the relationship between paternal exposure to solvents and NTDs and from which 2×2 tables could be extracted. The OR for all NTDs was statistically significant, 1.86 (95% CI: 1.40–2.46). The chance of anencephaly in offspring of exposed fathers was two-fold higher than that of unexposed fathers (OR: 2.18, 95%: 1.52–3.11, based on 107,761 participants). For spina bifida (96,517 participants) there was an increased risk, but the risk was not statistically significant (OR: 1.59, 95% CI: 0.99–2.56). Logman et al. (2005) warn that conclusions should be interpreted with caution. *Organic solvents* is a broad term including a variety of chemical substances. Consequently, all studies may not have examined the same chemical classes. It is also possible that retrospective studies may have been subject to response bias and/or recall bias. Another major problem in these studies was the assessment of exposure to the organic solvents. In these types of epidemiologic studies, it is difficult to quantify the actual exposure, the duration, and the timing. With these limitations, it is not always possible to ascertain that the risk is actually caused by the organic solvent exposure or is due to other (unmeasured) risk factors. However, this meta-analysis clearly shows that until the exact relationship is determined, not only women but also men who wish to have children should minimize their exposure to organic solvents in the 3 months (or longer, depending on the kinetics of the particular solvent) prior to the planned conception date.

Mercury

In Sikorski et al.'s (1987) study of women working in dentistry, metallic mercury exposure was determined through levels in scalp and pubic hair and was found to differ statistically significantly from that of a control group. More spontaneous abortions, stillbirths, and congenital defects occurred in dentists and dental assistants compared with the control group (24% and 11%, respectively), and five out of six malformations were spina bifida.

Agricultural Workers

English gardeners and groundsmen, who are likely to handle the herbicide 2,4,5,-T, experienced increased ratios for children with spina bifida, anencephaly, and facial clefts [observed/expected ratios (O/E) were 123, 117, and 142, respectively], while other agricultural workers had increased ratios for spina bifida and facial clefts (O/E ratio of 128 and 127, respectively) (Balarajan and McDowall, 1983). Brender and Suarez (1990) found an association between pesticide exposure and a slightly increased risk of spina bifida (OR: 1.3, 95% CI: 0.8–2.1). However, exposure was inferred from the occupational title and was not assessed by means of detailed exposure information.

Occupations Involving Ionizing Radiation Exposure

Exposure of employees of a nuclear power plant to low-level ionizing radiation and the risk of congenital malformations in offspring was investigated by Sever et al. (1988). When all malformations were analyzed as a group, no evidence of any association was found. Analyses of fathers' cumulative exposure showed positive but nonsignificant trends; a statistically significant association was seen only for NTDs (mean exposure 24.2 mSv compared to an expected mean value of 13.4 mSv, $p = .04$), even on the basis of a small number of cases.

Health-Care Workers

Offspring of mothers employed in nursing were found to be at statistically significantly increased risk of having, among others, anencephaly or spina bifida (RR: 2.0, 95% CI: 1.0–4.3) (Fedrick, 1976). However, the finding of several statistically significant RR was expected because the RRs were estimated for a large number of associations.

OTHER FACTORS

Socioeconomic Inequalities

The presence, as well as the extent, of socioeconomic inequalities in the prevalence of congenital anomalies can be an important etiological factor, especially in regard to nutrition (Little and Elwood, 1991) and also adds potential for environmental confounding factors, such as residence near industrial sites (Dolk et al., 1998) and smoking during pregnancy (Vrijheid et al., 2000). Analysis of socioeconomic inequalities in congenital anomaly prevalence is an important component of the needs assessment and of effective service targeting, such as periconceptional FA supplementation, and provides valuable information for the evaluation of population interventions. For example, Dawson et al. (2001) conducted a survey from April to July 1996 among women attending the genetics clinic at an Ottawa pediatric hospital. All women attending the clinic during the study period were given the option of completing the survey. The survey was completed anonymously by 342 (69%) of the 494 women who were approached. The authors found that level of education does not correlate with adequate FA supplementation. Contrary to the report of McDonnell et al. (1999), Dawson et al. (2001) found no association between SES and the use of FA, probably because of the skewed SES of their study population. Few studies have examined the presence of socioeconomic inequalities in specific congenital defects, with the exception of NTDs, for which a two- to fourfold higher increase in risk among lower social classes has been documented (Little and Elwood, 1991). A study in California from 1989 to 1991 noted an excess risk of NTDs in women from more deprived neighborhoods (Wasserman et al., 1998). In many of the classic studies of NTDs, occupation, particularly the father's occupation, was used as an indicator of social class or SES (Emanuel and Sever, 1973). Other variables used to define it include education and mean census track income. Despite the difficulty in assessing SES, further research is particularly important in evaluating the impact periconceptional FA supplementation recommendations may have in changing socioeconomic inequalities as a factor in the prevalence of NTDs (Achenson, 1998; de Walle et al., 1998).

Maternal and Paternal Age

A number of studies have reported the maternal age risk for NTDs to be U-shaped, that is, highest among the youngest and oldest women, while other studies have found the risk to decrease with increasing age or increase with decreasing age (Leck, 1974; Campbell et al., 1986; Little and Elwood, 1991; Hendricks et al., 1999; McDonnell et al., 1999; Owen et al., 2000) or show a clear maternal age trend (Forrester and Merz, 2000). Feldman et al. (1982) and Strassburg et al. (1983), for instance, reported a statistically significant increase in the risk of NTDs and anencephaly with increasing maternal age. Paternal age has not been clearly linked to NTD risk (Little and Elwood, 1991; Shaw et al., 1994), although one investigation identified an increased NTD risk in the lowest and highest paternal age groups (McIntosh et al., 1995). Similarly, the Kazaura et al. (2004) study of 1,869,388 Norwegian births demonstrated a 1.3-fold (95% CI: 1.1–1.5) risk for NTDs relative to the reference when the father was 20 to 24 years old. Therefore, a pattern of moderately higher risks for younger fathers seems to be consistent for NTDs.

Parity and Birth Order

As in age, both monotonic and U-shaped relationships with NTD risk (high prevalence in primiparas, low prevalence in second births, and increasing prevalence with increasing parity) have been found, the former occurring mainly in low-risk, the latter in high-risk areas (Campbell et al., 1986; Little and Elwood, 1991; Owen et al., 2000; Whiteman et al., 2000). Folic acid deficiency has been proposed as a possible cause of NTDs in multiparous women since, in the small group of pregnant women who were included in the second National Health and Nutrition Examination Survey, blood levels decreased with an increase in parity (Bailey, 1992).

In a recent meta-analysis of 20 studies, Vieira (2004) observed that increased birth order is associated with increasing risk for spina bifida (but not anencephaly), especially when the woman already had three children. This *birth order effect* has received considerable attention, although the results of the various studies are often contradictory (see Table 13.6). Both psychosocial and biological interpretations (such as maternal stress and young children carrying respiratory viral infections into a household) have been proposed for this effect (Vieira, 2004).

It should be pointed out, however, that grand multiparity (para > 4) is associated with low SES and low education, poorer prenatal care, smoking, and alcohol consumption, and that grand multiparas have a higher BMI and a higher rate of insulin-dependent gestational diabetes than multiparous (para 2–4) (Roman et al., 2004). Therefore, any putative association between increased parity and elevated risk for NTDs should account for these factors.

Prenatal Maternal Stress

Maternal anxiety (Crandon, 1979) and moderate to severe life events (Wadhwa et al., 1993; Lou et al., 1994) during pregnancy increase the risk of obstetric complications such as preeclampsia, fetal distress, preterm birth, and low birth weight and predict an increase in neonatal crying (Van den Bergh, 1990), acute health problems during the first year (Goldman and Owen, 1994), and behavioral and/or emotional problems at 4 years of age (O'Connor et al., 2002). Moreover, Apgar scores at 5 minutes are 2 standard deviations lower in newborns of anxious mothers (Crandon, 1979), indicating birth trauma. In studies of congenital malformations, maternal stress is often based either on a self-appraisal of *psychological or emotional stress* or on having experienced *stressors*—life events, such as a family death, job loss, accident, or divorce. Research has also focused on whether exogenous exposures to steroid hormones, normally produced in response to stress, are harmful to the developing fetus (Fraser and Fainstat, 1951; Lahti et al., 1972; Czeizel and Rockenbauer, 1997; Rodriguez-Pinilla and Martínez-Frías, 1998; Carmichael and Shaw, 1999). While the precise mechanism by which stress may affect neural tube development is unknown, it is also hypothesized that stress might cause women to smoke more, drink more alcohol, or eat poorly (Suarez et al., 2003), factors that also influence NTD risk.

Richards (1969) reported a twofold frequency of "accidents in pregnancy" during the first trimester in mothers of offspring with anencephaly compared with mothers of unaffected offspring. Carmichael and Shaw (2000) explored the relationship between certain life events during the periconceptional period and several types of congenital anomalies, and reported a modest association between NTD risk and experience of the death of a friend or family member, divorce, or job loss

TABLE 13.6. *Studies on Birth Order and Risk for Neural Tube Defects*

Source and Study Location	Number of Cases	Reported Results	OR (95% C.I.) Birth Order "1"	OR (95% C.I.) Birth Order "4 or more"
Anencephaly				
Frézal et al. (1964)—France	254	—	1.28 (0.93–1.75)	1.2 (0.83–1.72)
Fedrick (1970)—England, Scotland, and Wales	491	U-shaped association	1.82 (1.44–2.28)	1.89 (1.43–2.45)
Hay and Barbano (1972)—USA	2160	—	0.97 (0.88–1.07)	0.93 (0.84–1.03)
Imaizumi (1974)—Japan	2488	+ for birth order "1"	1.08 (0.99–1.18)	1.84 (1.54–2.21)
Granroth et al. (1978)—Finland	197	+ for birth order "4 or more"	1.07 (0.75–1.52)	1.96 (1.25–3.06)
Imaizumi (1979)—Japan	1815	+ for birth order "4 or more"	0.93 (0.84–1.03)	2.17 (1.78–2.64)
Feldman et al. (1982)—USA	88	+ for birth order "4 or more"	1.11 (0.63–1.98)	2.39 (1.32–4.31)
Sever (1982)—USA	446	—	0.97 (0.77–1.24)	1.36 (1.05–1.77)
Brender et al. (1989)—USA	706	—	1.04 (0.87–1.24)	1.3 (1.02–1.65)
*Mean effect size delta (95% CI)**			*0.061 (0.025–0.097)*	*0.092 (0.013–0.171)*
Spina Bifida				
Hay and Barbano (1972)—USA	5,834	+ for birth order "1"	1.24 (1.17–1.32)	1.07 (1.0–1.14)
Imaizumi (1974)—Japan	176	—	0.98 (0.7–1.38)	2.24 (1.21–4.16)
Granroth et al. (1978)—Finland	238	+ for birth order "4 or more"	1.41 (1.03–1.94)	1.65 (1.07–2.57)
Nesbit and Ziter (1979)—USA	115	—	1.2 (0.69–2.08)	1.52 (0.87–2.65)
Feldman et al. (1982)—USA	82	—	0.83 (0.47–1.47)	1.82 (1.02–3.27)
Sever (1982)—USA	441	—	1.07 (0.84–1.37)	1.27 (0.97–1.68)
Mean effect size delta (95% CI)			*0.041 (−0.073–0.156)*	*0.352 (0.178–0.524)*
Neural Tube Defects				
Horowitz and McDonald (1969)—Canada	1353	+ for birth order "1"	1.34 (1.15–1.57)	1.17 (1.01–1.36)
Czeizel and Révész (1970)—Hungary	958	+ for birth order "3 or more"	1.75 (1.49–2.04)	1.07 (0.83–1.37)
Naggan (1971)—Israel	776	+ for birth order "5 or more"	0.94 (0.78–1.13)	1.43 (1.22–1.68)
Field (1978)—Australia	1572	+ for birth order "4 or more"	1.22 (1.08–1.38)	1.37 (1.17–1.61)
Feldman et al. (1982)—USA	177	—	0.99 (0.67–1.47)	2.07 (1.38–3.13)
Sever (1982)—USA	959	Not tested	1.08 (0.92–1.27)	1.37 (1.14–1.65)
Bower et al. (1984)—Australia	1060	—	0.85 (0.73–0.98)	1.63 (1.37–1.94)
Kulkarni et al. (1989)—India	40	—	1.18 (0.53–2.63)	1.29 (0.51–3.28)
Airede (1992)—Nigeria	5977	+ for birth order "4 or more"	0.84 (0.36–1.94)	2.58 (1.07–6.24)
Dudin (1997)—Palestine	148	—	1.83 (1.01–3.35)	3.17 (1.58–6.37)
Owen et al. (2000)—Australia	944	+ for birth order "3 or more"	0.98 (0.83–1.16)	1.24 (1.03–1.49)
Nazer et al. (2001)				
Chile	583	U-shaped association	1.18 (0.99–1.42)	1.49 (1.2–1.86)
ECLAMC (without Chile)†	4581	U-shaped association	1.08 (1.01–1.16)	1.14 (1.07–1.23)
Mean effect size delta (95% CI)			*0.110 (0.077–0.113)*	*0.287 (0.237–0.337)*

— = no association, + = positive association.

*Mean effect size delta and 95% confidence intervals (CI) calculated by Vieira (2004). Effect sizes can be thought of as the average percentile standing of the average treated (or experimental) group relative to the average untreated (or control) group. An effect size of 0.0 indicates that the mean effect size delta of the treated group is at the 50th percentile of the untreated group. An effect size of 0.8 indicates that the mean effect size delta of the treated group is at the 79th percentile of the untreated group. An effect size of 1.7 indicates that the mean of the treated group is at the 95.5 percentile of the untreated group.

†ECLAMC is the Latin American Collaborative Study of Congenital Malformations and comprises data from hospitals in Argentina, Bolivia, Brazil, Chile, Colombia, Costa Rica, Dominican Republic, Ecuador, Peru, Uruguay, Paraguay, and Venezuela.

Source: Modified from Vieira (2004).

during the periconceptional period (OR: 1.51; 95% CI: 1.1–2.1). These associations tended to be restricted to women who were not obese and to women with a high school education or less. More recently, Suarez et al. (2003) examined whether maternal stress and lack of social support contributed to NTD risk in 184 Mexican-American case mothers with NTD-affected pregnancies compared to 225 controls. Maternal stress was measured by tallying the number of job changes, residential moves, and major injuries occurring during the year before conception. Social support was measured using social integration and perceived emotional support scales. Mothers who experienced one or more stressful life events during the year before conception had an increased risk for NTDs (OR: 2.9, 95% CI: 1.8–4.7) compared with mothers experiencing no such events. Mothers who scored low on emotional support had an elevated risk compared with those who scored high (OR: 4.6, 95% CI: 2.2–9.7). Social support measures, such as network size and satisfaction, group interactions, and church attendance, were unrelated to NTD risk. The estimated effects were not modified or confounded by age, education, country of birth, income, obesity, vitamin supplements, dietary folate, cigarette smoking, or alcohol consumption.

Environmental Pollution

People living near landfill sites may be exposed to chemicals released into the air, water, or soil (Upton, 1989). Dolk et al. (1998) studied the risk of congenital anomalies associated with residences near European hazardous-waste landfill sites using a sample of 1089 live births, stillbirths, and terminations of pregnancy with nonchromosomal congenital anomalies and 2366 controls without malformation; residence within 3 km of a landfill site was associated with a significantly raised risk of congenital anomaly (295 cases/511 controls living 0–3 km from landfill sites, 794/1855 living 3–7 km from landfill sites with a combined OR of 1.33 [95% CI 1.11–1.59], adjusted for maternal age and SES). There was a fairly consistent decrease in risk with increased distance from the sites. A significantly raised OR for residence within 3 km of a landfill site was found for NTDs (OR: 1.86, 95% CI: 1.24–2.79). Shaw et al. (1992) were unable to confirm these findings in California. Elliott et al.'s (2001) findings in Great Britain in populations living within 2 km of 9565 landfill sites operational between 1982 and 1997 (from a total of 19,196 sites) demonstrated an adjusted RR for all anomalies of residents near landfill sites (all waste types) that was marginally significant: 1.01 (99% CI: 1.005–1.023) or one extra anomaly among 5903 who were exposed (against the baseline population risk of one anomaly among each 59 individuals). The adjusted RR for NTDs was 1.05 (99% CI: 1.01–1.10) or one extra defect among 35,714 exposed people (against the baseline risk of one per 1786 in the general population). Extending this further, one can calculate the number of the total population among whom one extra anomaly will be produced by the presence of landfill sites (to which 55% of the population are exposed within 2 km) or the *population impact number* (Heller and Dobson, 2000). For all anomalies it is 10,733 and for spina bifida it is 64,935 (Heller, 2001). Like Shaw et al. (1992), Dummer et al. (2003a) found no evidence to suggest an increased risk of NTDs among British babies whose mothers lived closer to hazardous industrial sites.

Despite concern over the health effects of emissions from incinerators (Mukarjee, 1998) and crematoriums (Maloney et al., 1998), there is little information concerning pregnancy outcomes for mothers living in their vicinity. Identification of possible health effects of incinerators is important given the growth of incineration as a method of waste disposal (Hu and Shy, 2001) and its widespread use for the disposal of animal carcasses during the 2001 outbreak of foot and mouth disease in the United Kingdom (Hunter, 2001). Dummer et al. (2000b) studied a total of 3234 stillbirths, 2663 neonatal deaths, and 1569 lethal congenital anomalies among the 244,758 British births between 1956 and 1993. After adjustment for social class, year of birth, birth order, and multiple births, there was an increased risk of lethal spina bifida (OR: 1.17, 95% CI: 1.07–1.28) for the mothers living near incinerators but no increased risk for the mothers living near crematoriums. In view of the scarcity of published data and our use of a distance function to represent potential exposure, it is difficult to assess whether the statistical association between maternal proximity to incinerators and increased risk for lethal spina bifida in the offspring reflects a causal effect. However, investigation in all areas—including miscarriages, abortions, and nonlethal congenital anomalies—should continue.

Nitrosatable Drugs

The *N*-nitroso compounds (NOCs) are a group of chemical compounds that includes nitrosamines (R_1NNOR_2) and nitrosamides ($R_1NNO.COR_2$). Endogenous formation of NOC in the maternal stomach and subsequent transplacental transmission to the fetus is the most likely source of significant prenatal exposure to these agents (McKean-Cowdin et al., 2003). Studies show that both nitrosamides and nitrosamines can be formed in vivo from their chemical precursors (amides, amines, and nitrites) under normal acidic conditions of the stomach (Lijinsky and Epstein, 1970) and that a single transplacental dose of ethylnitrosourea (a type of nitrosamide) is sufficient to induce central and peripheral nervous system tumors in 100% of the offspring of mice (Kleihues et al., 1982). Some therapeutic drugs provide concentrated sources of amides or amines that, in the presence of nitrites in the stomach from the diet or in the saliva, can form NOCs (Mirvish, 1995). These products may act locally or circulate in the bloodstream to act in distant tissues, including the central nervous system (Kleihues et al., 1976; Kleihues et al., 1982; Magee, 1989). Many common drugs such as phenylpropanolamine, clorpheniramine, beta-blocking agents, and some antibiotics are nitrosatable. Several NOCs have been found in animal models to induce congenital malformations, including NTDs (von Kreybig and Schmidt, 1967; Givelber and

DiPaolo, 1969; Koyama et al., 1970; Pfaffenroth et al., 1974; Inouye and Murakami, 1976). However, few studies have been conducted in humans; they suggest increased risks for craniosynostosis (Olshan and Faustman, 1989; Gardner et al., 1998) and meningomyelocele/meningocele, hydrocephaly, and abnormalities of the eye and gastrointestinal system (Olshan and Faustman, 1989). In a study, Olshan and Faustman found that women who took nitrosatable drugs during the first 4 months of pregnancy were 4.6 times more likely to give birth to a child with meningomyelocele or meningocele (95% CI: 0.7–31.6); they found no positive association between these drug exposures and anencephaly. Croen et al. (2001) essentially found no association (OR: 1.2, 95% CI: 0.8–1.8) between nitrosatable drug exposure and NTDs in California drinking water. Brender et al. (2004) interviewed 184 Mexican-American women with NTD-affected pregnancies and 225 women with normal live births, asking about periconceptional drug exposures and dietary intake. For 110 study participants, nitrate was also measured in the usual source of drinking water. Women who reported taking drugs classified as nitrosatable were 2.7 times more likely to have an NTD-affected pregnancy than women without this exposure (95% CI: 1.4–5.3). The OR's for anencephaly (2.5, 95% CI: 1.1–5.5) and for spina bifida (2.7, 95% CI: 1.2–5.8) were similar, although the OR for encephalocele was somewhat lower (1.8, 95% CI: 0.3–9.3). The effect of nitrosatable drugs was observed only in women with higher intakes of dietary nitrite and total nitrite (dietary nitrite + 5% dietary nitrate). Women within the highest tertile (>10.5 mg/day) of total nitrite were 7.5 times more likely to have an NTD-affected pregnancy if they took nitrosatable drugs (95% CI: 1.8–45.4). This might explain the discrepancy of results with the study of Croen et al. (2001), since in the California study the estimated daily intake of nitrite was considerably lower than that in Texas. The highest dietary nitrite intake in the Croen et al. study was 3.9 mg/day compared with 12.6 mg/day in the Brender study. Restricting Brender's study to women whose dietary nitrite intake was 3.9 mg/day or less resulted in an estimate similar to that of Croen et al. (OR: 1.3, 95% CI: 0.5–3.4). In summary, the evidence suggests that the effects of nitrosatable drug exposure on risk for NTDs in offspring could be influenced by dietary nitrite and total nitrite intake.

CONCLUSION

This is an exciting time in the study of NTDs: in the past two decades, a lot has been learned. Yet the most challenging issues still have to be addressed. Determination of the relative contributions of environmental and genetic factors of complex diseases is difficult, complicated by gene–environment interactions. That is, the genetic contribution to a disease may vary by a person's level of environmental exposure; conversely, environmental exposure may have different effects, depending on one's genetic background. Valuable insights into the causation of complex diseases such as the NTDs will be revealed as we continue to dissect these complicated gene–environment relationships.

Novel studies need to be developed to better assess the etiology of those NTDs not prevented by supplemental FA. These studies should involve physiological and molecular models useful not only to characterize individual susceptibilities, but also to elucidate the effect of specific genetic mutations. It is expected that the results of these future studies will provide information that will eventually enable physicians to practice predictive and preventive medicine.

REFERENCES

Abrams BF, Laros RK Jr (1986). Prepregnancy weight, weight gain, and birth weight. Am J Obstet Gynecol 154:503–509.

Achenson D (1998). *Independent Inquiry into Inequalities in Health*. London: HM Stationary Office.

Airede KI (1992). Neural tube defects in the middle belt of Nigeria. J Trop Pediatr 38:27–30.

Alsdorf R, Wyszynski DF (2005). Teratogenicity of sodium valproate. Expert Opin Drug Saf 4:345–353.

Andrews J, McGarry JM (1972). A community study of smoking in pregnancy. J Obstet Gynaecol Br Commonw 79:1057–1073.

Aschengrau A, Zierler S, Cohen A (1993). Quality of community drinking water and the occurrence of late adverse pregnancy outcomes. Arch Environ Health 48:105–113.

Astrup P, Olsen HM, Trolle D, Kjeldsen K (1972). Effect of moderate carbon-monoxide exposure on fetal development. Lancet 2:1220–1222.

Bailey L (1992). Evaluation of a new Recommended Dietary Allowance for folate. J Am Diet Assoc 92:463–468, 471.

Baird D (1980). Environment and reproduction. Br J Obstet Gynaecol 87:1057–1067.

Balarajan R, McDowall M (1983). Congenital malformations and agricultural workers. Lancet 1:1112–1113.

Becerra JE, Khoury MJ, Cordero JF, Erickson JD (1990). Diabetes mellitus during pregnancy and the risks for specific birth defects: a population-based case-control study. Pediatrics 85:1–9.

Beech JA, Diaz R, Ordaz C, Palomeque B (1980). Nitrates, chlorates and trihalomethanes in swimming pool water. Am J Public Health 70:79–82.

Beemster P, Groenen P, Steegers-Theunissen R (2002). Involvement of inositol in reproduction. Nutr Rev 60:80–87.

Berry RJ, Li Z, Erickson JD, Li S, Moore CA, Wang H, et al. (1999). Prevention of neural-tube defects with folic acid in China. China–U.S. Collaborative Project for Neural Tube Defect Prevention. N Engl J Med 341:1485–1490.

Bjerkedal T, Czeizel A, Goujard J, Källen B, Mastroiacovo P, Nevin N (1982). Valproic acid and spina bifida. Lancet 2:1096.

Blatter BM, Hermens R, Bakker M, Roeleveld N, Verbeek AL, Zielhuis GA (1997). Paternal occupational exposure around conception and spina bifida in offspring. Am J Ind Med 32:283–291.

Block G, Hartman AM, Dresser CM, Carroll MD, Gannon J, Gardner L (1986). A data-based approach to diet questionnaire design and testing. Am J Epidemiol 124:453–469.

Bove FJ, Fulcomer MC, Klotz JB, Esmart J, Dufficy EM, Savrin JE (1995). Public drinking water contamination and birth outcomes. Am J Epidemiol 141:850–862.

Bower C, Hobbs M, Carney A, Simpson D (1984). Neural tube defects in Western Australia 1966–81 and a review of Australian data 1942–81. J Epidemiol Commun Health 38:208–213.

Brender JD, Carmichael L, Preece MJ, Larimer GC, Suarez L (1989). Epidemiology of anencephaly in Texas, 1981–1986. Tex Med 85:33–35.

Brender JD, Olive JM, Felkner M, Suarez L, Marckwardt W, Hendricks KA (2004). Dietary nitrites and nitrates, nitrosatable drugs, and neural tube defects. Epidemiology 15:330–336.

Brender JD, Suarez L (1990). Paternal occupation and anencephaly. Am J Epidemiol 131:517–521.

Brodie MJ, Dichter MA (1997). Established antiepileptic drugs. Seizure 6:159–174.

Brown AS, Susser ES (1997). Sex differences in prevalence of congenital neural defects after periconceptional famine exposure. Epidemiology 8:55–8.

Burger GC, Drummond JC, Sandstead HR, eds (1948). *Malnutrition and Starvation in Western Netherlands, September 1944–July 1945*. The Hague, The Netherlands: General State Printing Office.

Campbell LR, Dayton DH, Sohal GS (1986). Neural tube defects: a review of human and animal studies on the etiology of neural tube defects. Teratology 34:171–187.

Carmichael SL, Shaw GM (1999). Maternal corticosteroid use and risk of selected congenital anomalies. Am J Med Genet 86:242–244.

Carmichael SL, Shaw GM (2000). Maternal life event stress and congenital anomalies. Epidemiology 11:30–35.

Carmichael SL, Shaw GM, Schaffer DM, Laurent C, Selvin S (2003). Dieting behaviors and risk of neural tube defects. Am J Epidemiol 158:1127–1131.

Carter M, Ulrich S, Oofuji Y, Williams DA, Ross ME (1999). Crooked tail (Cd) models human folate-responsive neural tube defects. Hum Mol Genet 8:2199–2204.

Cavalli P, Copp AJ (2002). Inositol and folate resistant neural tube defects. J Med Genet 39:E5.

Cedergren MI, Källén BA (2003). Maternal obesity and infant heart defects. Obes Res 11:1065–1071.

Chambers CD, Johnson KA, Dick LM, Felix RJ, Jones KL (1998). Maternal fever and birth outcome: a prospective study. Teratology 58:251–257.

Chang TI, Loeken MR (1999). Genotoxicity and diabetic embryopathy: impaired expression of developmental control genes as a cause of defective morphogenesis. Semin Reprod Endocrinol 17:153–165.

Christianson RE (1980). The relationship between maternal smoking and the incidence of congenital anomalies. Am J Epidemiol 112:684–695.

Christo GG, Urala MS, Duvvi HV, Venkatesh A (1987). Maternal hyperthermia as a teratogenic agent. Indian Pediatr 24:597–600.

Chung CS, Myrianthopoulos NC (1975a). Factors affecting risks of congenital malformations. I. Analysis of epidemiologic factors in congenital malformations. Report from the Collaborative Perinatal Project. Birth Defects Orig Artic Ser 11:1–22.

Chung CS, Myrianthopolous NC (1975b). Factors affecting risks of congenital malformations. II. Effect of maternal diabetes on congenital malformations. Birth Defects Orig Artic Ser 11:23–38.

Cnattingius S (2004). The epidemiology of smoking during pregnancy: smoking prevalence, maternal characteristics, and pregnancy outcomes. Nicotine Tob Res 6(Suppl 2):S125–S140.

Coffey VP, Jessop WJ (1959). Rubella and incidence of congenital abnormalities. Ir J Med Sci 172:1–11.

Cogram P, Tesh S, Tesh J, Wade A, Allan G, Greene ND, Copp AJ (2002). D-Chiro-inositol is more effective than myo-inositol in preventing folate-resistant mouse neural tube defects. Hum Reprod 17:2451–2458.

Cogswell ME, Serdula MK, Hungerford DW, Yip R (1995). Gestational weight gain among average-weight and overweight women—what is excessive? Am J Obstet Gynecol 172:705–712.

Cole PV, Hawkins LH, Roberts D (1972). Smoking during pregnancy and its effects on the fetus. J Obstet Gynaecol Br Commonw 79:782–787.

Correa A, Botto L, Liu Y, Mulinare J, Erickson JD (2003). Do multivitamin supplements attenuate the risk for diabetes-associated birth defects? Pediatrics 111:1146–1151.

Crandon AJ (1979). Maternal anxiety and obstetric complications. J Psychosom Res 23:109–111.

Croen LA, Todoroff K, Shaw GM (2001). Maternal exposure to nitrate from drinking water and diet and risk for neural tube defects. Am J Epidemiol 153:325–331.

Czeizel AE, Dudas I (1992). Prevention of the first occurrence of neural-tube defects by periconceptional vitamin supplementation. N Engl J Med 327:1832–1835.

Czeizel AE, Kodaj I, Lenz W (1994). Smoking during pregnancy and congenital limb deficiency. BMJ 308:1473–1476.

Czeizel A, Revesz C (1970). Major malformations of the central nervous system in Hungary. Br J Prev Soc Med 24:205–222.

Czeizel AE, Rockenbauer M (1997). Population-based case-control study of teratogenic potential of corticosteroids. Teratology 56:335–340.

Davis H, Gergen PJ (1994). The weights and heights of Mexican-American adolescents: the accuracy of self-reports. Am J Public Health 84:459–462.

Dawson LE, Pham B, Hunter AG (2001). Low rate of adequate folic acid supplementation in well-educated women of high socioeconomic status attending a genetics clinic. CMAJ 164:1149–1150.

de Walle HE, van der Pal KM, de Jong-van den Berg LT, Schouten J, de Rover CM, Buitendijk SE, Cornel MC (1998). Periconceptional folic acid in The Netherlands in 1995. Socioeconomic differences. J Epidemiol Community Health 52:826–827.

Dodds L, King WD (2001). Relation between trihalomethane compounds and birth defects. Occup Environ Med 58:443–446.

Dodds L, King W, Woolcott C, Pole J (1999). Trihalomethanes in public water supplies and adverse birth outcomes. Epidemiology 10:233–237.

Dolk H, Vrijheid M, Armstrong B, Abramsky L, Bianchi F, Garne E, Nelen V, Robert E, Scott JE, Stone D, Tenconi R (1998). Risk of congenital anomalies near hazardous-waste landfill sites in Europe: the EUROHAZCON study. Lancet 352:423–427.

Doria A, Warram JH, Krolewski AS (1995). Genetic susceptibility to nephropathy in insulin-dependent diabetes: from epidemiology to molecular genetics. Diabetes Metab Rev 11:287–314.

Dudin A (1997). Neural tube defect among Palestinians: a hospital-based study. Ann Trop Paediatr 17:217–222.

Dummer TJ, Dickinson HO, Parker L (2003a). Prevalence of adverse pregnancy outcomes around hazardous industrial sites in Cumbria, north-west England, 1950–93. Paediatr Perinat Epidemiol 17:250–255.

Dummer TJ, Dickinson HO, Parker L (2003b). Adverse pregnancy outcomes around incinerators and crematoriums in Cumbria, north-west England, 1956–93. J Epidemiol Community Health 57:456–461.

Elliott P, Briggs D, Morris S, de Hoogh C, Hurt C, Jensen TK, Maitland I, Richardson S, Wakefield J, Jarup L (2001). Risk of adverse birth outcomes in populations living near landfill sites. BMJ 323:363–368.

Elwood JH, Elwood JM (1984). Investigation of area differences in the prevalence at birth of anencephalus in Belfast. Int J Epidemiol 13:45–52.

Emanuel I, Sever LE (1973). Questions concerning the possible association of potatoes and neural-tube defects, and an alternative hypothesis relating to maternal growth and development. Teratology 8:325–332.

Ericson A, Källén B, Lofkvist E (1988). Environmental factors in the etiology of neural tube defects: a negative study. Environ Res 45:38–47.

Ericson A, Källén B, Westerholm P (1979). Cigarette smoking as an etiologic factor in cleft lip and palate. Am J Obstet Gynecol 135:348–351.

Eriksson UJ, Borg LAJ, Forsberg H, Siman CM, Suzuki N, Yang X (1996). Can fetal loss be prevented? The biochemical basis of diabetic embryopathy. Diabetes Rev 4:49–69.

Evans DR, Newcombe RG, Campbell H (1979). Maternal smoking habits and congenital malformations: a population study. Br Med J 2:171–173.

Fedrick J (1970). Anencephalus: variation with maternal age, parity, social class and region in England, Scotland and Wales. Ann Hum Genet 34:31–38.

Fedrick J (1976). Anencephalus in the Oxford Record Linkage Study area. Dev Med Child Neurol 18:643–656.

Feldman JG, Stein SC, Klein RJ, Kohl S, Casey G (1982). The prevalence of neural tube defects among ethnic groups in Brooklyn, New York. J Chronic Dis 35:53–60.

Field B (1978). Neural tube defects in New South Wales, Australia. J Med Genet 15:329–338.

Fine E, Horal M, Chang T, Fortin G, Loeken M (1999). Hyperglycemia is responsible for altered gene expression, apoptosis, and neural tube defects associated with diabetic pregnancy. Diabetes 48:2454–2462.

Flegal KM, Carroll MD, Kuczmarski RJ, Johnson CL (1998). Overweight and obesity in the United States: prevalence and trends, 1960–1994. Int J Obesity 22:39–47.

Flegal KM, Carroll MD, Ogden CL, Johnson CL (2002). Prevalence and trends in obesity among US adults, 1999–2000. JAMA 288:1723–1727.

Fleming A, Copp AJ (1998). Embryonic folate metabolism and mouse neural tube defects. Science 280:2107–2109.

Forrester MB, Merz RD (2000). Epidemiology of neural tube defects, Hawaii, 1986–1997. Hawaii Med J 323–327, 341.

Fraser FC, Fainstat TD (1951). Production of congenital defects in the offspring of pregnant mice treated with cortisone. Pediatrics 8:527–533.

Gallagher MD, Nuckols JR, Stallones L, Savitz DA (1998). Exposure to trihalomethanes and adverse pregnancy outcomes. Epidemiology 9:484–489.

Galtier-Dereure F, Boegner C, Bringer J (2000). Obesity and pregnancy: complications and cost. Am J Clin Nutr 71:1242S–1248S.

Garbaciak JA, Richter MD, Miller S, Barton JJ (1985). Maternal weight and pregnancy complications. Am J Obstet Gynecol 152:238–245.

Gardner JS, Guyard-Boileau B, Alderman BW, Fernbach SK, Greene C, Mangione EJ (1988). Maternal exposure to prescription and non-prescription pharmaceuticals or drugs of abuse and risk of craniosynostosis. Int J Epidemiol 27:64–67.

Givelber HM, DiPaolo JA (1969). Teratogenic effects of *N*-ethyl-*N*-nitrosourea in the Syrian hamster. Cancer Res 29:1151–1155.

Goldman SL, Owen MT (1994). The impact of parental trait anxiety on the utilization of health care services in infancy: a prospective study. J Pediatr Psychol 19:369–381.

Granroth G, Haapakoski J, Hakama M (1978). Defects of the central nervous system in Finland. II. Birth order, outcome of previous pregnancies and family history. Teratology 17:213–222.

Greene MF (1993). Prevention and diagnosis of congenital anomalies in diabetic pregnancies. Clin Perinatol. 20:533–547.

Greene NDE, Copp AJ (1997). Inositol prevents folate-resistant neural tube defects in the mouse. Nat Med 3:60–66.

Groenen PM, Klootwijk R, Schijvenaars MM, Straatman H, Mariman EC, Franke B, Steegers-Theunissen RP (2004a). Spina bifida and genetic factors related to myo-inositol, glucose, and zinc. Mol Genet Metab 82:154–161.

Groenen PM, Peer PG, Wevers RA, Swinkels DW, Franke B, Mariman EC, Steegers-Theunissen RP (2003). Maternal myo-inositol, glucose, and zinc status is associated with the risk of offspring with spina bifida. Am J Obstet Gynecol 189:1713–1719.

Groenen PM, van Rooij IA, Peer PG, Ocke MC, Zielhuis GA, Steegers-Theunissen RP (2004b). Low maternal dietary intakes of iron, magnesium, and niacin are associated with spina bifida in the offspring. J Nutr 134:1516–1522.

Haddow JE, Kloza EM, Knight GJ, Smith DE (1981). Relation between maternal weight and serum alpha-fetoprotein concentration during the second trimester. Clin Chem 27:133–134.

Hales BF, Smith S, Robaire B (1986). Cyclophosphamide in the seminal fluid of treated males: transmission to females by mating and effect on pregnancy outcome. Toxicol Appl Pharmacol 84:423–430.

Hammond FG, Canache MF (1991). Some epidemiological aspects of neural tube defects in Barquisimeto, Venezuela (abstract). Am J Hum Genet 49(Suppl):470.

Hay S, Barbano H (1972). Independent effects of maternal age and birth order on the incidence of selected congenital malformations. Teratology 6:271–279.

Hearey CD, Harris JA, Usatin MS, Epstein DM, Ury HK, Neutra RR (1984). Investigation of a cluster of anencephaly and spina bifida. Am J Epidemiol 120:559–564.

Heller D (2001). Risks from landfill sites can be presented in alternative ways. BMJ 323:1365

Heller RF, Dobson AJ (2000). Disease impact number and population impact number: a population perspective to measures of risk and benefit. BMJ 321:950–952

Hemminki K, Mutanen P, Luoma K, Saloniemi I (1980). Congenital malformations by the parental occupation in Finland. Int Arch Occup Environ Health 46:93–98.

Hemminki K, Mutanen P, Saloniemi I (1983). Smoking and the occurrence of congenital malformations and spontaneous abortions: multivariate analysis. Am J Obstet Gynecol 145:61–66.

Hemminki K, Mutanen P, Saloniemi I, Luoma K (1981). Congenital malformations and maternal occupation in Finland: multivariate analysis. J Epidemiol Community Health 35:5–10.

Hendricks KA, Nuno OM, Suarez L, Larsen R (2001). Effects of hyperinsulinemia and obesity on risk of neural tube defect among Mexican Americans. Epidemiology 12:630–635.

Hendricks KA, Simpson JS, Larsen RD (1999). Neural tube defects along the Texas–Mexico border, 1993–1995. Am J Epidemiol 149:1119–1127.

Hernández-Díaz S, Werler MM, Walker AM, Mitchell AA (2001). Neural tube defects in relation to use of folic acid antagonists during pregnancy. Am J Epidemiol 153:961–968.

Hoet JJ, Beard RW (1979). Clinical perspectives in the care of the pregnant diabetic patient. In Pregnancy metabolism, diabetes and the fetus. Ciba Foundation Series 63. Excerpta Med 283–300.

Holmberg PC, Nurminen M (1980). Congenital defects of the central nervous system and occupational factors during pregnancy. A case-referent study. Am J Ind Med 1:167–176.

Honein MA, Moore CA, Watkins ML (2003). Subfertility and prepregnancy overweight/obesity: possible interaction between these risk factors in the etiology of congenital renal anomalies. Birth Defects Res Part A Clin Mol Teratol 67:572–577.

Horowitz I, McDonald AD (1969). Anencephaly and spina bifida in the Province of Quebec. Can Med Assoc J 100:748–755.

Hotzel D (1986). Suboptimal nutritional status in obesity (selected nutrients). Bibl Nutr Dieta 37:36–41.

Hu SW, Shy SM (2001). Health effects of waste incineration: a review of epidemiologic studies. J Air Waste Manag Assoc 51:1100–1109.

Hunter AG (1984). Neural tube defects in Eastern Ontario and Western Quebec: demography and family data. Am J Med Genet 19:45–63.

Hunter M (2001). Public health concerns grow over foot and mouth outbreak. BMJ 322:881.

Hwang BF, Magnus P, Jaakkola JJ (2002). Risk of specific birth defects in relation to chlorination and the amount of natural organic matter in the water supply. Am J Epidemiol 156:374–382

Imaizumi Y (1974). Statistical analysis on anencephaly, spina bifida and congenital hydrocephaly in Japan. Jinrui Idengaku Zasshi 19:115–135.

Imaizumi Y (1979). Anencephaly in Japan: paternal age, maternal age and birth order. Ann Hum Genet 42:445–455.

Inouye M, Murakami U (1976). Teratogenic effect of *N*-methyl-*N′*-nitro-*N*-nitrosoguanidine in mice. Mutat Res 38:337–338.

Institute of Medicine, National Academy of Sciences (1990). *Nutrition during Pregnancy.* Washington, DC: National Academy Press.

Jaakkola JJ, Magnus P, Skrondal A, Hwang BF, Becher G, Dybing E (2001). Foetal growth and duration of gestation relative to water chlorination. Occup Environ 58:437–442.

Källén K (1997a). Maternal smoking and orofacial clefts. Cleft Palate Craniofac J 34:11–16.

Källén K (1997b). Maternal smoking during pregnancy and limb reduction malformations in Sweden. Am J Public Health 87:29–32.

Källén K (1997c). Maternal smoking and urinary organ malformations. Int J Epidemiol 26:571–574.

Källén K (1998). Maternal smoking, body mass index, and neural tube defects. Am J Epidemiol 147:1103–1111.

Kalter H, Warkany J (1959). Experimental production of congenital malformations in mammals by metabolic procedure. Physiol Rev 69–115.

Kanitz S, Franco Y, Patrone V, Caltabellotta M, Raffo E, Riggi C, Timitilli D, Ravera G (1996). Association between drinking water disinfection and somatic parameters at birth. Environ Health Perspect 104:516–520.

Karabiber H, Sonmezgoz E, Ozerol E, Yakinci C, Otlu B, Yologlu S (2003). Effects of valproate and carbamazepine on serum levels of homocysteine, vitamin B_{12}, and folic acid. Brain Dev 25:113–115.

Kaufman NJ, Nichter M (2001). The marketing of tobacco to women: global perspectives. In Samet JM, Yoon SY (eds): *Women and the Tobacco Epidemic: Challenges for the 21st Century.* Geneva: World Health Organization, pp. 69–98.

Kazaura M, Lie RT, Skjaerven R (2004). Paternal age and the risk of birth defects in Norway. Ann Epidemiol 14:566–570.

Kelsey JL, Dwyer T, Holford TR, Bracken MB (1978). Maternal smoking and congenital malformations: an epidemiological study. J Epidemiol Community Health 32:102–107.

Khoury MJ, Gomez-Farias M, Mulinare J (1989). Does maternal cigarette smoking during pregnancy cause cleft lip and palate in offspring? Am J Dis Child 143:333–337.

King WD, Dodds L, Armson BA, Allen AC, Fell DB, Nimrod C (2004). Exposure assessment in epidemiologic studies of adverse pregnancy outcomes and disinfection byproducts. J Expo Anal Environ Epidemiol 14:466–472.

Kleihues P, Lantos P, Magee P (1976). Chemical carcinogenesis in the nervous system. Int Rev Exp Pathol 15:94–153.

Kleihues P, Patzschke K, Doerjer G (1982). DNA modification and repair in the experimental induction of nervous system tumors by chemical carcinogens. Ann NY Acad Sci 381:290–303.

Klotz JB, Pyrch LA (1999). Neural tube defects and drinking water disinfection by-products. Epidemiology 10:383–390.

Koyama T, Handa J, Handa H, Matsumoto S (1970). Methylnitrosourea-induced malformations of brain in SD-JCL rat. Arch Neurol 22:342–347.

Kramer MD, Lynch CF, Isacson P, Hanson JW (1992). The association of waterborne chloroform with intrauterine growth retardation. Epidemiology 3:407–413.

Kucera J (1971). Rate and type of congenital anomalies among offspring of diabetic women. J Reprod Med 7:61–70.

Kulkarni ML, Mathew MA, Reddy V (1989). The range of neural tube defects in southern India. Arch Dis Child 64:201–204.

Lahti A, Antila E, Saxen L (1972). The effect of hydrocortisone on the closure of the palatal shelves in two inbred strains of mice in vivo and in vitro. Teratology 6:37–41.

Lampen A, Siehler S, Ellerbeck U, Gottlicher M, Nau H (1999). New molecular bioassays for the estimation of the teratogenic potency of valproic acid derivatives in vitro: activation of the peroxisomal proliferator-activated receptor (PPARdelta). Toxicol Appl Pharmacol 160:238–249.

Layde PM, Edmonds LD, Erickson JD (1980). Maternal fever and neural tube defects. Teratology 21:105–108.

Leck I (1974). Causation of neural tube defects: clues from epidemiology. Br Med Bull 30:158–163.

Levesque B, Ayotte P, LeBlanc A, Dewailly E, Prud'Homme D, Lavoie R, Allaire S, Levallois P (1994). Evaluation of dermal and respiratory chloroform exposure in humans. Environ Health Perspect 102:1082–1087.

Lewis DP, Van Dyke DC, Stumbo PJ, Berg MJ (1998). Drug and environmental factors associated with adverse pregnancy outcomes. Part II: Improvement with folic acid. Ann Pharmacother 32:947–961.

Li DK, Mueller BA, Hickok DE, Daling JR, Fantel AG, Checkoway H, Weiss NS (1996). Maternal smoking during pregnancy and the risk of congenital urinary tract anomalies. Am J Public Health 86:249–253.

Lijinsky W, Epstein SS (1970). Nitrosamines as environmental carcinogens. Nature 225:21–23.

Lindhout D, Meinardi H (1984). Spina bifida and in-utero exposure to valproate. Lancet 2:396.

Lindhout D, Omtzigt JG, Cornel MC (1992). Spectrum of neural-tube defects in 34 infants prenatally exposed to antiepileptic drugs. Neurology 42:111–118.

Lindstrom AB, Pleil JD, Beerkoff DC (1997). Alveolar breath sampling and analysis to assess trihalomethane exposures during competitive swimming training. Environ Health Perspect 105:636–642.

Little J, Cardy A, Munger RG (2004). Tobacco smoking and oral clefts: a meta-analysis. Bull World Health Organ 82:213–218.

Little J, Elwood JM (1991). Epidemiology of neural tube defects. In Kiley M (ed): *Reproductive and Perinatal Epidemiology.* Boston: CRC Press, pp. 251–336.

Logman JF, de Vries LE, Hemels ME, Khattak S, Einarson TR (2005). Paternal organic solvent exposure and adverse pregnancy outcomes: a meta-analysis. Am J Ind Med 47:37–44.

Lou HC, Hansen D, Nordentoft M, Pryds O, Jensen F, Nim J, Hemmingsen R (1994). Prenatal stressors of human life affect fetal brain development. Dev Med Child Neurol 36:826–832.

Lynberg MC, Khoury MJ, Lu X, Cocian T (1994). Maternal flu, fever, and the risk of neural tube defects: a population-based case-control study. Am J Epidemiol 140:244–255.

Magee PN (1989). The experimental basis for the role of nitroso compounds in human cancer. Cancer Surv 8:207–39.

Magee PN, Montesano R, Preussman R (1976). *N*-Nitroso compounds and related carcinogens. In Searle CE (ed.): *ACS Monograph Series No. 173, Chemical Carcinogens.* Washington, DC: American Chemical Society, pp. 491–625.

Magnus P, Jaakkola JJ, Skrondal A, Alexander J, Becher G, Krogh T, Dybing E (1999). Water chlorination and birth defects. Epidemiology 10:513–517.

Malloy MH, Kleinman JC, Bakewell JM, Schramm WF, Land GH (1989). Maternal smoking during pregnancy: no association with congenital malformations in Missouri 1980–83. Am J Public Health 79:1243–1246.

Maloney SR, Phillips CA, Mills A (1998). Mercury in the hair of crematoria workers. Lancet 352:1602.

Martinez-Frias ML (1994). Epidemiological analysis of outcomes of pregnancy in diabetic mothers: identification of the most characteristic and most frequent congenital anomalies. Am J Med Genet 51:108–113.

McDonald AD, Armstrong BG, Sloan M (1992). Cigarette, alcohol, and coffee consumption and congenital defects. Am J Public Health 82:91–93.

McDonald AD, McDonald JC, Armstrong B, Cherry NM, Nolin AD, Robert D (1989). Fathers' occupation and pregnancy outcome. Br J Ind Med 46:329–333.

McDonnell R, Johnson Z, Doyle A, Sayers G (1999). Determinants of folic acid knowledge and use among antenatal women. J Public Health Med 21:145–149.

McIntosh GC, Olshan AF, Baird PA (1995). Paternal age and the risk of birth defects in offspring. Epidemiology 6:282–288.

McKean-Cowdin R, Pogoda JM, Lijinsky W, Holly EA, Mueller BA, Preston-Martin S (2003). Maternal prenatal exposure to nitrosatable drugs and childhood brain tumours. Int J Epidemiol 32:211–217.

McKone T (1993). Linking a PBPK model for chloroform with measured breath concentrations in showers: implications for dermal exposure models. J Expo Anal Environ Epidemiol 3:339–365.

Miller P, Smith DW, Shepard TH (1978). Maternal hyperthermia as a possible cause of anencephaly. Lancet 1:519–521.

Mills JL (1982). Malformations in infants of diabetic mothers. Teratology 25:385–394.

Mills JL, Knopp RH, Simpson JL, Jovanovic-Peterson L, Metzger BE, Holmes LB, Aarons JH, Brown Z, Reed GF, Bieber FR, et al (1988). Lack of relation of increased malformation rates in infants of diabetic mothers to glycemic control during organogenesis. N Engl J Med 318:671–676.

Milunsky A, Alpert E, Kitzmiller JL, Younger MD, Neff RK (1982). Prenatal diagnosis of neural tube defects. VIII. The importance of serum alpha-fetoprotein screening in diabetic pregnant women. Am J Obstet Gynecol 142:1030–1032.

Milunsky A, Jick H, Jick SS, Bruell CL, MacLaughlin DS, Rothman KJ, Willett W (1989). Multivitamin/folic acid supplementation in early pregnancy reduces the prevalence of neural tube defects. JAMA 262:2847–2852.

Milunsky A, Ulcickas M, Rothman KJ, Willett W, Jick SS, Jick H (1992). Maternal heat exposure and neural tube defects. JAMA 268:882–885.

Mirvish SS (1995). Role of *N*-nitroso compounds (NOC) and *N*-nitrosation in etiology of gastric, esophageal, nasopharyngeal and bladder cancer and contribution to cancer of known exposures to NOC. Cancer Lett 93:17–48.

MMWR (1982). International notes valproic acid and spina bifida: a preliminary report—France. MMWR 31:565–566.

Mokdad AH, Bowman BA, Ford ES, Vinicor F, Marks JS, Koplan JP (2001). The continuing epidemics of obesity and diabetes in the United States. JAMA 286:1195–1200.

Mokdad AH, Ford ES, Bowman BA, Dietz WH, Vinicor F, Bales VS, Marks JS (2003). Prevalence of obesity, diabetes, and obesity-related health risk factors, 2001. JAMA 289:76–79.

Moore LL, Singer MR, Bradlee ML, Rothman KJ, Milunsky A (2000). A prospective study of the risk of congenital defects associated with maternal obesity and diabetes mellitus. Epidemiology 11:689–694.

Morrow JI, Russell AJC, Irwin B, Guthrie E, Morrison P, Parsons L, Robertson I, Craig J (2004). The safety of antiepileptic drugs in pregnancy: results from the UK epilepsy and pregnancy registry. Epilepsia 45(Suppl 3):57.

Mukarjee D (1998). Health impacts of polychlorinated dibenzo-p-dioxins: a critical review. J Air Waste Manag Assoc 48:157–65.

Mulinare J, Cordero JF, Erickson JD, Berry RJ (1998). Periconceptual use of multivitamins and the occurrence of neural tube defects. JAMA 260:3141–3145.

Naeye RL (1990). Maternal body weight and pregnancy outcome. Am J Clin Nutr 52:273–279.

Naggan L (1971). Anencephaly and spina bifida in Israel. Pediatrics 47:577–586.

Nau H, Scott WJ Jr (1986). Weak acids may act as teratogens by accumulating in the basic milieu of the early mammalian embryo. Nature 323:276–278.

Nazer J, Lopez-Camelo J, Castilla EE (2001). ECLAMC: 30-year study of epidemiological surveillance of neural tube defects in Chile and Latin America. Rev Med Chile 129:531–539.

Nesbit DE, Ziter FA (1979). Epidemiology of myelomeningocele in Utah. Dev Med Child Neurol 21:754–757.

Nieuwenhuijsen MJ, Toledano MB, Eaton NE, Fawell J, Elliott P (2000). Chlorination disinfection by-products in water and their association with adverse reproductive outcomes: a review. Occup Environ Med 57:73–85

O'Connor TG, Heron J, Golding J, Beveridge M, Glover V (2002). Maternal antenatal anxiety and children's behavioural/emotional problems at 4 years. Report from the Avon Longitudinal Study of Parents and Children. Br J Psychiatry 180:502–508.

Olsen J (1983). Risk of exposure to teratogens amongst laboratory staff and painters. Dan Med Bull 30:24–28.

Olshan AF, Faustman EM (1989). Nitrosatable drug exposure during pregnancy and adverse pregnancy outcome. Int J Epidemiol 18:891–899.

Olshan AF, Teschke K, Baird PA (1991). Paternal occupation and congenital anomalies in offspring. Am J Ind Med 20:447–475.

Omtzigt JG, Los FJ, Grobbee DE, Pijpers L, Jahoda MG, Brandenburg H, Stewart PA, Gaillard HL, Sachs ES, Wladimiroff JW, et al (1992). The risk of spina bifida aperta after first-trimester exposure to valproate in a prenatal cohort. Neurology 42:119–125.

Owen TJ, Halliday JL, Stone CA (2000). Neural tube defects in Victoria, Australia: potential contributing factors and public health implications. Aust NZ J Public Health 24:584–589.

Pani L, Horal M, Loeken MR (2002). Polymorphic susceptibility to the molecular causes of neural tube defects during diabetic embryopathy. Diabetes 51:2871–2874.

Pederson LM, Tygstrup I, Pederson J (1964). Congenital malformations in newborn infants of diabetic women. Lancet 1:1124–1126.

Pfaffenroth MJ, Das GD, McAllister JP (1974). Teratologic effects of ethylnitrosourea on brain development in rats. Teratology 9:305–315.

Reece EA, Hobbins JC (1986). Diabetic embryopathy: pathogenesis, prenatal diagnosis and prevention. Obstet Gynecol Surv 41:325–335.

Reece EA, Wu Y-K (1997). Prevention of diabetic embryopathy in offspring of diabetic rats with use of a cocktail of deficient substrates and an antioxidant. Am J Obstet Gynecol 176:790–798.

Richards ID (1969). Congenital malformations and environmental influences in pregnancy. Br J Prev Soc Med 23:218–225.

Rodriguez-Pinilla E, Martinez-Frias ML (1998). Corticosteroids during pregnancy and oral clefts: a case-control study. Teratology 58:2–5.

Roman H, Robillard PY, Verspyck E, Hulsey TC, Marpeau L, Barau G (2004). Obstetric and neonatal outcomes in grand multiparity. Obstet Gynecol 103:1294–1299.

Rook J (1974). Formation of haloforms during chlorination of natural waters. Water Treat Exam 23:90–92.

Rosa FW (1991). Spina bifida in infants of women treated with carbamazepine during pregnancy. N Engl J Med 324:674–677.

Rosner B, Prineas R, Loggie J, Daniels SR (1998). Percentiles for body mass index in U.S. children 5 to 17 years of age. J Pediatr 132:211–222.

Samren EB, van Duijn CM, Koch S, Hiilesmaa VK, Klepel H, Bardy AH, Mannagetta GB, Deichl AW, Gaily E, Granstrom ML, Meinardi H, Grobbee DE, Hofman A, Janz D, Lindhout D (1997). Maternal use of antiepileptic drugs and the risk of major congenital malformations: a joint European prospective study of human teratogenesis associated with maternal epilepsy. Epilepsia 38:981–990.

Savitz DA, Andrews KW, Pastore LM (1995). Drinking water and pregnancy outcome in Central North Carolina: source, amount and trihalomethane levels. Environ Health Perspect 103:592–596.

Schnitzer PG, Olshan AF, Erickson JD (1995). Paternal occupation and risk of birth defects in offspring. Epidemiology 6:577–583.

Schorah CJ, Wild J, Hartley R, Sheppard S, Smithells RW (1983). The effect of periconceptional supplementation on blood vitamin concentrations in women at recurrence risk for neural tube defect. Br J Nutr 49:203–211.

Seidman DS, Ever-Hadani P, Gale R (1990). Effect of maternal smoking and age on congenital anomalies. Obstet Gynecol 76:1046–1050.

Seller MJ (1994). Vitamins, folic acid, and the cause and prevention of neural tube defects. Ciba Found Symp 181:161–179.

Seller MJ, Nevin NC (1984). Periconceptional vitamin supplementation and the prevention of neural tube defects in south-east England and Northern Ireland. J Med Genet 21:325–330.

Sever LE (1982). An epidemiologic study of neural tube defects in Los Angeles County II. Etiologic factors in an area with low prevalence at birth. Teratology 25:323–334.

Sever LE (1995). Looking for causes of neural tube defects: where does the environment fit in? Environ Health Perspect 103:165–171.

Sever LE, Emanuel I (1981). Is there a connection between maternal zinc deficiency and congenital malformations of the central nervous system in man? Teratology 7:117.

Sever LE, Emanuel I (1981). Intergenerational factors in the etiology of anencephalus and spina bifida. Dev Med Child Neurol 23:151–154.

Sever LE, Gilbert ES, Hessol NA, McIntyre JM (1988). A case-control study of congenital malformations and occupational exposure to low-level ionizing radiation. Am J Epidemiol 127:226–242.

Shaw GM, Croen LA, Todoroff K, Tolarova MM (2000a). Periconceptional intake of vitamin supplements and risk of multiple congenital anomalies. Am J Med Genet 93:188–193.

Shaw GM, Jensvold NG, Wasserman CR, Lammer EJ (1994). Epidemiologic characteristics of phenotypically distinct neural tube defects among 0.7 million California births, 1983–87. Teratology 49:143–149.

Shaw GM, Quach T, Nelson V, Carmichael SL, Schaffer DM, Selvin S, Yang W (2003). Neural tube defects associated with maternal periconceptional dietary intake of simple sugars and glycemic index. Am J Clin Nutr 78:972–978.

Shaw GM, Schulman J, Frisch JD, Cummins SK, Harris JA (1992). Congenital malformations and birthweight in areas with potential environmental contamination. Arch Environ Health 47:147–154.

Shaw GM, Todoroff K, Carmichael SL, Schaffer DM, Selvin S (2001). Lowered weight gain during pregnancy and risk of neural tube defects among offspring. Int J Epidemiol 30:60–65.

Shaw GM, Todoroff K, Finnell RH, Lammer EJ (2000b). Spina bifida phenotypes in infants or fetuses of obese mothers. Teratology 61:376–381.

Shaw GM, Todoroff K, Schaffer DM, Selvin S (1999). Periconceptional nutrient intake and risk for neural tube defect-affected pregnancies. Epidemiology 10:71171–71176.

Shaw GM, Todoroff K, Schaffer DM, Selvin S (2000c). Maternal height and prepregnancy body mass index as risk factors for selected congenital anomalies. Paediatr Perinat Epidemiol 14:234–239.

Shaw GM, Todoroff K, Velie EM, Lammer EJ (1998). Maternal illness, including fever and medication use as risk factors for neural tube defects. Teratology 57:1–7.

Shaw GM, Velie EM, Morland KB (1996a). Parental recreational drug use and risk for neural tube defects. Am J Epidemiol 144:1155–1160.

Shaw GM, Velie EM, Schaffer D (1996b). Risk of neural tube defect-affected pregnancies among obese women. JAMA 275:1093–1096.

Shaw GM, Velie EM, Schaffer DM (1997). Is dietary intake of methionine associated with a reduction in risk for neural tube defect-affected pregnancies? Teratology 56:295–299.

Shin JH, Shiota K (1999). Folic acid supplementation of pregnant mice suppresses heat-induced neural tube defects in the offspring. J Nutr 129:2070–2073.

Shiono PH, Klebanoff MA, Berendes HW (1986). Congenital malformations and maternal smoking during pregnancy. Teratology 34:65–71.

Shiota K (1982). Neural tube defects and maternal hyperthermia in early pregnancy: Epidemiology in a human embryo population. Am J Med Genet 12:281–288.

Siega-Riz AM, Adair LS, Hobel CJ (1994). Institute of Medicine maternal weight gain recommendations and pregnancy outcome in a predominantly Hispanic population. Obstet Gynecol 84:565–573.

Sikorski R, Juszkiewicz T, Paszkowski T, Szprengier-Juszkiewicz T (1987). Women in dental surgeries: reproductive hazards in occupational exposure to metallic mercury. Int Arch Occup Environ Health 59:551–557.

Siman CM, Eriksson UJ (1997). Vitamin E decreases the occurrence of malformations in the offspring of diabetic rats. Diabetes 46:1054–1061.

Smithells RW, Nevin NC, Seller MJ, Sheppard S, Harris R, Read AP, Fielding DW, Walker S, Schorah CJ, Wild J (1983). Further experience of vitamin supplementation for prevention of neural tube defect recurrences. Lancet 1:1027–1031.

Smithells RW, Sheppard S, Wild J, Schorah CJ (1989). Prevention of neural tube defect recurrences in Yorkshire: final report. Lancet 2:498–499.

Strassburg MA, Greenland S, Portigal LD, Sever LE (1983). A population-based case-control study of anencephalus and spina bifida in a low-risk area. Dev Med Child Neurol 25:632–641.

Suarez L, Cardarelli K, Hendricks K (2003). Maternal stress, social support, and risk of neural tube defects among Mexican Americans. Epidemiology 14:612–6.

Substance Abuse and Mental Health Services Administration (2003). *Results from the 2002 National Survey on Drug Use and Health: National Findings, Tobacco Use.* Rockville, MD: Substance Abuse and Mental Health Services Administration, Office of Applied Studies. 2003. Available at http://www.oas.samhsa.gov/NHSDA/2k2NSDUH/Results/2k2results.htm.

Susser E, Hoek HW, Brown A (1998). Neurodevelopmental disorders after prenatal famine: The story of the Dutch Famine Study. Am J Epidemiol 147:213–216.

Swan SH, Waller K (1998). Disinfection by-products and adverse pregnancy outcomes: what is the agent and how should it be measured? Epidemiology 9:479–481.

Swan SH, Waller K, Hopkins B, Windham G, Fenster L, Schaefer C, Neutra RR (1998). A prospective study of spontaneous abortion: relation to amount and source of drinking water consumed in early pregnancy. Epidemiology 9:126–133.

Taffel SM, Keppel KG, Jones GK (1993). Medical advice on maternal weight gain and actual weight gain. Results from the 1988 National Maternal and Infant Health Survey. Ann N Y Acad Sci 678:293–305.

Tibbets J (1995). What's in the water: the disinfection dilemma. Environ Health Perspect 103:30–34.

Upton AC (1989). Public health aspects of toxic chemical disposal sites. Annu Rev Public Health 10:1–25.

Van den Bergh BR (1990). The influence of maternal emotions during pregnancy on fetal and neonatal behavior. Preperinat Psychol 5:119–130.

Van Den Eeden SK, Karagas MR, Daling JR, Vaughan TL (1990). A case-control study of maternal smoking and congenital malformations. Paediatr Perinat Epidemiol 4:147–155.

van Rooij IA, Groenen PM, van Drongelen M, Te Morsche RH, Peters WH, Steegers-Theunissen RP (2002). Orofacial clefts and spina bifida: *N*-acetyltransferase phenotype, maternal smoking, and medication use. Teratology 66:260–266.

van Straaten HW, Copp AJ (2001). *Curly tail:* a 50-year history of the mouse spina bifida model. Anat Embryol (Berl) 203:225–237.

Velie EM, Block G, Shaw GM, Samuels SJ, Schaffer DM, Kulldorff M (1999). Maternal supplemental and dietary zinc intake and the occurrence of neural tube defects in California. Am J Epidemiol 150:605–616.

Viana M, Herrera, Bonet B (1996). Teratogenic effects of diabetes mellitus in the rat. Prevention by vitamin E. Diabetologia 39:1041–1046.

Vieira AR (2004). Birth order and neural tube defects: a reappraisal. J Neurol Sci 217:65–72.

von Kreybig T, Schmidt W (1967). Chemically induced fetopathies in the rat. Experimental studies on the effect of cyclophosphamide and *N*-methyl-*N*-nitroso-urea after administration on day 15 or 16 of gestation. Arzneimittelforschung 17:1093–1100.

Vrijheid M, Dolk H, Stone D, Abramsky L, Alberman E, Scott JE (2000). Socioeconomic inequalities in risk of congenital anomaly. Arch Dis Child 82:349–352.

Wadhwa PD, Sandman CA, Porto M, Dunkel-Schetter C, Garite TJ (1993). The association between prenatal stress and infant birth weight and gestational age at birth: a prospective investigation. Am J Obstet Gynecol 169:858–865.

Wald N, Sneddon J, Densem J, Frost C, Stone R, MRC Vitamin Study Research Group (1991). Prevention of neural tube defects: results of the Medical Research Council Vitamin Study. MRC Vitamin Study Research Group. Lancet 338:131–137.

Waller DK, Mills JL, Simpson JL, Cunningham GC, Conley MR, Lassman MR, Rhoads GG (1994). Are obese women at higher risk for producing malformed offspring? Am J Obstet Gynecol 170:541–548.

Waller K, Swan SH, DeLorenze G, Hopkins B (1998). Trihalomethanes in drinking water and spontaneous abortion. Epidemiology 9:134–140.

Wasserman CR, Shaw GM, O'Malley CD, Tolarova MM, Lammer EJ (1996). Parental cigarette smoking and risk for congenital anomalies of the heart, neural tube, or limb. Teratology 53:261–267.

Wasserman CR, Shaw GM, Selvin S, Gould JB, Syme SL (1998). Socioeconomic status, neighborhood social conditions, and neural tube defects. Am J Public Health 88:1674–1680.

Watkins ML, Botto LD (2001). Maternal prepregnancy weight and congenital heart defects in offspring. Epidemiology 12:439–446.

Watkins ML, Rasmussen SA, Honein MA, Botto LD, Moore CA (2003). Maternal obesity and risk for birth defects. Pediatrics 111:1152–1158.

Watkins ML, Scanlon KS, Mulinare J, Khoury MJ (1996). Is maternal obesity a risk factor for anencephaly and spina bifida? Epidemiology 7:507–512.

Weisel CP, Jo WK (1996). Ingestion, inhalation and dermal exposure to chloroform and trichloroethane from tap water. Environ Health Perspect 104:48–51.

Weisel CP, Kim H, Haltmeier P, Klotz JB (1999). Related Exposure estimates to disinfection by-products of chlorinated drinking water. Environ Health Perspect 107:103–110.

Werler MM (2002). Exposure assessment in studies of oral clefts. In Wyszynski DF (ed): *Cleft Lip and Palate. From Origin to Treatment.* New York: Oxford University Press, pp. 108–116.

Werler MM, Shapiro S, Mitchell AA (1993). Periconceptional folic acid exposure and risk of occurrent neural tube defects. JAMA 269:1257–1261.

Werler MM, Louik C, Shapiro S, Mitchell AA (1996). Prepregnant weight in relation to risk of neural tube defects. JAMA 275:1089–1092.

Whiteman D, Murphy M, Hey K, O'Donnell M, Goldacre M (2000). Reproductive factors, subfertility, and risk of neural tube defects: a case-control study based on the Oxford Record Linkage Study Register. Am J Epidemiol 152:823–828.

Wright JM, Schwartz J, Dockery DW (2003). Effect of trihalomethane exposure on fetal development. Occup Environ Med 60:173–180.

Wyszynski DF, Duffy DL, Beaty TH (1997). Maternal cigarette smoking and oral clefts: a meta-analysis. Cleft Palate Craniofac J 34:206–210.

Wyszynski DF, Nambisan M, Surve T, Alsdorf RM, Reilly C, Holmes LB (2005). Increased rate of major malformations in offspring exposed to valproate during pregnancy. Neurology 64:961–965.

Wyszynski DF, Wu T (2000). Use of U.S. birth certificate data to estimate the risk of maternal cigarette smoking for oral clefting. Cleft Palate Craniofac J 39:188–192.

Yerby MS (2003). Management issues for women with epilepsy: neural tube defects and folic acid supplementation. Neurology 61:S23–26.

Yerushalmy J (1971). The relationship of parents' cigarette smoking to outcome of pregnancy—implications as to the problem of inferring causation from observed associations. Am J Epidemiol 93:443–456.

Zacharias JF, Jenkins JH, Marion JP (1984). The incidence of neural tube defects in the fetus and neonate of the insulin-dependent diabetic woman. Am J Obstet Gynecol 150:797–798.

Zhao Q, Behringer RR, De Crombrugghe B (1996). Prenatal folic acid treatment suppresses acrania and meroanencephaly in mice mutant for the *Cart1* homeobox gene. Nat Genet 13:275–83.

IV

Genetics of Neural Tube Defects

14

Nonsyndromic Neural Tube Defects: Genetic Basis and Genetic Investigations

EVADNIE RAMPERSAUD
ELIZABETH C. MELVIN
MARCY C. SPEER

The majority of human neural tube defect (NTD) cases are nonsyndromic, meaning that the NTD is the only defect, not just one feature of an identified syndrome such as trisomy 13 or Meckel-Gruber syndrome. The etiology of nonsyndromic NTDs is considered to be complex or multifactorial, with both environmental and genetic factors implicated. In fact, it is likely that multiple genes and environmental factors interact in order for complex disorders such as NTDs to occur. The genetic factors may make the fetus susceptible, with the environmental factors providing the trigger or catalyst for the development of the NTD. A multifactorial threshold model, in which the liability to this complex disorder follows a normal distribution pattern, is often used to illustrate the concept of complex disease inheritance (Edwards, 1969). In this threshold model, when the additive effects of several genetic and environmental factors cumulate to increase the liability to disease, the phenotype is expressed (Fig. 14.1).

The goal of this chapter is to provide evidence for a genetic contribution to nonsyndromic NTDs that do not follow a Mendelian pattern of inheritance, along with a discussion of the various approaches for identifying such genes. An overview of the molecular and statistical methods frequently used to study candidate genes is presented, along with a brief summary of the major research completed to date in studies of human NTDs.

EVIDENCE FOR A GENETIC FACTOR IN NEURAL TUBE DEFECTS

Several lines of evidence suggest a genetic component to NTDs. First, NTDs are known to be associated with established genetic syndromes, including Meckel-Gruber syndrome, Currarino syndrome, and Mohr syndrome, in addition to others. These syndromic forms of NTDs are considered separately in Chapter 16. The NTDs can also be associated with various chromosome rearrangements and anomalies, the most common of which include trisomy 13, trisomy 18, tetraploidy, and deletions involving chromosomes 2, 3, 11, 13, and 22. It has been estimated that less than 10% of NTDs are associated with chromosomal abnormalities (O'Reilly and Shields, 2000).

Additionally, in NTDs occurring independently of other syndromic features, the recurrence risk for siblings is approximately 2%–5%, giving a λ_s (Risch, 1990) value between 20 and 50, which represents up to a 50-fold increased risk over that observed in the general population (e.g., Penrose, 1946; Czeizel and Bodnar, 1970; Carter and Evans, 1973; Lippman-Hand et al., 1978; summarized in Elwood et al., 1992). Data are inconsistent about the recurrence risk in second- and third-degree relatives, but in general, recurrences tend to be lower than those in first-degree relatives (Toriello and Higgins, 1985). Some studies have suggested that the risk to extended family

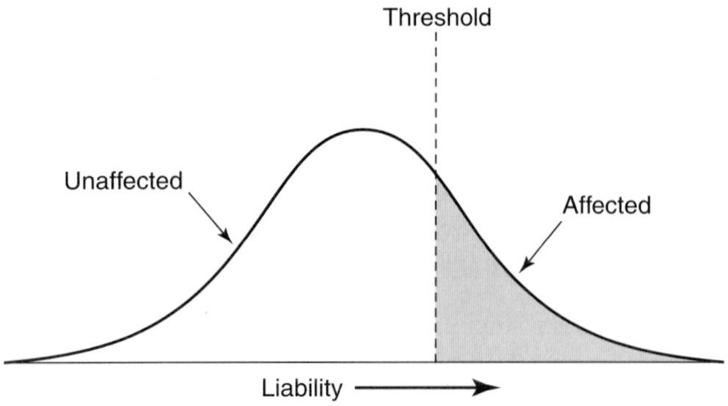

FIGURE 14.1. The multifactorial threshold model.

members is no greater than the general population prevalence (Williamson, 1965; Czeizel and Bodnar, 1970; Nevin and Johnston, 1980), while others suggest that it may be elevated (Carter et al., 1968; Lippman-Hand et al., 1978; Khoury et al., 1982).

The presence of a positive family history of NTDs supports the genetic hypothesis of NTDs. For example, a positive family history in two related German families with five out of eight children having an NTD implied an autosomal recessive inheritance model (Fuhrmann, 1971). In another study, a positive family history of 8.5% was found (Partington and McLone, 1995). Inspection of these multiplex NTD families shows that affected parent–child pairs are rare and that most affected relative pairs are related at either the second or third degree, thus suggesting oligogenic inheritance. Other studies have provided evidence suggesting a Mendelian form of NTDs segregating in large extended families; however, no gene has been identified to date (Banta and Nichols, 1969; Fellous et al., 1982). Formal segregation analysis demonstrating evidence of a major gene has been performed in a series of NTD families, one demonstrating evidence for a major dominant gene (Fineman et al., 1982) and another for a major gene with a recessive effect (Demenais et al., 1982). These studies are admittedly small, however, and suffer from common biases of ascertainment.

Twin studies of NTDs are also sparse, comparing concordance in same-sex versus opposite-sex twins instead of the more accurate comparison in which zygosity is confirmed clinically or molecularly. These data have been summarized thoroughly (Elwood et al., 1992). They indicate that while the concordance rate is relatively low among cotwins of affected cases, the concordance rate is higher in same-sex (monozygotic and dizygotic) than opposite-sex twins (only dizygotic), a trend consistent with a genetic hypothesis. Specifically, among 609 reported cases of anencephaly, the concordance rate is 6.1% in same-sex twins and 3.9% in opposite-sex twins; among 275 cases of spina bifida, the concordance rate is 7.7% in same-sex twins and 2.2% in opposite-sex twins. When the type of NTD in the cotwin is allowed to be different from that of the proband, the concordance in same-sex twins is 7.7% and in opposite-sex twins it is 4.0% (Elwood et al., 1992).

The occurrence of NTDs differs by ethnic group and geographical location. It is not clear whether this variation in rates is due to population-specific differences in risk-associated alleles or to ethnically specific dietary habits or other geographically related exposures. Internationally, there is marked geographical variability, with the highest reported incidence occurring in northern China (7 per 1000 births) and the lowest in Japan (0.1 to 0.6 per 1000). In Caucasian populations, the highest rate occurs in Ireland (3 per 1000) and the lowest in continental Europe. The marked decrease in incidence seen in Ireland between 1974 (6 to 8 per 1000) and 1984 (3.3 per 1000) has been correlated with a substantial increase in dietary folate in that population. The incidence in eastern Mediterranean (with the exception of Israeli Jews) and Indian populations is also high; however, anencephaly tends to be more common than spina bifida. In India, the rates in northern states are the highest (3.9 to 9 per 1000), particularly among the Sikh population. A high incidence has also been seen in Guatemala; however, it has been attributed to fumonisin B1 (FB1) contamination of maize, a dietary staple in that population; the correlation between FB1 contamination of maize and the development of NTDs was first found in a study along the Texas–Mexico border in the United States (Suarez et al., 2000). The data in Africa are sparse; however, studies in South Africa report a higher incidence in rural versus urban areas. Among racial groups in the United States, the incidence is highest among Hispanics (around 9–16 per 10,000 live births) (Cragan et al., 1995; Harris and Shaw, 1995). The overall incidence pattern in the United States shows an increase from the West Coast to the East Coast, with the highest rates seen in the Appalachia regions. It is likely that currently reported rates are underestimated since these figures might not have accounted for prenatally diagnoses cases, stillbirths, and miscarriages. Thus, extensive epidemiologic studies are still needed to characterize accurately the incidence of NTDs worldwide. A review of the epidemiologic evidence from data collected internationally on NTD rates is given in Chapter 13.

Another important line of evidence for a genetic basis for NTDs comes from numerous mouse models (summarized in Juriloff and Harris, 2000). Since early developmental processes are hypothesized to be highly conserved across species, the fact that known genetic mutations have been identified in the mouse suggests that mutations in the same gene or genes within the implicated pathway(s) may be involved in human pathogenesis. Mouse models of NTDs are described in more detail in Chapter 17.

THE IMPORTANCE OF CLINICAL ASSESSMENTS AND DETAILED PHENOTYPES

Although it is well established there is a definite genetic component to NTDs, the exact genetic factors remain unclear. For studies aimed at elucidating genetic influences in NTDs, careful phenotypic definitions will be of paramount importance.

The term *neural tube defect* represents a broad spectrum of abnormalities including open defects, such as myelomeningocele and anencephaly, and closed defects, such as lipomyelomeningocele (see Chapter 6). Thus, detailed clinical evaluations to ensure accurate diagnosis are crucial for gene identification studies and can lead to useful stratifications of the data. Ultimately, comprehensive clinical data allow more accurate correlations of genotype with phenotype once the genetic association or linkage is identified. Such data were invaluable, for example, in separating Parkinson-type Alzheimer's disease from non-Parkinson Alzheimer's disease, leading to significant refinement of a disease gene interval on chromosome 12 (Scott et al., 1998).

In addition to characterizing the type of lesion, another critical clinical assessment of NTDs concerns the level of the lesion. One of the longest controversies, still unsettled, is whether NTDs at different levels represent different defects (Hall and Keena, 1986; Seller, 1990; Park et al., 1992; Van Allen et al., 1993; George et al., 1996). In other words, are higher-level defects, those generally considered to be above thoracic level 11/12, different in etiology from lower-level defects? Is anencephaly genetically different from spina bifida? Scoring and databasing these data are critical in the eventual ability to sort out the mechanisms of gene action and expression.

Neural tube defects tend to breed true within families; in other words, recurrences in families in which the case is affected with spina bifida tend to be spina bifida, and recurrences in families in which the case is anencephaly tend to be anencephaly (Toriello and Higgins, 1985; Hall and Keena, 1986; Frecker et al., 1988; Drainer et al., 1991; Garabedian and Fraser, 1993). However, between 30% and 40% of recurrences involve an NTD phenotype that is different from the case phenotype. This intrafamily heterogeneity may represent the pleiotropic effect of a common underlying gene or may suggest that different phenotypic presentations may result from different underlying genes. These different phenotypes must be documented carefully in clinical studies of NTDs. Cytogenetic studies, often indicated clinically in the assessment of a prenatally identified or newborn NTD case, can also be useful in characterizing NTDs. Cytogenetic studies are frequently warranted when dysmorphic features are present in an NTD case. A compelling example of the utility of chromosome studies in complex disease comes from the study of autistic disorder. A genomic screen (Pericak-Vance et al., 1998) identified a large area of chromosome 7 with a high likelihood of harboring a gene predisposing to autistic disorder. The process of identifying a gene in the interval was enhanced significantly by the availability of a paracentric inversion on 7q in a family segregating the disorder (Pericak-Vance et al., 1998).

In summary, careful clinical assessments including level and extent of the lesion, cytogenetic studies, and dysmorphic assessments (particularly to identify syndromic cases) are necessary for long-range studies of this complicated disorder. Using such an approach will be key to sorting out the genetic influences of NTDs and understanding their phenotypic consequences.

IDENTIFICATION OF CANDIDATE GENES IN NONSYNDROMIC NEURAL TUBE DEFECTS

Candidate genes for NTDs can be classified into two categories—biological and positional—according to how they are identified. Candidate genes identified based on biological plausibility have physiological relevance to the disorder being studied. A plethora of genes have resulted from research done in experimental animals, most notably from mouse models, and from known biological pathways thought to be important for NTDs. For example, genes identified as having a role in neural development or in folate metabolism are plausible biological candidates for NTDs. Candidate genes can also be identified through positional techniques via chromosomal anomalies/rearrangements in NTD-affected individuals or genomic screens with associated linkage analysis.

GENES FROM EXPERIMENTAL SYSTEMS

Candidate genes gleaned from research done in experimental systems have been extremely valuable in the study of human genetic disease. The mouse model remains one of the most well studied animal models for NTDs. More than 60 candidate genes have been identified through this model system (Juriloff and Harris, 2000). There are both naturally occurring and induced strains of mice with varying NTD phenotypes. The two most common mouse phenotypes are (*1*) exencephaly comparable to anencephaly in humans and (*2*) exencephaly occurring in conjunction with spina bifida. The mouse system is useful for the study of NTDs because the genetic map of the mouse is known, the function of many mouse genes has been identified, and many of the human homologues are known. The mouse also has a shorter gestation period and does not require the same ethical considerations as the study of humans. Another advantage is that both genetic and environmental factors can be studied in the mouse. For example, three mouse mutants have shown a reduced risk for NTDs in response to folic acid supplementation: *crooked* (*Cd*), *splotch* (*Sp*), and *cartilage homeoprotein 1* (*Cart1*). Of the three, only the *Pax3* gene (*splotch* mutant) has been studied in humans, and, although it is not directly involved in the folate metabolism pathway, it is still considered a potentially important candidate in folate-related NTDs (Juriloff and Harris, 2000). Studies in *curly tail* mice have shown that another important nutrient, inositol, reduces the risk for NTDs in non-folate-responsive mutants (Seller, 1994; Greene and Copp, 1997). *Curly tail* has been mapped to mouse chromosome 4, which is equivalent to 1p36-1pter in humans; however, no human gene homologue has been identified to date.

There are obvious differences in NTDs between mice and humans, so it is likely that the genes that contribute to NTDs in mice may not always do so in humans. One major difference involves the genetic model for mouse versus human NTDs. The majority of human NTDs appears to be nonsyndromic and caused by complex multifactorial inheritance. In contrast, many mouse models are lethal in the homozygous knockout state, and the NTDs are part of a larger syndrome (Juriloff and Harris, 2000). There is also a discrepancy regarding the number of closure sites in mice compared to humans. While substantial work has been performed to characterize neural tube closure in the mouse (Macdonald et al., 1989; Sakai, 1989; Golden and Chernoff, 1993), limited work has been done in humans, primarily because of the early developmental stage at which the neural tube closes. This makes obtaining relevant human tissue very difficult. Mice have a well-defined four-site model neural tube fusion, and the rationale for the study of model systems has been that such an early and crucial developmental process should have substantial homogeneity between mouse and human. However, the position and number of sites of initial fusion of the neural tube are points of dispute among embryologists. It has recently been established that the closure sites in mouse and human differ (Sulik et al., 1998; O'Rahilly and Muller, 2002), although there is general agreement on the presence of the rostral and caudal closures sites.

The human homologues to many mouse candidate genes have been studied to determine their role in the development of human NTDs. The selection of a mouse candidate gene to study in humans can be a complicated process, and the relevance of the mouse phenotype to the human phenotype must be considered. Researchers must also consider the function of the candidate gene, how it may be involved in the developmental pathway, and the size of the gene or the ease of studying it in the laboratory. None of the mouse mutations with known human homology identified to date represent a major risk factor for NTDs in humans; however, few have actually been investigated extensively.

A handful of studies have revealed modest evidence of positive associations in mouse candidate genes. For example, several groups (Chatkupt et al., 1995; Hol et al., 1996; Trembath et al., 1999; Volcik et al., 2002) have studied the *PAX* gene family, the paired box containing genes that encode for specific DNA binding transcription factors important in regulating embryonic development. The only positive finding to date is from a study primarily of Hispanics, which examined transmission of alleles in three *PAX* genes from parents to their children (Volcik et al., 2002). No mutation has actually been identified in any of the *PAX* genes studies; however, it is possible that these genes may be in linkage disequilibrium with a true genetic variant in another gene. Another possibility is that unexamined variations in intronic or promoter regions of *PAX* genes may actually confer a risk for NTDs. Current studies are underway to determine if there is a true association between *PAX* genes and the risk for NTDs.

Another mouse candidate gene that has been studied and found to be potentially significant in causing NTDs is the *Sonic hedgehog (Shh)* gene, considered important in patterning of the ventral neural tube (Echlard et al., 1993). One study found abnormal expression of *Shh,* based on in situ hybridization, in the floor plate in one human embryo with craniorachischisis and in two embryos with spina bifida (Kirillova et al., 2000). These results suggest that abnormal *Shh* expression in the floor plate might be associated with an open NTD; however, additional studies in other embryos must be carried out before any substantial conclusions can be reached.

Several studies have examined the human homologue (T) of the mouse T (*Brachyury*) gene, believed to be important as a transcription factor that regulates genes involved in notochord differentiation. A modest association was found in the human T locus in an Irish sample (Shields et al., 2000) and in a mixed Dutch and British sample (Morrison et al., 1998); however, similar studies in other populations have failed to replicate this finding (Trembath et al., 1999; Richter et al., 2002; Speer et al., 2002).

While the most commonly studied animal model for NTDs is the mouse, other systems can be used including the sea urchin and zebrafish. The sea urchin (*Lytechinus variegatus*) is a model system that has been used historically to study early development and gastrulation. This model has several unique advantages, including the transparency of the eggs and early embryos and the highly synchronous development of fertilized eggs. As an example, the T-locus product as a critical factor for gastrulation has been studied using sea urchin models (Gross and McClay, 2001).

The zebrafish (*Brachydanio rerio*) is a cost-effective model system for studying NTDs since fertilized eggs can develop rapidly as transparent embryos, allowing all stages of vertebrate development to be visualized easily

(Udvadia and Linney, 2003). Examples of zebrafish research include investigations of spinal cord development (Papan and CamposOrtega, 1997) and studies of genes that position and metabolize retinoic acid in the developing embryo (Perz-Edwards et al., 2001). The soon-to-be-completed sequencing of the zebrafish genome will lead to the identification of NTD candidate genes that can eventually be tested in human populations.

Studies in chick models have long been carried out to investigate genes thought to be involved in early developmental processes. One candidate gene from the chick model that has been tested in a human population is *NCAM1*, a neural cell adhesion molecule that controls cell migration in neural cells. The study found significant evidence for an association in an American Caucasian population primarily of lumbosacral myelomeningocele cases and families (Bastress et al., 2003). Further studies are being conducted towards identifying a causal mutation in this gene.

GENES FROM THE FOLATE PATHWAY

Because of the 50%–70% reduction in NTDs resulting from periconceptional folic acid supplementation (Milunsky et al. 1991; MRC Vitamin Study Research Group, 1991; Centers for Disease Control and Prevention, 1992), any of the genes in the folate metabolic pathway are feasible candidates. One of the best-studied genes in this pathway is methylenetetrahydrofolate reductase (*MTHFR*). Past studies have implicated homozygosity for the C677T thermolabile variant of the *MTHFR* gene as a risk factor for NTDs (Frosst et al., 1995; Ou et al., 1995; van der Put et al., 1995; Whitehead et al., 1995; Shields et al., 1999). Other reports have failed to demonstrate this association (Papapetrou et al., 1996; Mornet et al., 1997; Speer et al., 1997; Koch et al., 1998; Shaw et al., 1998, 1999; Rampersaud et al., 2003a). Another study has suggested that the effect may be dependent on the level of the lesion (Volcik et al., 2002). In addition, some researchers have looked at other mutations in the *MTHFR* gene, including *A1298C*, and other genes, such as cystathionine β-synthase (CBS), that, in combination with the *C677T* allele, may increase the risk for NTDs (van der Put et al., 1998; Speer et al., 1999; Rampersaud et al., 2003a). While the role of *MTHFR* in NTD development has not been fully elucidated, it is possible that this gene is involved in interactions with other genes to confer a risk for the development of NTDs. Alternatively, *MTHFR* may be involved in causing NTDs only in persons with certain ethnic backgrounds or may be important in producing specific NTD phenotypes. Chapters 4 and 15 describe the studies of candidate genes gleaned from the folate metabolic pathway and also examine evidence for gene–gene and gene–environment interactions.

CHROMOSOMAL REARRANGEMENTS

Neural tube defects can be caused by chromosome rearrangements. Chromosome abnormalities, specifically aneuploidy, can be found in 5%–17% of cases of NTD (Hume et al., 1996; Kennedy et al., 1998; Philipp and Kalousek, 2002). The identification of individuals with both an NTD and a chromosomal rearrangement can provide clues in identifying candidate genes. In chromosomal translocations, deletions, duplications, and insertions, the breakpoint of these rearrangements could disrupt genes important in NTD development. These genes may not be otherwise identified as candidate genes except when an affected individual with an NTD is identified as also having an abnormal karyotype. Furthermore, the addition or deletion of genetic material may point to a dosage effect. In many cases, individuals with chromosomal rearrangements are syndromic (i.e., have other features in addition to the NTDs), as discussed in more detail in Chapter 16. For example, NTDs can be a major feature in both trisomy 13 and trisomy 18. As another example, one or more genes in the critical region of 13q33–34 have been implicated in NTDs with the 13q deletion syndrome (Luo et al., 2000). Deletion of 22q11 has also been reported as an infrequent cause of NTDs (Nickel and Magenis, 1996).

GENOMIC SCREENING

The tried-and-true approach for identifying positional candidate genes is through a genomic screen, in which genetic markers at known locations throughout the genome are tested in families with two or more affected individuals (*multiplex* pedigrees). Because of advances in the density and polymorphism of genetic markers, high-throughput genotyping methods, and innovations in statistical genetic linkage analysis, it is now possible to perform large-scale investigations of complex human traits such as NTDs. The general approach involves testing for allele sharing above what is expected by chance alone. This type of analysis is performed using either a parametric lod-score approach, in which components of the genetic model (dominant or recessive, disease allele frequency and penetrance, etc.) are specified, or a nonparametric approach, which requires fewer assumptions. Regions of the genome with excess sharing of alleles among affected individuals are considered to be regions of interest and may harbor genes that predispose to NTDs.

Typically, as many multiplex pedigrees as can be identified are included in genomic screens for common complex disorders. In the case of NTDs, high morbidity and mortality rates are associated with the disorder, and pregnancy terminations following case identification are not uncommon. These factors limit the ascertainment of families with two or more living affected individuals (Melvin et al., 1998; Harris, 2001). Historically, a few families have been identified with multiple individuals having an NTD (Williamson, 1965; Carter et al., 1968; Nevin and Johnston, 1980). One study of anencephaly done in an Icelandic pedigree to evaluate the X-chromosome used a genomic screening approach. Using numerous markers and haplotype analysis, linkage to the X chromosome was excluded in this kindred (Newton et al., 1994). A deletion study of *ZIC2* (which maps to 13q32) was also carried out in a sample with a range of NTD phenotypes including anencephaly, myelomeningocele, and encephalocele (Brown et al., 2002). Definitive conclusions could not be drawn because of the small sample size, but it appears that *ZIC2* mutations are infrequent causes of NTDs.

The first genome-wide screen for NTDs was performed on 44 multiplex NTD Caucasian American families (Rampersaud et al., in press). This study found linkage to chromosomes 7 and 10, both with maximum parametric multipoint LOD scores (MLOD) > 2.0. The linkage results on chromosome 7 were attributed mainly to a large multigenerational pedigree. Two candidate genes (Meox2, Twist1) were identified on chromosome 7, and three candidates (FGFR2, GFRA1, Pax2) were found in the region on chromosome 10. Further investigation of the linkage results are ongoing.

MOLECULAR APPROACHES TO STUDYING CANDIDATE GENES

Once a candidate gene has been identified, the molecular approach to evaluating it needs to be determined. In general, from a laboratory perspective, there are three approaches for assessing candidate genes. Each approach varies in terms of cost, ease of study, and completeness of mutation identification. The gold standard involves sequencing the gene itself to look specifically for variants that may have functional significance. This approach is sensitive but expensive.

The second approach involves using one of a variety of screening tools for variation detection. Today the most common approach involves the application of denaturing high-performance liquid chromatography. This approach is particularly appealing when there is a gene with a few small exons. The detection of variants is based on the differences in melting temperatures between homozygous double-stranded templates and mismatched, heterozygous templates. Polymerase chain reaction products of candidate genes, derived from both alleles, are melted and allowed to reanneal, as in heteroduplex analysis. If there are sequence differences between the reannealed strands, then the heteroduplex strands melt and separate under denaturing conditions faster than homoduplexes. The system can detect more than 90% of mutations in fragments ≤500 bp. It may be used on fragments of up to 1200 bp, but accuracy levels decrease with these greater sizes.

The third approach uses known or predicted polymorphisms within genes (e.g., microsatellite repeat markers or single nucleotide polymorphisms) to characterize allelic association and/or linkage disequilibrium within a gene. The data generated are subjected to a statistical test (see below), depending on whether the study design has a case-control or family-based control design.

STATISTICAL APPROACHES TO STUDYING CANDIDATE GENES

At the candidate gene level, statistical tests are employed to assess evidence of allelic association, which is different from testing for genetic linkage. Evidence for linkage implies physical proximity between a marker and a disease locus based on segregation patterns within a family. However, the particular marker allele segregating with the disease phenotype can vary from pedigree to pedigree. In contrast, allelic association is population-specific, meaning that allele frequency differences in various ethnic or clinically heterogeneous groups can impact association results. There are two general methods of testing for allelic association in NTD candidate genes: case-control and family-based. These approaches, and nuances associated with them, are outlined in Figure 14.2.

Traditionally, NTD candidate gene studies have employed case-control study methods where the allele frequencies in an unrelated set of affected cases are compared to a set of unrelated controls (van der Put et al., 1995; Papapetrou et al., 1996). However, this study design can be flawed if the controls are not appropriately matched with respect to age or other factors like gender. The resulting *population admixture* can produce spurious associations, even in unassociated loci. Family-based association studies, on the other hand, control for such problems by comparing the frequency of the alleles transmitted by a parent to an affected child to that of the alleles not transmitted. In this way, the nontransmitted alleles serve as an internal control. Compared with the case-control method, the family-based study design has several advantages. First, it is a test of linkage disequilibrium, which is a measure of both linkage and association. When there is linkage disequilibrium, multiple pedigrees show excess transmission of the same allele to affected individuals. Second, the added family information provides a means of reducing genotyping errors since genotypes of

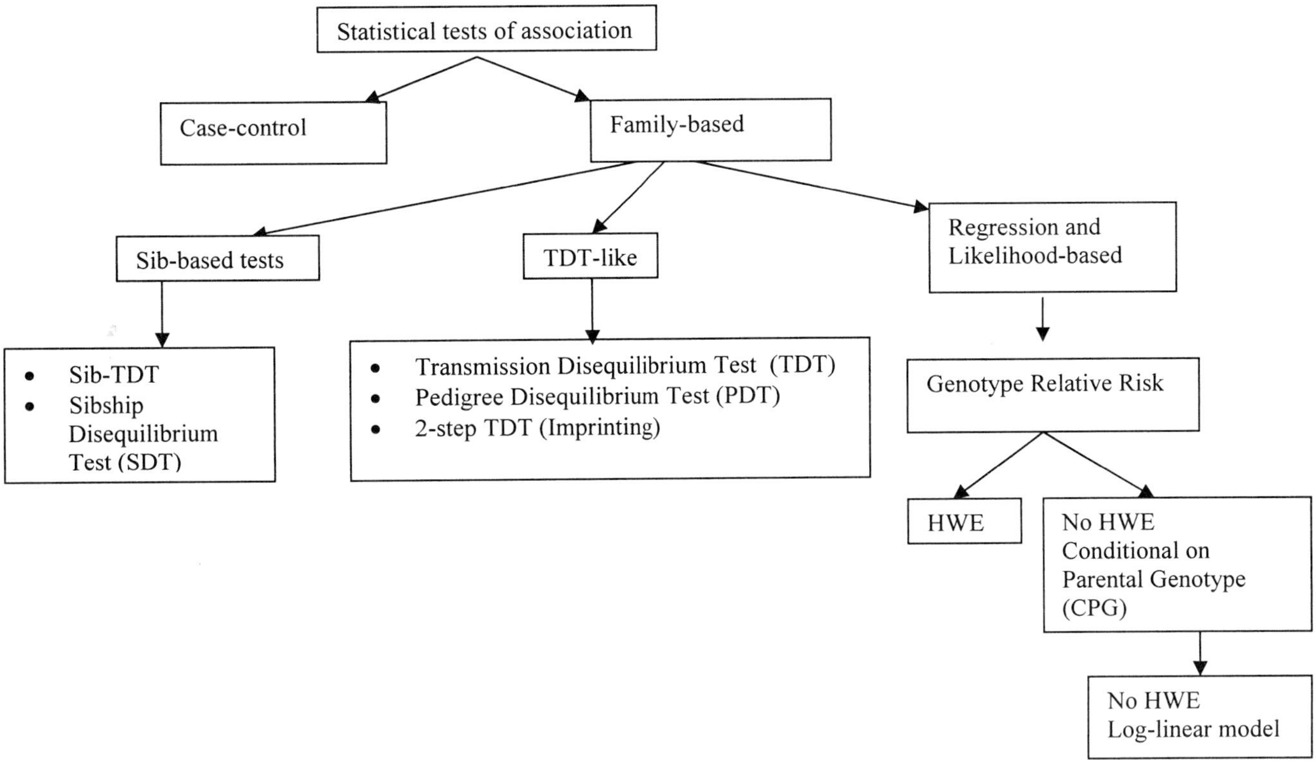

FIGURE 14.2. Single-marker tests of association in candidate genes.

affected children can be checked against those of their parents. Third, maternal and paternal genotype effects can also be detected using some family-based methods.

The most widely used family-based association test is the transmission disequilibrium test (TDT), which is a valid test of linkage in the presence of association, even when there is population admixture (Spielman et al., 1993) or one of a variety of extensions. In a two-allele marker system where *M* represents the variant disease-associated allele and *N* represents the normal allele, the TDT compares the number of *M* versus *N* alleles transmitted from a heterozygous parent to an affected offspring (Table 14.1). A chi-square TDT statistic tests for departure from the expected equal transmission rate of *M* and *N* alleles from the heterozygous parents under the null hypothesis of no linkage or no association. If there is linkage between the marker and disease, as well as allelic association, then the number of times alleles *M* and *N* are transmitted will differ. In studies of candidate genes, TDT results have often failed to replicate the significant results found in case-control analyses (Speer et al., 1999; Trembath et al., 1999; Volcik et al., 2002). Since the same data set was sometimes used, this might indicate initial false-positive results.

TABLE 14.1. *Contingency Table for the Transmission Disequilibrium Test*

	Nontransmitted Allele		
Transmitted Allele	*M*	*N*	Total
M	*A*	*B*	*a+b*
N	C	*D*	*c+d*
Total	*a+c*	*b+d*	*2n*

where $*TDT:\chi_1^2 = \dfrac{(b-c)^2}{(b-c)}$

*Chi-square test with 1 df.

A limitation of the TDT is that it cannot be used as a valid test of association if related nuclear families and/or sibships from larger pedigrees are used. The pedigree disequilibrium test (PDT) was developed as a valid test of linkage disequilibrium that can use data from related nuclear families and discordant sibships (DSP) from extended families (Martin et al., 2000). It has been used to find significant associations in studies of ischemic heart disease, type 1 diabetes, and bipolar disease (Sale et al., 2002; Spence et al., 2002; Toyota et al., 2002), as well as in a study of *MTHFR* and NTDs (Rampersaud et al., 2003a). The PDT can be valuable in situations where multiple affected NTD cases of varying relationships have been ascertained in large families. If all of the information in a pedigree is used, the chance of finding an association at a candidate gene can be improved.

Epigenetic factors such as parent-of-origin or maternal genotype effects have been implicated in NTDs (Chatkupt et al., 1992; Byrne et al., 1996). For example, a parent-of-origin effect can occur if the phenotype results from parent-specific transmission of a gene. These factors cannot be measured directly using the traditional TDT method. As a result, the two-step TDT test was developed to test for maternal genotype effects; however, this test requires DNA from maternal grandparents (Mitchell, 1997).

As an alternative to the TDT, likelihood-based tests have been developed for candidate gene association studies. These tests are flexible and allow the researcher to examine gene–gene and gene–environment interactions, as well as parent-of-origin and maternal effects. An added advantage is that relative risk estimates can be calculated when the child has either a single copy of the gene or two copies. In this way, researchers can even look for dose-dependent effects. Additionally, only nuclear family members are required for sampling, even when testing for parent-of-origin effects. The Genotype Relative Risk (GRR) model is an example of a likelihood-based association test (Schaid and Sommer, 1993). When Hardy Weinberg equilibrium (HWE) cannot be assumed, the GRR is functionally equivalent to the TDT and has been shown to perform better than the TDT in a dominant or recessive model. Another likelihood-based test, the log-linear method (Weinberg et al., 1998), is conceptually similar to the GRR model when HWE is not assumed. It should be noted that the assumption of HWE can be made with certainty only if there has been random mating in a population and no selection, migration, or mutation has occurred. In many studies of complex diseases such as NTDs, it is difficult to make such a strong assumption, and deviations from HWE can have a major impact on analysis results. The log-linear model has the added benefit of being easily generalized to test for maternal effects as well as parent-of-origin effects. The model has been further extended to test for gene–environment interactions (Umbach and Weinberg, 2000) in a diallelic autosomal candidate gene and a two-level exposure variable. Another proposed extension will improve the estimations in the model by allowing unaffected siblings to be used when parental data are missing (Rampersaud et al., 2003b).

Situations may exist where parents are unavailable for sampling; in this case, unaffected siblings can also be used as controls. Several test statistics have been proposed, including the Sib Transmission/Disequilibrium Test (S-TDT) and the Sibship Disequilibrium Test (SDT) (Curtis 1997; Horvath and Laird, 1998). Generally speaking, these tests compare marker allele frequencies in affected and unaffected siblings. In a study of insulin dependent diabetes, it was shown that the results of the Czeizel and Bodnar (1970) test and the TDT were almost identical (Spielman and Ewens, 1998). While this may not be a global finding, the example illustrates the fact that the S-TDT can be used as an alternative to the TDT when parents are unavailable. Traditionally, sib-based association tests have not been used in birth defect studies like NTDs, but may prove useful in situations where parents are difficult or impossible to sample.

The selection of the appropriate statistical test depends on multiple factors, primarily the structure of the data set at hand and whether or not environmental information has been collected. In the case of the latter, likelihood-based tests allow these factors to be incorporated into the analysis. If parents are available in most families, then the traditional TDT approach is valid; otherwise, sib-based or likelihood methods are preferable. In recent years, many new extensions of statistical algorithms have been developed to tackle the complicated analysis of complex disorders like NTDs—for example, by using a haplotype approach instead of relying on single-marker tests of association (Clayton, 1999; Rabinowitz and Laird, 2000). These and other approaches are helping to redefine the statistical tools researchers can use in the search for genes that may be important in the etiology of NTDs.

NEW FRONTIERS IN IDENTIFICATION OF CANDIDATE GENES: EXPRESSION ANALYSES

Laboratory and statistical technology has greatly increased the ability to identify candidate genes. The Human Genome Project has led to the identification of thousands of genes whose functions are under study. DNA microarray (the gene "chip") and the SAGE (serial analysis of gene expression) technique are laboratory techniques that aim to identify genes expressed in a given tissue at a given time in development. The techniques differ in that microarrays have a pre-established set of genes on the matrix, limiting the genes studied to those on the microarray, whereas SAGE identifies potentially novel genes. These techniques can theoretically be used on either human tissue or tissue from NTD animal models to identify potential candidate genes. The utility of these techniques in humans is limited due to the relative paucity of available human tissue in very early embryological development. However, the study and comparison of gene expression in normal tissue versus NTD tissue in animal systems could be very useful in identifying candidate genes for study in humans.

COMBINED STRATEGIES IN HUMAN NEURAL TUBE DEFECT GENE IDENTIFICATION

The most successful strategy to identify genes that contribute to the cause of human NTDs is likely to be one

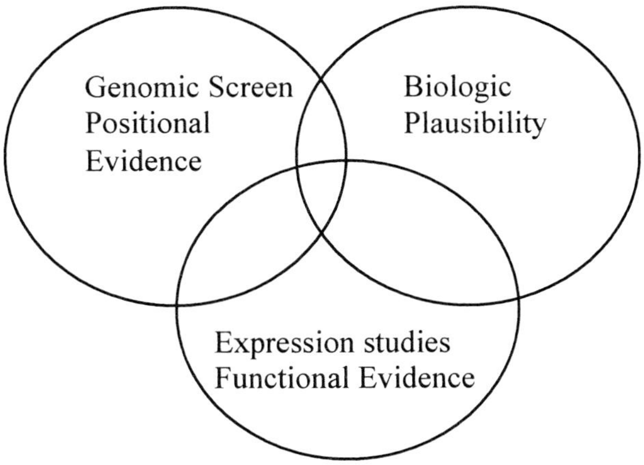

FIGURE 14.3. Combined strategy for gene identification in neural tube defects.

that combines the use of candidate genes from many different sources. Candidate genes identified from the intersection of animal models, biological plausibility such as those from the folate metabolic pathway, expression studies, and positional candidate genes from genomic screening and/or cytogenetic rearrangements can narrow the field of potential candidate genes to be studied in humans (Fig. 14.3) (Hauser et al., 2003).

A directed candidate gene analysis provides a systematic, integrated method for prioritizing candidate genes, allowing the genetic factors contributing to NTDs to be more readily identified. Once genes implicated in the development of NTDs are identified, it will be essential to understand how these genes interact with other genes and the environment to cause spina bifida, anencephaly, and the other NTD phenotypes, and ultimately the relationship between the nonsyndromic and syndromic forms of NTDs. As technology progresses and is improved and as major genetic effects are identified, unraveling the gene–environment interactions will prove to be the next frontier.

REFERENCES

Banta JV, Nichols O (1969). Sacral agenesis. J Bone Joint Surg Am 51(4):693–703.

Bastress KL, Melvin EC, Siegel D, Gilbert JR, Enterline DS, George TM, Speer MC (2003). A SNP in *NCAM1* shows association with human neural tube defects. Am J Hum Genet 73:531.

Brown LY, Hodge SE, Johnson WG, Guy SG, Nye JS, Brown S (2002). Possible association of NTDs with a polyhistidine tract polymorphism in the *ZIC2* gene. Am J Med Genet 108(2):128–131.

Byrne J, Cama A, Reilly M, Vigliarolo M, Levato L, Boni L, Lavia N, et al (1996). Multigeneration maternal transmission in Italian families with neural tube defects. Am J Med Genet 66(3):303–310.

Carter CO, David PA, Laurence KM (1968). A family study of major central nervous system malformations in South Wales 1. J Med Genet 5(2):81–106.

Carter CO, Evans K (1973). Spina bifida and anencephalus in greater London 1. J Med Genet 10(3):209–234.

Centers for Disease Control and Prevention (1992). Recommendations for the use of folic acid to reduce the number of cases of spina bifida and other neural tube defects. MMWR 41:1–7.

Chatkupt S, Hol FA, Shugart YY, Geurds MPA, Stenroos ES, Koenigsberger MR, Hamel BCJ, et al (1995). Absence of linkage between familial neural tube defects and *PAX3* gene. J Med Genet 32(3):200–204.

Chatkupt S, Lucek PR, Koenigsberger MR, Johnson WG (1992). Parental sex effect in spina bifida: a role for genomic imprinting? Am J Med Genet 44(4):508–512.

Clayton D (1999). A generalization of the transmission/disequilibrium test for uncertain-haplotype transmission. Am J Hum Genet 65:1170–1177.

Cragan JD, Roberts HE, Edmonds LD, Khoury MJ, Kirby RS, Shaw GM, Velie EM, et al (1995). Surveillance for Anencepahly and Spina Bifida and the impact of prenatal diagnosis—United States, 1985–1994. MMWR 44, 1–13.

Curtis D (1997). Use of siblings as controls in case-control association studies. Ann Hum Genet 61:319–333.

Czeizel E, Bodnar L (1970). [Congenital developmental anomalies and genetics]. Orv Hetil 111(35):2091–2093.

Demenais F, Le Merrer M, Briard ML, Elston RC (1982). Neural tube defects in France: segregation analysis. Am J Med Genet 11:287–298.

Drainer E, May HM, Tolmie JL (1991). Do familial neural tube defects breed true? J Med Genet 28(9):605–608.

Echlard Y, Epstein DJ, St-Jacques B, Shen L, Mohler J, McMahon JA, McMahon AP (1993). *Sonic hedgehog,* a member of a family of putative signaling molecules, is implicated in the regulation of CNS polarity. Cell 75:1417–1430.

Edwards JH (1969). Inheritance of chronic granulomatous disease. Lancet 2(7625):850–851.

Elwood JM, Little J, Elwood JH (1992). *Epidemiology and Control of Neural Tube Defects.* Oxford: Oxford University Press.

Fellous M, Boue J, Malbrunot C, Wollman E, Sasportes M, Van Cong N, Marcelli A, et al (1982). A five-generation family with sacral agenesis and spina bifida: possible similarities with the mouse T-locus. Am J Med Genet 12:465–487.

Fineman RM, Jorde LB, Martin RA, Hasstedt SJ, Wing SD, Walker ML (1982). Spinal dysraphia as an autosomal dominant defect in four families. Am J Med Genet 12:457–464.

Frecker MF, Fraser FC, Heneghan WD (1988) Are "upper" and "lower" neural tube defects aetiologically different? J Med Genet 25(7):503–504.

Frosst P, Blom HJ, Milos R, Goyette P, Sheppard CA, Matthews RG, Boers GJH, et al (1995). A candidate genetic risk factor for vascular disease: a common mutation in methylenetetrahydrofolate reductase. Nat Genet 10:111–113.

Fuhrmann W (1971). [Genetic counseling as a problem of pediatric practice. Introduction]. Monatsschr Kinderheilkd 119(4):154–156.

Garabedian BH, Fraser FC (1993). Upper and lower neural tube defects: an alternate hypothesis. J Med Genet 30(10):849–851.

George TM, Wolpert CM, Worley G, Mackey JF, Fuchs HE, Speer MC (1996). Variable presentation of neural tube defects in three families. Am J Hum Genet 59:A93.

Golden JA, Chernoff GF (1993). Intermittent pattern of neural tube closure in two strains of mice. Teratology 47:73–80.

Greene ND, Copp AJ (1997). Inositol prevents folate-resistant neural tube defects in the mouse. Nat Med 3(1):60–66.

Gross JM, McClay DR (2001). The role of *Brachyury* (*T*) during gastrulation movements in the sea urchin *Lytechinus variegatus.* Dev Biol 239(1):132–147.

Hall JG, Keena BA (1986). Adjusting recurrence risks for neural tube defects based on B.C. data. Am J Hum Genet 39:A64.

Harris JA, Shaw GM (1995). Neural tube defects—why are rates high among populations of Mexican descent? Environ Health Perspect 103(Suppl 6):163–164.

Harris MJ (2001). Why are the genes that cause risk of human neural tube defects so hard to find? Teratology 63(5):165–166.

Hauser MA, Li YJ, Takeuchi S, Walters R, Noureddine M, Maready M, Darden T, et al (2003). Genomic convergence: identifying candidate genes for Parkinson's disease by combining serial analysis of gene expression and genetic linkage. Hum Mol Genet 12(6):671–677.

Hol FA, Geurds MPA, Chatkupt S, Shugart YY, Balling R, Schrander Stumpel CTR, Johnson WG, et al (1996). *PAX* genes and human neural tube defects: an amino acid substitution in *PAX1* in a patient with spina bifida. J Med Genet 33(8):655–660.

Horvath SM, Laird NM (1998). A discordant-sibship test for disequilibrium and linkage: no need for parental data. Am J Hum Genet 63:1886–1897.

Hume RF, Drugan A, Reichler A, Lampinen J, Martin LS, Johnson MP, Evans MI (1996). Aneuploidy among prenatally detected neural tube defects. Am J Med Genet 61:171–173.

Juriloff DM, Harris MJ (2000). Mouse models for neural tube closure defects. Hum Mol Genet 9(6):993–1000.

Kennedy D, Chitayat D, Winsor EJT, Silver M, Toi A (1998). Prenatally diagnosed neural tube defects: ultrasound, chromosome, and autopsy or postnatal findings in 212 cases. Am J Med Genet 77:317–321.

Khoury MJ, Erickson JD, James LM (1982). Etiologic heterogeneity of neural tube defects. II. Clues from family studies. Am J Hum Genet 34:980–987.

Kirillova I, Novikova I, Galaganova L, Augé J, Audollent S, Crosnier C, Esnault D, et al (2000). Comparative expression of the *SHH, GL13* and *JAG1* genes in normal and neural tube defects human embryos. Am J Hum Genet 67(4):168:888A.

Koch MC, Stegmann K, Ziegler A, Schroter B, Ermet A (1998). Evaluation of the MTHFR *C677T* allele and the *MTHFR* gene locus in a German spina bifida population. Eur J Pediatr 157:487–492.

Lippman-Hand A, Fraser FC, Biddle CJ (1978). Indications for prenatal diagnosis in relatives of patients with neural tube defects. Obstet Gynecol 51(1):72–76.

Luo J, Balkin N, Stewart JF, Sarwark JF, Charrow J, Nye JS (2000). Neural tube defects and the 13q deletion syndrome: evidence for a critical region in 13q33–34. Am J Med Genet 91(3):227–230.

Macdonald KB, Juriloff DM, Harris MJ (1989). Developmental study of neural tube closure in a mouse stock with a high incidence of exencephaly. Teratology 39(2):195–213.

Martin ER, Monks SA, Warren LL, Kaplan NL (2000). A test for linkage and association in general pedigrees: the pedigree disequilibrium test. Am J Hum Genet 67(1):146–154.

Melvin EC, Drake CR, Franklin AD, Mackey JF, George TM, Viles KD, Worley G, et al (1998). Neural tube defects and the search for the genetic cause: the dilemma of multiplex families. Am J Hum Genet 63(4):A113.

Milunsky A, Jick H, Jick SS, Bruell CL, MacLaughlin DS, Rothman KJ, Willett W (1991). Multivitamin/folic acid supplementation in early pregnancy reduces the prevalence of neural tube defects. JAMA 262:2847–2852.

Mitchell LE (1997). Differentiating between fetal and maternal genotypic effects, using the transmission test for linkage disequilibrium. Am J Hum Genet 60(4):1006–1007.

Mornet E, Muller F, Lenvoise-Furet A, Delezoide AL, Col JY, Simon-Bouy B, and Serre JL (1997). Screening of the *C677T* mutation on the methylenetetrahydofolate redustase gene in French patients with neural tube defects. Hum Genet 100:512–514.

Morrison K, Papapetrou C, Hol FA, Mariman EC, Lynch SA, Burn J, Edwards YH (1998). Susceptibility to spina bifida: an association study of five candidate genes. Ann Hum Genet 62(Pt 5):379–396.

MRC Vitamin Study Research Group (1991). Prevention of neural tube defects: results of the Medical Research Council Vitamin Study. Lancet 338:131–137.

Nevin NC, Johnston WP (1980). A family study of spina bifida and anencephalus in Belfast, Northern Ireland (1964 to 1968). J Med Genet 17(3):203–211.

Newton R, Stanier P, Loughna S, Henderson DJ, Forbes SA, Farrall M, Jensson O, et al (1994). Linkage analysis of 62 X-chromosomal loci excludes the X chromosome in an Icelandic family showing apparent X-linked recessive inheritance of neural tube defects. Clin Genet 45:241–249.

Nickel RE, Magenis RE (1996). Neural tube defects and deletions of 22q11. Am J Med Genet 66:25–27.

O'Rahilly R, Muller F (2002). The two sites of fusion of the neural folds and the two neuropores in the human embryo. Teratology 65(4):162–170.

O'Reilly GC, Shields LE (2000). Karyotyping for isolated neural tube defects. A report of two cases. J Reprod Med 45(11):950–952.

Ou CY, Stevenson RE, Brown VK, Schwartz CE, Allen WP, Khoury MJ, Oakley GP Jr, et al (1995). *C677T* homozygosity associated with thermolabile 5, 10 methylenetetrahydrofolate reductase as a risk factor for neural tube defects. Am J Hum Genet 57(4):A223.

Papan C, CamposOrtega JA (1997). A clonal analysis of spinal cord development in the zebrafish. Dev Genes Evol 207(2):71–81.

Papapetrou C, Lynch SA, Burn J, Edwards YH (1996). Methylenetetrahydrofolate reductase and neural tube defects. Lancet 348:58.

Park CH, Stewart W, Khoury MJ, Mulinare J (1992). Is there etiologic heterogeneity between upper and lower neural tube defects? Am J Epidemiol 136(12):1493–1501.

Partington MD, McLone DG (1995). Hereditary factors in the etiology of neural tube defects. Pediatr Neurosurg 23:311–316.

Penrose LS (1946). Familial data on 144 cases of anencephaly, spina bifida and congenital hydrocephaly. Ann Eugen 13:73–98.

Pericak-Vance MA, Wolpert CM, Menold MM, Bass MP, Hauser ER, Donnelly SL, Ravan SA, et al (1998). Chromosome 7 and autistic disorder (AD). Am J Hum Genet 63(4):A16.

Perz-Edwards A, Hardison NL, Linney E (2001). Retinoic acid–mediated gene expression in transgenic reporter zebrafish. Dev Biol 229(1):89–101.

Philipp T, Kalousek DK (2002). Neural tube defects in missed abortions: embryoscopic and cytogenetic findings. Am J Med Genet 107(1):52–57.

Rabinowitz D, Laird N (2000). A unified approach to adjusting association tests for population admixture with arbitrary pedigree structure and arbitrary missing marker information. Hum Hered 50:211–223.

Rampersaud E, Bassuk AG, Enterline DS, Siegel MG, Melvin EC, Aben J, Allen J et al. (in press). Whole genome-wide linkage screen for neural tube defects reveals regions of interest on chromosomes 7 and 10. J Med Genet.

Rampersaud E, Melvin EC, Siegel D, Mehltretter L, Dickerson ME, George TM, Enterline D, et al (2003a). Updated investigations of the role of *MTHFR* in human neural tube defects. Clin Genet 63(3):210–214.

Rampersaud E, Speer MC, Martin ER (2003b). Improved inference of missing parental data in a log-linear test of association by inclusion of unaffected siblings. Am J Hum Genet (S)73 (5):617.

Richter B, Schultealbert AH, Koch MC (2002). Human *T* and risk for neural tube defects. J Med Genet 39(3):E14.

Risch N (1990). Linkage strategies for genetically complex traits. II. The power of affected relative pairs. Am J Hum Genet 46(2):229–241.

Sakai Y (1989). Neurulation in the mouse: manner and timing of neural tube closure. Anat Rec 223(2):194–203.

Sale MM, FitzGerald LM, Charlesworth JC, Bowden DW, Rich SS (2002). Evidence for a novel type 1 diabetes susceptibility locus on chromosome 8. Diabetes 51:S316–S319.

Schaid DJ, Sommer SS (1993). Genotype relative risks: methods for design and analysis of candidate- gene association studies. Am J Hum Genet 53(5):1114–1126.

Scott WK, Yamaoka LH, Bass MP, Gaskell PC, Conneally PM, Small GW, Farrer LA, et al (1998). No genetic association between the LRP receptor and sporadic or late-onset familial Alzheimer disease. Neurogenetics 1:179–183.

Seller MJ (1990). Neural tube defects: are neurulation and canalization forms causally distinct? Am J Med Genet 35:394–396.

Seller MJ (1994). Vitamins, folic acid and the cause and prevention of neural tube defects. Ciba Found Symp 181:161–173.

Shaw GM, Todoroff K, Finnell RH, Rozen R, Lammer EJ (1999). Maternal vitamin use, infant *C677T* mutation in *MTHFR,* and isolated cleft palate risk. Am J Med Genet 85(1):84–85.

Shaw SH, Carrasquillo MM, Kashuk C, Puffenberger EG, Chakravarti A (1998). Allele frequency distributions in pooled DNA samples: applications to mapping complex disease genes. Genome Res 8:111–123.

Shields DC, Kirke PN, Mills JL, Ramsbottom D, Molloy AM, Burke H, Weir DG, et al (1999). The "thermolabile" variant of methylenetetrahydrofolate reductase and neural tube defects: an evaluation of the genetic risk and the relative importance of the genotypes of the embryo and the mother. Am J Hum Genet 64:1045–1055.

Shields DC, Ramsbottom D, Donoghue C, Pinjon E, Kirke PN, Molloy AM, Edwards YH, et al (2000). Association between historically high frequencies of neural tube defects and the human *T* homologue of mouse *T* (*Brachyrury*). Am J Med Genet 92:206–211.

Speer MC, Melvin EC, Viles KD, Bauer KA, Rampersaud E, Drake C, George TM, et al (2002). *T* locus shows no evidence for linkage disequilibrium or mutation in American Caucasian neural tube defect families. Am J Med Genet 110(3):215–218.

Speer MC, Melvin E, Worley G, Fuchs HE, George TM (1997). Search for major candidate genes for human neural tube defects. Paper presented at the annual meeting of the AANS/CNS Section on Pediatric Neurological Surgery, April 1997, Denver.

Speer MC, Nye J, McLone D, Worley G, Melvin EC, Viles KD, Franklin A, et al (1999). Possible interaction of genotypes at cystathionine beta-synthase and methylenetetrahydrofolate reductase (*MTHFR*) in neural tube defects. NTD Collaborative Group. Clin Genet 56(2):142–144.

Speer MC, Rampersaud E, Melvin EC, George TM, Allen J, Floyd LE, Dickerson M, et al (2003). Genomic screening and testing of candidate genes in human neural tube defects. Paper presented at the International Neural Tube Defects Conference, October 2003, Houston.

Spence MS, McGlinchey PG, Patterson CC, Belton C, Murphy G, McMaster D, Fogarty DG, et al (2002). Family-based investigation of the *C677T* polymorphism of the methylenetetrahydrofolate reductase gene in ischaemic heart disease. Atherosclerosis 165(2):293–299.

Spielman RS, Ewens WJ (1998). A sibship test for linkage in the presence of association: the sib transmission/disequilibrium test. Am J Hum Genet 62(2):450–458.

Spielman RS, McGinnis RE, Ewens WJ (1993). Transmission test for linkage disequilibrium: the insulin gene region and insulin-dependent diabetes mellitus (IDDM). Am J Hum Genet 52(3):506–516.

Suarez L, Hendricks KA, Cooper SP, Sweeney AM, Hardy RJ, Larsen RD (2000). Neural tube defects among Mexican Americans living on the U.S.–Mexico border: effects of folic acid and dietary folate. Am J Epidemiol 152(11):1017–1023.

Sulik KK, Zucker RM, Dehart DB, et al (1998). Normal patterns of neural tube closure differ in the human and mouse. Proc Greenwood Genet Ctr 18:129–130.

Toriello HV, Higgins JV (1985). Possible causal heterogeneity in spina bifida cystica. Am J Med Genet 21:13–20.

Toyota T, Yamada K, Saito K, Detera-Wadleigh SD, Yoshikawa T (2002). Association analysis of adenylate cyclase type 9 gene using pedigree disequilibrium test in bipolar disorder. Mol Psychiatry 7(5):450–452.

Trembath D, Sherbondy AL, Vandyke DC, Shaw GM, Todoroff K, Lammer EJ, Finnell RH, et al (1999). Analysis of select folate pathway genes, *PAX3,* and human *T* in a Midwestern neural tube defect population. Teratology 59(5):331–341.

Udvadia AJ, Linney E (2003). Windows into development: historic, current, and future perspectives on transgenic zebrafish. Dev Biol 256(1):1–17.

Umbach DM, Weinberg C (2000). The use of case–parent triads to study joint effects of genotype and exposure. Am J Hum Genet 66:251–261.

Van Allen MI, Kalousek DK, Chernoff GF, Juriloff D, Harris M, McGillivray BC, Yong SL, et al (1993). Evidence for multi-site closure of the neural tube in humans. Am J Med Genet 47:723–743.

van der Put NM, Gabreels F, Stevens EM, Smeitink JA, Trijbels FJ, Eskes TK, van den Heuvel LP, et al (1998). A second common mutation in the methylenetetrahydrofolate reductase gene: an additional risk factor for neural-tube defects? Am J Hum Genet 62:1044–1051.

van der Put NM, Steegers-Theunissen RPM, Frosst P, Trijbels FJM, Eskes TKAB, van den Heuvel LP, Mariman ECM, et al (1995). Mutated methylenetetrahydrofolate reductase as a risk factor for spina bifida. Lancet 346:1070–1071.

Volcik KA, Blanton SH, Kruzel MC, Townsend IT, Tyerman GH, Mier RJ, Northrup H (2002). Testing for genetic associations with the *PAX* gene family in a spina bifida population. Am J Med Genet 110(3):195–202.

Weinberg CR, Wilcox AJ, Lie RT (1998). A log-linear approach to case–parent–triad data: assessing effects of disease genes that act either directly or through maternal effects and that may be subject to parental imprinting. Am J Hum Genet 62:969–978.

Whitehead AS, Gallagher P, Mills JL, Kirke PN, Burke H, Molloy AM, Weir DG, et al (1995). A genetic defect in 5,10 methylenetetrahydrofolate reductase in neural tube defects. Q J Med 88:763–766.

Williamson EM (1965). Incidence and family aggregation of major congential malformations of central nervous system. J Med Genet 2:161–172.

15

Genetic Risk Factors for Neural Tube Defects: Variants in Folate Metabolism

RIMA ROZEN

Neural tube defects (NTDs) are multifactorial disorders that are influenced by genetic and nongenetic factors. Inadequate dietary folate has been recognized for some time as an important nongenetic contributor to the risk for NTD. In contrast, the identification of genetic factors that alter NTD risk is a relatively newer area of investigation. One sequence change, at bp 677 in the gene encoding a folate-metabolizing enzyme, methylenetetrahydrofolate reductase (MTHFR), has emerged as the first genetic risk factor for NTD. However, the expectation for complex traits is that combinations of genetic polymorphisms and environmental modifiers will influence the disease risk; a polymorphism is a mutation (base change or sequence variant) with a prevalence >1%. Consequently, other variants in MTHFR and sequence changes in other genes involved in folate metabolism are being explored as possible genetic risk factors for NTD, but additional data are required for these candidates before their role can be confirmed. This chapter will present an overview of folate metabolism, discuss the findings on MTHFR as a risk factor for NTD, and summarize the information on some of the other candidate genes in folate metabolism that have been investigated as potential risk factors.

OVERVIEW OF FOLATE METABOLISM

Folates consist of a pterin moiety and *p*-aminobenzoic acid linked to a variable number of glutamic acid residues. Dietary folates have to undergo several steps before they can be utilized intracellularly, including hydrolysis to monoglutamate forms in the intestine before absorption, transport across the luminal membrane, and release across the basolateral membrane into the portal circulation. Two different types of transport systems have been described for folate entry into cells. Within the cell, folates require polyglutamylation and entry into the mitochondria. Interconversion of folate derivatives is catalyzed by several enzymes in both the cytosol and mitochondria. All these processes, which prepare the folate for various biochemical reactions, require many different genes and gene products, not all of which have been described (Rosenblatt and Fenton, 2001).

The actual biochemical reactions in which folates participate are transfers of single-carbon units in several critical pathways (Rosenblatt and Fenton, 2001). These pathways include synthesis or catabolism of amino acids (serine, glycine, histidine, and methionine) and synthesis of nucleotides (thymidine and purines). Through their role in methionine synthesis, folates are also critical for the methylation cycle since methionine is the precursor of *S*-adenosylmethionine (SAM). *S*-adenosylmethionine is the major methyl donor for many important methylation reactions including DNA methylation and synthesis of creatine, phospholipids, and neurotransmitters.

Of particular relevance for this chapter is the conversion of 5,10-methylenetetrahydrofolate (5,10-methyleneTHF) to 5-methyltetrahydrofolate (5-methylTHF), the primary circulatory form of folate, through the action of MTHFR (Daubner and Matthews, 1982) (Fig. 15.1). 5-MethylTHF provides the methyl group for the vitamin B_{12}-catalyzed remethylation of homocysteine to methionine by methionine synthase; the gene encoding methionine synthase has been designated *MTR* (Leclerc et al., 1996). Methionine synthase requires reactivation after a certain number of cycles; this step is catalyzed by methionine synthase reductase, for which the gene symbol is *MTRR* (Leclerc et al., 1998).

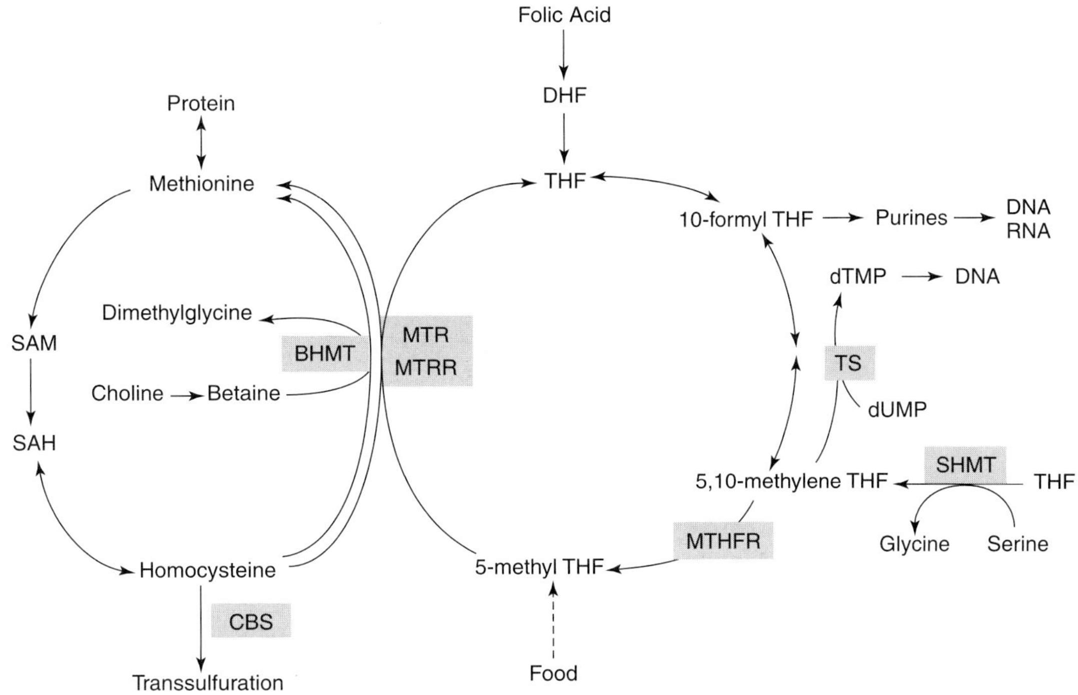

FIGURE 15.1. The relationship between folate and homocysteine metabolism, indicating the genes/enzymes that are discussed in the text. BHMT, betaine homocysteine methyltransferase; CBS, cystathionine β-synthase; DHF, dihydrofolate; dTMP, thymidine-5′-phosphate; dUMP, deoxyuridine-5′-phosphate; MTHFR, methylenetetrahydrofolate reductase; MTR, methionine synthase; MTRR, methionine synthase reductase; SAH, S-adenosylhomocysteine; SAM, S-adenosylmethionine; SHMT, serine hydroxymethyltransferase; THF, tetrahydrofolate; TS, thymidylate synthase. *Source:* A. Lawrance, McGill University.

Folate-dependent conversion of homocysteine to methionine (via MTHFR and methionine synthase) begins early in development and is present in all tissues (Gaull et al., 1973) These enzymatic reactions provide a link between folate and homocysteine metabolism. An elevation of plasma homocysteine, mild hyperhomocysteinemia, has become recognized as a risk factor for cardiovascular disease (Graham et al., 1997; Clarke et al., 2002), but disturbances in homocysteine metabolism may be equally relevant for NTD since hyperhomocysteinemia has also been observed in NTD families (Steegers-Theunissen et al., 1994; Mills et al., 1995) and since mutations in MTHFR result in hyperhomocysteinemia and an increased risk for NTD (van der Put et al., 1995; Botto and Yang, 2000). An understanding of other homocysteine outflow pathways is therefore important for identification of other enzymes that might contribute to the NTD risk.

Homocysteine remethylation to methionine can also be performed through the action of betaine homocysteine methyltransferase (BHMT), which uses betaine as a methyl donor instead of folate, but this reaction is largely limited to liver and kidney; betaine is a product of choline oxidation (Mudd et al., 2001). This reaction provides a link between folate and choline metabolism. Homocysteine can also undergo transsulfuration to generate cysteine; the first enzyme in the transsulfuration pathway is cystathionine-β-synthase (CBS). The transsulfuration pathway can also result in conversion of cysteine to other sulfur derivatives, such as glutathione or taurine, but it is the primary degradative pathway for homocysteine through the generation of inorganic sulfate (Mudd et al., 2001).

Homocysteine metabolism is approximately equally distributed between the remethylation and transsulfuration pathways. However, this distribution can be altered by SAM, highlighting the importance of methylation reactions to homocysteine and folate metabolism. When dietary protein/methionine intake is high, SAM inhibits MTHFR and folate-dependent remethylation and activates CBS to increase degradation of homocysteine through the transsulfuration pathway (Finkelstein, 2001). Deficiency of SAM has been reported to induce BHMT in an attempt to maintain methionine synthesis (Park et al., 1997).

5,10-MethyleneTHF, the substrate of MTHFR, is also a substrate of thymidylate synthase. Thymidylate synthase catalyzes the conversion of deoxyuridine-5′-phosphate (dUMP) to thymidine-5′-phosphate (dTMP), providing thymidine for DNA synthesis. 5,10-MethyeneTHF can also be interconverted to generate 10-formyltetrahydrofolate (10-formylTHF), which donates carbons to generate the purine ring (Rosenblatt and Fenton, 2001). When MTHFR activity is decreased (by SAM or by mutation), more 5,10-methyleneTHF should be available for synthesis of thymidine and purines (Bagley and Selhub, 1998).

Even though only some of the folate-dependent reactions have been described above, it is evident that inadequate folate intake or genetic disturbances in folate metabolism may disrupt not only folate-dependent reactions, but also the metabolism of several other critical compounds including methionine, choline, and nucleotides.

METHYLENETETRAHYDROFOLATE REDUCTASE DEFICIENCY

Methylenetetrahydrofolate reductase converts 5,10-methyleneTHF to 5-methylTHF, the methyl donor for homocysteine conversion to methionine. Severe deficiency of MTHFR has been recognized as a cause of homocystinuria since the 1970s. This inborn error of metabolism is associated with markedly elevated levels of homocysteine in plasma and urine; patients display a wide variety of neurological and vascular complications (Rosenblatt and Fenton, 2001). The hypothesis that mild elevations in homocysteine might increase the risk of vascular disease was largely based on the observation that these homocystinuric patients with dramatic elevations in homocysteine frequently had thrombotic episodes (McCully, 1969). Although homocystinuria and severe deficiency of MTHFR are rare, a more common MTHFR deficiency, with a thermolabile enzyme, was reported in 1988 in a group of coronary artery disease patients. This type of deficiency was observed after heating lymphocyte extracts at 46°C for 5 minutes and measuring residual MTHFR activity after heating (Kang et al., 1988).

The isolation of the cDNA/gene for MTHFR in 1994 (Goyette et al., 1994) first enabled the identification of mutations in patients with severe MTHFR deficiency. Shortly thereafter, Frosst et al. (1995) identified a C→T substitution at bp 677, which converted an alanine residue to a valine residue. Biochemical studies confirmed that this mutation encoded the previously reported thermolabile variant, characterized by reduced residual activity after heating as well as by reduced specific activity at 37°C. Of greater interest, however, was the reported association of this polymorphism with increased plasma homocysteine. The MTHFR 677C→T variant is extremely common, with homozygosity frequencies ranging between 5% and 15% in many studied populations (Botto and Yang, 2000). It is even more common in Hispanic populations in California and Colombia, with approximately 20%–25% homozygosity (Botto and Yang, 2000), and has been reported to reach 34% homozygosity in a study in Mexico (Mutchinick et al., 1999). The genotype is infrequent in some American black and African black populations (Botto and Yang, 2000).

The association of the mutant 677 MTHFR genotype with hyperhomocysteinemia occurs only in individuals with low folate status. Stratification of a group of 365 Americans by their median plasma folate value (15 nM) demonstrated that only those with the 677TT genotype and folate values below the median were predisposed to hyperhomocysteinemia; the mutant genotype had no effect on homocysteine levels when the folate status was adequate (Jacques et al., 1996). Folate has been shown to stabilize the mutant human enzyme, as well as the wild-type enzyme; consequently, with higher folate levels, the mutant enzyme may be able to function relatively normally and provide adequate amounts of 5-methylTHF for homocysteine metabolism (Guenther et al., 1999). These initial studies using crude human enzyme preparations (Guenther et al., 1999) have been extended to the purified human enzyme generated in a baculovirus expression system (Yamada et al., 2001), with similar conclusions. These observations suggested, and subsequent studies showed, that folate supplementation should prevent hyperhomocysteinemia in mutant individuals (Malinow et al., 1997).

The mutant enzyme is also stabilized by flavin adenine dinucleotide (FAD), the cofactor for MTHFR (Guenther et al., 1999). Since riboflavin is the precursor for FAD, the influence of riboflavin levels on plasma homocysteine has also been examined in mutant individuals; three studies have suggested that the higher homocysteine levels in 677TT individuals may also be due to a lower riboflavin status (Rozen, 2002). A recent study has reported that 677TT mutant individuals respond to homocysteine lowering with riboflavin supplementation (McNulty et al., 2003).

Although the best-characterized biochemical disturbance in mild MTHFR deficiency is an elevation in plasma homocysteine (Frosst et al., 1995; Jacques et al., 1996; Meleady et al., 2003), other alterations reported in human studies include decreased plasma folate (van der Put et al., 1995; Meleady et al., 2003), increased levels of nonmethylfolates (Bagley and Selhub, 1998), and decreased DNA methylation (Friso et al., 2002). The effect of the variant on red blood cell folates has been inconsistent among studies, possibly due to the different assays currently in use (van der Put et al., 1995; Molloy et al., 1997; Bagley and Selhub, 1998). A mouse model for mild *MTHFR* deficiency, generated by a heterozygous knockout of the MTHFR gene, also displays hyperhomocysteinemia, decreased plasma folate, and decreased DNA methylation in some tissues (Chen et al., 2001). In addition, studies with this mouse model have revealed that liver betaine levels are decreased, presumably due to enhanced flux of homocysteine through the betaine-dependent BHMT pathway, when folate-dependent remethylation is disturbed (Schwahn et al., 2003). A negative correlation in humans between plasma homocysteine and plasma betaine levels suggests that the enhanced flux through BHMT may also be present in mild hyperhomocysteinemia in humans (Schwahn et al., 2003).

A second common variant in MTHFR is an A to C substitution at bp 1298, which converts a glutamate residue to an alanine residue (van der Put et al., 1998; Weisberg et al., 1998). This mutation is not as well characterized as the 677 variant. The frequency of homozygotes ranges from 7% to 13% in European populations; it is somewhat lower in Asians (Robien and Ulrich, 2003). Homozygotes for the mutant enzyme have slightly reduced specific activity in lymphocyte extracts, consistent with the findings for the recombinant mutant human enzyme expressed in bacteria (Weisberg et al., 2001). However, this decrease in activity does not appear to be sufficient to elevate plasma homocysteine or lower plasma folate in homozygous mutant individuals (van der Put et al., 1998; Weisberg et al., 1998). Furthermore, the purified recombinant human enzyme with this mutation did not exhibit catalytic properties different from those of the wild-type enzyme (Yamada et al., 2001).

The 1298 mutation is in strong linkage disequilibrium with the 677 variant, such that the 1298C and 677T changes are rarely seen on the same allele. It is therefore likely that the two mutations arose independently, on distinct alleles, and the physical distance between them is too small to expect frequent recombination events. However, the two mutations can occur on separate alleles in the same individual; these individuals may be predisposed to hyperhomocysteinemia, particularly if the folate status is low (Weisberg et al., 2001). Heterozygosity for both variants occurs in 15%–20% of the North American and European populations that have been studied.

Other polymorphisms have been identified in MTHFR, but many of these are silent changes that do not affect the coding sequence or they occur deep within introns (Leclerc et al., 2004). In any case, functional assessment of polymorphisms through biochemical studies has been performed only for the 677 and 1298 changes. Consequently, until proven otherwise, these additional variants may not have any impact on the activity or stability of the enzyme.

METHYLENETETRAHYDROFOLATE REDUCTASE DEFICIENCY AND NEURAL TUBE DEFECTS

Decreased folate in pregnant women is an established risk factor for having a child with an NTD (Kirke et al., 1993). Folate supplementation has been shown to reduce the occurrence and recurrence of NTD (MRC Vitamin Study Research Group, 1991; Czeizel and Dudas, 1992). These observations underscore the importance of adequate dietary folate for prevention of these birth defects. However, in addition to lower folate status, mothers of children with NTD had been suspected of having a metabolic abnormality in folate metabolism. These observations, as well as reports demonstrating that mothers of NTD children had mild hyperhomocysteinemia (Steegers-Theunissen et al., 1994; Mills et al., 1995), led to the investigation of the MTHFR 677C→T variant as a genetic risk factor for NTD. Van der Put et al (1995) first reported a positive association of this variant with the NTD risk in children with spina bifida and in their parents. The odds ratios in this study of Dutch families were 3.7 (95% CI 1.5–9.1) for mothers with the TT genotype, 2.9 (95% CI 1.0–7.9) for the children, and 2.2 (95% CI 0.8–6.3) for the fathers.

Subsequent to this initial report, many, but not all, studies around the world have reported similar conclusions. Meta-analyses were performed in 1997 (van der Put et al., 1997a) and 2000 (Botto and Yang, 2000). The latter study reported a pooled odds ratio of 2.0 (95% CI 1.5–2.8) for the maternal 677TT genotype and 1.8 (95% CI 1.4–2.2) for the child's mutant genotype. The father's genotype was not associated with an increased risk.

The suggestion has been made that the incidence of NTDs in different populations may correlate with the frequency of the MTHFR variant. One such study, in the Mexican population, reported a homozygosity frequency of 34.8%; the prevalence of NTD in Mexico may be as high as 1/250 (Mutchinick et al., 1999).

Since folate status is critical for manifestation of the consequences of the mutant genotype (Jacques et al., 1996), the maternal folate status during pregnancy is an important variable. Unfortunately, no reports have assessed maternal folate status in the first month of pregnancy, the time of development of the neural tube, in combination with the MTHFR genotype. Some of the inconsistencies in the literature regarding the influence of the MTHFR 677 genotype may be related to this issue.

The 1298 variant has also been examined for its role in NTD. In the first report, the homozygous mutant genotype of the child, mother, and father did not significantly affect the NTD risk (van der Put et al., 1998). A subsequent meta-analysis reached the same conclusion (Botto and Yang, 2000). However, compound heterozygosity for the 1298C and 677T alleles has been suggested to increase the risk, although the results have been conflicting (van der Put et al., 1998; Trembath et al., 1999; Richter et al., 2001).

The epidemiologic evidence for the MTHFR 677 variant as a risk factor for NTD is quite convincing. Additional biological evidence of a role for MTHFR in the development of the neural tube has been obtained from antisense studies. When gestational day 8 mouse embryos were cultured in the presence of antisense oligonucleotides that inhibit expression of MTHFR, there was an increase in the frequency of embryos with NTD (Hansen et al., 2001). The mechanisms by which MTHFR mutation or inhibition delays neural tube closure are not known, although several possibilities exist: (*1*) the increased homocysteine itself may be toxic to the embryo (Rosenquist et al., 1996); (*2*) homocysteine accumulation may lead to increased oxidative stress or endoplasmic reticulum stress, as suggested by studies investigating hyperhomocysteinemia and vascular disease (Welch and Loscalzo, 1998; Werstuck et al., 2001); (*3*) altered distribution of folates (Bagley and Selhub, 1998) may affect other folate-related processes, such as DNA synthesis; (*4*) decreased availability of SAM (Friso et al., 2002) may disrupt methylation reactions; the multitude of SAM-dependent methylation reactions makes it difficult to identify the specific methyltransferase that might be critical for neural tube development, but potential candidates are DNA methyltransferase reactions that would affect DNA methylation and gene expression, or methylation reactions in phospholipid biosynthesis or neurotransmitter metabolism.

OTHER GENETIC VARIANTS IN FOLATE AND HOMOCYSTEINE METABOLISM

The MTHFR 677 variant has been suggested to account for approximately 10% of the NTD risk (Botto and Yang, 2000). Since up to 70% of NTD may be folate responsive, the search continues for polymorphisms in other genes involved in folate or homocysteine metabolism. Thus far, the results have been disappointing. Although some variants appear promising, there are too few studies thus far, with conflicting results in many cases; additional studies are clearly warranted. Furthermore, it is likely that these variants interact to increase the risk. This necessitates the analysis of even larger cohorts for proper evaluation of interactive effects. The list below provides a brief overview of the variants that have been studied, but many of the results should be considered to be somewhat preliminary.

1. *Methionine synthase.* Methionine synthase, a vitamin B_{12}-dependent enzyme, utilizes 5-methyltetrahydrofolate, generated by MTHFR, for homocysteine remethylation to methionine. A polymorphism in the methionine synthase gene (*MTR;* 2756A→G) results in the substitution of an aspartic acid by a glycine residue (D919G) (Leclerc et al., 1996). It is not as common as the MTHFR variants, with a homozygosity frequency of less than 5%. The functional impact of this substitution on the human enzyme has not been examined. Several studies have examined the impact of the variant on the NTD risk, but the majority have not reported a significant association (van der Put et al., 1997b; Morrison et al., 1998; Brody et al., 1999; Christensen et al., 1999; Trembath et al., 1999; Akar et al., 2000; Johanning et al., 2000), although a report using the transmission disequilibrium test has suggested an impact of the maternal mutant genotype (Doolin et al., 2002).
2. *Methionine synthase reductase.* Methionine synthase reductase catalyzes the reductive activation of methionine synthase. A common variant in this gene (*MTRR;* 66A→G) converts the isoleucine residue at codon 22 into a methionine residue (I22M) (Wilson et al., 1999). The isoleucine allele appears to be as common as the methionine allele in North American populations (allele frequency ~ 0.5), but the isoleucine residue has been designated as the wild-type or ancestral allele based on comparison with related proteins (Wilson et al., 1999). A recent study suggests that this substitution may affect the interaction of the reductase with the methionine synthase (Olteanu et al., 2002).

   The first study to examine this variant in NTD reported a nonsignificant increase in the odds ratio for mothers and children. However, the risk for mothers increased to an odds ratio of 4.8 (95% CI 1.5–15.8) when the genotype effect was examined in conjunction with low vitamin B_{12} (Wilson et al., 1999). The interaction between a mutant genotype and nutrient status is interesting considering the aforementioned interactions between MTHFR and folate status; furthermore, the maternal vitamin B_{12} level has been suggested to be an independent risk factor for NTD (Kirke et al., 1993). Other studies have also suggested that mothers (Doolin et al., 2002; Zhu et al., 2003) or children (Gueant-Rodriguez et al., 2003; Zhu et al., 2003) with the mutant I22M genotype have an increased risk for NTD, but interaction with nutrients has not been examined. Although most of the above studies involved small numbers of families, of note is one positive report (Doolin et al., 2002) with a larger cohort that used the transmission disequilibrium test to obtain a maternal risk of 2.05 (95% CI 1.05–3.99).
3. *Cystathionine beta-synthase (CBS).* Cystathionine beta-synthase catalyzes the first step in the transsulfuration pathway of homocysteine metabolism. The allele frequency of a 68-bp insertion in exon 8 of the *CBS* gene was reported to be approximately 12% in a North American study (Tsai et al., 1996), but a deleterious effect of the mutation on enzyme function has not been demonstrated (Romano et al., 2002). This variant on its own does not appear to be associated with an increased NTD risk in several studies (Ramsbottom et al., 1997; Morrison et al., 1998; Speer et al., 1999).

4. *Reduced folate carrier (RFC1).* A common variant in the gene for the reduced folate carrier, which transports 5-methyltetrahydrofolate across the plasma membrane (80A→G), converts a histidine into an arginine residue at codon 27 (H27R). The frequency of the RR mutant genotype is quite high, approximately 25% in the studied North American and European populations (Shaw et al., 2002; Morin et al., 2003a). A recent study (Morin et al., 2003a) reported that mothers with the homozygous mutant RR genotype, with low red blood cell folate, were at increased risk for having a child with a NTD (odds ratio = 4.6; 95% CI = 1.47–14.37). A nonsignificant increase in risk was also reported in a group of California newborns whose mothers had not used vitamins (Shaw et al., 2002). As discussed previously, the interaction between genotype and nutritional status is consistent with the multifactorial nature of NTD. Additional studies of this variant are clearly warranted.
5. *Folate receptors.* This group of genes ($FR\alpha$, β, and γ), which bind folate and bring it into the cell, were considered good candidates for a folate-responsive disorder, but several studies have failed to identify common variants that influence the NTD risk (Heil et al., 1999; Trembath et al., 1999; Barber et al., 2000; O'Leary et al., 2003).
6. *Transcobalamin II (TCII).* Several genetic polymorphisms have been identified in TCII, a protein that internalizes vitamin B_{12} into peripheral cells (Afman et al., 2002). Reduced vitamin B_{12} binding by TCII has been reported to increase the risk of NTD (Afman et al., 2001). However, only two genetic studies have been published thus far, with conflicting results and small cohorts (Afman et al., 2002; Gueant-Rodriguez et al., 2003).
7. *Glutamate carboxypeptidase II (GCPII).* This enzyme, located in the jejunum, catalyzes the deconjugation of folate polyglutamates to monoglutamates prior to absorption. The variant, a histidine to tyrosine change at codon 475 (H475Y), is relatively rare and, in a limited number of studies, does not appear to be associated with an increased NTD risk (Vieira et al., 2002; Afman et al., 2003; Morin et al., 2003a).
8. *Single reports of other variants.* Betaine homocysteine methyltransferase catalyzes homocysteine remethylation to methionine using betaine as the methyl donor. A recent study has suggested that the QQ homozygous mutant genotype, of the R239Q polymorphism in BHMT, is associated with decreased odds ratios for the NTD risk in mothers and children, but the decrease was not significant (Morin et al., 2003b). Two variants have been examined in serine hydroxymethyltransferase, the enzyme that generates most of the 5,10-methyleneTHF derivative, but an increased risk for NTD was not observed (Heil et al., 2001). One study has reported a polymorphism (R653Q) in the trifunctional enzyme (methylenetetrahydrofolate dehydrogenase/methenyltetrahydrofolate cyclohydrolase/formyltetrahydrofolate synthetase) that interconverts folate derivatives and found that the *Q* allele was associated with an increased NTD risk in mothers (Brody et al., 2002).
9. *Gene–gene interactions.* The interaction between genetic polymorphisms in the folate-homocysteine metabolic pathway is an important area of investigation, since it is likely that a single variant will contribute only a modest increase in risk. Furthermore, these types of studies may uncover a role for some genetic mutations that, by themselves, did not yield significant results. For example, children who were homozygous for the MTHFR mutant genotype in combination with the CBS mutant genotype had a five-fold greater risk of NTD; the MTHFR mutation alone had a two-fold increased risk, whereas there was no detectable increased risk for the CBS genotype alone (Botto and Mastroiacovo, 1998). Other studies on this interaction have suggested a positive trend (Speer et al., 1999) or reached a negative conclusion (Richter et al., 2001). The MTRR mutant genotype combined with the MTHFR mutant genotype showed a significant four-fold increase in risk for children, whereas the MTRR genotype alone did not show an increased risk (Wilson et al., 1999). An interaction between the MTR mutant genotype and the MTHFR mutant genotype has been reported in a study of mothers of NTD offspring (Morrison et al., 1998), but a second study did not reach the same conclusion (Johanning et al., 2000). An interaction of MTR and MTRR genotypes has also recently been proposed (Zhu et al., 2003).

SUMMARY

Although there are many different mutations in mice that can result in NTDs (Linder and Davisson, 1994), there appears to be only one well-characterized genetic risk factor for human NTD, the 677C→T change in *MTHFR*. Yet even this risk factor explains only a small percentage of human NTD. Over a dozen polymorphisms in genes encoding different proteins involved in folate transport or metabolism have been identified, but the data are not yet convincing for most or all of them. Many studies of single genetic polymorphisms or of gene–gene interactions have been limited by sample size or by the lack of nutritional information. As clearly shown for MTHFR, the genetic risk may manifest itself more readily in individuals with suboptimal nutrient levels. The interaction between genetic and nongenetic factors is clearly an important area of investigation that requires even larger, well-characterized cohorts.

The cloning of genes is often followed by studies of regulatory regions and of interacting proteins, as well as by generation of mouse models with knockouts or of transgenic mice with high expression of their respective gene products. The investigation of folate and homocysteine metabolism is no exception. Mouse models with knockouts of genes for MTHFR (Chen et al., 2001), MTR (Swanson et al., 2001), folate receptors or binding proteins (Wlodarczyk et al., 2001; Tang and Finnell, 2003), reduced folate carrier (Zhao et al., 2001), and CBS are available (Watanabe et al., 1995) and should identify ancillary pathways or regulatory proteins that may impact the NTD risk. There are also many nutrients and metabolic intermediates directly or indirectly involved in folate-dependent pathways—vitamin B_{12}, riboflavin, methionine/SAM, thymidine, and choline/betaine. Studies of the genes involved in the transport, metabolism, or utilization of these compounds should provide an ever-expanding list of candidate risk factors.

REFERENCES

Afman LA, Lievers KJ, van der Put NM, Trijbels FJ, Blom HJ (2002). Single nucleotide polymorphisms in the transcobalamin gene: relationship with transcobalamin concentrations and risk for neural tube defects. Eur J Hum Genet 10:433–438.

Afman LA, Trijbels FJ, Blom HJ (2003). The H475Y polymorphism in the glutamate carboxypeptidase II gene increases plasma folate without affecting the risk for neural tube defects in humans. J Nutr 133:75–77.

Afman LA, van der Put NM, Thomas CM, Trijbels JM, Blom HJ (2001). Reduced vitamin B_{12} binding by transcobalamin II increases the risk of neural tube defects. Q J Med 94:159–166.

Akar N, Akar E, Deda G, Arsan S (2000). Spina bifida and common mutations at the homocysteine metabolism pathway. Clin Genet 57:230–231.

Bagley PJ, Selhub J (1998). A common mutation in the methylenetetrahydrofolate reductase gene is associated with an accumulation of formylated tetrahydrofolates in red blood cells. Proc Natl Acad Sci USA 95:13217–13220.

Barber R, Shalat S, Hendricks K, Joggerst B, Larsen R, Suarez L, Finnell R (2000). Investigation of folate pathway gene polymorphisms and the incidence of neural tube defects in a Texas Hispanic population. Mol Genet Metab 70:45–52.

Botto LD, Mastroiacovo P (1998). Exploring gene–gene interactions in the etiology of neural tube defects. Clin Genet 53:456–459.

Botto LD, Yang Q (2000). 5,10-Methylenetetrahydrofolate reductase gene variants and congenital anomalies: A HuGE review. Am J Epidemiol 9:862–877.

Brody LC, Baker PJ, Chines PS, Musick A, Molloy AM, Swanson DA, Kirke PN, et al (1999). Methionine synthase: high-resolution mapping of the human gene and evaluation as a candidate locus for neural tube defects. Mol Genet Metab 67:324–333.

Brody LC, Conley M, Cox C, Kirke PN, McKeever MP, Mills JL, Molloy AM, et al (2002). A polymorphism, *R653Q*, in the trifunctional enzyme methylenetetrahydrofolate dehydrogenase/methenyltetrahydrofolate cyclohydrolase/ formyltetrahydrofolate synthetase is a maternal genetic risk factor for neural tube defects: report of the Birth Defects Research Group. Am J Hum Genet 71:1207–1215.

Chen Z, Karaplis AC, Ackerman SL, Pogribny IP, Melnyk S, Lussier-Cacan S, Pai A, John S, et al (2001). Mice deficient in methylenetetrahydrofolate reductase exhibit hyperhomocysteinemia and decreased methylation capacity, with neuropathology and aortic lipid deposition. Hum Mol Genet 10:433–443.

Christensen B, Arbour L, Tran P, Leclerc D, Sabbaghian N, Platt R, Gilfix BM, et al (1999). Genetic polymorphisms in methylenetetrahydrofolate reductase and methionine synthase, folate levels in red blood cells, and risk of neural tube defects. Am J Med Genet 84:151–157.

Clarke R, Collins R, Lewington S, Donald A, Alfthan G, Tuomilehto J, Arnesen E, et al, and the Homocysteine Studies Collaboration (2002). Homocysteine and risk of ischemic heart disease and stroke. A meta-analysis. JAMA 288:2015–2023.

Czeizel AE, Dudas I (1992). Prevention of the first occurrence of neural-tube defects by periconceptional vitamin supplementation. N Engl J Med 327:1832–1835.

Daubner SC, Matthews RG (1982). Purification and properties of methylenetetrahydrofolate reductase from pig liver. J Biol Chem 257:140–145.

Doolin M-T, Barbaux S, McDonnell M, Hoess K, Whitehead AS, Mitchell LE (2002). Maternal genetic effects, exerted by genes involved in homocysteine remethylation, influence the risk of spina bifida. Am J Hum Genet 71:1222–1226.

Finkelstein JD (2001). Regulation of homocysteine metabolism. In Carmel R, Jacobsen DW (eds): *Homocysteine in Health and Disease.* Cambridge: Cambridge University Press, pp. 92–99.

Friso S, Choi SW, Girelli D, Mason JB, Dolnikowski GG, Bagley PJ, Olivieri O, et al (2002). A common mutation in the 5,10-methylenetetrahydrofolate reductase gene affects genomic DNA methylation through an interaction with folate status. Proc Natl Acad Sci USA 99:5605–5611.

Frosst P, Blom HJ, Milos R, Goyette P, Sheppard CA, Matthews RG, Boers GJH, et al (1995). A candidate genetic risk factor for vascular disease: a common mutation in methylenetetrahydrofolate reductase. Nat Genet 10:111–113.

Gaull GE, Von Berg W, Raiha NC, Sturman JA (1973). Development of methyltransferase activities of human fetal tissues. Pediatr Res 7:527–533.

Goyette P, Sumner JS, Milos R, Duncan AMV, Rosenblatt DS, Matthews RG, Rozen R (1994). Human methylenetetrahydrofolate reductase: isolation of cDNA, mapping and mutation identification. Nat Genet 7:195–200.

Graham IM, Daly LE, Refsum HM, Robinson K, Brattstrom LE, Ueland PM, Palma-Reis RJ, et al, and the European Concerted Action Project (1997). Plasma homocysteine as a risk factor for vascular disease. JAMA 277:1775–1781.

Guéant-Rodriguez RM, Rendeli C, Namour B, Venuti L, Romano A, Anello G, Bosco P, et al (2003). Transcobalamin and methionine synthase reductase mutated polymorphisms aggravate the risk of neural tube defects in humans. Neurosci Lett 334:189–192.

Guenther BG, Sheppard CA, Tran P, Rozen R, Matthews RG, Ludwig ML (1999). The structure and properties of methylenetetrahydrofolate reductase from *Escherichia coli:* a model for the role of folate in ameliorating hyperhomocysteinemia in humans. Nat Struct Biol 6:359–365.

Hansen DK, Barbee SA, Grafton TF, Gu Y, Streck RD (2001). Antisense modulation of 5,10-methylenetetrahydrafolate reductase expression produces neural tube defects in mouse embryos. Reprod Toxicol 15:21–29.

Heil SG, van der Put NM, Trijbels FJ, Gabreels FJ, Blom HJ (1999). Molecular genetic analysis of human folate receptors in neural tube defects. Eur J Hum Genet 7:393–396.

Heil SG, van der Put NM, Waas ET, den Heijer M, Trijbels FJ, Blom HJ (2001). Is mutated serine hydroxymethyltransferase (SHMT) involved in the etiology of neural tube defects? Mol Genet Metab 73:164–172.

Jacques PF, Bostom AG, Williams RR, Ellison RC, Eckfeldt JH, Rosenberg IH, Selhub J, et al (1996). Relation between folate status, a common mutation in methylenetetrahydrofolate reductase, and plasma homocysteine concentrations. Circulation 93:7–9.

Johanning GL, Tamura T, Johnston KE, Wenstrom KD (2000). Comorbidity of 5,10-methylenetetrahydrofolate reductase and methionine synthase gene polymorphisms and risk for neural tube defects. J Med Genet 37:949–951.

Kang S-S, Wong PWK, Zhou J, Sora J, Lessick M, Ruggie N, Grcevich G (1988). Thermolabile methylenetetrahydrofolate reductase in patients with coronary artery disease. Metabolism 37:611–613.

Kirke PN, Molloy AM, Daly LE, Burke H, Weir DG, Scott JM (1993). Maternal plasma folate and vitamin B_{12} are independent risk factors for neural tube defects. Q J Med 86:703–708.

Leclerc D, Campeau E, Goyette P, Adjalla CE, Christensen B, Ross M, Eydoux P, et al (1996). Human methionine synthase:cDNA cloning, chromosomal localization, and identification of mutations in patients of the *cblG* complementation group of folate/cobalamin disorders. Hum Mol Genet 5:1867–1874.

Leclerc D, Sibani S, Rozen R (2004). Molecular biology of methylenetetrahydrofolate reductase (MTHFR) and overview of mutations/polymorphisms. In Ueland PM, Rozen R (eds): *MTHFR Polymorphisms and Disease.* Georgetown, TX: Landes Bioscience Press. pp. 1–20.

Leclerc D, Wilson A, Dumas R, Gafuik C, Song D, Watkins D, Heng HHQ, et al (1998). Cloning and mapping of a cDNA for methionine synthase reductase, a flavoprotein defective in patients with homocystinuria. Proc Natl Acad Sci USA 95:3059–3064.

Linder CC, Davisson MT (1994). Mouse models for studying neural tube defects. Bar Harbor, ME: Neurology News, The Jackson Laboratory.

Malinow MR, Nieto FJ, Kruger WD, Duell PB, Hess DL, Gluckman RA, Block PC, et al (1997). The effects of folic acid supplementation on plasma total homocysteine are modulated by multivitamin use and methylenetetrahydrofolate reductase genotypes. Arterioscler Thromb Vasc Biol 17:1157–1162.

McCully KS (1969). Vascular pathology of homocysteinemia: implications for the pathogenesis of arteriosclerosis. Am J Pathol 56:111–128.

McNulty H, Dowey LC, Scott JM, Molloy AM, McAnena LB, Hughes JP, Ward M, et al (2003). Riboflavin supplementation lowers plasma homocysteine in individuals homozygous for the MTHFR *C677T* polymorphism. J Inherit Metab Dis 26(Suppl 1):12.

Meleady R, Ueland PM, Blom H, Whitehead AS, Refsum H, Daly LE, Vollset SE et al, and the EC Concerted Action Project. (2003). Thermolabile methylenetetrahydrofolate reductase, homocysteine, and cardiovascular disease risk: the European Concerted Action Project. Am J Clin Nutr 77:63–70.

Mills JL, McPartlin JM, Kirke PN, Lee YJ, Conley MR, Weir DG, Scott JH (1995). Homocysteine metabolism in pregnancies complicated by neural-tube defects. Lancet 345:149–151.

Molloy AM, Daly S, Mills JL, Kirke PN, Whitehead AS, Ramsbottom D, Conley MR, et al (1997). Thermolabile variant of 5,10-methylenetetrahydrofolate reductase associated with low red-cell folates: implications for folate intake recommendations. Lancet 349:1591–1593.

Morin I, Devlin AM, Leclerc D, Sabbaghian N, Halsted CH, Finnell R, Rozen R (2003a). Evaluation of genetic variants in the reduced folate carrier and in glutamate carboxypeptidase II for spina bifida risk. Mol Genet Metab 79:197–200.

Morin I, Platt R, Weisberg I, Sabbaghian N, Wu Q, Garrow TA, Rozen R (2003b). A common variant in betaine-homocysteine methyltransferase (BHMT) and risk for spina bifida. Am J Med Genet 119A:172–176.

Morrison K, Papapetrou C, Hol FA, Mariman ECM, Lynch SA, Burn J, Edwards YH (1998). Susceptibility to spina bifida; an association study of five candidate genes. Ann Hum Genet 62:379–396.

MRC Vitamin Study Research Group (1991). Prevention of neural-tube defects: results of the Medical Research Council vitamin study. Lancet 338:131–137.

Mudd SH, Levy HL, Kraus JP (2001). Disorders of transsulfuration. In Scriver CR, Beaudet AL, Sly WS, Valle D (eds): *The Metabolic and Molecular Bases of Inherited Disease,* 8th ed. New York: McGraw-Hill, pp. 2007–2056.

Mutchinick OM, Lopêz MA, Luna L, Waxman J, Babinsky VE, and the RYVEMCE Collaborative Group (1999). High prevalence of the thermolabile methylenetetrahydrofolate reductase variant in Mexico: a country with a very high prevalence of neural tube defects. Mol Genet Metab 68:461–467.

O'Leary VB, Mills JL, Kirke PN, Parle-McDermott A, Swanson DA, Weiler A, Pangilinan F, et al (2003). Analysis of the human folate receptor beta gene for an association with neural tube defects. Mol Genet Metab 79:129–133.

Olteanu H, Munson T, Banerjee R (2002). Differences in the efficiency of reductive activation of methionine synthase and exogenous electron acceptors between the common polymorphic variants of human methionine synthase reductase. Biochemistry 41:13378–13385.

Park EI, Renduchintala MS, Garrow TA (1997). Diet-induced changes in hepatic betaine-homocysteine methyltransferase activity are mediated by changes in the steady-state level of its mRNA. J Nutr Biochem 8:541–545.

Ramsbottom D, Scott JM, Molloy A, Weir DG, Kirke PN, Mills JL, Gallagher PM, et al (1997). Are common mutations of cystathionine β-synthase involved in the aetiology of neural tube defects? Clin Genet 51:39–42.

Richter B, Stegmann K, Roper B, Boddeker I, Ngo ET, Koch MC (2001). Interaction of folate and homocysteine pathway genotypes evaluated in susceptibility to neural tube defects (NTD) in a German population. J Hum Genet 46:105–109.

Robien K, Ulrich CM (2003). 5,10-Methylenetetrahydrofolate reductase polymorphisms and leukemia risk: a HuGE minireview. Am J Epidemiol 157:571–582.

Romano M, Marcucci R, Buratti E, Ayala YM, Sebastio G, Baralle FE (2002). Regulation of the 3′ splice site selection in the 844ins68 polymorphism of the cystathionine β-synthase gene. J Biol Chem 277:43821–43829.

Rosenblatt DS, Fenton W (2001). Inherited disorders of folate and cobalamin transport and metabolism. In Scriver CR, Beaudet AL, Sly WS, Valle D (eds): *The Metabolic and Molecular Bases of Inherited Disease,* 8th ed. New York: McGraw-Hill, pp. 3897–3933.

Rosenquist TH, Ratashak SA, Selhub J (1996). Homocysteine induces congenital defects of the heart and neural tube: effect of folic acid. Proc Natl Acad Sci USA 93:15227–15232.

Rozen R (2002). MTHFR: a link between folate and riboflavin? Am J Clin Nutr 76:301–302.

Schwahn BC, Chen Z, Laryea MD, Wendel U, Lussier-Cacan S, Genest J Jr, Mar M-H, et al (2003). Homocysteine–betaine interactions in a murine model of 5,10-methylenetetrahydrofolate reductase deficiency. FASEB J Express 17:512–514.

Shaw GM, Lammer EJ, Zhu H, Baker MW, Neri E, Finnell RH (2002). Maternal periconceptional vitamin use, genetic variation of infant reduced folate carrier (A80G), and risk of spina bifida. Am J Med Genet 108:1–6.

Speer MC, Nye J, McLone D, Worley G, Melvin EC, Viles KD, Franklin A, et al, and the NTD Collaborative Group. (1999). Possible interaction of genotypes at cystathionine β-synthase and methylenetetrahydrofolate reductase (MTHFR) in neural tube defects. Clin Genet 56:142–144.

Steegers-Theunissen RPM, Boers GHJ, Trijbels FJM, Finkelstein JD, Blom HJ, Thomas CMG, Borm GF, et al (1994). Maternal hyperhomocysteinemia: a risk factor for neural-tube defects? Metabolism 43:1475–1480.

Swanson DA, Liu ML, Baker PJ, Garrett L, Stitzel M, Wu J, Harris M, et al (2001). Targeted disruption of the methionine synthase gene in mice. Mol Cell Biol 21:1058–1065.

Tang LS, Finnell RH (2003). Neural and orofacial defects in Folbp1 knockout mice. Birth Defects Res Part A Clin Mol Teratol 67:209–218.

Trembath D, Sherbondy AL, Vandyke DC, Shaw GM, Todoroff K, Lammer EJ, Finnell RH, et al (1999). Analysis of select folate pathway genes, *PAX3* and human *T* in a Midwestern neural tube defect population. Teratology 59:331–341.

Tsai MY, Bignell M, Schwichtenberg K, Hanson NQ (1996). High prevalence of a mutation in the cystathionine beta-synthase gene. Am J Hum Genet 59:1262–1267.

van der Put NMJ, Eskes TKAB, Blom HJ (1997a). Is the common 677C → T mutation in the methylenetetrahydrofolate reductase gene a risk factor for neural tube defects? A meta-analysis. Q J Med 90:111–115.

van der Put NMJ, Gabreels F, Stevens EMB, Smeitink JAM, Trijbels FJM, Eskes TKAB, van den Heuvel LP, et al (1998). A second common mutation in the methylenetetrahydrofolate reductase gene: an additional risk factor for neural-tube defects? Am J Hum Genet 62:1044–1051.

van der Put NMJ, Steegers-Theunissen RPM, Frosst P, Trijbels FJM, Eskes TKAB, van den Heuvel LP, Mariman ECM, et al (1995). Mutated methylenetetrahydrofolate reductase as a risk factor for spina bifida. Lancet 346:1070–1071.

van der Put NMJ, van der Molen EF, Kluijtmans LAJ, Heil SG, Trijbels JMF, Eskes TKAB, van Oppenraaij-Emmerzaal D, et al (1997b). Sequence analysis of the coding region of human methionine synthase: relevance to hyperhomocysteinaemia in neural-tube defects and vascular disease. Q J Med 90:511–517.

Vieira AR, Trembath D, Vandyke DC, Murray JC, Marker S, Lerner G, Bonner E, et al (2002). Studies with His475Tyr glutamate carboxipeptidase II polymorphism and neural tube defects. Am J Med Genet 111:218–219.

Watanabe M, Osada J, Aratani Y, Kluckman K, Reddick R, Malinow M, Maeda N (1995). Mice deficient in cystathionine beta-synthase: animal models for mild and severe homocyst(e)inemia. Proc Natl Acad Sci USA 92:1585–1589.

Weisberg IS, Jacques PF, Selhub J, Bostom AG, Chen Z, Ellison RC, Eckfeldt JH, et al (2001). The 1298A → C polymorphism in methylenetetrahydrofolate reductase (MTHFR): in vitro expression and association with homocysteine. Atherosclerosis 56:409–415.

Weisberg I, Tran P, Christensen B, Sibani S, Rozen R (1998). A second genetic polymorphism in methylenetetrahydofolate reductase (MTHFR) associated with decreased enzyme activity. Mol Genet Metab 64:169–172.

Welch GN, Loscalzo J (1998). Homocysteine and atherothrombosis. N Engl J Med 338:1042–1050.

Werstuck GH, Lentz SR, Dayal S, Hossain GS, Sood SK, Shi YY, Zhou J, et al (2001). Homocysteine-induced endoplasmic reticulum stress causes dysregulation of the cholesterol and triglyceride biosynthetic pathways. J Clin Invest 107:1263–1273.

Wilson A, Platt R, Wu Q, Leclerc D, Christensen B, Yang H, Gravel R, et al (1999). A common variant in methionine synthase reductase combined with low cobalamin (vitamin B_{12}) increases risk for spina bifida. Mol Genet Metab 67:317–323.

Wlodarczyk B, Spiegelstein O, Gelineau-van Waes J, Vorce RL, Lu X, Le CX, Finnell RH (2001). Arsenic-induced congenital malformations in genetically susceptible folate binding protein-2 knockout mice. Toxicol Appl Pharmacol 177:238–246.

Yamada K, Chen Z, Rozen R, Matthews R (2001). Effects of common polymorphisms on the properties of recombinant human methylenetetrahydrofolate reductase. Proc Natl Acad Sci USA 98:14853–14858.

Zhao R, Russell RG, Wang Y, Liu L, Gao F, Kneitz B, Edelmann W, et al (2001). Rescue of embryonic lethality in reduced folate carrier–deficient mice by maternal folic acid supplementation reveals early neonatal failure of hematopoietic organs. J Biol Chem 276:10224–10228.

Zhu H, Wicker NJ, Shaw GM, Lammer EJ, Hendricks K, Suarez L, Canfield M, et al (2003). Homocysteine remethylation enzyme polymorphisms and increased risks for neural tube defects. Mol Genet Metab 78:216–221.

16

Genetics of Syndromic Neural Tube Defects

SONJA A. RASMUSSEN
JAIME L. FRÍAS

The etiology of neural tube defects (NTDs) is known to be heterogeneous (Holmes et al., 1976; Khoury et al., 1982a, 1982b; Martin et al., 1983). In the majority of infants with NTDs, a multifactorial mode of determination (a combination of multiple genetic and environmental factors) is believed to be involved. The NTDs in these infants are isolated, meaning that no other major unrelated malformations or conditions of known etiology, such as single-gene disorders or chromosome abnormalities, are present (Rasmussen et al., 2003a). In these isolated cases, empiric figures (detailed in Chapter 28) are used to counsel families regarding their risk for recurrence because of the current lack of understanding of the genetic and environmental factors involved. However, for a significant proportion of infants with NTDs, empiric recurrence risks are not applicable. It is essential that health-care providers of patients with NTDs and their families recognize situations in which the use of empiric recurrence risk figures are inappropriate and other, more specific recurrence risk information should be provided.

The NTDs for which empiric recurrence risk figures are not applicable fall into two categories: those with unrecognized patterns of multiple birth defects and those with specific syndromes. Infants in whom both an NTD and another unrelated major defect are present (in the absence of a syndrome of known etiology) are classified as having *multiple birth defects* (Khoury et al., 1982b; Rasmussen et al., 2003a). For example, a child with an NTD and a congenital heart defect, but without a chromosome abnormality or a single-gene condition, has multiple birth defects. Infants with NTDs and additional unrelated birth defects have been shown to be epidemiologically, and presumably etiologically, different from those who have isolated NTDs. In one study, infants with isolated NTDs had the well-known epidemiologic characteristics of NTDs (e.g., predominance of females and whites and decreasing rates over time), while those with other associated major defects were epidemiologically different (Khoury et al., 1982b). In addition, siblings of infants with multiple birth defects were shown to have a lower precurrence rate (the rate of defects among siblings born before the proband with an NTD) than those with isolated birth defects, both for NTDs (0.0% vs. 2.0%) and for any major birth defect (2.9% vs. 20.0%) (Khoury et al., 1982a). A study in Utah showed similar findings (Martin et al., 1983). Although the numbers in that study were small, the recurrence risk for infants with isolated NTDs was 3.2%, while the recurrence risk in families with other major malformations in addition to NTDs was 0%. Thus, it appears that the risk to siblings of infants with NTDs associated with additional unrelated major defects is lower than the empiric recurrence risk figures typically cited for isolated NTDs.

Empiric recurrence risk figures are also not applicable for infants with syndromes. In this chapter, we use the term *syndrome* to refer to a recognizable pattern of multiple malformations that is known or presumed to have a specific cause, such as a single-gene condition, chromosome abnormality, or teratogenic exposure. Identification of infants with syndromes is important because information provided to the family may vary significantly based on the diagnosis of a syndrome. Recurrence risks associated with syndromes can vary from no increased risk to as high as 50% and are often significantly different from the 3% recurrence risk figure provided to families with a child with an isolated NTD. In addition, options for dealing with the increased recurrence risk may be available; for example, in the case of an autosomal recessive condition in which the gene has been identified and diagnostic testing is available, preimplantation genetic diagnosis (Harper and Bui, 2002) would be available to the family, an option not available to families with a child with an isolated NTD. Prognostic information may also be very different for an infant with a syndrome compared to an infant with an isolated NTD. Finally, better understanding of syndromes associated with NTDs may provide insight into the causation of isolated NTDs.

CONTRIBUTION OF MULTIPLE BIRTH DEFECTS AND SYNDROMES TO NEURAL TUBE DEFECTS

The proportion of infants with NTDs classified as isolated, multiple birth defects, and syndromes varies widely among different studies, depending on the study methodology and the type of NTD studied (Roberts and Powell, 1975; David and Nixon, 1976; Holmes et al., 1976; David et al., 1983; Martin et al., 1983; Khoury et al., 1982b; Baird and Sadovnick, 1984; Hunter, 1984; Sadovnick and Baird, 1985; Martínez-Frías et al., 1990; Simpson et al., 1991). Some factors that can affect these proportions include case ascertainment methods (e.g., ascertainment through hospital discharge diagnoses versus active review of hospital or autopsy records); whether spontaneous abortions and stillborns are included in the study; the frequency with which autopsies are performed on infants who die; and the frequency of the use of laboratory tests, such as cytogenetic analyses. A study by Källén and coworkers (1998) may illustrate the difference in classification of infants as having isolated NTDs, multiple birth defects, or syndromes based on study methodology. Using encephalocele as an example, 77% of infants ascertained from a registry in France were classified as having an isolated NTD, 18% as having multiple birth defects, and 5% as having syndromic NTDs (chromosomal, single-gene, or teratogenic syndromes). In contrast, 44% of infants with encephaloceles ascertained by the California Birth Defects Monitoring Program were classified as isolated, 43% as having multiple birth defects, and 13% as having syndromic NTDs. At least part of the difference seen between these populations may be related to the frequency of prenatal diagnosis followed by pregnancy termination (Källén et al., 1998) and whether information on pregnancy terminations was included in the surveillance system (other possible reasons include differences in population ethnicity). Information on pregnancy terminations was included in the French registry but not in the California program. Based on several studies, the proportion of all NTDs that are isolated ranges from 79% to 94% (Holmes et al., 1976; Khoury et al., 1982b; Martin et al., 1983; Hunter, 1984; Simpson et al., 1991). Conversely, those classified as syndromic NTDs constitute a small proportion of cases (0.4%–5.6%) (Holmes et al., 1976; Khoury et al., 1982b; Martin et al., 1983). However, it is likely that these studies underestimate the true proportion of infants with syndromes, because cytogenetic analyses and genetic evaluations were not routinely performed.

The classification of infants with NTDs as isolated, multiple, or syndromic also varies by type of NTD. Several studies have suggested that the proportion of infants classified as having isolated defects is highest for anencephaly and spina bifida and lower for encephalocele. In a study by Khoury and colleagues (1982b), 82.1% of cases of nonsyndromic anencephaly and 79.0% of cases of spina bifida were isolated compared to 71.9% of cases of encephalocele. In another study, the proportion of cases of anencephaly and spina bifida classified as having isolated NTDs was similar (83.3% and 82.3%, respectively) compared to 46.2% of cases of encephalocele (Hunter, 1984). In a study of nonsyndromic NTDs (Hall et al., 1988), 85.3% of infants with anencephaly, 89.9% with spina bifida, and 70% with encephalocele were classified as isolated. Among liveborn infants with NTDs from birth defects surveillance systems in California and Illinois, 90.6% of cases of anencephaly and 85.5% of cases of spina bifida were classified as isolated compared to 77.1% with encephalocele (Simpson et al., 1991). Among infants with NTDs but without a chromosome abnormality, 86% of those with anencephaly, 65% with encephalocele, 77% with upper spina bifida, and 86% with lower spina bifida had isolated NTDs (Källén et al., 1994). In another study (Martínez-Frías et al., 1990), an isolated NTD was found in 94.3% of infants with anencephaly and 82.5% of infants with spina bifida, in contrast to 66.1% of those with encephalocele. Neural tube defects other than anencephaly, spina bifida, and encephalocele have not been as well studied, although one study on iniencephaly showed that a large proportion of infants (84%) had other malformations outside the nervous system (David and Nixon, 1976). In one study of craniorachischisis (Hall et al., 1988), 38% of infants were classified as having an isolated NTD, whereas all three cases were classified as isolated in another study (Simpson et al., 1991). The study of these less frequent types of NTDs is hampered by small numbers.

The proportion of infants with each type of NTD classified as syndromic also varies by study. In one study, none of the infants with anencephaly were recognized as having a syndrome compared to 4.3% of those with spina bifida (most had chromosome abnormalities) and 21% of infants with encephalocele (the majority of these had single-gene conditions) (Martínez-Frías et al., 1990). Using data from the California Birth Defects Monitoring Program, 1.6% of infants with anencephaly were classified as having a syndrome (single-gene, teratogenic, or chromosomal) compared to 4.9% of those with spina bifida and 13.2% of those with encephalocele (Källén et al., 1998).

It is important that fetuses or infants with syndromic NTDs be appropriately identified to allow families to receive accurate genetic counseling for future pregnancies. Clinical information about syndromes that are associated with NTDs is summarized in Chapter 7. We focus here on the genetics of syndromes associated with NTDs and have divided the chapter into two parts, focusing on chromosome abnormalities and single-gene conditions.

CHROMOSOME ABNORMALITIES

The contribution of chromosome abnormalities to the etiology of NTDs has not been well documented. In a study of 106 infants with NTDs (Holmes et al., 1976), only 1 infant (or less than 1%) had a chromosome abnormality; however, karyotyping was performed in only 17 infants. In another study using data from three different birth defects surveillance systems, the proportion of cases with chromosome abnormalities varied from 0.9% (France) to 1.2% (Sweden) to 2.9% (California) (Källén et al., 1998). These percentages also varied by the type of NTD. Using data from the California Birth Defects Monitoring Program, 1.4% of infants with anencephaly, 3.3% with spina bifida, and 5.4% with encephalocele had chromosome abnormalities (Källén et al., 1998). However, not all infants were karyotyped in these studies, probably resulting in an underestimation of the contribution of chromosome abnormalities to NTDs.

Some studies using prenatally diagnosed cases and with increased use of chromosome analyses have shown a much higher occurrence of chromosome abnormalities. In a study of prenatally diagnosed meningomyelocele (Babcook et al., 1995), 17% of fetuses in whom karyotyping was performed had chromosome abnormalities. In a study by Hume et al. (1996), 10 of 145 cases (7%) with prenatally diagnosed NTDs had a chromosome abnormality. In another study of prenatally diagnosed NTDs (Kennedy et al., 1998), 13 of 200 fetuses who were karyotyped successfully (6.5%) had a chromosome abnormality. The contribution of chromosome abnormalities differed by the type of NTD: 2.3% of cases of anencephaly had a chromosome abnormality compared to 7.1% of cases of encephalocele and 10.2% of cases of meningomyelocele. Although fetuses whose ultrasound examinations showed additional findings were more likely to have a chromosome abnormality, absence of additional abnormalities on ultrasound was not predictive of a fetus with a normal karyotype (2.4% of fetuses with isolated NTDs had chromosome abnormalities) (Kennedy et al., 1998). Several factors contribute to the higher rate of chromosome abnormalities among prenatally diagnosed cases, including the following: (*1*) the proportion of cases with cytogenetic analysis is higher than in other studies; (*2*) some fetuses diagnosed prenatally, especially those with more severe defects such as chromosome abnormalities, would be lost prior to delivery and thus would not be included in studies of liveborn infants; and (*3*) those diagnosed prenatally might be more likely than liveborn infants to have additional malformations that led to prenatal ultrasonographic diagnosis, and cases with additional malformations are more likely to have chromosome abnormalities. In addition, these studies were not population-based; instead, they were based on the results of studies performed by specific clinics or hospitals. The high rate of chromosome abnormalities found in some studies has led authors to recommend cytogenetic analysis when an NTD is detected prenatally (Babcook et al., 1995; Kennedy et al., 1998).

Neural tube defects have been associated with a wide variety of chromosome abnormalities. In a study of prenatally diagnosed meningomyelocele, abnormalities identified included trisomy 18, trisomy 13, triploidy, and an unbalanced translocation (Babcook et al., 1995). In a study of prenatally diagnosed NTDs (Kennedy et al., 1998), several different types of chromosome abnormalities were identified, including trisomy 18, trisomy 9, triploidy, Turner syndrome, and inherited and sporadic chromosome rearrangements. In a study by Källén and colleagues (1998), among a total of 73 liveborn and stillborn infants with NTDs and chromosome abnormalities, the most frequently observed abnormality was trisomy 18 (in 31), followed by trisomy 13 (in 14). Other frequently observed abnormalities were deletions (in seven infants), unbalanced translocations (in five infants), and triploidy and Down syndrome (each seen in four infants). A detailed list of chromosome abnormalities associated with NTDs is beyond the scope of this chapter; however, for anencephaly and spina bifida, associated chromosome abnormalities have been summarized in a recent paper (Melvin et al., 2000). Because chromosome abnormalities have previously led to the identification of genes involved in isolated birth defects (Belloni et al., 1996), it has been proposed that these loci be examined for genes possibly involved in the etiology of NTDs.

A significant proportion of cases with trisomy 13, trisomy 18, and triploidy have NTDs; in one study of midtrimester fetuses, 8% with trisomy 13, 24% with trisomy 18, and 23% with triploidy had NTDs. Based on that and other studies, when an NTD was present, it was most frequently sacral or lumbosacral spina bifida (Seller, 1995).

Neural tube defects have also been reported in association with deletion of chromosome 22q11. Three unrelated children with NTDs were found to have 22q11 deletion, two with velocardiofacial syndrome and one with DiGeorge syndrome (Nickel et al., 1994). Subsequently, 295 patients with NTDs were identified by chart review (Nickel and Magenis, 1996). Twenty-two patients with at least one clinical trait of 22q11 deletion (congenital heart defect, minor facial anomalies, thymic hypoplasia, cleft lip and/or palate, or hypocalcemia) or a positive family history of an NTD, congenital heart defect, or cleft lip and/or palate were identified. Of these 22, 16 were tested (including the initial 3 patients discussed previously). Other than the three cases previously identified, no additional cases with 22q11 deletion and NTDs were found, suggesting that 22q11 deletion infrequently contributes to the causation of spina bifida. Two infants with 22q11 deletion described by Botto and colleagues (2003) also had meningomyelocele; both infants also had heart defects. The family originally described by Kousseff and having the syndrome subsequently called *Kousseff syndrome* (MIM 245210), characterized by meningomyelocele and conotruncal heart defects, has recently been shown to have a 22q11 deletion by fluorescence in situ hybridization (FISH) analysis (Forrester et al., 2002). A fetus with lumbosacral spina bifida and myeloschisis was found to have a de novo X/22q translocation (Fryns et al., 1996). The 22q11 region was shown to be intact by FISH, and the breakpoint in chromosome 22 was located just distal to 22q11, leading Fryns and colleagues to suggest that a gene in the region distal to the 22q11 region might be important in the development of the neural tube (Fryns et al., 1996). Based on these studies, it has been proposed that patients with NTDs associated with other anomalies, such as conotruncal heart defects (Forrester et al., 2002), or a family history of findings consistent with 22q11 deletion be evaluated for 22q deletions (Nickel and Magenis, 1996). The contribution of 22q11 deletion to the etiology of isolated NTDs has not been studied. Of note, a 22q11 deletion will not be detected with routine chromosome analysis; instead, FISH testing for 22q deletion must be specifically requested.

Identification of a chromosome abnormality in a fetus or infant with an NTD significantly alters the information provided to parents. The information on outcome also differs, depending on whether a chromosome abnormality is identified. For example, an infant with an isolated sacral NTD has an excellent prognosis, but the prognosis is drastically changed if the infant has trisomy 18, a condition associated with a high degree of mortality (Rasmussen et al., 2003b). Similarly, the recurrence risk information provided will vary, sometimes dramatically, when the diagnosis of a chromosome abnormality is made (Gardner and Sutherland, 1996) compared to the use of empiric recurrence risk figures. For example, the recurrence risk for trisomy 18 or trisomy 13 is about 1% (Stene et al., 1984), less than the empiric risk figures typically cited for NTDs. In contrast, the recurrence risk of 22q11 deletion can be 50% if one of the parents also has the deletion.

SINGLE-GENE CONDITIONS

Single-gene conditions associated with NTDs are inherited in an autosomal recessive, autosomal dominant, X-linked recessive, and X-linked dominant manner. Brief clinical and molecular genetic data on disorders associated with NTDs in which autosomal dominant, autosomal recessive, or X-linked inheritance is documented are contained in Tables 16.1, 16.2, and 16.3. In addition, mitochondrial mutations have been associated with NTDs in two patients (Nye et al., 2000; Barisic et al., 2002). Recognition of these conditions is important because of the significant change in prognostic and genetic counseling information provided to the family when such a diagnosis is made. In some cases, a causative gene has been identified for these conditions. Because better understanding of these genes and how they function can provide insight into the genes that might be involved in isolated NTDs, we will describe the genes and their functions, when known, for single-gene disorders frequently associated with NTDs.

Autosomal Recessive Conditions

Several autosomal recessive conditions have been identified that are associated with NTDs (Table 16.1). Because the recurrence risk for families with a child with one of these conditions is 25%, clinicians need to be aware of them so that they can be recognized and families counseled appropriately.

The most common single-gene cause of NTDs is Meckel syndrome, an autosomal recessive condition characterized by occipital encephalocele, polycystic kidneys, and polydactyly. Meckel syndrome is known to be genetically heterogeneous (Paavola et al., 1997; Roume et al., 1997), with linkage to three distinct chromosome locations in different families: chromosomes 17q21–24 (Paavola et al., 1995), 11q13 (Roume et al., 1998), and 8q24 (Morgan et al., 2002). Specific genes associated with Meckel syndrome have not yet been identified.

In some autosomal recessive conditions, the responsible gene has been identified. One of the genes for Knobloch syndrome, characterized by early onset of high myopia, vitrioretinal degeneration, retinal detachment, and encephalocele or meningocele, has been identified as the *COL18A1* gene (Sertie et al., 2000). *COL18A1* maps to 21q22.3 and codes for type XVIII collagen. These results suggest that type XVIII collagen plays a role in embryonic cell proliferation or migration, either as a primary or a secondary effect (Sertie et al., 2000). However, because some patients examined have not had mutations in the *COL18A1* gene and linkage to this locus has been excluded in at least one family (Suzuki et al., 2002; Menzel et al., 2004), Knobloch syndrome is believed to be genetically heterogeneous.

TABLE 16.1. *Autosomal Recessive Conditions Associated with Neural Tube Defects*

Condition (MIM No.*)	Type of Neural Tube Defect	Other Clinical Features	Chromosome Location	Gene (If Known)	Reference
Acrocallosal syndrome (MIM 200990)	Anencephaly	Macrocephaly, absent corpus callosum, hypertelorism, postaxial polydactyly, duplicated hallux, mental retardation			Kedar et al. (1996)
Acromelic frontonasal dysostosis (MIM 603671)	Encephalocele/meningocele	Frontonasal dysplasia, preaxial polydactyly of the feet, postaxial polydactyly, agenesis of the corpus callosum, Dandy-Walker malformation, epibulbar dermoid			Slaney et al. (1999)
Arima syndrome (MIM # not available)	Occipital cephalocele	Cerebellar vermis hypoplasia, cystic dysplastic kidney, retinopathy, Dandy-Walker malformation, liver fibrosis			Satran et al. (1999)
Cerebellar vermis hypo/aplasia, oligophrenia, congenital ataxia, ocular coloboma, and hepatic fibrosis (COACH syndrome) (MIM 216360)	Occipital cephalocele	Cerebellar vermis hypoplasia, congenital ataxia, coloboma, hepatic fibrosis, nephronophthisis			Satran et al. (1999)
Craniotelencephalic dysplasia (MIM 218670)	Encephalocele	Craniosynostosis, frontal bone protrusion, lissencephaly			Hughes et al. (1983)
DK-phocomelia (von Voss-Cherstvoy syndrome) (MIM 223340)	Variable—occipital encephalocele, meningocele, iniencephaly, meningoencephalocele	Phocomelia, thrombocytopenia, urogenital abnormalities	mosaic del 13q12 in one case		Lubinsky et al. (1994)
Dyssegmental dysplasia (Rolland-Desbuquois syndrome) (MIM 224400)	Encephalocele	Neonatal chondrodystrophy, abnormally segmented vertebrae, micromelia, cleft palate, hydrocephalus, hypertrichosis			Cohen and Lemire (1982), Aleck et al. (1987)
Dyssegmental dysplasia (Silverman-Hanmaker type) (MIM 224410)	Encephalocele	Lethal short-limb dwarfism, abnormal vertebral segmentation (anisospondyly), narrow chest, cleft palate	1p36.1	*HSPG2*	Cohen and Lemire (1982), Aleck et al. (1987)
Fraser cryptophthalmos syndrome (MIM 219000)	Meningomyelocele, encephalocele	Cryptophthalmos, cutaneous syndactyly, renal agenesis, genital anomalies	4q21	*FRAS1*	Slavotinek and Tifft (2002), McGregor et al. (2003)
Frontofacionasal dysplasia (MIM 229400)	Encephalocele	Brachycephaly, blepharophimosis, cleft lip, midfacial hypoplasia			Gollop et al. (1984)
Fryns anophthalmia syndrome (MIM 600776)	Open sacral neural tube defect, frontal encephalocele	Anophthalmia/microphthalmia, cleft lip/palate, uterus unicornis			Warburg et al. (1997)
Fukuyama congenital muscular dystrophy (MIM 253800)	Encephalocele	Congenital muscular dystrophy, mental retardation, optic atrophy, retinal detachment, cerebral and cerebellar micropolygyria, hydrocephalus, focal interhemispheric fusion	9q31	*FKTN* (mutations maintain residual fukutin activity)	Yoshioka and Kuroki (1994)

(*continued*)

TABLE 16.1. *Autosomal Recessive Conditions Associated with Neural Tube Defects (Continued)*

Condition (MIM No.*)	Type of Neural Tube Defect	Other Clinical Features	Chromosome Location	Gene (If Known)	Reference
Hydrolethalus (MIM 236680)	Anencephaly, encephalocele	Hydrocephaly, absent midline structures of brain, micrognathia, postaxial polydactyly (hands), preaxial polydactyly (feet), malformations of midline structures	11q23–q25		Aughton and Cassidy (1987), Visapaa et al. (1999)
Joubert syndrome (MIM 213300)	Cranial meningocele, occipital meningo-encephalocele	Agenesis of the cerebellar vermis, developmental delay, hypotonia, abnormal eye movements, ataxia, episodic apnea-hyperpnea	9q34.3		Maria et al. (1999)
Knobloch syndrome (MIM 267750)	Occipital encephalocele	Myopia, vitreoretinal degeneration, retinal detachment	21q22.3	*COL18A1*	Kliemann et al. (2003)
Meckel (Meckel-Gruber) syndrome (MKS1—MIM 249000; MKS2—MIM 603194; MKS3—MIM 607361)	Encephalocele	Encephalocele, polycystic kidneys, hepatic ductal dysplasia, postaxial polydactyly	MKS1 17q22–23, MKS2 11q13, MKS3 8q24		Paavola et al. (1997)
Mohr syndrome (MIM 252100)	Occipital meningocele	Preaxial polydactyly of feet, broad nasal tip, lingular tumors, conductive deafness, absence of skin			Reardon et al. (1989)
Neu-Laxova syndrome (MIM 256520)	Spina bifida, anencephaly	Severe intrauterine growth retardation, microcephaly, protruding eyes, abnormal skin, limb defects			Naveed et al. (1990), Rode et al. (2001)
PHAVER syndrome (MIM 261575)	Meningomyelocele	Pterygia, heart defects, segmentation defects of the spine, radio-ulnar synostosis, abnormal position of ears			Powell et al. (1993)
Roberts syndrome (MIM 268300)	Anterior encephalocele, meningocele	Phocomelia, hypertelorism, midface capillary hemangioma, cloudy corneas or cataracts, bilateral cleft lip and palate, premature centromere separation			Van Den Berg and Francke (1993)
Short rib-polydactyly syndrome (type II) (MIM 263520)	Anencephaly	Short limbs, narrow thorax, short ribs, polydactyly, cleft lip, perinatal lethality			Martínez-Frías et al. (1993)
VACTERL with hydrocephalus (MIM 276950)	Occipital encephalocele	Vertebral, anal, cardiac, renal, and limb abnormalities, tracheoesophageal fistula, aqueductal stenosis, dysplastic ears, an/microphthalmia			Corsello and Giuffre (1994)
Walker-Warburg syndrome (HARD+/–E syndrome) (MIM 236670)	Encephalocele	Hydrocephaly, agyria (lissencephaly), retinal dysplasia	9q34.1; 9q31	*POMT, FKTN* (mutations result in complete loss of fukutin activity)	Beltran-Valero de Bernabe et al. (2002, 2003)
XK aprosencephaly (MIM 207770)	Anencephaly	Holoprosencephaly, radial aplasia, oligodactyly			Townes et al. (1988)

*Refers to the number given to the condition in the Online Mendelian Inheritance in Man database (see Electronic Database Information).

TABLE 16.2. *Autosomal Dominant Conditions Associated with Neural Tube Defects*

Condition (MIM No.*)	Type of Neural Tube Defect	Other Clinical Features	Chromosome Location	Gene (If Known)	Reference
Apert syndrome (MIM 101200)	Encephalocele	Acrobrachycephaly, flat face, prognathism, syndactyly of the hands and feet, mental retardation	10q26	*FGFR2*	Cohen and Kreiborg (1994)
Boomerang dysplasia (MIM 112310)	Encephalocele/meningocele	Boomerang-shaped long bones, absent long bones, characteristic facial appearance, deficient spine ossification, large iliac wings, small iliac bodies			Odent et al. (1999)
Cerebrocostomandibular syndrome (MIM 117650)	Meningomyelocele	Posterior gap in ossification of ribs, severe micrognathia with Robin sequence			van den Ende et al. (1998)
Cerebro-oculonasal syndrome (MIM 605627)	Anterior encephalocele/meningocele	Macrocephaly, brachycephaly, anophthalmia, nasal midline groove, skin appendages, low-set and posteriorly rotated ears			Guion-Almeida et al. (2000)
Split-hand with obstructive uropathy, spina bifida, and diaphragmatic defects (MIM 183802)	Spina bifida occulta, spina bifida cystica	Obstructive uropathy, cutaneous syndactyly, split-hand/foot, diaphragmatic hernia			Czeizel and Losonci (1987)
Goldenhar (facio-auricular-vertebral) syndrome (MIM 164210)	Encephalocele/ meningocele	Asymmetric facial abnormalities, microtia, preauricular ear tags, macrostomia, epibulbar dermoid, vertebral anomalies, cardiac defects			Kelberman et al. (2001)
Osteosclerosis with abnormalities of the nervous system and meninges (MIM 130720)	Multiple meningoceles	Osteosclerosis, short stature, empty sella turcica, facial dysmorphism			Lehman et al. (1977)
Waardenburg syndrome type I (MIM 193500)	Meningomyelocele	White forelock, heterochromia irides, sensorineural deafness, dystopia canthorum, high nasal bridge	2q35	*PAX3*	Chatkupt and Johnson (1993)
Waardenburg syndrome type III (Klein-Waardenburg syndrome) (MIM 148820)	Meningomyelocele	Dystopia canthorum, white forelock, hearing loss, upper limb anomalies	2q35	*PAX3*	Nye et al. (1998)
Weissenbacher-Zweymuller syndrome (MIM 277610)	Meningocele, parieto-occipital encephalocele	Rhizomelia, dumbbell-shaped long bones, myopia, micrognathia, cleft palate, midface hypoplasia	6p21.3	*COL11A2*	Ramer et al. (1993)

*Refers to the number given to the condition in the Online Mendelian Inheritance in Man database (see Electronic Database Information).

TABLE 16.3. *X-linked Conditions Associated with Neural Tube Defects*

Condition (MIM No.*)	Type of Neural Tube Defect	Other Clinical Features	Chromosome Location	Gene (If Known)	Reference
Congenital hemidysplasia with ichthyosiform erythroderma and limb defects (CHILD syndrome) (MIM 308050)	Meningomyelocele	Unilateral ichthyosiform skin lesions, ipsilateral limb anomalies and abnormalities of the internal organs, punctate calcifications of epiphyses	Xq28	NAD(P)H Steroid Dehydrogenase-like protein (*NSDHL*)	Hebert et al. (1987), Grange et al. (2000)
Focal dermal hypoplasia (MIM 305600)	Meningomyelocele	Male lethality, atrophy and linear pigmentation of the skin, papillomas of skin and mucosae, ocular defects, hypoplastic teeth, digital anomalies			Almeida et al. (1988), Temple et al. (1990)
X-linked laterality sequence (MIM 306955)	Meningomyelocele	Abdominal situs inversus, complex cardiac defects, asplenia, polysplenia	Xq26.2	*ZIC3*	Mathias et al. (1987), Gebbia et al. (1997)
X-linked midline defect (MIM 313850)	Anencephaly	Hydrocephalus, cleft lip, congenital heart defect, renal agenesis, hypospadias in different family members	Xq25–26.1		Toriello and Higgins (1985)
X-linked neural tube defects (MIM 301410)	Anencephaly, spina bifida	—	? Linkage analysis of one family excludes X linkage		Newton et al. (1994)

*Refers to the number given to the condition in the Online Mendelian Inheritance in Man database (see Electronic Database Information).

Another example of an autosomal recessive disorder often associated with an NTD for which the gene is known is Walker-Warburg syndrome, also known as HARD+/– E (hydrocephalus, agyria, retinal dysplasia with or without encephalocele). Walker-Warburg syndrome is characterized by severe brain malformations (including lissencephaly and, sometimes, encephalocele), muscular dystrophy, and eye abnormalities. In some patients with Walker-Warburg syndrome, a mutation has been identified in the *POMT1* gene, a gene that codes for O-mannosyltransferase 1. This enzyme is believed to catalyze the first step in O-mannosyl glycan synthesis and suggests that O-mannosylation is important in neuronal migration (Beltran-Valero de Bernabe et al., 2002). At least two patients with phenotypes consistent with Walker-Warburg syndrome have been found to have mutations in the *FKTN* gene (also known as the *FCMD* gene), which codes for fukutin (Beltran-Valero de Bernabe et al., 2003; Silan et al., 2003), previously associated with a similar but milder phenotype (Fukuyama congenital muscular dystrophy) (Kobayashi et al., 1998). Both patients with Walker-Warburg syndrome had homozygous nonsense mutations in the *FKTN* gene, predicted to result in a complete loss of fukutin activity, whereas patients with the milder phenotype (Fukuyama congenital muscular dystrophy) had mutations predicted to maintain residual fukutin activity (Beltran-Valero de Bernabe et al., 2003). Fukutin is believed to be an enzyme that modifies cell-surface glycoproteins or glycolipids (Takeda et al., 2003).

Autosomal Dominant Conditions

Only a few autosomal dominant conditions have been postulated to be associated with NTDs (Table 16.2). One of these is Waardenburg syndrome, a condition characterized by dystopia canthorum, broad nasal root, heterochromia irides, and sensorineural hearing loss and caused by mutations in the *PAX3* gene. Several lines of evidence suggest that Waardenburg syndrome could be associated with meningomyelocele. These include pedigrees with Waardenburg syndrome in which family members have been shown to have meningomyelocele (Pantke and Cohen, 1971; Moline and Sandlin, 1993), several patients with both Waardenburg syndrome and meningomyelocele (Arnvig, 1959; Pantke and Cohen, 1971; de Saxe et al., 1984; Narod et al., 1988; Begleiter and Harris, 1992; Carezani-Gavin et al., 1992; Chatkupt and Johnson, 1993), including two in the same sibship (Chatkupt and Johnson, 1993); and the fact that a mouse model of NTDs (known as Splotch) has mutations in the gene homologous to *PAX3* in humans (the gene responsible for Waardenburg syndrome). In addition, the *PAX3* gene is expressed in the neural folds, dorsal neural tube, and early neural crest (Tassabehji et al., 1994), consistent with the hypothesis that *PAX3* is involved in some cases of NTDs. These findings have led some authors to suggest that prenatal screening for meningomyelocele be considered in pregnancies in which the fetus is at risk for Waardenburg syndrome (Carezani-Gavin et al., 1992; Chatkupt and Johnson, 1993).

Mutations in *PAX3* have been identified in some patients with Waardenburg syndrome and NTDs. Hol et al. (1995) screened 39 patients with familial NTDs for mutations in the *PAX3* gene and found 1 patient with a lumbosacral meningomyelocele with a 5-bp deletion in exon 5, which results in a frameshift and premature protein truncation. The patient also had mild signs of Waardenburg syndrome type I. In a study conducted in a large spina bifida clinic, 515 children were screened for neural crest anomalies, such as those seen in patients with Waardenburg syndrome, to determine the contribution of these conditions to NTDs (Nye et al., 1999). To screen for these anomalies, the investigators asked questions about the presence or absence of hearing loss; hand or foot defects; colon defects; heart defects; cleft lip or palate; neural tube defects; and pigmentary defects of the hair, eyebrows, eyelashes, irises, or skin in the proband and any relative. When an anomaly was noted, further information was obtained to determine if the defect was congenital and to confirm the family member affected. Neural crest anomalies were seen in 62 patients (12.2%), including 9 with Waardenburg-like syndromes (6 with type I, 2 with type III and 1 with type IV). The two patients with Waardenburg syndrome type III were studied further (Nye et al., 1998). Both were found to have de novo interstitial deletions of chromosome 2, including the *PAX3* gene. Nye et al. (1998) suggested that another genetic or environmental event, in addition to the cytogenetic deletion, must be necessary, since previous deletions in the region have not been associated with NTDs. The authors hypothesized that the second event may involve a single gene (consistent with a digenic mechanism of inheritance) since interaction of certain genes has been shown to result in NTDs in animal models (Nye et al., 1998).

Studies of the *PAX3* gene in individuals with NTDs, but without signs of Waardenburg syndrome, have been performed. Linkage analysis on 17 American and 14 Dutch families with NTDs showed no evidence of linkage to *PAX3* (Chatkupt et al., 1995). In addition, the multiallelic transmission disequilibrium test using an intragenic polymorphism of *PAX3* was applied in 78 families in which the proband had lumbosacral meningomyelocele. These results suggested that *PAX3* did not play a major role in the etiology of NTDs in these families (Melvin et al., 2000). However, these studies do not exclude the possibility that *PAX3* is involved in a subgroup of NTDs.

Another autosomal dominant condition associated with NTDs is Weissenbacher-Zweymuller syndrome, characterized by short stature with rhizomelic shortening at birth, improvement in growth rate beginning at age

2–3 years, and subsequent normalization of radiographical abnormalities. A set of identical twins, both with Weissenbacher-Zweymuller syndrome, were also found to have NTDs (one had a meningocele and the other had a parieto-occipital encephalocele) (Ramer et al., 1993). The gene for Weissenbacher-Zweymuller syndrome has been identified as *COL11A2* (Pihlajamaa et al., 1998). Given that these twins are the only patients in whom Weissenbacher-Zweymuller syndrome has been observed with NTDs, the possibility that these conditions occurred together by chance cannot be ruled out.

X-Linked Conditions

Several X-linked conditions include NTDs as part of their phenotype, two X-linked dominant disorders (congenital hemidysplasia with ichthyosiform erythroderma and limb defects or CHILD syndrome, and focal dermal hypoplasia) and three X-linked recessive disorders (Table 16.3). At least four families with isolated NTDs have been reported in which the pedigree is consistent with an X-linked recessive mode of inheritance. These were a four-generation pedigree with five affected males with anencephaly or spina bifida (Toriello et al., 1980); a three-generation pedigree with three males affected with spina bifida (Toriello, 1984); a two-generation pedigree with six males affected with encephalocele or spina bifida (Baraitser and Burn, 1984); and a three-generation pedigree with five affected males with spina bifida, anencephaly, or encephalocele (Jensson et al., 1988). The finding of a female fetus with a terminal deletion Xp and anencephaly supports the role of an X-linked gene in NTDs (Plaja et al., 1994). However, linkage analysis performed on one of the four families using markers from 62 informative loci on the X chromosome excluded X linkage (Newton et al., 1994). That study raised the question of whether an X-linked form of NTDs exists; however, the authors noted that the exclusion of linkage to the X chromosome relies on several assumptions, including that the disease phenotype is fully penetrant and that a single recessive gene is responsible for NTDs in all affected members of the family (Newton et al., 1994). Thus, involvement of an X-linked gene in NTDs remains a possibility.

Mitochondrial Mutations

Mitochondrial mutations have been observed in at least two patients with NTDs (Barisic et al., 2002; Nye et al., 2000). One patient had mitochondrial encephalopathy, lactic acidosis, and stroke-like episodes consistent with MELAS syndrome, as well as a ventricular septal defect and meningocele. She was identified as having a mitochondrial point mutation at nucleotide 3271 (Barisic et al., 2002). In another family, the proband had a myelocystocele, Arnold-Chiari type I malformation, cloacal exstrophy, and hearing loss; other family members had sensorineural hearing loss, along with minor pigmentary, digital, and spinal anomalies. The family was identified as having a mitochondrial mutation (*A1555G* mutation in the *12S rRNA* gene). To examine the contribution of the mitochondrial A1555G mutation to the etiology of NTDs, the authors screened 218 persons with NTDs for the *A1555G* mutation. None had this mutation, suggesting that the mutation is unlikely to be a common factor in NTD etiology (Nye et al., 2000).

The possibility that the mitochondrial mutations and NTDs in these two patients may have occurred by chance cannot be ruled out. However, NTDs in these patients could be explained by the effect of abnormal respiratory chain function secondary to mitochondrial mutations on sensitive cells involved in neural tube formation at a critical time during embryogenesis (Barisic et al., 2002). This mechanism and its effect on neural crest cells could also account for the neural crest–related anomalies observed in other family members with the mitochondrial mutation reported by Nye et al. (2000).

IDENTIFICATION OF SYNDROMES ASSOCIATED WITH NEURAL TUBE DEFECTS

As discussed previously, recognition of the presence of a chromosome abnormality or single-gene-determined syndrome is necessary to provide appropriate prognostic information and genetic counseling to the family. To allow recognition of these conditions, referral to a clinical geneticist with expertise in dysmorphology is important. An infant may appear to have an isolated NTD to a health-care provider without dysmorphology training, since the minor dysmorphic features associated with a specific syndrome might otherwise be overlooked. A careful history including a detailed pregnancy history and three-generation pedigree should be obtained. Questions should be asked specifically about a family history of NTDs, other birth defects, spontaneous abortions, stillbirths, and neonatal deaths. The health-care provider should ask specifically about consanguinity, because its presence can provide a clue that the condition is inherited in an autosomal recessive manner. In the event of fetal or infant death, a complete autopsy should be conducted to identify other defects that might have been missed by external examination, and chromosome analysis should be attempted (chromosome studies are often successful if tissue specimens are obtained within several hours of death) (Holmes et al., 1976; Urioste, 1993). Likewise, for prenatally diagnosed cases, thorough ultrasonographic and cytogenetic evaluations should be performed, particularly if a destructive method of pregnancy termination is planned (Main and Mennuti, 1986; Simpson et al., 1991). If the child is liveborn, a physical examination by a clinical geneticist familiar with syndromes associated with NTDs should be conducted. In addition, appropriate laboratory tests, including cytogenetic evaluation, should be performed, depending on the findings of the physical examination. As more genes are identified and molecular genetic studies become more readily available, these studies will also become an integral part of the evaluation of children with NTDs who might have a syndrome of single-gene etiology.

Families who require genetic counseling with a history of a previous pregnancy with an NTD in which the fetus or infant is no longer available for examination present a particular challenge. If a careful examination and appropriate laboratory evaluation were not performed, the family must be counseled that recurrence risk estimates could be significantly altered, because a syndromic NTD cannot be excluded.

CONCLUSIONS

A multifactorial mode of determination and empiric recurrence risk figures apply to most, but not all, families with NTDs. A significant proportion of infants have NTDs associated with either a chromosome abnormality or a single-gene disorder. Clinicians need to recognize infants with these syndromes so that their families can be provided with accurate prognostic and recurrence risk information. Study of infants with chromosome abnormalities could lead to the identification of new genes involved in the causation of NTDs. In addition, investigation of single-gene conditions associated with NTDs could provide insight into the pathogenesis and causation of these common birth defects.

ELECTRONIC DATABASE INFORMATION

Online Mendelian Inheritance in Man (OMIM). McKusick-Nathans Institute for Genetic Medicine, Johns Hopkins University (Baltimore) and National Center for Biotechnology Information, National Library of Medicine (Bethesda, MD), 2000. World Wide Web URL: http://www.ncbi.nlm.nih.gov/omim/

REFERENCES

Aleck KA, Grix A, Clericuzio C, Kaplan P, Adomian GE, Lachman R, Rimoin DL (1987). Dyssegmental dysplasias: clinical, radiographic, and morphologic evidence of heterogeneity. Am J Med Genet 27:295–312.

Almeida L, Anyane-Yeboa K, Grossman M, Rosen T (1988). Myelomeningocele, Arnold-Chiari anomaly and hydrocephalus in focal dermal hypoplasia. Am J Med Genet 30:917–923.

Arnvig J (1959). The syndrome of Waardenburg. Acta Genet 9:41–46.

Aughton DJ, Cassidy SB (1987). Hydrolethalus syndrome: report of an apparent mild case, literature review, and differential diagnosis. Am J Med Genet 27:935–942.

Babcook CJ, Goldstein RB, Filly RA (1995). Prenatally detected fetal myelomeningocele: is karyotype analysis warranted? Radiology 194:491–494.

Baird PA, Sadovnick AD (1984). Survival in infants with anencephaly. Clin Pediatr (Phila) 23:268–271.

Baraitser M, Burn J (1984). Brief clinical report: neural tube defects as an X-linked condition. Am J Med Genet 17:383–385.

Barisic N, Kleiner IM, Malcic I, Papa J, Boranic M (2002). Spinal dysraphism associated with congenital heart disorder in a girl with MELAS syndrome and point mutation at mitochondrial DNA nucleotide 3271. Croat Med J 43:37–41.

Begleiter ML, Harris DJ (1992). Waardenburg syndrome and meningocele. Am J Med Genet 44:541.

Belloni E, Muenke M, Roessler E, Traverso G, Siegel-Bartelt J, Frumkin A, Mitchell HF, et al. (1996). Identification of *Sonic hedgehog* as a candidate gene responsible for holoprosencephaly. Nat Genet 14:353–356.

Beltran-Valero de Bernabe D, Currier S, Steinbrecher A, Celli J, van Beusekom E, van der Zwaag B, Kayserili H, et al. (2002). Mutations in the O-mannosyltransferase gene *POMT1* give rise to the severe neuronal migration disorder Walker-Warburg syndrome. Am J Hum Genet 71:1033–1043.

Beltran-Valero de Bernabe D, van Bokhoven H, van Beusekom E, Van den Akker W, Kant S, Dobyns WB, Cormand B, et al. (2003). A homozygous nonsense mutation in the *Fukutin* gene causes a Walker-Warburg syndrome phenotype. J Med Genet 40:845–848.

Botto LD, May K, Fernhoff PM, Correa A, Coleman K, Rasmussen SA, Merritt RK, et al. (2003). A population-based study of the 22q11.2 deletion: phenotype, incidence, and contribution to major birth defects in the population. Pediatrics 112:101–107.

Carezani-Gavin M, Clarren SK, Steege T (1992). Waardenburg syndrome associated with meningomyelocele. Am J Med Genet 42:135–136.

Chatkupt S, Hol FA, Shugart YY, Geurds MP, Stenroos ES, Koenigsberger MR, Hamel BC, et al. (1995). Absence of linkage between familial neural tube defects and *PAX3* gene. J Med Genet 32:200–204.

Chatkupt S, Johnson WG (1993). Waardenburg syndrome and myelomeningocele in a family. J Med Genet 30:83–84.

Cohen MM Jr, Kreiborg S (1994). Unusual cranial aspects of the Apert syndrome. J Craniofac Genet Dev Biol 14:48–56.

Cohen MM Jr, Lemire RJ (1982). Syndromes with cephaloceles. Teratology 25:161–172.

Corsello G, Giuffre L (1994). VACTERL with hydrocephalus: a further case with probable autosomal recessive inheritance. Am J Med Genet 49:137–138.

Czeizel A, Losonci A (1987). Split hand, obstructive urinary anomalies and spina bifida or diaphragmatic defect syndrome with autosomal dominant inheritance. Hum Genet 77:203–204.

David TJ, McCrae FC, Bound JP (1983). Congenital malformations associated with anencephaly in the Fylde peninsula of Lancashire. J Med Genet 20:338–341.

David TJ, Nixon A (1976). Congenital malformations associated with anencephaly and iniencephaly. J Med Genet 13:263–265.

de Saxe M, Kromberg JG, Jenkins T (1984). Waardenburg syndrome in South Africa. Part I. An evaluation of the clinical findings in 11 families. S Afr Med J 66:256–261.

Forrester S, Kovach MJ, Smith RE, Rimer L, Wesson M, Kimonis VE (2002). Kousseff syndrome caused by deletion of chromosome 22q11–13. Am J Med Genet 112:338–342.

Fryns JP, Devriendt K, Moerman P (1996). Lumbosacral spina bifida and myeloschizis in a female foetus with de novo X/autosomal translocation (t(X;22)(q27;q121)). Genet Couns 7:159–160.

Gardner RJ, Sutherland GR (1996). *Chromosome Abnormalities and Genetic Counseling*. New York: Oxford University Press.

Gebbia M, Ferrero GB, Pilia G, Bassi MT, Aylsworth A, Penman-Splitt M, Bird LM, et al. (1997). X-linked situs abnormalities result from mutations in *ZIC3*. Nat Genet 17:305–308.

Gollop TR, Kiota MM, Martins RM, Lucchesi EA, Alvarenga Filho E (1984). Frontofacionasal dysplasia: evidence for autosomal recessive inheritance. Am J Med Genet 19:301–305.

Grange DK, Kratz LE, Braverman NE, Kelley RI (2000). CHILD syndrome caused by deficiency of 3beta-hydroxysteroid-delta8, delta7-isomerase. Am J Med Genet 90:328–335.

Guion-Almeida ML, Kokitsu-Nakata NM, Richieri-Costa A (2000). Clinical variability in cerebro-oculo-nasal syndrome: report on two additional cases. Clin Dysmorphol 9:253–257.

Hall JG, Friedman JM, Kenna BA, Popkin J, Jawanda M, Arnold W (1988). Clinical, genetic, and epidemiological factors in neural tube defects. Am J Hum Genet 43:827–837.

Harper JC, Bui TH (2002). Pre-implantation genetic diagnosis. Best Pract Res Clin Obstet Gynaecol 16:659–670.

Hebert AA, Esterly NB, Holbrook KA, Hall JC (1987). The CHILD syndrome. Histologic and ultrastructural studies. Arch Dermatol 123:503–509.

Hol FA, Hamel BC, Geurds MP, Mullaart RA, Barr FG, Macina RA, Mariman EC (1995). A frameshift mutation in the gene for *PAX3* in a girl with spina bifida and mild signs of Waardenburg syndrome. J Med Genet 32:52–56.

Holmes LB, Driscoll SG, Atkins L (1976). Etiologic heterogeneity of neural-tube defects. N Engl J Med 294:365–369.

Hughes HE, Harwood-Nash DC, Becker LE (1983). Craniotelencephalic dysplasia in sisters: further delineation of a possible syndrome. Am J Med Genet 14:557–565.

Hume RF Jr, Drugan A, Reichler A, Lampinen J, Martin LS, Johnson MP, Evans MI (1996). Aneuploidy among prenatally detected neural tube defects. Am J Med Genet 61:171–173.

Hunter AG (1984). Neural tube defects in Eastern Ontario and Western Quebec: demography and family data. Am J Med Genet 19:45–63.

Jensson O, Arnason A, Gunnarsdottir H, Petursdottir I, Fossdal R, Hreidarsson S (1988). A family showing apparent X linked inheritance of both anencephaly and spina bifida. J Med Genet 25:227–229.

Källén B, Cocchi G, Knudsen LB, Castilla EE, Robert E, Daltveit AK, Lancaster PL, et al (1994). International study of sex ratio and twinning of neural tube defects. Teratology 50:322–331.

Källén B, Robert E, Harris J (1998). Associated malformations in infants and fetuses with upper or lower neural tube defects. Teratology 57:56–63.

Kedar I, Amiel A, Fejgin M, Drugan A (1996). Recurrent anencephaly as a primary manifestation of the acrocallosal syndrome. Am J Med Genet 62:415–416.

Kelberman D, Tyson J, Chandler DC, McInerney AM, Slee J, Albert D, Aymat A, et al (2001). Hemifacial microsomia: progress in understanding the genetic basis of a complex malformation syndrome. Hum Genet 109:638–645.

Kennedy D, Chitayat D, Winsor EJ, Silver M, Toi A (1998). Prenatally diagnosed neural tube defects: ultrasound, chromosome, and autopsy or postnatal findings in 212 cases. Am J Med Genet 77:317–321.

Khoury MJ, Erickson JD, James LM (1982a). Etiologic heterogeneity of neural tube defects. II. Clues from family studies. Am J Hum Genet 34:980–987.

Khoury MJ, Erickson JD, James LM (1982b). Etiologic heterogeneity of neural tube defects: clues from epidemiology. Am J Epidemiol 115:538–548.

Kliemann SE, Waetge RT, Suzuki OT, Passos-Bueno MR, Rosemberg S (2003). Evidence of neuronal migration disorders in Knobloch syndrome: clinical and molecular analysis of two novel families. Am J Med Genet 119A:15–19.

Kobayashi K, Nakahori Y, Miyake M, Matsumura K, Kondo-Iida E, Nomura Y, Segawa M, et al (1998). An ancient retrotransposal insertion causes Fukuyama-type congenital muscular dystrophy. Nature 394:388–392.

Lehman RA, Stears JC, Wesenberg RL, Nusbaum ED (1977). Familial osteosclerosis with abnormalities of the nervous system and meninges. J Pediatr 90:49–54.

Lubinsky MS, Kahler SG, Speer IE, Hoyme HE, Kirillova IA, Lurie IW (1994). von Voss-Cherstvoy syndrome: a variable perinatally lethal syndrome of multiple congenital anomalies. Am J Med Genet 52:272–278.

Main DM, Mennuti MT (1986). Neural tube defects: issues in prenatal diagnosis and counselling. Obstet Gynecol 67:1–16.

Maria BL, Boltshauser E, Palmer SC, Tran TX (1999). Clinical features and revised diagnostic criteria in Joubert syndrome. J Child Neurol 14:583–590; discussion 590–591.

Martin RA, Fineman RM, Jorde LB (1983). Phenotypic heterogeneity in neural tube defects: a clue to causal heterogeneity. Am J Med Genet 16:519–525.

Martínez-Frías ML, Bermejo E, Urioste M, Egues J, Lopez Soler JA (1993). Short rib-polydactyly syndrome (SRPS) with anencephaly and other central nervous system anomalies: a new type of SRPS or a more severe expression of a known SRPS entity? Am J Med Genet 47:782–787.

Martínez-Frías ML, Frias JL, Salvador J (1990). Clinical/epidemiological analysis of malformations. Am J Med Genet 35:121–125.

Mathias RS, Lacro RV, Jones KL (1987). X-linked laterality sequence: situs inversus, complex cardiac defects, splenic defects. Am J Med Genet 28:111–116.

McGregor L, Makela V, Darling SM, Vrontou S, Chalepakis G, Roberts C, Smart N, et al (2003). Fraser syndrome and mouse blebbed phenotype caused by mutations in *FRAS1/Fras1* encoding a putative extracellular matrix protein. Nat Genet 34:203–208.

Melvin EC, George TM, Worley G, Franklin A, Mackey J, Viles K, Shah N, et al (2000). Genetic studies in neural tube defects. NTD Collaborative Group. Pediatr Neurosurg 32:1–9.

Menzel O, Bekkeheien RC, Reymond A, Fukai N, Boye E, Kosztolanyi G, Aftimos S, et al (2004). Knobloch syndrome: novel mutations in *COL18A1,* evidence for genetic heterogeneity, and a functionally impaired polymorphism in endostatin. Hum Mutat 23:77–84.

Moline ML, Sandlin C (1993). Waardenburg syndrome and meningomyelocele. Am J Med Genet 47:126.

Morgan NV, Gissen P, Sharif SM, Baumber L, Sutherland J, Kelly DA, Aminu K, et al (2002). A novel locus for Meckel-Gruber syndrome, MKS3, maps to chromosome 8q24. Hum Genet 111:456–461.

Narod SA, Siegel-Bartelt J, Hoffman HJ (1988). Cerebellar infarction in a patient with Waardenburg syndrome. Am J Med Genet 31:903–907.

Naveed M, Manjunath CS, Sreenivas V (1990). New manifestations of Neu-Laxova syndrome. Am J Med Genet 35:55–59.

Newton R, Stanier P, Loughna S, Henderson DJ, Forbes SA, Farrall M, Jensson O, et al (1994). Linkage analysis of 62 X-chromosomal loci excludes the X chromosome in an Icelandic family showing apparent X-linked recessive inheritance of neural tube defects. Clin Genet 45:241–249.

Nickel RE, Magenis RE (1996). Neural tube defects and deletions of 22q11. Am J Med Genet 66:25–27.

Nickel RE, Pillers DA, Merkens M, Magenis RE, Driscoll DA, Emanuel BS, Zonana J (1994). Velo-cardio-facial syndrome and DiGeorge sequence with meningomyelocele and deletions of the 22q11 region. Am J Med Genet 52:445–459.

Nye JS, Balkin N, Lucas H, Knepper PA, McLone DG, Charrow J (1998). Myelomeningocele and Waardenburg syndrome (type 3) in patients with interstitial deletions of 2q35 and the *PAX3* gene: possible digenic inheritance of a neural tube defect. Am J Med Genet 75:401–408.

Nye JS, Hayes EA, Amendola M, Vaughn D, Charrow J, McLone DG, Speer MC, et al (2000). Myelocystocele-cloacal exstrophy in a pedigree with a mitochondrial 12S rRNA mutation, aminoglycoside-induced deafness, pigmentary disturbances, and spinal anomalies. Teratology 61:165–171.

Nye JS, McLone DG, Charrow J, Hayes EA (1999). Neural crest anomaly syndromes in children with spina bifida. Teratology 60:179–189.

Odent S, Loget P, Le Marec B, Delezoide AL, Maroteaux P (1999). Unusual fan shaped ossification in a female fetus with radiological features of boomerang dysplasia. J Med Genet 36:330–332.

Paavola P, Salonen R, Baumer A, Schinzel A, Boyd PA, Gould S, Meusburger H, et al (1997). Clinical and genetic heterogeneity in Meckel syndrome. Hum Genet 101:88–92.

Paavola P, Salonen R, Weissenbach J, Peltonen L (1995). The locus for Meckel syndrome with multiple congenital anomalies maps to chromosome 17q21-q24. Nat Genet 11:213–215.

Pantke OA, Cohen MM Jr (1971). The Waardenburg syndrome. Birth Defects Orig Artic Ser 7:147–152.

Pihlajamaa T, Prockop DJ, Faber J, Winterpacht A, Zabel B, Giedion A, Wiesbauer P, et al (1998). Heterozygous glycine substitution in the *COL11A2* gene in the original patient with the Weissenbacher-Zweymuller syndrome demonstrates its identity with heterozygous OSMED (nonocular Stickler syndrome). Am J Med Genet 80:115–120.

Plaja A, Vendrell T, Sarret E, Toran N, Mediano C (1994). Terminal deletion of Xp in a dysmorphic anencephalic fetus. Prenat Diagn 14:410–412.

Powell CM, Chandra RS, Saal HM (1993). PHAVER syndrome: an autosomal recessive syndrome of limb pterygia, congenital heart anomalies, vertebral defects, ear anomalies, and radial defects. Am J Med Genet 47:807–811.

Ramer JC, Eggli K, Rogan PK, Ladda RL (1993). Identical twins with Weissenbacher-Zweymuller syndrome and neural tube defect. Am J Med Genet 45:614–618.

Rasmussen SA, Olney RS, Holmes LB, Lin AE, Keppler-Noreuil KM, Moore CA, and the National Birth Defects Prevention Study (2003a). Guidelines for case classification for the National Birth Defects Prevention Study. Birth Defects Res (Pt A) 67:193–201.

Rasmussen SA, Wong LY, Yang Q, May KM, Friedman JM (2003b). Population-based analyses of mortality in trisomy 13 and trisomy 18. Pediatrics 111:777–784.

Reardon W, Harbord MG, Hall-Craggs MA, Kendall B, Brett EM, Baraitser M (1989). Central nervous system malformations in Mohr's syndrome. J Med Genet 26:659–663.

Roberts CJ, Powell RG (1975). Interrelation of the common congenital malformations: some aetiological implications. Lancet 2:848–850.

Rode ME, Mennuti MT, Giardine RM, Zackai EH, Driscoll DA (2001). Early ultrasound diagnosis of Neu-Laxova syndrome. Prenat Diagn 21:575–580.

Roume J, Genin E, Cormier-Daire V, Ma HW, Mehaye B, Attie T, Razavi-Encha F, et al (1998). A gene for Meckel syndrome maps to chromosome 11q13. Am J Hum Genet 63:1095–1101.

Roume J, Ma HW, Le Merrer M, Cormier-Daire V, Girlich D, Genin E, Munnich A (1997). Genetic heterogeneity of Meckel syndrome. J Med Genet 34:1003–1006.

Sadovnick AD, Baird PA (1985). Congenital malformations associated with anencephaly in liveborn and stillborn infants. Teratology 32:355–361.

Satran D, Pierpont ME, Dobyns WB (1999). Cerebello-oculo-renal syndromes including Arima, Senior-Loken and COACH syndromes: more than just variants of Joubert syndrome. Am J Med Genet 86:459–469.

Seller MJ (1995). Neural tube defects, chromosome abnormalities and multiple closure sites for the human neural tube. Clin Dysmorphol 4:202–207.

Sertie AL, Sossi V, Camargo AA, Zatz M, Brahe C, Passos-Bueno MR (2000). Collagen XVIII, containing an endogenous inhibitor of angiogenesis and tumor growth, plays a critical role in the maintenance of retinal structure and in neural tube closure (Knobloch syndrome). Hum Mol Genet 9:2051–2058.

Silan F, Yoshioka M, Kobayashi K, Simsek E, Tunc M, Alper M, Cam M, et al (2003). A new mutation of the fukutin gene in a non-Japanese patient. Ann Neurol 53:392–396.

Simpson JL, Mills J, Rhoads GG, Cunningham GC, Conley MR, Hoffman HJ (1991). Genetic heterogeneity in neural tube defects. Ann Genet 34:279–286.

Slaney SF, Goodman FR, Eilers-Walsman BL, Hall BD, Williams DK, Young ID, Hayward RD, et al (1999). Acromelic frontonasal dysostosis. Am J Med Genet 83:109–116.

Slavotinek AM, Tifft CJ (2002). Fraser syndrome and cryptophthalmos: review of the diagnostic criteria and evidence for phenotypic modules in complex malformation syndromes. J Med Genet 39:623–633.

Stene J, Stene E, Mikkelsen M (1984). Risk for chromosome abnormality at amniocentesis following a child with a non-inherited chromosome aberration. A European Collaborative Study on Prenatal Diagnoses 1981. Prenat Diagn 4 Spec No:81–95.

Suzuki OT, Sertie AL, Der Kaloustian VM, Kok F, Carpenter M, Murray J, Czeizel AE, et al (2002). Molecular analysis of collagen XVIII reveals novel mutations, presence of a third isoform, and possible genetic heterogeneity in Knobloch syndrome. Am J Hum Genet 71:1320–1329.

Takeda S, Kondo M, Sasaki J, Kurahashi H, Kano H, Arai K, Misaki K, et al (2003). Fukutin is required for maintenance of muscle integrity, cortical histiogenesis and normal eye development. Hum Mol Genet 12:1449–1459.

Tassabehji M, Newton VE, Leverton K, Turnbull K, Seemanova E, Kunze J, Sperling K, et al (1994). *PAX3* gene structure and mutations: close analogies between Waardenburg syndrome and the *Splotch* mouse. Hum Mol Genet 3:1069–1074.

Temple IK, MacDowall P, Baraitser M, Atherton DJ (1990). Focal dermal hypoplasia (Goltz syndrome). J Med Genet 27:180–187.

Toriello HV (1984). Report of a third kindred with X-linked anencephaly/spina bifida. Am J Med Genet 19:411–412.

Toriello HV, Higgins JV (1985). X-linked midline defects. Am J Med Genet 21:143–146.

Toriello HV, Warren ST, Lindstrom JA (1980). Brief communication: possible X-linked anencephaly and spina bifida—report of a kindred. Am J Med Genet 6:119–121.

Townes PL, Reuter K, Rosquete EE, Magee BD (1988). XK aprosencephaly and anencephaly in sibs. Am J Med Genet 29:523–528.

Urioste M (1993). Chromosome cultures from human cartilage. Am J Med Genet 46:123–125.

Van Den Berg DJ, Francke U (1993). Roberts syndrome: a review of 100 cases and a new rating system for severity. Am J Med Genet 47:1104–1123.

van den Ende JJ, Schrander-Stumpel C, Rupprecht E, Meinecke P, Maroteaux P, de Die-Smulders C, Hamel BC (1998). The cerebro-costo-mandibular syndrome: seven patients and review of the literature. Clin Dysmorphol 7:87–95.

Visapaa I, Salonen R, Varilo T, Paavola P, Peltonen L (1999). Assignment of the locus for hydrolethalus syndrome to a highly restricted region on 11q23–25. Am J Hum Genet 65:1086–1095.

Warburg M, Jensen H, Prause JU, Bolund S, Skovby F, Miranda MJ (1997). Anophthalmia-microphthalmia-oblique clefting syndrome: confirmation of the Fryns anophthalmia syndrome. Am J Med Genet 73:36–40.

Yoshioka M, Kuroki S (1994). Clinical spectrum and genetic studies of Fukuyama congenital muscular dystrophy. Am J Med Genet 53:245–250.

17

Mouse Mutants as Models of Neural Tube Defects

ANDREW J. COPP
NICHOLAS D.E. GREENE
JENNIFER N. MURDOCH

While most animals have a central nervous system (CNS), the process of neurulation, in which neural folding and fusion create a closed neural tube (reviewed in Chapter 2), occurs only in higher vertebrates. Embryos with an abnormal open neural tube are seen, therefore, only in higher animals, including amphibians, birds, and mammals. This fact has precluded advances in our understanding of the genetic basis of neural tube defects (NTDs) from studies of lower organisms. Genetic studies in the fruit fly *Drosophila,* and in the nematode worm *Caenorhabditis elegans,* have unraveled the mechanisms underlying many developmental events, including the specification, differentiation, and programmed death of CNS neurons (Ellis and Horvitz, 1986; Gaiano and Fishell, 2002). In contrast, invertebrate studies have not contributed directly to an understanding of the morphogenetic process of neurulation or the molecular basis of NTDs.

NTDs have an important genetic component (reviewed in Chapter 14), and it is vital, therefore, that research is aimed at determining the mechanistic basis of this genetic etiology. Among the higher vertebrates that exhibit neurulation, only two have well-understood genetics: the human and the mouse. Studies of human genetics in relation to NTDs are reviewed elsewhere in this volume (see Chapter 14), and the present chapter concentrates on the contribution made by studies of mouse genetics. The benefits of mouse genetics for an understanding of NTDs are, first, the wealth of available mouse strains in which NTDs are a prominent feature of the mutant phenotype and, second, that as standard laboratory animals, mouse models of NTD permit experimental studies designed specifically to reveal the principles of NTD etiology and pathogenesis. Experimental studies are not possible in humans for ethical reasons, making mouse research of key significance.

TYPES OF MOUSE MUTANTS THAT EXHIBIT NEURAL TUBE DEFECTS AND THEIR ORIGIN

A large number of mouse mutant strains exhibit NTDs (Harris and Juriloff, 1997, 1999; Juriloff and Harris, 2000). Table 17.1 shows the growing list of mouse mutants at the time of writing. The mutants have arisen from a variety of sources, as reflected by the classification in the table. Spontaneous, mutagen-induced, and gene trap–induced mutations (Table 17.1, sections A–C) are all examples of random genetic events that disrupt the function of an unknown gene, thereby causing NTDs. These mutant strains were isolated and preserved because of their interesting phenotypes; subsequently, genetic studies identified the disrupted gene in some cases. Hence, these types of mutant have arisen via a *phenotype-driven* process. In contrast, NTD mutants that have arisen through transgene misexpression or gene targeting are the by-products of a *gene-driven* process in which an already identified and characterized gene is manipulated to alter/abolish its function (Table 17.1, sections D, E). Once NTDs are observed in the phenotype of such transgenic mice, a relationship is immediately established between the mutated gene and neurulation.

TABLE 17.1. *Mouse Mutant Models of Neural Tube Defects*

Mutant Name	Neural Tube Defect*	Gene Mutated†	Chr‡	Function of Protein	Reference
A. Spontaneous					
Axial defects (Axd)	Sb	n.d.	n.d.	n.d.	Essien et al. (1990)
Bent-tail (Bn)	Ex + Sb	*Zic3*	X	Transcription factor	Carrel et al. (2000), Klootwijk et al. (2000), Purandare et al. (2002)
Circletail (Crc)	CRN	*Scrb1*	15	Cytoplasmic protein with role in apicobasal polarity	Murdoch et al. (2003)
Crooked tail (Cd)	Ex	n.d.	6	n.d.	Borello et al. (1999)
Curly tail (ct)	Ex + Sb	n.d.	4	n.d.	Van Straaten and Copp (2001)
Doublefoot (Dbf)	Ex	n.d.	1	n.d.	Lyon et al. (1996)
Exencephaly (xn)	Ex	n.d.	n.d.	n.d.	Wallace et al. (1978)
Extra-toes	Ex	*Gli3*	13	Transcription factor	Hui and Joyner (1993), Franz (1994)
Eye blebs (eb)	Ex	n.d.	n.d.	n.d.	Swiergiel et al. (2000)
Fused (fu)	Ex + Sb	*Axin*	17	Regulator of G-proteins in Wnt signaling	Zeng et al. (1997)
Head blebs (heb)	Ex	n.d.	4	n.d.	Varnum and Fox (1981)
Loop-tail (Lp)	CRN	*Vangl2*	1	Transmembrane protein (strabismus) with role in planar cell polarity	Strong and Hollander (1949), Murdoch et al. (2001a)
No turning (nt)		n.d.	n.d.	n.d.	Melloy et al. (1998)
Open brain (opb)	Ex + Sb	*Rab23*	1	Rab family of vesicle transport proteins	Günther et al. (1994), Eggenschwiler et al. (2001)
Patch, PDGFαR	Ex	*Pdgfra*	5	Growth factor receptor	Morrison-Graham et al. (1992), Soriano (1997)
Rib fusions (Rf)	Ex	n.d.	n.d.	n.d.	Theiler and Stevens (1960)
Splotch (Sp, Sp^{2H})	Ex + Sb	*Pax3*	1	Transcription factor	Epstein et al. (1991)
Tail short (Ts)	Ex	n.d.	11	n.d.	Johnson (1976)
Vacuolated lens (vl)	Sb	n.d.	1	n.d.	Wilson and Wyatt (1986)
B. Mutagen-Induced					
Blebs (my)	Ex	n.d.	3	n.d.	Carter (1959)
Crash (Crsh)	CRN	*Celsr1*	15	Transmembrane nonclassical cadherin with function in planar cell polarity	Curtin et al. (2003)
Exma	Ex	n.d.	X	n.d.	Cunningham et al. (2002)
Nucleosome assembly protein-1-like 2 (Nap1l2)	Ex + Sb	*Nap1l2*	X	Nucleosome assembly	Rogner et al. (2000)
C. Gene Trap					
Jumonji	Ex	*jmj*	13	Retinoblastoma-binding protein homologue	Takeuchi et al. (1995)
Mdm4	Ex	*Mdm4*	1	p53-dependent cell cycle regulation	Migliorini et al. (2002)
Shroom	Ex + Sb	*shrm*	5	PDZ-containing cytoskeletal protein	Hildebrand and Soriano (1999)
D. Transgene Misexpression					
ATRX	Ex	*Xnp*	X	Member of SWI/SNF chromatin remodeling family	Berube et al. (2002)
Connexin 43	Ex	*Cx43* (also called *Gja1*)	10	Gap junction component	Ewart et al. (1997)
Glial cells missing-1	Sb	*Gcm1*	9	Transcription factor	Nait-Oumesmar et al. (2002)
Msx2	Ex	*Msx2*	13	Transcription factor	Winograd et al. (1997)

(continued)

TABLE 17.1. *Mouse Mutant Models of Neural Tube Defects (Continued)*

Mutant Name	Neural Tube Defect*	Gene Mutated†	Chr‡	Function of Protein	Reference
Notch 3	Ex	*Notch3*	17	Cell surface receptor for delta ligands	Lardelli et al. (1996)
Sonic hedgehog	Ex	*Shh*	5	Signalling peptide regulating nervous system dorsoventral patterning	Echelard et al. (1993)
E. Gene Knockout					
Abl/Arg double mutant	Ex	*Abl1, Abl2*	2 & 1	Nonreceptor tyrosine kinases	Koleske et al. (1998)
AP2α	Ex	*AP2α* (also called *Tcfap2a*)	13	Transcription factor	Schorle et al. (1996), Zhang et al. (1996), Kohlbecker et al. (2002)
Apaf1 and *forebrain overgrowth (fog,* mutation of the *Apaf1* gene)	Ex or Sb	Apaf1	10	Protease-activating factor in the caspase-dependent apoptosis pathway	Harris et al. (1997), Cecconi et al. (1998), Yoshida et al. (1998), Honarpour et al. (2001)
Apolipoprotein B	Ex	*Apob*	12	Plasma lipoprotein	Farese et al. (1995), Homanics et al. (1995)
Bcl10	Ex	*Bcl10*	3	CARD-containing anti-apoptotic protein	Ruland et al. (2001)
Bmp5/Bmp7 double mutant	Ex	*Bmp5,Bmp7*	9,2	Members of the bone morphogenetic protein family of signaling proteins	Solloway and Robertson (1999)
Brca1	Ex + Sb	*Brca1*	11	Transcription factor	Gowen et al. (1996)
Brg1	Ex	Smarca4	9	Chromatin remodeling protein	Bultman et al. (2000)
Calreticulin	Ex	Calr	8	Calcium binding protein	Rauch et al. (2000)
Cart1 (cartilage homeoprotein 1)	Ex	*Cart1*	10	Transcription factor	Zhao et al. (1996)
Caspase 3	Ex	*Casp3*	8	Enzyme of apoptosis pathway	Kuida et al. (1998)
Caspase 9	Ex	*Casp9*	4	Enzyme of apoptosis pathway	Hakem et al. (1998), Kuida et al. (1998)
CBP	Ex	*Crebbp*	17	Transcriptional coactivator	Yao et al. (1998)
Cited2	Ex	*Cited2*	10	Transcriptional coactivator	Bamforth et al. (2001), Martinez-Barbera et al. (2002), Yin et al. (2002)
CYP26	Ex + Sb	*Cyp26A1*	19	Retinoic acid metabolic enzyme	Abu-Abed et al. (2001), Sakai et al. (2001), Niederreither et al. (2002)
CYPOR	Ex	*Por*	5	NADPH-cytochrome P450 reductase	Shen et al. (2002)
Dlx5	Ex	*Dlx5*	6	Homeodomain protein	Acampora et al. (1999)
Dnmt3b	Ex	*Dnmt3b*	2	DNA methyltransferase	Okano et al. (1999)
Eph-A7	Ex	*Epha7*	4	Receptor tyrosine kinase	Holmberg et al. (2000)
Ephrin-A5	Ex	*Efna5*	17	Ligand for Eph receptor tyrosine kinase	Holmberg et al. (2000)
Fibroblast growth factor receptor 1	Sb	*Fgfr1*	8	Growth factor receptor	Deng et al. (1997)
FKBP12	Ex	*Fkbp1a*	2	Cis-trans prolyl isomerase	Shou et al. (1998)
Folate binding protein 1	Ex	*Folbp1*	7	Folate binding protein enabling folate entry into cells	Piedrahita et al. (1999)
Hairy and enhancer of split 1	Ex	*Hes1*	16	Transcription factor	Ishibashi et al. (1995)
Hes1/Hes3 double mutant	Ex	*Hes1, Hes3*	16, 4	Transcription factors	Hirata et al. (2001)
Hic1	Ex	*Hic1*	11	POZ-domain transcription factor	Carter et al. (2000)

TABLE 17.1. *Mouse Mutant Models of Neural Tube Defects (Continued)*

Mutant Name	Neural Tube Defect*	Gene Mutated†	Chr‡	Function of Protein	Reference
Jnk1/Jnk2 double mutant	Ex	*Mapk8, Mapk9*	14	*c*-Jun-*N*-terminal kinases	Sabapathy et al. (1999)
KIF3B	Ex	*Kif3b*	2	Kinesin superfamily protein	Nonaka et al. (1998)
Laminin a5	Ex	*Lama5*	2	Extracellular protein component of basement membranes	Miner et al. (1998)
MARCKS (myristoylated alanine rich C-kinase subtrate)	Ex	*Marcks*	10	Cytoskeleton-related protein with function in signal transduction	Stumpo et al. (1995)
MARCKS-related protein, Mrp	Ex with or without Sb	*Mlp*	4	Cytoskeleton-related protein with function in signal transduction	Wu et al. (1996)
Mena/profilin I double mutant	Ex	*Enah/Pfn1*	1, 11	Regulation of actin polymerization	Lanier et al. (1999)
Mf3 (mesoderm/mesenchyme forkhead 3)	Ex	*Foxb1*	9	Transcription factor	Labosky et al. (1997)
Neurofibromin	Ex	*Nf1*	11	Negative regulator of $p21^{ras}$	Lakkis et al. (1999)
Nf1/Pax3 double mutant	Ex with or without Sb	*Nf1, Pax3*	11, 1	As *Nf1*	Lakkis et al. (1999)
Noggin	Ex + Sb, or CRN	*Nog*	11	BMP antagonist	McMahon et al. (1998)
Nucleoporin	Ex	*Nup50*	15	Nuclear pore protein binding to $p27^{Kip1}$	Smitherman et al. (2000)
Numb	Ex	*Numb*	12	Protein participating in asymmetric cell division	Zhong et al. (2000)
p300	Ex	*Ep300*	n.d.	Transcriptional integrator	Yao et al. (1998)
p53 (transformation-related protein 53)	Ex	*Trp53*	11	Tumor suppressor	Sah et al. (1995)
Patched1	Ex or CRN	*Ptch1*	13	Transmembrane receptor for Sonic Hedgehog peptide	Goodrich et al. (1997), Milenkovic et al. (1999)
Pax7Pax3 double mutant	Ex + Sb	*Pax3/Pax7*	1, 4	Transcription factors	Mansouri and Gruss (1998)
Perlecan	Ex	*Hspg2*	4	Heparan sulfate proteoglycan, component of basement membranes	Arikawa-Hirasawa et al. (1999)
Pitx2	Ex	*Pitx2*	3	Homeodomain transcription factor	Aghi et al. (1999)
Protein kinase a sub units Cα/Cβ1 double mutant	Ex	*Prkaca; Prkacb*	8; 3	Protein kinase A	Huang et al. (2002)
RBP-Jκ	Ex	*Rbpsuh*	5	Transcription factor	Oka et al. (1995)
Retinoic acid receptors α/γ double mutant	Ex	*Rara, Rarg*	11, 15	Nuclear retinoid receptors	Lohnes et al. (1994)
RhoGAP P190	Ex	*Grlf1*	n.d.	Rho GTPase activating protein	Brouns et al. (2000)
Ski	Ex	*ski*	4	Transcription factor and proto-oncogene	Berk et al. (1997)
Srg3	Ex	*Smarcc1*	9	Subunit of SWI/SNF complex, involved in chromatin remodeling	Wechsler-Reya (2001)
Squalene synthase	Ex	*Fdft1*	14	Cholesterol biosynthesis	Naus and Bani-Yaghoub (1998)
Treacle	Ex	*Tcof1*	18	Nucleolar phosphoprotein	Dixon et al. (2000)
Telomerase RNA, mTR	Ex + Sb	*Terc*	3	Maintains telomeres on chromosomes	Herrera et al. (1999)
Tumour necrosis factor receptor–associated factor 4	Sb	*Traf4*	11	Intracellular signaling adaptor	Regnier et al. (2002)

(continued)

TABLE 17.1. *Mouse Mutant Models of Neural Tube Defects (Continued)*

Mutant Name	Neural Tube Defect*	Gene Mutated†	Chr‡	Function of Protein	Reference
Tumour necrosis factor receptor–associated factor 6	Ex	*Traf6*	2	Intracellular signaling adaptor	Lomaga et al. (2000)
Tubby-like protein 3	Ex + Sb	*Tulp3*	6	Not known	Ikeda et al. (2001)
Twist	Ex	*Twist*	12	Transcription factor	Chen and Behringer (1995)
Vinculin	Ex	Vcl	14	Cytoskeletal protein	Xu et al. (1998)
Yin Yang 1	Ex	*YY1*	12	Transcription factor	Donohoe et al. (1999)
Wnt3a	Sb	*Wnt3a*		Extracellular signaling factor	Takada et al. (1994)
ZIC2	Ex + Sb	*Zic2*	14	Transcription factor	Nagai et al. (2000)

* Neural tube defect phenotypes: CRN, craniorachischisis; Ex, exencephaly; Sb, spina bifida.
† Gene mutated: n.d., not determined.
‡ Mouse chromosome position: n.d., not determined.
BMP, bone morphogenetic protein; CARD, caspase-associated recruitment domain; GTPase, guanosine triphosphatase; NADPH, reduced nicotinamide adenine dinucleotide phosphate; PDZ, *P*ostsynaptic density, protein *D*iscs-large, protein *z*O-1; SWI/SNF, yeast protein *s*ucrose *non*fermenting
POZ = *Po*x virus, *Z*inc finger proteins

A variety of spontaneous and mutagen-induced mouse mutants exist, including some of the models that most closely resemble human NTDs. For example, all of the single-gene models of craniorachischisis, the severest NTDs, fall within this category (*loop-tail, circletail,* and *crash*), as do the well-studied *splotch* and *curly tail* mutants, which exhibit exencephaly and spina bifida. Considerable research effort has been expended recently on intensive mutagenesis of the mouse genome using ethylnitrosourea (ENU), which induces point mutations with high frequency (Anderson, 2000). Of the many ENU-induced mutations identified so far, *opb*[2] (Eggenschwiler et al., 2001), has proven particularly illuminating in revealing the role of the *Sonic hedgehog* signaling pathway in neural tube closure (see below for further details).

The gene trap method involves insertion of a reporter (e.g., *lacZ*) transgene into the genome of embryonic stem (ES) cells as a result of recombination between splice site sequences in the transgene and those at the exon-intron boundaries of endogenous genes (Joyner, 1991). Transgene integration not only "traps" endogenous genes but also disrupts their DNA sequence, potentially yielding functional mutations. Embryonic stem cells containing gene trap insertions can be selected and expanded in vitro before being injected into mouse preimplantation embryos in order to create liveborn chimeric mice. In some cases, chimeras produce ES cell–derived germ cells that can yield offspring hemizygous for the gene trap integration. Intercrossing hemizygotes then yields litters containing homozygotes for the gene trap integration, enabling the phenotype of the gene trap to be determined. Of the many gene trap–induced mutant phenotypes produced to date, *jumonji* is a model of cranial NTDs (Takeuchi et al., 1999).

Generating misexpression of mouse genes is usually achieved by injection of a transgene directly into the male pronucleus of the fertilized oocyte, where the transgene sequence integrates randomly into the host genome. In some cases, the transgene is expressed in a manner that differs from endogenous gene expression (either in amount, timing in development, or tissue of localization), yielding a transgene misexpression model. Misexpression of the gap junction protein connexin 43 has produced a model of cranial NTDs (Ewart et al., 1997).

Quantitatively, the most prolific source of mouse genetic NTD models is gene targeting (i.e., gene knockout technology). Homologous recombination is performed in ES cells, whereby a copy of a specific endogenous gene is replaced with an engineered version of the same gene lacking a critical component or incorporating a mutation (Capecchi, 1989). After ES cells that exhibit the new mutation are selected, chimeras are produced and the new mutation is passed through the germ line of these individuals to yield heterozygous mice, which can be interbred to produce homozygotes. Hundreds of gene-targeted strains have been constructed since the technology was introduced in the late 1980s and, of these, a proportion exhibit NTDs. The great majority of these gene disruptions yield the cranial NTD exencephaly, although a number also exhibit spinal defects (Table 17.1). The NTD phenotype of most mutants has been subjected to preliminary analysis, often in only a single study. Nevertheless, the large number of mouse mutants that exhibit NTDs demonstrates the genetic complexity that must underlie early development of the CNS. The normal functioning of many genes appears to be necessary for the neural tube to close correctly.

RANGE OF NEURAL TUBE DEFECTS EXHIBITED BY THE MOUSE MUTANTS

The spectrum of NTDs in humans encompasses extensive lesions such as craniorachischisis, in which the neural tube is open throughout part of the cranial region as well as the whole of the spine, and more localized lesions affecting the cranial region (anencephaly) or spinal region (open spina bifida). All of these NTD types are represented among the mouse genetic models (Table 17.1). A small number of mutants, *loop-tail, circletail,* and *crash,* and the *dishevelled-1/2* double mutant, exhibit craniorachischisis (Fig. 17.1*A*), and embryonic studies in these mice demonstrate that the basic defect is a failure of initiation of neural tube closure at the hindbrain/cervical boundary when the embryo has six or seven somites (8.5 days of gestation) (Copp et al., 1994; Murdoch et al., 2001b; Hamblet et al., 2002; Curtin et al., 2003). This initial closure event, so-called Closure 1, is required for the subsequent events of midbrain, hindbrain, and spinal closure to be successfully completed. Interestingly, however, forebrain closure is achieved in the mutants with craniorachischisis (Greene et al., 1998), as in many human embryos with this NTD. This probably results from the relatively normal occurrence of Closure 2, which takes place in most strains at the boundary between the future midbrain and forebrain and which does not appear to require the normal functioning of the *Lp, Crc, Crsh,* and *Dvl* genes.

Cranial NTDs, in the absence of spinal defects, are observed in a large number of mouse mutants (Table 17.1). Initially, such embryos exhibit a failure of one or more of the cranial closure events (reviewed in Chapter 2), so that the neural folds bulge out from the developing brain, a condition termed *exencephaly* (Fig. 17.1*B*). As gestation progresses, however, the delicate neuroepithelium that is exposed to the amniotic fluid in the exencephalic lesion undergoes degeneration, resulting, by birth in the mouse, in the "flat skull" appearance of anencephaly (Wood and Smith, 1984) that is typical of human cranial NTDs. Hence, exencephaly and anencephaly are successive stages in the development of the NTD lesion that results from failure of cranial closure.

Spinal closure begins at Closure 1 and spreads caudally, following the progressive growth of the spinal region, until it is completed with closure of the posterior (caudal) neuropore in embryos with 28–30 somites (10 days of gestation). Delay of spinal closure is seen in a number of mutants, with the effect that the posterior neuropore appears increasingly enlarged as spinal development proceeds (Van Straaten et al., 1992). An enlarged neuropore in embryos with 28–30 somites is compatible with two possible developmental outcomes. Severe delay precludes completion of closure and the spinal neural tube remains open, as spina bifida (equivalent to the early stage of myelocele or myelomeningocele in humans). A more minor delay in neuropore closure may be compatible with eventual closure but is often associated with a dorsal bend of the tail, yielding a curled-tail phenotype (Copp, 1985). Hence, tail flexion defects are frequent findings in mouse mutants with spinal NTDs.

Development of the caudal nervous system proceeds by so-called secondary neurulation, following closure of the posterior neuropore (reviewed in Chapter 2). This process yields a neural tube without neural folding, so defects are never open but instead involve tethering of the neural tube to surrounding tissues. This is the primary finding in many low (dysraphic) human spinal defects, which may require surgery to free the spinal cord from surrounding vertebral and other tissues. Because of the difficulty of identifying mouse mutants with these rather subtle defects, there are few mouse models.

Tethering of the spinal cord to surrounding tissues can also occur in open NTDs, for example where an open spina bifida lesion maintains its contact with the surface epidermis (Stiefel et al., 2003). Spinal tethering limits the

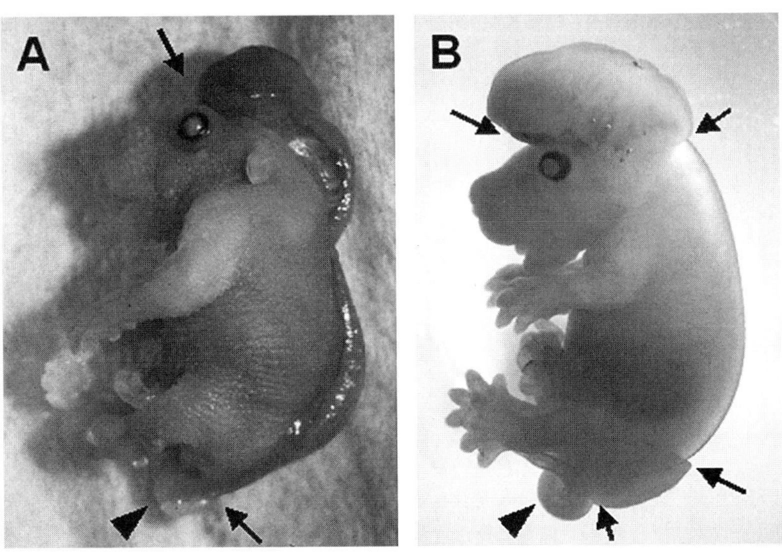

FIGURE 17.1. Appearance of the main types of neural tube defects (NTDs), as seen in the mouse mutant models and in humans. (*A*) Craniorachischisis in an E16.5 fetus doubly heterozygous for the *loop-tail* and *circletail* mutations. This severe NTD encompasses the entire axial region between the midbrain and low spine (between the *arrows*). (*B*) Exencephaly and spina bifida in an E16.5 fetus homozygous for the *curly tail* mutation. Exencephaly involves the midbrain and anterior hindbrain (between the upper pair of *arrows*), while spina bifida affects the low lumbar and sacral regions (between the lower pair of *arrows*). The neural tube between the two NTD lesions has closed normally. Note the presence of a curled tail in both fetuses (*arrowheads* in *A* and *B*).

physiological ascent of the spinal cord during development and may be instrumental in causing the Chiari type II malformation, in which part of the brain stem herniates through the foramen magnum and which is often present in association with hydrocephalus in spinal NTDs (Harding and Copp, 2002).

We have seen that the range of NTDs in the mouse genetic models covers much of the conditions observed in humans, indicating that mouse mutants provide appropriate models for human NTDs. Importantly, the fact that the various mouse mutants develop NTDs at different levels of the body axis indicates a specific genetic requirement for each phase of neurulation. Moreover, the penetrance of NTDs in mouse models is frequently affected by both genetic background and environmental influences. Hence, it is unrealistic to expect a single cause of NTDs in humans. Rather, these malformations must be viewed as a heterogeneous collection of defects, with varying etiology and pathogenic mechanisms.

LETHAL EMBRYONIC MUTANTS MASQUERADING AS NEURAL TUBE DEFECT MODELS

A particular problem in establishing whether a mouse mutant gene provides a model for NTDs is presented by the coexistence of embryonic lethality. Many genetic defects are lethal, with the stage of lethality corresponding to the type of defect that occurs. For example, cardiac defects are often lethal in the second half of mouse gestation, whereas CNS defects, including NTDs, become lethal only in the perinatal period (Copp, 1995). A functioning CNS is not necessary for in utero survival in the mouse. Hence, the finding of embryonic/fetal lethality in a mouse mutant with NTDs must indicate a coexisting pathology, probably involving the cardiovascular, hemopoietic, or placental systems. If embryos die during the period in which the neural tube closes (8–10 days of gestation), this poses a particular problem of interpretation. Does a persistently open neural tube in an embryo that is dying from a defect in another system constitute an NTD? Clearly, if the embryo does not survive long enough in utero to close its neural tube, then the fact that the neural tube is open cannot be taken as evidence of an NTD. Notwithstanding this argument, a number of mutants have been suggested to exhibit NTDs in such circumstances. For instance, embryos lacking an active *csk* gene die at around 9 days of gestation, when their cranial neural tube has not yet closed, although prolonged survival might have been compatible with successful closure (Imamoto and Soriano, 1993). Similarly, embryos homozygous for a null mutation in the *telomerase* gene die with open neural tube, although there appears to be widespread degeneration occurring at the time of neurulation (Herrera et al., 1999). Hence, before concluding that a given mouse mutant exhibits NTDs, care must be taken to ensure that embryonic lethality and/or degenerative processes are not likely to be responsible for preventing normal development beyond neurulation.

It is becoming increasingly feasible to circumvent embryonic lethality in gene knockouts by use of *conditional* gene targeting (Cohen-Tannoudji and Babinet, 1998). For example, if a gene mutation causes lethal defects in cardiac development, it is now possible to "activate" the mutant version of the gene in the CNS cell lineage but not in the developing heart. This can be achieved by placing loxP sites around the portion of the gene that needs to be excised to yield the mutant allele. The bacterial enzyme Cre recombines adjacent loxP sites, enabling intervening sequence to be excised, with a single loxP site left in its place. Hence, expression of Cre from a CNS-specific gene promoter in an independent coexisting transgene has the effect of inducing a null allele of the gene in question only in the developing CNS. Cardiac lethality is avoided and the requirement of the gene for neural tube closure can be fully evaluated.

USES OF MOUSE MUTANTS AS NEURAL TUBE DEFECT MODELS—EVIDENCE FROM THE *ct* AND *Sp^{2H}* MUTANTS

A variety of experimental studies can be conducted using mouse models that are not possible in humans. As a result, considerable information is emerging on various aspects of NTD etiology and pathogenesis, as summarized below.

Identification of Gene–Gene Interactions

The mouse mutant genes listed in Table 17.1 produce NTDs, for the most part, when they are homozygous. An important extension of this genetic work has been the identification of interactions between genes that also result in the development of NTDs. Hence, while mice of genotypes *ct/ct* and *Sp^{2H}/Sp^{2H}* each develop spina bifida, double heterozygotes (*ct/+; Sp^{2H}/+*) also have NTDs in a proportion of cases, and embryos of genotype *ct/ct; Sp^{2H}/+* exhibit particularly severe spina bifida (Estibeiro et al., 1993). Other examples of this so-called digenic inheritance have been described in the mutant combinations *Lp/Crc, Nf1/Sp^{2H}, Abl/Arg, un/Ptch,* and *Dvl1/Dvl2* (Helwig et al., 1995; Koleske et al., 1998; Lakkis et al., 1999; Murdoch et al., 2001b; Hamblet et al., 2002). Since the great majority of the mutant combinations have yet to be tested, it is possible that a relatively large number of gene–gene interactions may promote the development of NTDs. Translated to the human situation, it seems possible that a relatively large number of gene variants predisposing toward NTD could be present in populations at relatively low frequencies. Neural tube defects would arise occasionally in homozygotes for a single-gene variant, but this would be a rare event. More commonly, the coming together of two or more different genetic variants in a single individual would provide the interaction necessary to disturb neurulation. A relatively sporadic occurrence of NTDs would result, with one or a few cases in a family, before the causative genetic variants segregated apart in subsequent generations, reducing the risk of subsequent NTD recurrence. Because of the large number of possible combinations of genetic variants that interact to produce NTDs, the sporadic occurrence would be relatively frequent. This accurately describes the natural history of human NTDs.

Influence of Genetic Background on Mutant Gene Effects

Not only do interactions occur between mutant genes of *major effect* (i.e., those capable of causing NTDs when homozygous), but *modifier* genes that make up the genetic background also have potent effects in modulating the severity and frequency of NTDs. This role of the genetic background is suspected in humans but has been demonstrated unequivocally in the mouse NTD models. Genetic backgrounds can be studied in pure form in mouse inbred strains, where all individuals are identical genetically. Different inbred backgrounds promote a different frequency and severity of NTDs in response to a variety of genetic and environmental influences. For example, the *curly tail* (*ct*) mutant gene, when crossed onto different inbred backgrounds, yields widely differing frequencies of spina bifida (Embury et al., 1979; Neumann et al., 1994), and a similar finding applies to the frequency of cranial NTDs resulting from the *splotch* (Sp^{2H}) mutant gene (Fleming and Copp, 2000). In the latter case, research has focused on the aspect of embryonic development that is governed by variation in genetic background, which appears directly responsible for modulating the ability of the Sp^{2H} mutation to produce exencephaly. Inbred strains differ in the precise position along the rostrocaudal axis of the developing brain at which Closure 2 occurs (Juriloff et al., 1991) (see Chapter 2 for further details). While the majority of strains exhibit Closure 2 at the midbrain/forebrain boundary, in others this event occurs more caudally within the midbrain (e.g., the DBA/2 strain) or more rostrally within the forebrain (e.g., the NZW strain). Experimental studies have shown that when the Sp^{2H} mutation is bred onto the DBA/2 background, midbrain closure is enhanced and the frequency of exencephaly in Sp^{2H}/Sp^{2H} embryos is reduced from 80% to around 40% (Fleming and Copp, 2000). On the other hand, breeding to the NZW strain maintains the high exencephaly rate seen in the splotch parent strain (which has a Closure 2 position similar to that of NZW). Hence, the precise position of Closure 2, dictated by the genetic background, modulates the effect of a major mutant gene such as Sp^{2H}. Clearly, the human population, with its continuously varying genetic background, provides enormous scope for background effects on NTD occurrence.

Gene–Environment Interactions

The gene–gene and gene–background interactions, reviewed in the preceding sections, operate in the context of the nongenetic milieu in which the embryo develops (here called the *environment*). A wide variety of exogenous agents, when applied to embryos developing either in utero or in vitro, exert teratogenic effects with the production of abnormalities that include NTDs. While the majority of the known NTD-causing agents are drugs, chemicals, or other substances extraneous to pregnancy, a smaller number of molecules derived from metabolism, particularly in maternal disease conditions, also cause NTDs (Copp et al., 1990). For example, elevated glucose and ketone body concentrations, as found in diabetes mellitus, increase the risk of NTDs (Sadler, 1980), and an excess or a deficiency of retinol (vitamin A), and particularly its active metabolite, retinoic acid (RA), are potent causes of NTDs (Shenefelt, 1972). In addition, physical factors such as hyperthermia can induce NTDs. As with major gene effects, different inbred mouse strains exhibit varying susceptibility to NTD-causing teratogenic agents. The polymorphism in the rostrocaudal position of Closure 2 (see above) affects susceptibility to exencephaly induced by the separate application in vitro of valproic acid and hyperthermia (Finnell et al., 1986, 1988). Strains with Closure 2 in the midbrain are relatively resistant to teratogenic influence, as they are to the influence of the Sp^{2H} genetic effect. Conversely, strains with Closure 2 in the forebrain are highly susceptible to both teratogenic and genetic influences. Hence, both exogenous agents and genetic mutations act by mechanisms that are equally and similarly affected by the genetic background.

Teratogens are also known to interact directly with genetic mutant effects in the causation of NTDs. Thus, the low natural frequency of exencephaly in the *curly tail* strain is elevated by administration of all-trans-RA (Seller et al., 1979), although, interestingly, the frequency of spina bifida in this strain is actually reduced by low-dose RA (Chen et al., 1994). This case demonstrates that environmental agents can exert sharply contrasting effects, either exacerbating or ameliorating, upon interaction with a genetic predisposition. The basis of this interaction can be understood by reference to the molecular mechanisms of action of the exogenous agent and the genetic mutation. In the case of the interaction between RA and the *curly tail* gene mutation, the available evidence implicates the well-established "downstream" signaling pathway of RA (Leid et al., 1992). Retinoic acid is synthesized physiologically in embryonic tissues from retinol by the action of retinaldehyde dehydrogenase and then bound by cellular retinoic acid binding protein (CRABP) which presents it to nuclear receptors. Retinoic acid binds to nuclear retinoic acid receptors (RARs), stimulating them to act as transcription factors, regulating the expression of other genes, and initiating cascades of molecular events. Excess RA administration can produce malformations by a mechanism that involves upregulation of the expression of RARs, especially the β-isoform (Fundele et al., 1990), presumably leading to supranormal stimulation of RAR pathways. In the case of the *curly tail* mouse, low-dose RA administration up-regulates RARβ in the hindgut within the caudal embryonic region (Chen et al., 1995), which is a known site of subnormal cell proliferation, leading to spina bifida in this strain (Copp et al., 1988a). Hence, the ameliorating effect of RA on spinal NTDs in this strain may occur through stimulation of proliferation via enhanced RARβ signaling in the hindgut tissue. The mechanism underlying the *teratogenic* effect of RA in increasing the frequency of exencephaly in the *curly tail* mutant strain is not yet understood.

Prevention of Neural Tube Defects by Vitamins

Any exogenous agent that ameliorates a genetic predisposition to NTDs is a candidate therapeutic agent for NTD prevention, although molecules such as RA are not applicable for clinical use during pregnancy owing to their known teratogenic effects. Emphasis in recent years has been placed heavily on folic acid as the most likely preventive agent for human NTD models. Several mouse NTD mutants, including Sp^{2H}, *Cart1, Cd,* and *Cited2* (Zhao et al., 1996; Fleming and Copp, 1998; Carter et al., 1999; Martinez-Barbera et al., 2002), have been shown to interact with folic acid, exhibiting a reduction in NTD frequency that mimics the phenomenon in humans. The existence of folate-preventable mouse NTD mutants reproduces, in an animal model, the observation made previously only in humans that folic acid exerts a preventive effect on NTDs. Moreover, it demonstrates that primary prevention of NTD can occur by normalization of neurulation, not by promotion of the death of affected fetuses (so-called terathanasia), as was suggested for human NTD prevention (Hook and Czeizel, 1997). Finally, the mouse mutants offer a route towards experimental analysis of the phenomenon of folic acid prevention of NTDs, whose underlying mechanism remains poorly understood (see Chapters 15 and 29).

A significant finding has been that several mouse NTD strains, including *curly tail, Axd,* and the *EphA7* knockout (Essien and Wannberg, 1993; Seller, 1994; Holmberg et al., 2000), do not exhibit a reduction in NTD frequency following folic acid administration. Hence, not all mouse models respond similarly to folic acid, coinciding with the prevailing view that some but not all human NTDs are likely to be folate-responsive. This leaves a proportion of NTDs (of unknown size) that require another type of preventive therapy. Examination of additional exogenous agents is indicated, therefore, to identify factors that might also exert a preventive action on NTDs and could perhaps complement the effects of folic acid clinically.

Inositol has proven highly effective in preventing the spinal NTDs observed in the folate-resistant *curly tail* mutant, an action that operates via stimulation of protein kinase C activity in embryonic cells (Greene and Copp, 1997). The ultimate effect is probably stimulation of cell proliferation within the caudal embryonic region, which is known to be defective in the *curly tail* strain. Expression of RARβ is up-regulated in inositol-treated embryos (Greene and Copp, 1997), similar to the preventive effect of low-dose RA (as discussed above). Moreover, in a comparison of two different enantiomeric forms, *myo*-inositol and D-*chiro*-inositol, both had NTD preventive activity but D-*chiro*-inositol exhibited greater potency (Cogram et al., 2002). Neither agent produced significant side effects in a fetal pathological analysis. In a single case study, a woman with two previous NTD-affected fetuses, despite high-dose folic acid supplementation in both pregnancies, took inositol in a third pregnancy with no reported side effects and had a normal fetal outcome (Cavalli and Copp, 2002). Hence, evidence is accumulating to suggest that inositol may offer a potentially useful adjunct to folic acid therapy to prevent a further proportion of NTDs that may be folate-resistant.

Developmental Mechanisms

The embryonic mechanisms that underlie NTDs can be established only through experimental analysis, making the mouse genetic models particularly valuable. Mouse embryos can be maintained in vitro throughout the stages of neurulation using the method of whole embryo culture (New, 1978). Using this experimental approach, it was established that, in the *curly tail* mutant, spinal NTDs develop owing to a genetically determined imbalance in cell proliferation in the caudal embryonic region (Fig. 17.2). Ventral tissues, the hindgut and notochord, proliferate abnormally slowly compared to the neuroepithelium dorsally, which proliferates normally (Copp et al., 1988a). In fact, this imbalance in proliferation has its origin earlier in development, with cells in the ventral part of the embryonic tail bud growing abnormally slowly (Peeters et al., 1998). The imbalance of cell proliferation leads to ventral curvature of the entire caudal region that opposes mechanically the dorsal apposition of the neural folds,

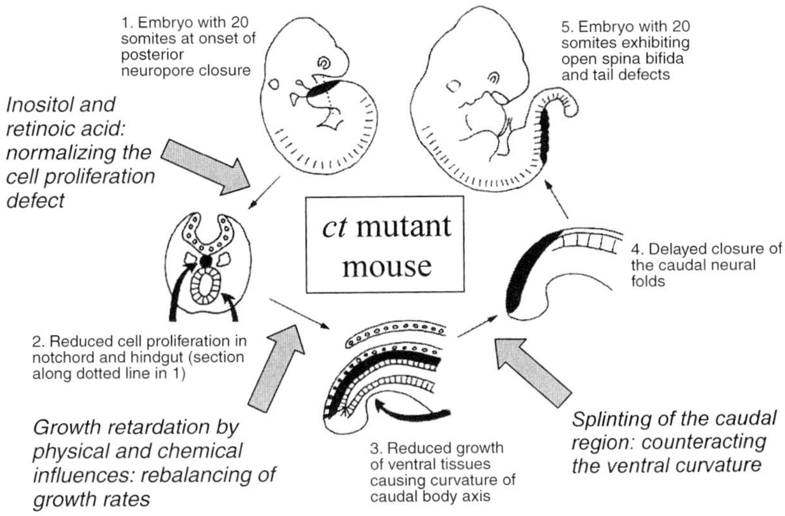

FIGURE 17.2. The pathogenic sequence of embryonic events in the *curly tail* mutant leading to development of spina bifida. Indicated in italics are the various experimental interventions that have been developed that lead to normalization of neural tube closure and prevention of spina bifida in this mouse model. Each intervention can be related to a specific event in the pathogenic sequence and, in several cases, was designed specifically as a result of our understanding of embryonic pathogenesis.

resulting in delay or total failure of closure of the posterior neuropore (Brook et al., 1991).

With this mechanism in mind, spinal NTDs in the *curly tail* mutant can now be prevented by several strategies, all designed to alleviate different aspects of the pathogenic sequence (Fig. 17.2). Hence, the cell proliferation imbalance can be rectified by increasing the rate of proliferation within the hindgut, which has been found to occur following inositol or low-dose RA treatment, or by slowing the growth of the entire embryo using maternal food deprivation, mild hyperthermia in vitro, or cytotoxic drug therapy (Seller and Perkins, 1986; Copp et al., 1988b; Cogram et al., 2004). Overall growth retardation affects the rapidly growing neuroepithelium to a greater extent than the slow-growing hindgut, leading to an effective rebalancing of tissue growth rates. An entirely different approach is to combat the ventral curvature that results from the proliferation imbalance. Physical splinting of the caudal region prevents curvature from developing and normalizes neuropore closure (Brook et al., 1991). Hence, knowledge of the pathogenic sequence enables a series of preventive measures to be developed for each model of NTDs.

A completely different pathogenic mechanism has recently been established for craniorachischisis, the severe NTD that develops in the *Lp, Crc, Crsh,* and *Dvl1/2* mutants. This defect arises from failure of Closure 1, the initiating event of neurulation in both mice and humans. While the neural folds elevate apparently normally at the site of Closure 1, the folds are spaced widely apart and cannot appose in the dorsal midline, preventing closure (Greene et al., 1998). This failure to initiate neural tube closure precludes closure at lower levels of the spinal axis, and also in the hindbrain and parts of the midbrain. On the other hand, Closures 2 and 3 occur apparently normally, leading to relatively normal formation of the forebrain and anterior midbrain.

Recent attention has focused on the shaping of the neural plate, which occurs by the process of cellular convergent extension (Keller et al., 2000). A polarized rearrangement of cells occurs within the plane of the neural plate and in the underlying mesoderm, with net cell movement in a medial direction and intercalation of cells in the midline. This process lengthens the body axis while narrowing the mediolateral dimension, converting the initially elliptical embryonic disc into the typical narrow, elongated embryonic shape. Experimental disturbance of convergent extension in *Xenopus* yields a relatively short, broad neural plate that fails, either totally or partially, to complete neural tube closure (Wallingford and Harland, 2002). The *Lp* and *Crc* mutations also exhibit a short, broad neural plate, suggesting that a defect in convergent extension may underlie the NTDs in these mutants. Significantly, the genes mutated in the *Lp, Crc, Crsh,* and *Dvl1/2* mutants (*Vangl2, Scrb1, Celsr1,* and *Dishevelled*) are all homologues of *Drosophila* genes that are involved in establishing cellular polarity, particularly via the so-called planar cell polarity (PCP) pathway (Murdoch et al., 2001a, 2003; Curtin et al., 2003). Recent examination of the inner ear of the mutants has shown that *Vangl2, Scrb1,* and *Celsr1* are indeed required for the establishment of PCP in the mammalian embryo (Curtin et al., 2003; Montcouquioi et al., 2003). Moreover, disruption of homologous PCP genes in *Xenopus* and zebrafish yields defects of convergent extension (Park and Moon, 2001; Wallingford and Harland, 2001; Darken et al., 2002; Goto and Keller, 2002; Jessen et al., 2002). Hence, the PCP signaling pathway is implicated in the early shaping of the neural plate, a process that appears vital for the correct initiation of neural tube closure.

Molecular Mechanisms

As reviewed above and summarized in Table 17.1, many of the genes that are disturbed in the NTD mutant mouse models are now being identified. With the completion of the Human and Mouse Genome Projects, it seems likely that the identity of all the genes listed in Table 17.1 will be determined over the next few years. This will enable an emerging molecular framework for neurulation to be developed in which the essential signaling pathways and other crucial molecular events are identified. The recent work on the PCP pathway exemplifies this approach, in which a single integrated pathway is determined to be essential for a particular neurulation event. Further consideration of this topic is beyond the scope of this chapter but has been the subject of a recent review (Copp et al., 2003).

WHY DO SO MANY MOUSE MUTANTS PRODUCE NEURAL TUBE DEFECTS, AND YET THE HUMAN GENES ARE DIFFICULT TO IDENTIFY?

It is striking that, despite the wealth of genetic information on mouse NTDs, very few genes have been positively identified as contributing to human NTD etiology (reviewed in Chapter 14). Several aspects of the mouse genetic regulation of neurulation, as reviewed in the earlier sections of this chapter, offer likely explanations for this apparent paradox. First, we have seen that in the great majority of mouse mutants, NTDs are observed only in homozygotes, with very few genes exhibiting haploinsufficiency. That is, NTD phenotypes are rare among the mouse heterozygotes. This contrasts with human genetic diseases, where haploinsufficiency is the most common cause of the clinical phenotype (Fisher and Scambler, 1994). Gene frequencies have to be very high in order to yield sufficient homozygotes to exhibit a common condition such as NTDs. On the other hand, we have seen that gene–gene interactions provide a powerful mechanism for producing high frequencies of NTDs despite potentially low frequencies of mutant alleles in the human population. A consequence of gene–gene interactions is genetic heterogeneity, a factor that is likely to preclude gene identification in humans, especially when conventional methods are used such as single-gene mutation screening within a group of patients with an apparently uniform phenotype. Clearly, an approach to identifying gene–gene interactions in human NTDs is to genotype a panel of NTD cases for a large number of the genes implicated in mouse NTDs. Multivariate analysis will then enable patterns of coexisting genetic variants to be discerned that can subsequently be tested, by constructing appropriate mouse genetic models, for their NTD-causing ability.

Embryonic lethality is another factor that characterizes many of the mouse mutant genes, and limits the likely role of these genes in human NTDs. Pregnancy wastage is extremely high in humans at all stages of development, so that disadvantaged embryos are unlikely to survive and contribute to the recorded cases of NTDs. This idea predicts that mutations in genes homologous to the mouse NTD mutants may be found among early human pregnancy losses, in which NTDs are known to be particularly plentiful.

Finally, the great majority of human genetic studies have concentrated on identifying protein coding mutations, while mutations that affect the regulation of the gene, rather than the function of the encoded protein, may give a similar phenotype. It remains to be seen, therefore, whether mutations in promoter/enhancer regions of genes that cause mouse NTDs will subsequently be identified among the human NTD cases.

CONCLUSIONS

A wealth of genetic information is now available from mouse studies concerning the genes that, when disrupted, yield NTDs. Taken to its logical conclusion, in a few years we should be able to identify every gene in the genome whose function is required for normal neurulation. A further level of complexity, requiring considerably more research effort, is to identify all possible combinations of these genes that, through gene–gene interaction, yield NTDs. Even more effort would then be needed to identify the critical modifying genes in the genetic background that modulate the effects of the major genes and the gene–gene interactions. Clearly, the genetic basis of NTDs is highly complex, particularly when interactions with nongenetic environmental factors are also taken into account. Nevertheless, this complexity, as emerging from the mouse studies, fits well with the multifactorial etiology of human NTDs as pointed out by Carter several decades ago (Carter, 1974). Not only do the mouse genetic models contribute to the emerging concept of NTD genetics in humans, they also provide the only realistic opportunity, within a mammalian system, to address issues of molecular and cellular pathogenesis in NTDs, and to conduct experimental studies on the action of agents such as folic acid and inositol in preventing NTDs. The mouse may be diminutive within the class Mammalia, but it is a giant among genetic models.

REFERENCES

Abu-Abed S, Dollé P, Metzger D, Beckett B, Chambon P, Petkovich M (2001). The retinoic acid–metabolizing enzyme, *CYP26A1*, is essential for normal hindbrain patterning, vertebral identity, and development of posterior structures. Genes Dev 15:226–240.

Acampora D, Merlo GR, Paleari L, Zerega B, Postiglione MP, Mantero S, Bober E, Barbieri O, Simeone A, Levi G (1999). Craniofacial, vestibular and bone defects in mice lacking the *Distal-less*-related gene *Dlx5*. Development 126:3795–3809.

Aghi M, Kramm CM, Breakefield XO (1999). Folylpolyglutamyl synthetase gene transfer and glioma antifolate sensitivity in culture and *in vivo.* J Natl Cancer Inst 91:1233–1241.

Anderson KV (2000). Finding the genes that direct mammalian development—ENU mutagenesis in the mouse. Trends Genet 16:99–102.

Arikawa-Hirasawa E, Watanabe H, Takami H, Hassell JR, Yamada Y (1999). Perlecan is essential for cartilage and cephalic development. Nature Genet 23:354–358.

Bamforth SD, Braganta J, Eloranta JJ, Murdoch JN, Marques FIR, Kranc KR, Farza H, Henderson DJ, Hurst HC, Bhattacharya S (2001). Cardiac malformations, adrenal agenesis, neural crest defects and exencephaly in mice lacking *Cited2,* a new *Tfap2* coactivator. Nature Genet 29:469–474.

Berk M, Desai SY, Heyman HC, Colmenares C (1997). Mice lacking the ski proto-oncogene have defects in neurulation, craniofacial, patterning, and skeletal muscle development. Genes Dev 11:2029–2039.

Berube NG, Jagla M, Smeenk C, De Repentigny Y, Kothary R, Picketts DJ (2002). Neurodevelopmental defects resulting from *ATRX* overexpression in transgenic mice. Hum Mol Genet 11:253–261.

Borello U, Buffa V, Sonnino C, Melchionna R, Vivarelli E, Cossu G (1999). Differential expression of the Wnt putative receptors *Frizzled* during mouse somitogenesis. Mech Dev 89:173–177.

Brook FA, Shum ASW, Van Straaten HWM, Copp AJ (1991). Curvature of the caudal region is responsible for failure of neural tube closure in the *curly tail* (*ct*) mouse embryo. Development 113:671–678.

Brouns MR, Matheson SF, Hu KQ, Delalle I, Caviness VS Jr, Silver J, Bronson RT, Settleman J (2000). The adhesion signaling molecule p190 RhoGAP is required for morphogenetic processes in neural development. Development 127:4891–4903.

Bultman S, Gebuhr T, Yee D, La Mantia C, Nicholson J, Gilliam A, Randazzo F, Metzger D, Chambon P, Crabtree G, Magnuson T (2000). A Brg1 null mutation in the mouse reveals functional differences among mammalian SWI/SNF complexes. Mol Cell 6:1287–1295.

Capecchi MR (1989). Altering the genome by homologous recombination. Science 244:1288–1292.

Carrel T, Purandare SM, Harrison W, Elder F, Fox T, Casey B, Herman GE (2000). The X-linked mouse mutation *Bent tail* is associated with a deletion of the *Zic3* locus. Hum Mol Genet 9:1937–1942.

Carter CO (1974). Clues to the aetiology of neural tube malformations. Dev Med Child Neurol 16(Suppl. 32):3–15.

Carter M, Ulrich S, Oofuji Y, Williams DA, Ross ME (1999). *Crooked tail* (*Cd*) models human folate-responsive neural tube defects. Hum Mol Genet 8:2199–2204.

Carter MG, Johns MA, Zeng XB, Zhou L, Zink MC, Mankowski JL, Donovan DM, Baylin SB (2000). Mice deficient in the candidate tumor suppressor gene *Hic1* exhibit developmental defects of structures affected in the Miller-Dieker syndrome. Hum Mol Genet 9:413–419.

Carter TC (1959). Embryology of the Little and Bagg X-rayed mouse stock. J Genet 56:401–435.

Cavalli P, Copp AJ (2002). Inositol and folate-resistant neural tube defects. J Med Genet 39:e5.

Cecconi F, Alvarez-Bolado G, Meyer BI, Roth KA, Gruss P (1998). Apaf1 (CED-4 homolog) regulates programmed cell death in mammalian development. Cell 94:727–737.

Chen W-H, Morriss-Kay GM, Copp AJ (1994). Prevention of spinal neural tube defects in the *curly tail* mouse mutant by a specific effect of retinoic acid. Dev Dyn 199:93–102.

Chen W-H, Morriss-Kay GM, Copp AJ (1995). Genesis and prevention of spinal neural tube defects in the *curly tail* mutant mouse: involvement of retinoic acid and its nuclear receptors RAR-beta and RAR-gamma. Development 121:681–691.

Chen Z-F, Behringer RR (1995). *twist* is required in head mesenchyme for cranial neural tube morphogenesis. Genes Dev 9:686–699.

Cogram P, Hynes A, Dunlevy LPE, Greene NDE, Copp AJ (2004). Specific isoforms of protein kinase C are essential for prevention of folate-resistant neural tube defects by inositol. Hum Mol Genet 13:7–14.

Cogram P, Tesh S, Tesh J, Wade A, Allan G, Greene NDE, Copp AJ (2002). D-*chiro*-inositol is more effective than *myo*-inositol in preventing folate-resistant mouse neural tube defects. Hum Reprod 17:2451–2458.

Cohen-Tannoudji M, Babinet C (1998). Beyond "knock-out" mice: new perspectives for the programmed modification of the mammalian genome. Mol Hum Reprod 4:929–938.

Copp AJ (1985). Relationship between timing of posterior neuropore closure and development of spinal neural tube defects in mutant (*curly tail*) and normal mouse embryos in culture. J Embryol Exp Morphol 88:39–54.

Copp AJ (1995). Death before birth: clues from gene knockouts and mutations in the mouse. Trends Genet 11:87–93.

Copp AJ, Brook FA, Estibeiro JP, Shum ASW, Cockroft DL (1990). The embryonic development of mammalian neural tube defects. Prog Neurobiol 35:363–403.

Copp AJ, Brook FA, Roberts HJ (1988a). A cell-type-specific abnormality of cell proliferation in mutant (*curly tail*) mouse embryos developing spinal neural tube defects. Development 104:285–295.

Copp AJ, Checiu I, Henson JN (1994). Developmental basis of severe neural tube defects in the *loop-tail* (*Lp*) mutant mouse: use of microsatellite DNA markers to identify embryonic genotype. Dev Biol 165:20–29.

Copp AJ, Crolla JA, Brook FA (1988b). Prevention of spinal neural tube defects in the mouse embryo by growth retardation during neurulation. Development 104:297–303.

Copp AJ, Greene NDE, Murdoch JN (2003). The genetic basis of mammalian neurulation. Nat Rev Genet 4:784–793.

Cunningham D, Xiao Q, Chatterjee A, Sulik K, Juriloff D, Elder F, Harrison W, Schuster G, Overbeek PA, Herman GE (2002). *exma:* an X-linked insertional mutation that disrupts forebrain and eye development. Mamm Genome 13:179–185.

Curtin JA, Quint E, Tsipouri V, Arkell RM, Cattanach B, Copp AJ, Fisher EM, Nolan PM, Steel KP, Brown SDM, Gray IC, Murdoch JN (2003). Mutation of *Celsr1* disrupts planar polarity of inner ear hair cells and causes severe neural tube defects in the mouse. Curr Biol 13:1–20.

Darken RS, Scola AM, Rakeman AS, Das G, Mlodzik M, Wilson PA (2002). The planar polarity gene *strabismus* regulates convergent extension movements in *Xenopus.* EMBO J 21:976–985.

Deng CX, Bedford M, Li CL, Xu XL, Yang X, Dunmore J, Leder P (1997). Fibroblast growth factor receptor-1 (FGFR-1) is essential for normal neural tube and limb development. Dev Biol 185:42–54.

Dixon J, Brakebusch C, Fässler R, Dixon MJ (2000). Increased levels of apoptosis in the prefusion neural folds underlie the craniofacial disorder, Treacher Collins syndrome. Hum Mol Genet 9:1473–1480.

Donohoe ME, Zhang XL, McGinnis L, Biggers J, Li E, Shi Y (1999). Targeted disruption of mouse Yin Yang 1 transcription factor results in peri-implantation lethality. Mol Cell Biol 19:7237–7244.

Echelard Y, Epstein DJ, St-Jacques B, Shen L, Mohler J, McMahon JA, McMahon AP (1993). *Sonic hedgehog,* a member of a family of putative signaling molecules, is implicated in the regulation of CNS polarity. Cell 75:1417–1430.

Eggenschwiler JT, Espinoza E, Anderson KV (2001). Rab23 is an essential negative regulator of the mouse *Sonic hedgehog* signalling pathway. Nature 412:194–198.

Ellis HM, Horvitz HR (1986). Genetic control of programmed cell death in the nematode *C. elegans.* Cell 44:817–829.

Embury S, Seller MJ, Adinolfi M, Polani PE (1979). Neural tube defects in curly-tail mice. I. Incidence and expression. Proc R Soc Lond B 206:85–94.

Epstein DJ, Vekemans M, Gros P (1991). *splotch* (Sp^{2H}), a mutation affecting development of the mouse neural tube, shows a deletion within the paired homeodomain of Pax-3. Cell 67:767–774.

Essien FB, Haviland MB, Naidoff AE (1990). Expression of a new mutation (*Axd*) causing axial defects in mice correlates with maternal phenotype and age. Teratology 42:183–194.

Essien FB, Wannberg SL (1993). Methionine but not folinic acid or vitamin B_{12} alters the frequency of neural tube defects in *Axd* mutant mice. J Nutr 123:27–34.

Estibeiro JP, Brook FA, Copp AJ (1993). Interaction between splotch (*Sp*) and curly tail (*ct*) mouse mutants in the embryonic development of neural tube defects. Development 119:113–121.

Ewart JL, Cohen MF, Meyer RA, Huang GY, Wessels A, Gourdie RG, Chin AJ, Park SMJ, Lazatin BO, Villabon S, Lo CW (1997). Heart and neural tube defects in transgenic mice overexpressing the Cx43 gap junction gene. Development 124:1281–1292.

Farese RV Jr, Ruland SL, Flynn LM, Stokowski RP, Young SG (1995). Knockout of the mouse apolipoprotein B gene results in embryonic lethality in homozygotes and protection against diet-induced hypercholesterolemia in heterozygotes. Proc Natl Acad Sci USA 92:1774–1778.

Finnell RH, Bennett GD, Karras SB, Mohl VK (1988). Common hierarchies of susceptibility to the induction of neural tube defects in mouse embryos by valproic acid and its 4-propyl-4-pentenoic acid metabolite. Teratology 38:313–320.

Finnell RH, Moon SP, Abbott LC, Golden JA, Chernoff GF (1986). Strain differences in heat-induced neural tube defects in mice. Teratology 33:247–252.

Fisher E, Scambler P (1994). Human haploinsufficiency—one for sorrow, two for joy. Nature Genet 7:5–7.

Fleming A, Copp AJ (1998). Embryonic folate metabolism and mouse neural tube defects. Science 280:2107–2109.

Fleming A, Copp AJ (2000). A genetic risk factor for mouse neural tube defects: defining the embryonic basis. Hum Mol Genet 9:575–581.

Franz T (1994). Extra-toes (*Xt*) homozygous mutant mice demonstrate a role for the *Gli-3* gene in the development of the forebrain. Acta Anat 150:38–44.

Fundele RH, Norris ML, Barton SC, Fehlau M, Howlett SK, Mills WE, Surani MA (1990). Temporal and spatial selection against parthenogenetic cells during development of fetal chimeras. Development 108:203–211.

Gaiano N, Fishell G (2002). The role of Notch in promoting glial and neural stem cell fates. Annu Rev Neurosci 25:471–490.

Goodrich LV, Milenkovic L, Higgins KM, Scott MP (1997). Altered neural cell fates and medulloblastoma in mouse *patched* mutants. Science 277:1109–1113.

Goto T, Keller R (2002). The planar cell polarity gene *Strabismus* regulates convergence and extension and neural fold closure in *Xenopus*. Dev Biol 247:165–181.

Gowen LC, Johnson BL, Latour AM, Sulik KK, Koller BH (1996). *Brca1* deficiency results in early embryonic lethality characterized by neuroepithelial abnormalities. Nature Genet 12:191–194.

Greene NDE, Copp AJ (1997). Inositol prevents folate-resistant neural tube defects in the mouse. Nature Med 3:60–66.

Greene NDE, Gerrelli D, Van Straaten HWM, Copp AJ (1998). Abnormalities of floor plate, notochord and somite differentiation in the *loop-tail* (*Lp*) mouse: a model of severe neural tube defects. Mech Dev 73:59–72.

Günther T, Struwe M, Aguzzi A, Schughart K (1994). *open brain,* a new mouse mutant with severe neural tube defects, shows altered gene expression patterns in the developing spinal cord. Development 120:3119–3130.

Hakem R, Hakem A, Duncan GS, Henderson JT, Woo M, Soengas MS, Elia A, De la Pompa JL, Kagi D, Khoo W, Potter J, Yoshida R, Kaufman SA, Lowe SW, Penninger JM, Mak TW (1998). Differential requirement for caspase 9 in apoptotic pathways in vivo. Cell 94:339–352.

Hamblet NS, Lijam N, Ruiz-Lozano P, Wang J, Yang Y, Luo Z, Mei L, Chien KR, Sussman DJ, Wynshaw-Boris A (2002). *Dishevelled 2* is essential for cardiac outflow tract development, somite segmentation and neural tube closure. Development 129:5827–5838.

Harding BN, Copp AJ. (2002). Congenital malformations. In Graham Dl, Lantos PL (eds): *Greenfield's Neuropathology.* London: Arnold, pp. 357–483.

Harris BS, Franz T, Ullrich S, Cook S, Bronson RT, Davisson MT (1997). Forebrain overgrowth (*fog*): a new mutation in the mouse affecting neural tube development. Teratology 55:231–240.

Harris MJ, Juriloff DM (1997). Genetic landmarks for defects in mouse neural tube closure. Teratology 56:177–187.

Harris MJ, Juriloff DM (1999). Mini-review: toward understanding mechanisms of genetic neural tube defects in mice. Teratology 60:292–305.

Helwig U, Imai K, Schmahl W, Thomas BE, Varnum DS, Nadeau JH, Balling R (1995). Interaction between *undulated* and *Patch* leads to an extreme form of spina bifida in double-mutant mice. Nature Genet 11:60–63.

Herrera E, Samper E, Blasco MA (1999). Telomere shortening in mTR-/-embryos is associated with failure to close the neural tube. EMBO J 18:1172–1181.

Hildebrand JD, Soriano P (1999). *Shroom,* a PDZ domain-containing actin-binding protein, is required for neural tube morphogenesis in mice. Cell 99:485–497.

Hirata H, Tomita K, Bessho Y, Kageyama R (2001). *Hes1* and *Hes3* regulate maintenance of the isthmic organizer and development of the mid/hindbrain. EMBO J 20:4454–4466.

Holmberg J, Clarke DL, Frisén J (2000). Regulation of repulsion versus adhesion by different splice forms of an Eph receptor. Nature 408:203–206.

Homanics GE, Maeda N, Traber MG, Kayden HJ, Dehart DB, Sulik KK (1995). Exencephaly and hydrocephaly in mice with targeted modification of the apolipoprotein B (*Apob*) gene. Teratology 51:1–10.

Honarpour N, Gilbert SL, Lahn BT, Wang XD, Herz J (2001). *Apaf-1* deficiency and neural tube closure defects are found in fog mice. Proc Natl Acad Sci USA 98:9683–9687.

Hook EB, Czeizel AE (1997). Can terathanasia explain the protective effect of folic-acid supplementation on birth defects? Lancet 350:513–515.

Huang Y, Roelink H, McKnight GS (2002). Protein kinase A deficiency causes axially localized neural tube defects in mice. J Biol Chem 277:19889–19896.

Hui C, Joyner AL (1993). A mouse model of Greig cephalopolysyndactyly syndrome: the *extra-toes^J* mutation contains an intragenic deletion of the *Gli3* gene. Nature Genet 3:241–246.

Ikeda A, Ikeda S, Gridley T, Nishina PM, Naggert JK (2001). Neural tube defects and neuroepithelial cell death in *Tulp3* knockout mice. Hum Mol Genet 10:1325–1334.

Imamoto A, Soriano P (1993). Disruption of the *csk* gene, encoding a negative regulator of Src family tyrosine kinases, leads to neural tube defects and embryonic lethality in mice. Cell 73:1117–1124.

Ishibashi M, Ang S-L, Shiota K, Nakanishi S, Kageyama R, Guillemot F (1995). Targeted disruption of mammalian *hairy* and *Enhancer of split* homolog-1 (*HES-1*) leads to up-regulation of neural helix-loop-helix factors, premature neurogenesis, and severe neural tube defects. Genes Dev 9:3136–3148.

Jessen JR, Topczewski J, Bingham S, Sepich DS, Marlow F, Chandrasekhar A, Solnica-Krezel L (2002). Zebrafish trilobite identifies new roles for *Strabismus* in gastrulation and neuronal movements. Nat Cell Biol 4:610–615.

Johnson DR (1976). The interfrontal bone and mutant genes in the mouse. J Anat 121:507–513.

Joyner AL (1991). Gene targeting and gene trap screens using embryonic stem cells: new approaches to mammalian development. BioEssays 13:649–656.

Juriloff DM, Harris MJ (2000). Mouse models for neural tube closure defects. Hum Mol Genet 9:993–1000.

Juriloff DM, Harris MJ, Tom C, MacDonald KB (1991). Normal mouse strains differ in the site of initiation of closure of the cranial neural tube. Teratology 44:225–233.

Keller R, Davidson L, Edlund A, Elul T, Ezin M, Shook D, Skoglund P (2000). Mechanisms of convergence and extension by cell intercalation. Philos Trans R Soc Lond B:Biol Sci 355:897–922.

Klootwijk R, Franke B, Van der Zee CEEM, De Boer RT, Wilms W, Hol FA, Mariman ECM (2000). A deletion encompassing *Zic3* in Bent tail, a mouse model for X-linked neural tube defects. Hum Mol Genet 9:1615–1622.

Kohlbecker A, Lee AE, Schorle H (2002). Exencephaly in a subset of animals heterozygous for AP-2a mutation. Teratology 65:213–218.

Koleske AJ, Gifford AM, Scott ML, Nee M, Bronson RT, Miczek KA, Baltimore D (1998). Essential roles for the Abl and Arg tyrosine kinases in neurulation. Neuron 21:1259–1272.

Kuida K, Haydar TF, Kuan CY, Gu Y, Taya C, Karasuyama H, Su MS, Rakic P, Flavell RA (1998). Reduced apoptosis and cytochrome c–mediated caspase activation in mice lacking caspase 9. Cell 94:325–337.

Labosky PA, Winnier GE, Jetton TL, Hargett L, Ryan AK, Rosenfeld MG, Parlow AF, Hogan BLM (1997). The winged helix gene, *Mf3,* is required for normal development of the diencephalon and midbrain, postnatal growth and the milk-ejection reflex. Development 124:1263–1274.

Lakkis MM, Golden JA, O'Shea KS, Epstein JA (1999). Neurofibromin deficiency in mice causes exencephaly and is a modifier for *Splotch* neural tube defects. Dev Biol 212:80–92.

Lanier LM, Gates MA, Witke W, Menzies AS, Wehman AM, Macklis JD, Kwiatkowski D, Soriano P, Gertler FB (1999). Mena is required for neurulation and commissure formation. Neuron 22:313–325.

Lardelli M, Williams R, Mitsiadis T, Lendahl U (1996). Expression of the Notch 3 intracellular domain in mouse central nervous system progenitor cells is lethal and leads to disturbed neural tube development. Mech Dev 59:177–190.

Leid M, Kastner P, Chambon P (1992). Multiplicity generates diversity in the retinoic acid signalling pathways. Trends Biochem Sci 17:427–433.

Lohnes D, Mark M, Mendelsohn C, Dollé P, Dierich A, Gorry P, Gansmuller A, Chambon P (1994). Function of the retinoic acid receptors (RARs) during development. (I) Craniofacial and skeletal abnormalities in RAR double mutants. Development 120:2723–2748.

Lomaga MA, Henderson JT, Elia AJ, Robertson J, Noyce RS, Yeh WC, Mak TW (2000). Tumor necrosis factor receptor-associated factor 6 (TRAF6) deficiency results in exencephaly and is required for apoptosis within the developing CNS. J Neurosci 20:7384–7393.

Lyon MF, Quinney R, Glenister PH, Kerscher S, Guillot P, Boyd Y (1996). *Doublefoot:* a new mouse mutant affecting development of limbs and head. Genet Res 68:221–231.

Mansouri A, Gruss P (1998). Pax3 and Pax7 are expressed in commissural neurons and restrict ventral neuronal identity in the spinal cord. Mech Dev 78:171–178.

Martinez-Barbera JP, Rodriguez TA, Greene NDE, Weninger WJ, Simeone A, Copp AJ, Beddington R, Dunwoodie S (2002). Folic acid prevents exencephaly in *Cited2* deficient mice. Hum Mol Genet 11:283–293.

McMahon JA, Takada S, Zimmerman LB, Fan CM, Harland RM, McMahon AP (1998). Noggin-mediated antagonism of BMP signaling is required for growth and patterning of the neural tube and somite. Genes Dev 12:1438–1452.

Melloy PG, Ewart JL, Cohen MF, Desmond ME, Kuehn MR, Lo CW (1998). No *turning,* a mouse mutation causing left-right and axial patterning defects. Dev Biol 193:77–89.

Migliorini D, Denchi EL, Danovi D, Jochemsen A, Capillo M, Gobbi A, Helin K, Pelicci PG, Marine JC (2002). *Mdm4* (*Mdmx*) regulates *p53*-induced growth arrest and neuronal cell death during early embryonic mouse development. Mol Cell Biol 22:5527–5538.

Milenkovic L, Goodrich LV, Higgins KM, Scott MP (1999). Mouse *patched1* controls body size determination and limb patterning. Development 126:4431–4440.

Miner JH, Cunningham J, Sanes JR (1998). Roles for laminin in embryogenesis: exencephaly, syndactyly, and placentopathy in mice lacking the laminin alpha5 chain. J Cell Biol 143:1713–1723.

Montcouquioi M, Rachel RA, Lanford PJ, Copeland NG, Jenkins NA, Kelley MW (2003). Identification of *Vangl2* and *Scrb1* as planar polarity genes in mammals. Nature 423:173–177.

Morrison-Graham K, Schatteman GC, Bork T, Bowen-Pope DF, Weston JA (1992). A PDGF receptor mutation in the mouse (*Patch*) perturbs the development of a non-neuronal subset of neural crest- derived cells. Development 115:133–142.

Murdoch JN, Doudney K, Paternotte C, Copp AJ, Stanier P (2001a). Severe neural tube defects in the *loop-tail* mouse result from mutation of *Lpp1,* a novel gene involved in floor plate specification. Hum Mol Genet 10:2593–2601.

Murdoch JN, Henderson DJ, Doudney K, Gaston-Massuet C, Phillips HM, Paternotte C, Arkell R, Stanier P, Copp AJ (2003). Disruption of *scribble* (*Scrb1*) causes severe neural tube defects in the *circletail* mouse. Hum Mol Genet 12:87–98.

Murdoch JN, Rachel RA, Shah S, Beermann F, Stanier P, Mason CA, Copp AJ (2001b). *Circletail,* a new mouse mutant with severe neural tube defects: chromosomal localisation and interaction with the *loop-tail* mutation. Genomics 78:55–63.

Nagai T, Aruga J, Minowa O, Sugimoto T, Ohno Y, Noda T, Mikoshiba K (2000). *Zic2* regulates the kinetics of neurulation. Proc Natl Acad Sci USA 97:1618–1623.

Nait-Oumesmar B, Stecca B, Fatterpekar G, Naidich T, Corbin J, Lazzarini RA (2002). Ectopic expression of *Gcm1* induces congenital spinal cord abnormalities. Development 129:3957–3964.

Naus CCG, Bani-Yaghoub M (1998). Gap junctional communication in the developing central nervous system. Cell Biol Int 22:751–763.

Neumann PE, Frankel WN, Letts VA, Coffin JM, Copp AJ, Bernfield M (1994). Multifactorial inheritance of neural tube defects: localization of the major gene and recognition of modifiers in *ct* mutant mice. Nature Genet 6:357–362.

New DAT (1978). Whole-embryo culture and the study of mammalian embryos during organogenesis. Biol Rev 53:81–122.

Niederreither K, Abu-Abed S, Schuhbaur B, Petkovich M, Chambon P, Dollé P (2002). Genetic evidence that oxidative derivatives of retinoic acid are not involved in retinoid signaling during mouse development. Nature Genet 31:84–88.

Nonaka S, Tanaka Y, Okada Y, Takeda S, Harada A, Kanai Y, Kido M, Hirokawa N (1998). Randomization of left-right asymmetry due to loss of nodal cilia generating leftward flow of extraembryonic fluid in mice lacking KIF3B motor protein. Cell 95:829–837.

Oka C, Nakano T, Wakeham A, De la Pompa JL, Mori C, Sakai T, Okazaki S, Kawaichi M, Shiota K, Mak TW, Honjo T (1995). Disruption of the mouse *RBP-J* kappa gene results in early embryonic death. Development 121:3291–3301.

Okano M, Bell DW, Haber DA, Li E (1999). DNA methyltransferases Dnmt3a and Dnmt3b are essential for de novo methylation and mammalian development. Cell 99:247–257.

Park M, Moon RT (2001). The planar cell-polarity gene *stbm* regulates cell behaviour and cell fate in vertebrate embryos. Nat Cell Biol 4:20–25.

Peeters MCE, Schutte B, Lenders MHJN, Hekking JWM, Drukker J, Van Straaten HWM (1998). Role of differential cell proliferation in the tail bud in aberrant mouse neurulation. Dev Dyn 211:382–389.

Piedrahita JA, Oetama B, Bennett GD, Van Waes J, Kamen BA, Richardson J, Lacey SW, Anderson RGW, Finnell RH (1999). Mice lacking the folic acid–binding protein *Folbp1* are defective in early embryonic development. Nature Genet 23:228–232.

Purandare SM, Ware SM, Kwan KM, Gebbia M, Bassi MT, Deng JM, Vogel H, Behringer RR, Belmont JW, Casey B (2002). A complex syndrome of left-right axis, central nervous system and axial skeleton defects in *Zic3* mutant mice. Development 129:2293–2302.

Rauch F, Prud'homme J, Arabian A, Dedhar S, St-Arnaud R (2000). Heart, brain, and body wall defects in mice lacking calreticulin. Exp Cell Res 256:105–111.

Regnier CH, Masson R, Kedinger V, Textoris J, Stoll I, Chenard MP, Dierich A, Tomasetto C, Rio MC (2002). Impaired neural tube closure, axial skeleton malformations, and tracheal ring disruption in TRAF4-deficient mice. Proc Natl Acad Sci USA 99:5585–5590.

Rogner UC, Spyropoulos DD, Le Novère N, Changeux JP, Avner P (2000). Control of neurulation by the nucleosome assembly protein-1-like. Nature Genet 25:431–435.

Ruland J, Duncan GS, Elia A, Barrantes ID, Nguyen L, Plyte S, Millar DG, Bouchard D, Wakeham A, Ohashi PS, Mak TW (2001). Bcl10 is a positive regulator of antigen receptor-induced activation of NF-kappaB and neural tube closure. Cell 104:33–42.

Sabapathy K, Jochum W, Hochedlinger K, Chang LF, Karin M, Wagner EF (1999). Defective neural tube morphogenesis and altered apoptosis in the absence of both *JNK1* and *JNK2*. Mech Dev 89:115–124.

Sadler TW (1980). Effects of maternal diabetes on early embryogenesis: II. Hyperglycemia-induced exencephaly. Teratology 21:349–356.

Sah VP, Attardi LD, Mulligan GJ, Williams BO, Bronson RT, Jacks T (1995). A subset of *p53*-deficient embryos exhibit exencephaly. Nature Genet 10:175–180.

Sakai Y, Meno C, Fujii H, Nishino J, Shiratori H, Saijoh Y, Rossant J, Hamada H (2001). The retinoic acid–inactivating enzyme CYP26 is essential for establishing an uneven distribution of retinoic acid along the anterio-posterior axis within the mouse embryo. Genes Dev 15:213–225.

Schorle H, Meier P, Buchert M, Jaenisch R, Mitchell PJ (1996). Transcription factor AP-2 essential for cranial closure and craniofacial development. Nature 381:235–238.

Seller MJ (1994). Vitamins, folic acid and the cause and prevention of neural tube defects. In Bock G, Marsh J (eds): *Neural Tube Defects.* Ciba Foundation Symposium 181. Chichester: Wiley, pp. 161–173.

Seller MJ, Embury S, Polani PE, Adinolfi M (1979). Neural tube defects in curly-tail mice. II. Effect of maternal administration of vitamin A. Proc R Soc Lond B 206:95–107.

Seller MJ, Perkins KJ (1986). Effect of mitomycin C on the neural tube defects of the *curly-tail* mouse. Teratology 33:305–309.

Shen AL, O'Leary KA, Kasper CB (2002). Association of multiple developmental defects and embryonic lethality with loss of microsomal NADPH-cytochrome P450 oxidoreductase. J Biol Chem 277:6536–6541.

Shenefelt RE (1972). Morphogenesis of malformations in hamster caused by retinoic acid: relation to dose and stage at treatment. Teratology 5:103–108.

Shou WN, Aghdasi B, Armstrong DL, Guo QX, Bao SD, Charng MJ, Mathews LM, Schneider MD, Hamilton SL, Matzuk MM (1998). Cardiac defects and altered ryanodine receptor function in mice lacking FKBP12. Nature 391:489–492.

Smitherman M, Lee K, Swanger J, Kapur R, Clurman BE (2000). Characterization and targeted disruption of murine Nup50, a p27(Kip1)-interacting component of the nuclear pore complex. Mol Cell Biol 20:5631–5642.

Solloway MJ, Robertson EJ (1999). Early embryonic lethality in *Bmp5;Bmp7* double mutant mice suggests functional redundancy within the 60A subgroup. Development 126:1753–1768.

Soriano P (1997). The PDGFa receptor is required for neural crest cell development and for normal patterning of the somites. Development 124:2691–2700.

Stiefel D, Shibata T, Meuli M, Duffy P, Copp AJ (2003). Tethering of the spinal cord in mouse fetuses and neonates with spina bifida. J Neurosurg (Spine) 99:206–213.

Strong LC, Hollander WF (1949). Hereditary loop-tail in the house mouse. J Hered 40:329–334.

Stumpo DJ, Bock CB, Tuttle JS, Blackshear PJ (1995). MARCKS deficiency in mice leads to abnormal brain development and perinatal death. Proc Natl Acad Sci USA 92:944–948.

Swiergiel JJ, Funderburgh JL, Justice MJ, Conrad GW (2000). Developmental eye and neural tube defects in the *eye blebs* mouse. Dev Dyn 219:21–27.

Takada S, Stark KL, Shea MJ, Vassileva G, McMahon JA, McMahon AP (1994). *Wnt-3a* regulates somite and tailbud formation in the mouse embryo. Genes Dev 8:174–189.

Takeuchi T, Kojima M, Nakajima K, Kondo S (1999). *jumonji* gene is essential for the neurulation and cardiac development of mouse embryos with a C3H/He background. Mech Dev 86:29–38.

Takeuchi T, Yamazaki Y, Katoh-Fukui Y, Tsuchiya R, Kondo S, Motoyama J, Higashinakagawa T (1995). Gene trap capture of a novel mouse gene, *jumonji,* required for neural tube formation. Genes Dev 9:1211–1222.

Theiler K, Stevens LC (1960). The development of rib fusions, a mutation in the house mouse. Am J Anat 106:171–183.

Van Straaten HWM, Copp AJ (2001). Curly tail: a 50-year history of the mouse spina bifida model. Anat Embryol 203:225–237.

Van Straaten HWM, Hekking JWM, Copp AJ, Bernfield M (1992). Deceleration and acceleration in the rate of posterior neuropore closure during neurulation in the *curly tail* (*ct*) mouse embryo. Anat Embryol 185:169–174.

Varnum DS, Fox SC (1981). Head blebs: a new mutation on chromosome 4 of the mouse. J Hered 72:293.

Wallace ME, Knights PJ, Anderson JR (1978). Inheritance and morphology of exencephaly, a neonatal recessive with partial penetrance, in the house mouse. Genet Res 32:135–149.

Wallingford JB, Harland RM (2001). *Xenopus Dishevelled* signaling regulates both neural and mesodermal convergent extension: parallel forces elongating the body axis. Development 128:2581–2592.

Wallingford JB, Harland RM (2002). Neural tube closure requires *Dishevelled*-dependent convergent extension of the midline. Development 129:5815–5825.

Wechsler-Reya RJ (2001). Caught in the matrix: how vitronectin controls neuronal differentiation. Trends Neurosci 24:680–682.

Wilson DB, Wyatt DP (1986). Pathogenesis of neural dysraphism in the mouse mutant vacuolated lens (*vl*). J Neuropathol Exp Neurol 45:43–55.

Winograd J, Reilly MP, Roe R, Lutz J, Laughner E, Xu X, Hu L, Asakura T, Vander Kolk C, Strandberg JD, Semenza GL (1997). Perinatal lethality and multiple craniofacial malformations in *MSX2* transgenic mice. Hum Mol Genet 6:369–379.

Wood LR, Smith MT (1984). Generation of anencephaly: 1. Aberrant neurulation and 2. Conversion of exencephaly to anencephaly. J Neuropathol Exp Neurol 43:620–633.

Wu M, Chen DF, Sasaoka T, Tonegawa S (1996). Neural tube defects and abnormal brain development in F52-deficient mice. Proc Natl Acad Sci USA 93:2110–2115.

Xu WM, Baribault H, Adamson ED (1998). Vinculin knockout results in heart and brain defects during embryonic development. Development 125:327–337.

Yao TP, Oh SP, Fuchs M, Zhou ND, Ch'ng LE, Newsome D, Bronson RT, Li E, Livingston DM, Eckner R (1998). Gene dosage–dependent embryonic development and proliferation defects in mice lacking the transcriptional integrator p300. Cell 93:361–372.

Yin Z, Haynie J, Yang XM, Han BG, Kiatchoosakun S, Restivo J, Yuan SY, Prabhakar NR, Herrup K, Conlon RA, Hoit BD, Watanabe M, Yang YC (2002). The essential role of *Cited2*, a negative regulator for HIF-1a, in heart development and neurulation. Proc Natl Acad Sci USA 99:10488–10493.

Yoshida H, Kong YY, Yoshida R, Elia AJ, Hakem A, Hakem R, Penninger JM, Mak TW (1998). *Apaf1* is required for mitochondrial pathways of apoptosis and brain development. Cell 94:739–750.

Zeng L, Fagotto F, Zhang T, Hsu W, Vasicek TJ, Perry WL III, Lee JJ, Tilghman SM, Gumbiner BM, Costantini F (1997). The mouse fused locus encodes Axin, an inhibitor of the Wnt signaling pathway that regulates embryonic axis formation. Cell 90:181–192.

Zhang J, Hagopian-Donaldson S, Serbedzija G, Elsemore J, Plehn-Dujowich D, McMahon AP, Flavell RA, Williams T (1996). Neural tube, skeletal and body wall defects in mice lacking transcription factor AP-2. Nature 381:238–241.

Zhao Q, Behringer RR, De Crombrugghe B (1996). Prenatal folic acid treatment suppresses acrania and meroanencephaly in mice mutant for the *Cart1* homeobox gene. Nature Genet 13:275–283.

Zhong WM, Jiang MM, Schonemann MD, Meneses JJ, Pedersen RA, Jan LY, Jan YN (2000). Mouse *numb* is an essential gene involved in cortical neurogenesis. Proc Natl Acad Sci USA 97:6844–6849.

II

TREATMENT AND EDUCATION

18

Fetal Surgery for Myelomeningocele

KELLY A. BENNETT
GEORGE H. DAVIS
NOEL TULIPAN
JOSEPH P. BRUNER

Open fetal surgery was first performed in the 1980s (Crombleholme et al., 1988; Langer et al., 1989) following preliminary studies in animal models. Because the potential risks were significant and the likelihood of success was uncertain, these early open procedures were confined to the treatment of lethal malformations. As experience with the open technique improved, and as the maternal and fetal risks became better understood, intervention in nonlethal circumstances was considered (Harrison, 2001). Among these, the rationale for intervention in cases of myelomeningocele was among the easiest to make (Tulipan et al., 1999a).

Myelomeningocele is a congenital defect of the spine and spinal cord resulting from incomplete closure of the neural tube during the fourth week of fetal life. In most cases, it is associated with a Chiari type II malformation. Current neonatal management consists of prompt closure of the defect in an attempt to prevent further injury to the exposed neural elements. However, a growing body of experimental evidence from both animal and human studies suggests that antenatal repair of myelomeningocele potentially may help to preserve neurological function that might otherwise be lost during gestation, and to prevent or reverse elements of the spectrum of deformity responsible for much of the morbidity and mortality of this condition.

Building on several years of clinical and laboratory experience, a surgical procedure for intrauterine repair of myelomeningocele was developed at a small number of centers in the United States (Tulipan et al., 1999a). Preliminary evidence suggests that this procedure restores the cerebellum and brainstem to a more normal configuration, thus reducing the incidence of shunt-dependent hydrocephalus. Its benefit in preserving neurological function in the lower extremities as well as continence remains, at present, inconclusive. However, the surgery is not without risk to both the mother and the fetus, and it remains to be proved whether the benefits outweigh these risks.

CLINICAL MANIFESTATIONS OF MYELOMENINGOCELE

Open neural tube defects arise by failure of appropriate closure of the neural tube by the 28th day of embryonic development. The most common deformities at birth are myelomeningocele, characterized by the presence of a fluid-filled sac in the posterior midline that contains the herniated spinal cord, and myeloschisis, an open defect without a sac through which the spinal cord is exposed to the external environment. Less commonly, a deformity of similar origin can present as a meningocele, in which the neural tube is closed only by a thin, membranous covering but without involvement of neural elements. The spectrum and severity of deformities and neurological deficits correspond to the spinal cord level of the lesion, as well as to the extent of injury to the cord during pregnancy, birth, and development.

Incidence

Open neural tube defects are the most common congenital anomalies of the central nervous system, affecting approximately 1500 to 2000 fetuses annually, or 1 in every 2000 live births in the United States (March of Dimes, 2003), half of which are represented by myelomeningocele. The incidence of neural tube defects has seen a decreasing trend throughout the 1990s, with a 24% reduction in myelomeningocele specifically between 1996 and 2001 (Mathews et al., 2002). Undoubtedly, some of these gains are the result of improving public education about the preventive effect of folic acid supplementation. Another important source of this trend is likely to be the increasing reliance on prenatal diagnosis, leading some prospective parents to choose elective termination of pregnancy.

Burden of Illness

Societal and Economic Costs. The economic cost of caring for affected individuals was estimated at $480 million per year in 1999 (Bentley et al., 1999), and it can be expected to increase as the overall cost of delivering health care continued to rise sharply throughout the 1990s and into the new millennium. Substantial additional costs undoubtedly are incurred by families caring for children with myelomeningocele in terms of actual health-care expenditures, as well as lost income from employment and other opportunities not realized.

Life Expectancy. Myelomeningocele is associated with an infant mortality rate of approximately 10% (Shurtleff et al., 1994; Hunt, 1997). In a retrospective review of 101 children with myelomeningocele treated at a single institution between 1971 and 1981, 83 (82%) of the original patients considered were alive at an average follow-up period of over 13 years (range, 9–20 years) (Steinbok et al., 1992). Of 18 deaths in the complete cohort, 11 (61%) occurred during the first year of life. These patients constitute a heterogeneous group treated in a nonstandardized fashion on an individual basis, according to accepted practices of the era. The highest mortality rates were noted in the subset of patients selected to receive nonaggressive treatment, with 11 deaths among 21 patients who did not undergo repair of myelomeningocele (52%). Mortality was shown to decrease with age at repair, with only 2 deaths among 57 patients (3%) repaired in the first 48 hours of life. Other investigators have observed similar outcomes, with a mortality rate of approximately 14% by the age of 5 years in a cohort of 63 neonates with myelomeningocele (Worley et al., 1996). The observed mortality rates serve to confirm that myelomeningocele should be considered a nonfatal disorder; however, survivors are subject to any of several important lifelong disabilities and other sources of morbidity occurring throughout the developmental period and into adulthood.

Effects in Childhood and Development. The majority of neonates born with myelomeningocele will survive into childhood and beyond, but often will be afflicted with a constellation of important problems that will leave them at lifelong need for comprehensive care by specialists in neurosurgery, urology, orthopedics, plastic surgery, and pediatrics or general medicine. Their care will also often require the involvement of nursing specialists, occupational therapists and physiotherapists, and social workers. The care burden placed on an affected individual's family can be considerable and, in a minority of cases, may be manageable only by institutionalization. The following sections review the spectrum of clinical problems that may often be encountered in myelomeningocele, with a view to providing a framework from which to assess the results of antenatal surgical therapy.

Hindbrain herniation and hydrocephalus. It has been demonstrated that 80%–90% of children born with myelomeningocele also are affected with hindbrain herniation, an element of the Arnold-Chiari type II malformation (herniation of the cerebellar vermis, posterior cerebral hemispheres, and fourth ventricle through the foramen magnum), with kinking of the brainstem, "beaking" of the tectum, polygyria, a large massa intermedia, a small posterior cranial fossa, and luckenschadel of the skull (Rauzzino and Oakess, 1995). According to the most widely accepted theory, hindbrain herniation occurs in the setting of myelomeningocele as a result of an abnormal configuration of the hydrostatic forces within the cerebral ventricular system (McLone and Knepper, 1989). Loss of cerebrospinal fluid into the amniotic space results in collapse of the rhombencephalic vesicle. With a reduction in cerebrospinal fluid hydrodynamic pressure, which is essential to effective cranial molding, decreased filling of the ventricles results in a constriction of posterior fossa volume and ultimately leads to herniation of its contents.

Hindbrain herniation is symptomatic in approximately 20% of patients. Typically, it results from compression of the medulla oblongata and lower cranial nerves. Symptoms may include apnea, stridor, loss of the gag reflex, and respiratory arrest. Hydrocephalus with hindbrain herniation is thus the leading cause of death in children with myelomeningocele, with one-third to one-half of symptomatic patients dying from it, usually within the first 2 years of life (Rauzzino and Oakes, 1995; Worley et al., 1996; Bruner et al., 2001). Relief of upstream pressure within the cerebral ventricles, and thereby of herniation, is thus the focus of treatment for symptomatic patients. This can be effectively accomplished by ventriculoperitoneal shunting. Shunt dependence nonetheless carries a complication rate that is considerable, with an estimated yearly mortality risk of 1%, and constitutes an ongoing source of morbidity (Iskander et al., 1998).

In the review of 101 children with myelomeningocele described above, 93 were documented to have hydrocephalus, with 85 (84%) requiring ventriculoperitoneal shunting (Steinbok et al., 1992). Of these, 14% required no revisions, 54% between one and three shunt revisions for shunt dysfunction, and 32% more than three revisions. Most of these became necessary during the first year of life. The risk of central nervous system infection was 5% per shunt operation performed. The most common neurosurgical problem unrelated to hydrocephalus and shunting was tethered cord syndrome, requiring surgery in 13 patients.

Motor function and deformity. Motor ability in the lower extremities, and specifically the ability to walk, is importantly related to the spinal level of the lesion, with higher lesions producing a greater degree of disability. Of 83 surviving patients in the series considered, 48 (58%) were at one time able to ambulate without a wheelchair, but only 44 (53%) chose to do so (Steinbok et al., 1992). Four preferred to use a wheelchair due to social pressures, obesity, or a need for faster mobility. Twenty ambulators (24% of all survivors) could walk without aids, while 24 (29%) required various orthoses, braces, or walkers. The spinal level of the lesion, particularly quadriceps function, was an important determinant of walking ability, being present in 45 of 48 ambulators (94%) and in only three of 35 nonambulators (9%). Kyphosis or scoliosis was present in 42% of patients, and 16 required treatment with orthopedic instrumentation. Other deformations of the lower extremities, such as congenital clubfoot or joint contractures, may also occur. These data reflect the outcomes of children treated by a variety of means from 1971 to 1981. Certain more recent estimates suggest that with appropriate physical therapy begun at an early age, approximately 70% of children with myelomeningocele will be able to learn to walk, usually with the assistance of braces or crutches (March of Dimes, 2003). Newer estimates may reflect certain improvements in treatment, but the bias introduced by the increasing reliance on prenatal diagnosis and elective termination of pregnancy should also be considered.

Continence. Social continence of urine, defined as being dry most of the time without the use of a diaper, was achieved in 62 (75%) of 83 survivors, with 51 using intermittent catheterization (Steinbok et al., 1992). Thirty-seven of these used oxybutinin hydrochloride to assist urinary function, and 49 took prophylactic antibiotics, usually trimethoprim-sulfamethoxazole. Seventy-one (86%) were socially continent of stool, with 31 requiring no special additional techniques.

Cognitive function. In approximately 90% of children with myelomeningocele, hindbrain herniation will lead to hydrocephalus, which, if untreated, can lead to severe developmental delay with reduction in cognitive abilities or other neurological damage (March of Dimes, 2003). This deterioration of cognitive function can often be prevented with ventriculoperitoneal shunting such that patients with functioning shunts can often expect relatively normal cerebral development and cognitive function. Using school performance as an index of intellectual function, the review described above (Steinbok et al., 1992) reported that 48 survivors (58%) were attending or had attended normal classes at a grade level appropriate to their age, with some learning difficulties present in 19 (23%). Thirty-three (40%) were not at a grade-appropriate level or were in special classes. In another examination of the long-term outcome in a cohort of 117 neonates with myelomeningocele treated unselectively during the 1960s, it was demonstrated that 68% of long-term survivors (older than 16 years) had an IQ above 80 but that learning disabilities were common, with only 48% able to live without external assistance or supervision and only 25% being employable (Hunt, 1990). With improvements in treatment over the subsequent decades, especially the use of early closure of the spinal defect and improvements in ventriculoperitoneal shunting, it is probable that more favorable results can be expected from similar studies with long-term follow-up.

UTERINE ENVIRONMENT AND EFFECTS ON THE FETUS

Sonographic observations of fetuses with myelomeningocele early in gestation have revealed that lower extremity movement can be present as late as the 17th week of gestation and ceases thereafter (Epstein et al., 1976). It is therefore reasonable to postulate that the etiological forces that lead to the typical neural tissue destruction and dysfunction produce their effect at a later stage of development. Early thinking on the etiology of spinal dysraphism centered on the belief that the clinical findings of myelomeningocele were a product of an overall pattern of ineffective neurulation. Experiments in fetal monkeys (Michejda, 1984), rats (Heffez et al., 1990), pigs (Heffez et al., 1993), and sheep (Meuli et al., 1995a, 1995b; 1996) have demonstrated morphological changes in the spinal cords of animals that underwent surgically induced spinal dysraphism similar to those observed in human infants with myelomeningocele (Meuli et al., 1997), as well as a typical spectrum of neurological dysfunction and deformity, as seen in affected human children. Rather than suggesting that a predetermined congenital myelodysplasia exists in children with myelomeningocele, these studies implicate exposure of the developing spinal cord to the amniotic fluid environment as a cause of the development of damage to the cord. Several theories have been advanced to explain these findings, centering principally on three possible elements that may have an etiological role in degeneration of the spinal cord: potentially toxic products in amniotic fluid, erosive changes from direct trauma, and disruption of normal growth due to altered mechanical forces (Heffez et al., 1993; Meuli et al., 1995a, 1996).

Amniotic fluid is known to become more hypotonic and hyponatremic after the 20th week of gestation and may therefore possibly lead to osmotic swelling in exposed neural tissue (Drewek et al., 1997; Tubbs et al., 2003). Fetal urine makes an increasing contribution to amniotic fluid production as pregnancy advances. This may lead to a substantial increase in the amniotic concentration of urea and uric acid (Lind, 1978). An additional element that may implicate an environmental cause occurring during fetal development, rather than an innate congenital one, includes the successful surgical creation of animal models of myelomeningocele whose lesions resemble, grossly and histologically, those found in affected human fetuses and whose spectrum of disability mirrors that of human patients.

HISTORY/DEVELOPMENT OF FETAL SURGERY

Laboratory and Animal Studies

Early investigations included a study in which a myelomeningocele model in *Macaca mulatta* fetuses was created in eight animals by performing intrauterine lumbar laminectomy (L3–L5) and displacing the spinal cord from the central canal (Michejda, 1984). Five fetuses underwent in utero repair of the lesion, including a repair of the bony defect with allogeneic bone paste and reapproximation of soft tissues and skin over the lesion. Neonatal animals were assessed for neurological function and subsequently for morphological changes after cesarean delivery at near term. The three control animals whose lumbar lesions were left open demonstrated lower extremity paraplegia, somatosensory loss, and incontinence, as well as morphological degeneration of the spinal cord, while the five animals that had undergone repair showed normal neurological function.

While the lower extremity paralysis seen in myelomeningocele has at times widely been viewed as arising from congenital dysplasia of the spinal cord, histological studies of the spinal cords of children born with myelomeningocele have demonstrated erosions and necrosis of neural elements. This has led to a *two-hit* hypothesis wherein the effects of congenital myelodysplasia are augmented by the abnormal exposure to the amniotic fluid environment to produce injury to the spinal cord. In an experiment in fetal rats, a myelomeningocele model was created in utero by performing a dorsal midline skin incision, a two- to three-level laminectomy, and opening of the dura over the spinal cord, taking care to avoid injury to the cord itself (Heffez et al., 1990). In the experimental group wounds were left open, while in control animals the skin wound was then reclosed over the exposed cord. Fourteen experimental and nine control pups were liveborn, and were evaluated for motor function and wound healing. All animals left with an open spinal defect demonstrated some neurological impairment and deformity of the hindlimbs and tail, and had a persistently open spinal wound with exposure of the cord. One of these demonstrated severe kyphosis. In contrast, six control pups showed a completely healed wound at the surgical site and had normal motor function without deformity. In addition, three pups from the control group had suffered a dehiscence of their wounds, thus exposing the spinal cord to the amniotic fluid environment, and demonstrated weakness or deformity of the hindlimbs. On histological examination of spinal cord sections from experimental animals and from those having suffered wound dehiscence, prominent and extensive erosion and necrosis of the cord was evident. These findings were apparent in animals sacrificed as early as 48 hours after surgical creation of the open spinal defect. Sections from control animals, in contrast, showed no acute inflammatory response and essentially normal neural architecture.

In a related study, laminectomies were performed in fetal rats and pigs (Heffez et al., 1993). Compared with control pups that had their spinal wounds left open, experimental rat pups that underwent delayed primary closure after 1 day of exposure to the amniotic fluid environment showed partial protection from the deleterious effects of this exposure, with five of nine liveborn pups appearing entirely normal and four showing mild or moderate deformities and weakness of the hindlimbs and tail. In order to clarify the relative role of toxic exposure versus mechanical trauma, investigators sought to provide a mechanical barrier against trauma while still exposing the spinal cord to diffusible toxic components of the amniotic fluid. Accordingly, one group of eight pups underwent immediate closure of their wounds with a patch of peritoneum from the mother's abdominal wall. These pups demonstrated a lesser degree of spinal cord injury than that found in control pups, with two pups being grossly normal and six demonstrating less severe neurological deficits, deformities of the hindlimbs and tail, and histological damage. In fetal pigs, the experimental group was treated by coverage of the spinal wound with a patch of human cadaveric dura. In four control piglets, three demonstrated motor or sensory deficits without significant external deformity, while one was stillborn. Each of these demonstrated moderate or severe dorsal erosion of the spinal cord on histological examination. One piglet from the experimental group had dehiscence of the patch from the margin of the wound, allowing amniotic fluid exposure, and showed severe hindlimb deformities and spinal cord erosion. The two remaining liveborn experimental piglets showed well-healed wounds without sensory deficit, hindquarter deformity, or significant spinal cord erosion. These findings serve to consolidate further the hypothesis that the findings typical of myelomeningocele are created during intrauterine life as a result of the abnormal exposure of the spinal cord. However, they continue to allow that several elements may still contribute in varying degrees to damaging the developing spinal cord.

In order to better simulate spontaneous dysraphism, investigators in one study performed consecutive fetal surgery procedures in lambs with the surgical creation of a spinal lesion at midgestation (75 days' gestation), followed by definitive closure of the lesion 25 days later (Meuli et al., 1996). Of 12 lambs operated on in the initial creation of the model, 7 survived to undergo experimental closure of their spinal defect at 100 days' gestation. Four of these died in utero or were aborted. The three surviving lambs showed healed skin wounds. They demonstrated mild paraparesis but were able to stand, walk, and perform certain motor tests, and no incontinence was noted. Sensory function of the hindlimbs was preserved, as demonstrated by physical examination and electrophysiological testing. Histological examination of the spinal cord at the level of the lesion demonstrated deformation, but also revealed evidence of preservation of the expected gross structural landmarks and cytoarchitecture. This experiment confirms the potential for preventing degeneration of the structure and function of the spinal cord with antenatal repair of myelomeningocele but highlights the significant risk of fetal demise, with an average mortality rate of approximately 50% per operative stage.

In the majority of children born with myelomeningocele, the Arnold-Chiari type II malformation is present, with characteristic hydrocephalus and hindbrain herniation (Tulipan et al., 1998; Sutton et al., 1999). Hydrocephalus complicated by hindbrain herniation requires treatment with ventriculoperitoneal shunting in over 90% of children affected, an important source of morbidity, and is the principal cause of death in these children (Ruge et al., 1992). While prior animal experimentation had demonstrated that in utero repair of myelomeningocele preserved spinal cord morphology and distal neurological function and prevented deformity, investigators sought to determine whether repair had a beneficial effect on hindbrain herniation and hydrocephalus. In a fetal lamb model of myelomeningocele, 10 lambs at 75 days' gestation (the duration of term gestation is 147 days) underwent surgery as previously described, but with a modification of technique to open the central canal of the spinal cord, allowing free leakage of cerebrospinal fluid into the amniotic fluid environment (Paek et al., 2000). Six control and experimental animals survived to full term and were compared to a cohort of unoperated normal lambs. Of the six, a control group of two lambs had undergone creation of myelomeningocele, followed by sham surgery at 100 days' gestation. Both developed severe hindbrain herniation, as defined by herniation of the medulla oblongata and cerebellar vermis through the foramen magnum. In the experimental group, four fetuses had undergone in utero repair of myelomeningocele at 100 days' gestation. The lesion in one lamb was repaired in a standard fashion by a pediatric neurosurgeon and a pediatric plastic surgeon experienced in postnatal repair of myelomeningocele, while in the other three, spinal wounds were simply covered with Alloderm (LifeCell Corporation, Branchburg, NJ), an acellular cadaveric dermal allograft. No evidence of hindbrain herniation was noted in any of these animals, and magnetic resonance imaging confirmed the absence of hydrocephalus in all cases.

Certain investigators have explored the use of closure techniques as an alternative to the standard straightforward advancement and closure or bilateral bipedicled skin and subcutaneous tissue flap approach described below. As seen above, the use of exogenous biocompatible materials (such as an acellular dermal allograft) is a potentially successful approach to correcting this disorder using an in utero surgical approach. Other techniques have also been explored. In an experimental model of surgically created myelomeningocele in fetal sheep, the latissimus dorsi muscle flap was used to repair the lumbar spinal defect. Of the seven fetuses operated on, three survived to term. Among liveborn lambs, complete healing of the cutaneous wound was noted. More importantly, these lambs demonstrated normal function of the hindlimbs (Mueli-Simmen et al., 1995).

Experimental and Clinical Applications in Humans

Developments in the past two decades in fetal surgery experimentation on animals have begun to yield fruit by opening the door to clinical applications in human fetuses afflicted with a variety of conditions. This work has principally centered on conditions typically considered at high risk of mortality, such as congenital diaphragmatic hernia (Harrison et al., 1990), cystic adenomatoid malformation of the lung, and obstructive uropathies. Fetal surgery has also been employed in humans in the treatment of sacrococcygeal teratomas (Langer et al., 1989). An extensive literature has documented the progress made in these fields, which is outside the scope of the present chapter, and to which the interested reader is referred (Adzick and Harrison, 1994; Quinn and Adzick, 1997; Harrison, 2001).

Myelomeningocele. While the principal human indications to date have centered on fatal conditions, increasing experience with the techniques, as well as an improved understanding of the risks, has led to consideration of the use of fetal surgery for conditions considered typically nonfatal. While the majority of fetuses affected with myelomeningocele survive to term and into postnatal life, the very high incidence of severe disability, morbidity, and threat to later life have encouraged a number of investigators to explore the potential use of fetal surgery in the human patient.

Exposure of the spinal cord to the intrauterine environment during gestation appears to lead to significant injury to the neural elements, to progressive loss of function below the spinal cord level involved, and ultimately to the characteristic deformities of the posterior cranial fossa and hindbrain. Evidence exists that human fetuses with myelomeningocele exhibit lower limb movement early in the gestational period and lose this ability subsequently during gestation (Epstein et al., 1976; Korenromp et al., 1986), demonstrating the characteristic disability and deformity at the time of birth. Accordingly, a potential window of opportunity is open to allow for in utero correction of the deformity causing the subsequent spectrum of problems characteristic of myelomeningocele. As detailed above, several animal studies have demonstrated that a profound loss of neurological function occurs with exposure of the fetal spinal cord to the intrauterine environment, and that this dysfunction is potentially preventable by early repositioning of the spinal cord in its habitual anatomical location, with reconstitution of the normal separation between the subarachnoid space and the external environment. Preliminary investigations have been carried out primarily at four teaching institutions in the United States with a goal of transferring experience with in utero repair of myelomeningocele in animal models to the treatment of human fetuses.

SURGICAL THERAPY FOR MYELOMENINGOCELE

Diagnosis and Planning

Appropriate prenatal diagnosis is an essential component of the care of individuals with myelomeningocele. Optimal care of these patients should begin with prompt diagnosis as early as possible in gestation to allow appropriate counseling, planning, and communication between prospective parents and their physicians.

Prenatal Diagnosis. As a result of the increasingly widespread use of combined second-trimester maternal serum α-fetoprotein and obstetrical ultrasonography (U.S.) in the routine care of pregnant women, it should be possible in the majority of cases to make the diagnosis of myelomeningocele prenatally. The ability to make this diagnosis early in the gestational period confers several notable advantages and significantly increases the spectrum of options open to parents and physicians.

Counseling. Prenatal recognition of myelomeningocele early in the second trimester of pregnancy provides an opportunity to inform parents at an early stage, thus allowing, at a minimum, necessary time for psychological preparation and genetic counseling prior to the birth of the affected child.

The lead time provided by prenatal diagnosis also allows for discussion of the expected effects on the child and gives sufficient time for reflection before a number of important decisions are to be made. Perhaps most important, prospective parents must consider and weigh several facts concerning the expected duration and quality of life of their child, and face the difficult decision of whether to carry the pregnancy to term or opt for termination, a course that has been chosen in approximately 30% of cases in recent samples (Roberts et al., 1995; Velie and Shaw, 1996). The advent of an effective means of treating this disorder might have an important effect on prospective parents facing these choices.

Delivery. Histopathological examination of the spinal cords of animal and human fetuses born by spontaneous vaginal delivery have consistently revealed hemorrhages and other signs of recent trauma, postulated to result from passage of the neonate through the birth canal. Standard obstetrical care of women pregnant with fetuses with myelomeningocele has consequently evolved to recommend delivery via the cesarean route. Amniocentesis may be performed at term to document fetal lung maturity, after confirmation of which elective cesarean delivery is planned, with the hope of preventing further injury to the exposed spinal neural tissues as a result of the baby's passage through the birth canal. An important precaution necessary in this patient population is the need to perform cesarean delivery in a latex-free environment due to the high incidence of latex allergy in these patients.

Postnatal Surgical Repair

The current standard of care of patients with myelomeningocele is to perform neurosurgical repair postnatally, ideally within the first 48 hours of postnatal life, with a goal of preventing further traumatic and infectious injury to the exposed neural tissues. This was, until recently, the only available treatment option, and will likely remain an important component of care even if antenatal repair proves to be safe and effective, as in cases of failure of antenatal surgery, and in those not discovered through prenatal diagnosis but rather recognized only at the time of birth.

Repair consists in most cases of a layered closure by separation of the open dura mater from surrounding skin, reconstitution of the neural placode, posterior closure of the dura on itself whenever possible, and elevation and approximation of surrounding skin and subcutaneous tissues to cover the defect (Tubbs et al., 2003). Occasionally, this requires more extensive measures to permit closure, for which the assistance of a pediatric plastic surgical team may be useful. Available methods range from bilateral relaxing incisions and elevation of bipedicled flaps of skin and subcutaneous tissue to the transfer of muscle or composite tissue flaps or even the use of alloplastic materials such as an acellular cadaveric dermal allograft.

Antenatal Surgical Repair

Operative Technique. On the day of operation, the mother is taken to a standard obstetrical operating room. Systemic broad-spectrum antibiotics are administered prophylactically. A 50-mg indomethacin suppository is administered per rectum. An epidural catheter is placed, and after induction of general anesthesia, the patient is prepared as for a cesarean section. A combination of general and epidural anesthesia is used because evidence suggests that this is superior to either individually in preventing unwanted uterine contractions (Mangels et al., 2000). The indwelling epidural catheter also enables administration of epidural narcotics for postoperative analgesia.

The gravid uterus is exposed via a Pfannenstiel incision and exteriorized (Bruner et al., 2001). The fetus and placenta are then localized using a sterile ultrasound transducer. The primary surgeon chooses the hysterotomy location based on the location of the placenta. Initial uterine entry is accomplished using a modified Seldinger technique. Any amniotic fluid that spills from the amniotic sac is retained in warm sterile syringes. The footplate of a U.S. Surgical CS-57 autostapling device (United States Surgical Corporation, Norwalk, CT) is then passed into the uterine cavity. The tissue in the stapler is examined manually and with color Doppler ultrasonography to exclude the presence of fetal tissue. The stapler is then engaged to create a 6- to 8-cm uterine incision. The fetus is directly visualized and manually positioned within the uterus such that the myelomeningocele sac is in the center of the hysterotomy.

The fetus is exposed to many of the same anesthetic agents given to the mother, and additionally is given 20 μg/kg (estimated fetal weight) fentanyl by subcutaneous injection for additional analgesia during surgery. Proper positioning is maintained by grasping the fetal head and trunk through the relaxed uterine wall. During the procedure, fetal heart function is monitored by continuous sonographic visualization or by continuous electronic fetal monitoring (EFM).

The myelomeningocele is closed in two layers in routine neurosurgical fashion with the assistance of loupe magnification. The neural placode is sharply dissected from the surrounding arachnoidal tissue and allowed to drop into the spinal canal. Retubularization of the neural placode is performed if technically possible. The dura is then identified and freed from the skin and lumbodorsal fascia. It is reflected over the placode and closed using a running 7-0 Vicryl (Ethicon, Somerville, NJ) suture. Finally, the skin is mobilized and closed using a single 5-0 PDS (Ethicon, Somerville, NJ) suture. For patients without a well-formed myelomeningocele sac (myeloschisis), a modification of this approach is required (Mangels et al., 2000). Bilateral vertical relaxing incisions are performed in the flanks, allowing elevation of two straight bipedicled skin and subcutaneous tissue flaps. These are approximated centrally and closed over the spinal defect. The bilateral secondary soft tissue defects created by the transposition of the flaps are covered with an acellular cadaveric dermal allograft (Alloderm).

The uterus is closed in layers using No. 1 PDS (Ethicon, Somerville, NJ) suture. The first layer incorporates the absorbable polyglycolic acid staples left by the autostapling device. As the last stitches of this layer are placed, the reserved amniotic fluid or warmed sterile saline, mixed with 500 mg nafcillin, is returned to the uterus. Warm sterile saline is added until preoperative amniotic fluid pressure, as measured by manometry testing, is re-created or until uterine turgor, as determined by manual palpation, is restored to the preoperative level. Ultrasonography may also be performed to restore the amniotic fluid volume to the preoperative level. Next, fibrin glue (Tisseel fibrin sealant; Baxter Healthcare, Atlanta, GA) is applied to the suture line in an attempt to provide a watertight seal. Finally, an imbricating layer of No. 1 PDS suture is added. This layer is also treated with fibrin glue, and a sheet of Interceed absorbable adhesion barrier (Johnson & Johnson Medical, Arlington, TX) or mobilized omentum is attached over the uterine incision to prevent adhesion formation. The uterus is returned to the abdominal cavity. The anterior rectus sheath is closed in routine fashion, and dermis closed with a running subcuticular suture or staples. A second 50-mg suppository of indomethacin is placed per rectum before leaving the operating room. The fetus is monitored postoperatively using continuous EFM.

Postoperative uterine contractions are monitored using continuous EFM. Uterine contractions are initially controlled overnight with intravenous magnesium sulfate and oral or rectal indomethacin, and the next morning with subcutaneous terbutaline or oral nifedipine. The epidural catheter is removed on the first postoperative day when the patient begins oral feedings, and antibiotics are changed from the intravenous to the oral route of administration. Two days of prophylactic antibiotic therapy is prescribed. Patients are discharged from the hospital when they are walking freely, eating a regular diet, and tolerating their medications well. The mean length of stay at the Vanderbilt University Medical Center is 3.3 days. Upon discharge, patients are free to return to their community of origin for continued prenatal care. Each patient is discharged from the hospital with a subcutaneous terbutaline pump (Matria Healthcare, Atlanta, GA), supplemented by indomethacin as needed. The terbutaline pump is used because the lower dose administered in this fashion may delay the onset of β-adrenergic receptor desensitization or tachyphylaxis (Iams et al., 1988). Oral nifedipine may be used as an alternative. Use of tocolytics is planned until 37 weeks' gestation. Patients are monitored with weekly transabdominal ultrasonographic examinations. Each child is delivered via standard cesarean section, since evidence suggests that children with myelomeningocele who are delivered via this route have fewer neurological defects (Luthy et al., 1991; Kuller et al., 1996). Cesarean delivery is also necessitated by the presence of the fundal hysterotomy scar. The fetus is delivered earlier for the usual obstetric indications. Specific indications for delivery include the onset of labor or amniorrhexis at greater than 34 weeks' and 0 days' gestation, chorioamnionitis, suspected uterine rupture, placental abruption, nonreassuring fetal status, and fetal lung maturity.

HUMAN STUDIES AND OUTCOME OF TREATMENT

At the time of this writing, intrauterine repair of myelomeningocele has been carried out in over 300 human fetuses, principally at four U.S. university medical centers. Knowledge of the effectiveness and outcomes of this novel treatment modality is, at present, available only in the form of several published case series.

Outcomes

Hindbrain Herniation and Hydrocephalus. Present in 80%–90% of cases of myelomeningocele, hindbrain herniation associated with hydrocephalus requires ventriculoperitoneal shunting and is the leading cause of death among affected patients. Although it was previously believed to be simply a component of an overall pattern of cerebrospinal dysgenesis, more recent observations in animals and humans have led to the conclusion that hindbrain herniation and the associated hydrocephalus are instead secondary to the distal open spinal defect and are progressive during the later stages of gestation (Osaka et al., 1978; Babcook et al., 1994; Bannister et al., 1998). Initially an incidental finding, early experience with fetal surgery for myelomeningocele revealed a consistent improvement in hindbrain herniation in patients who had undergone in utero repair of their spinal lesion. At one major center, this salutary effect was noted in the first four fetal surgery patients (Tulipan et al., 1998). Postnatal sonographic examination and magnetic resonance imaging of the head were performed in each case. Sonograms were graded by a blinded reviewer according to the degree of posterior fossa herniation on a six-point (0–5) scale. These were compared to the sonograms of a consecutive cohort of 33 patients with isolated myelomeningocele who had been treated at the same center using standard postnatal closure and had been examined by ultrasound. In the retrospective cohort, the degree of cerebellar herniation spanned the range from grade 2 (asymmetry of the vermis above and below the fourth ventricle) to grade 5 (fourth ventricle at or below the foramen magnum), with only 6% classified as grade 2 and the mean of the grades being 3.3. All patients required ventriculoperitoneal shunting. By contrast, among patients who had undergone intrauterine repair, three were classified as grade 1 (normal, but with no visible cisterna magna) and one as grade 2. Ventriculoperitoneal shunting for symptomatic hydrocephalus was required in two of these patients at 3 weeks and 3 months of age, significantly later than in the majority of cases of hydrocephalus, where shunt placement is typically required in the first few days of life. Magnetic resonance imaging study findings of the four experimental patients were in keeping with the ultrasound results, showing an absence of significant hindbrain herniation, while other stigmata of the Chiari type II malformation remained. This experience is mirrored in case reports from other centers. In one early report, a fetus was found to have an open spinal lesion that extended from thoracic level 11 to sacral level 1 and was associated with an Arnold-Chiari type II malformation and borderline hydrocephalus (Adzick et al., 1998). Intrauterine repair was carried out at 23 weeks' gestation, followed by cesarean delivery for preterm labor at 30 weeks' gestation. Magnetic resonance imaging revealed resolution of the hindbrain herniation and hydrocephalus, obviating the need for ventriculoperitoneal shunting at the 6-month follow-up.

These early findings have since been supplemented by those of larger-scale studies examining the effect of intrauterine repair of myelomeningocele on hindbrain herniation and the need for ventriculoperitoneal shunting. In a series consisting of the 10 initial patients at one center, including 1 who was the subject of a previous case report (Adzick et al., 1998), 10 fetuses with myelomeningocele were treated with fetal surgery at 22–25 weeks' gestation. All were prospectively examined by fetal ultrasound and magnetic resonance imaging preoperatively, and at 3 weeks and 6 weeks postoperatively, to determine the severity of the posterior fossa deformity, which was graded on a four-point scale (0–3). Preoperative imaging revealed grade 3 hindbrain herniation (displacement of the cerebellum below the foramen magnum and obliteration of all posterior fossa cerebrospinal fluid spaces) in all cases. One neonate died of respiratory insufficiency at the age of 2 days after preterm birth at 25 weeks' gestation. The surgical closure was well healed in all cases, but one patient required reclosure at 1 week for cerebrospinal fluid leakage. Herniation had improved to a grade 1 configuration (no cerebellar displacement below the foramen magnum and both cisterna magna and fourth ventricle visible) in all nine surviving patients at 6-week postoperative and postnatal imaging. Frequent apneic episodes with mild ventriculomegaly led to the placement of a ventriculoperitoneal shunt in one patient at the age of 2 weeks, with resolution of symptoms. At 1 to 13 months of clinical follow-up, no infants were found to manifest signs or symptoms referable to the Chiari malformation (Sutton et al., 1999). These findings support improvement, rather than the expected progression, in the stigmata of hindbrain herniation following intrauterine myelomeningocele repair in this series, along with a less than expected need for ventriculoperitoneal shunting, although no comparison was offered to any untreated group or historical control. In a similar study that examined the initial nine patients who underwent intrauterine repair of myelomeningocele at another major U.S. center, eight of the nine demonstrated moderate to severe hindbrain herniation on intraoperative ultrasound scans performed during fetal surgery. Postnatal examinations in five patients revealed no herniation and only mild herniation in four, demonstrating a reversal of existing hindbrain herniation after intrauterine repair (Tulipan et al., 2003).

A recent review of a large series of 297 conventionally treated myelomeningocele patients has established that the spinal level of the lesion is an important determinant of the incidence of hydrocephalus, with 100% of thoracic, 88% of lumbar, and 68% of sacral anatomical level lesions requiring shunting (Rintoul et al., 2002). Concern existed that the results of antenatal repair might be skewed by the inclusion of a higher proportion of fetuses with lower-level and thus more functionally favorable lesions. This report has provided a useful historical control to which were subsequently compared the results of treatment of all patients treated at two of the principal U.S. fetal surgery centers (Tulipan et al., 2003). This cohort included all fetal surgery patients who had reached 1 year of age, after which the incidence of required ventriculoperitoneal shunting is minimal. The study examined the results of antenatal repair on the need for placement of a ventriculoperitoneal shunt or, equivalently, performance of third ventriculostomy, taking into account the anatomical spinal level of the lesion (as in historical controls), the estimated gestational age and ventricular size at the time of surgery, and the gestational age at delivery. Of 190 patients requiring intrauterine fetal repairs performed at the two centers until the close of data collection, 104 were still alive, older than 1 year, and had undergone postnatal spine evaluation with magnetic resonance imaging or plain radiography. Shunting was required in 86% of controls overall (Rintoul et al., 2002). A similar relationship of spinal level to shunt rate was noted in the experimental group, but at a rate that was significantly lower overall, with only 55% of the total group requiring shunting. This difference was statistically significant from controls for patients with lumbar (58%) and especially sacral lesions (27%), but not in the small number of patients ($n = 5$) with thoracic lesions (80%). The most substantial gains were therefore made in patients with the lowest-level lesions, with a sharp and significant drop in the shunt rate at approximately the L3 level; shunting was required in 90% of patients with L1–L2 lesions and only in 54% of L3–L5 patients.

Another important finding concerns the impact of gestational age at the time of repair. While fetuses who underwent repair after 25 weeks' gestational age had an overall shunt rate of 75%, not significantly different from that of controls, those operated on at or before 25 weeks' gestational age had a shunt rate of only 44%, significantly different from the rates in both the older group and controls, and representing approximately a 50% decrease in incidence compared to the latter. This evidently has an important impact on recommendations concerning the optimal timing of fetal repair; conceptually, a limited window of opportunity must exist before which the deleterious effects of amniotic fluid exposure of the spinal cord occur, producing the characteristic tissue destruction and neurological dysfunction seen in untreated cases at birth. These findings importantly serve to better delineate that boundary. That early closure of the spinal defect in myelomeningocele should result in prevention of the development of hindbrain herniation and improvement in the clinical spectrum of hydrocephalus is conceptually in keeping with other published studies that have documented progressive worsening of cerebellar compression and herniation as well as ventriculomegaly in the later stages of gestation and even into the postnatal period (Van den Hof et al., 1990; Ruge et al., 1992; Babcook et al., 1994). Confirmation and further delineation of any possible benefit in reducing the incidence of shunt-dependent hydrocephalus in human fetuses must now await the results of a formal randomized, controlled clinical trial.

Motor Function and Deformity. In the series of 10 early patients with intrauterine repair described above, all were prospectively examined by fetal ultrasound and magnetic resonance imaging and were confirmed to have leg and foot movement without clubfoot or any other leg deformity (Sutton et al., 1999). Among nine live-born neonates, five were reported as having better than expected function of the lower extremities by at least two spinal levels, based on the initial imaging, including three with thoracic or high lumbar lesions with function at the L5 level or better. However, no formal functional testing results were reported, and bowel and bladder continence were not evaluated. Clinically significant spinal cord tethering required release from overlying skin in the initial patient at the age of 7 months due to loss of leg function below the hips; function was not regained. Incidental cord tethering was also corrected in one neonate at the time of reclosure for cerebrospinal fluid leakage.

The prospect for preserving function of the lower limbs with antenatal repair of myelomeningocele had been shown to be encouraging in several animal models. Disturbingly, an early report of a small group of human fetuses treated with antenatal repair showed no significant improvement over controls treated with conventional postnatal repair (Tulipan et al., 1999a). In the most complete comparative examination to date of neurological function in the lower extremities of patients treated by intrauterine repair of myelomeningocele, a cohort of 37 consecutive patients treated at a principal U.S. fetal surgery center were compared prospectively to a control group of 40 patients treated contemporaneously at another large university medical center (Tubbs et al., 2003). Thoracic and lumbosacral radiographs of each arm were used to determine the anatomical level of the rostral end of the spinal lesion. Neurological examinations were recorded for all patients, then stripped of any identifying data and blindly assigned a neurological functional level by a single pediatric neurosurgeon. The difference between radiological and functional levels was calculated for each patient and assigned a numeric score according to whether the functional level was more caudal than expected based on the radiological level (better, assigned a negative score) or more rostral (worse, a positive score). The baseline radiological levels of lesions in the two groups were comparable overall, with those in the fetal surgery group having an average level of L4-L5 and those in the control group, an average level of L4. The proportions of patients in the fetal surgery group whose functional level was better (more caudal) than, in complete agreement with, and worse (more rostral) than the radiological level were 46%, 11%, and 43%, respectively. In the conventional repair group, the proportions were 50%, 23%, and 28%, respectively. These grouped proportions indicate no statistically significant difference in functional outcome between patients treated by in utero and conventional repair. Similarly, with surgical modalities compared by patients' quantitative difference between radiological and functional levels, published data allow the reader to calculate a mean improvement of −0.05 level for the fetal surgery group and −0.53 level for the conventional group, not significantly different ($p = .314$).

In a similar examination of lower extremity neurological function in a distinct cohort consisting of the first 50 patients treated with intrauterine repair of myelomeningocele at another major U.S. fetal surgery center, and considering the entire group of 47 liveborn patients, 51% demonstrated function that was better than, 30% in agreement with, and 19% worse than that expected based on the baseline radiological assessment of the spinal lesion level (Johnson et al., 2003). In this publication, neurological function was not explicitly compared to that of any control group, but even casual examination shows that the findings are quite comparable to those described in the control group in the study reported above (Tubbs et al., 2003). It is notable, however, that the greatest improvement appears to have been derived by patients with more proximal lesions, with 89% better than expected and 0% worse among patients with thoracic (T) and lumbar levels 1 and 2 lesions (L1, L2) ($n = 9$); 63% better versus 9% worse in those with L3 and L4 lesions ($n = 22$); and 13% better versus 44% worse in those with L5 and S1 lesions ($n = 16$). The data published in this report comparing radiological to functional levels allow the reader to calculate quantitatively, as above, a mean improvement of −0.94 level for the fetal surgery group. When compared to the same conventionally treated control group (Tubbs et al., 2003), again no significant difference between the groups is noted ($p = .323$). Therefore, current results indicate that no net functional improvement appears to be gained by antenatal closure of myelomeningocele in human fetuses overall, and imply that prospective parents considering the procedure should be advised accordingly so that they can make decisions based on appropriate expectations. It is noteworthy, however, to recognize the possibility of an as-yet unsubstantiated benefit in certain subgroups of patients with higher-level lesions.

Continence. Little information has been published to date addressing the potential effect of antenatal fetal repair on continence. Some anecdotal early reports suggest preservation of function in at least some patients treated, but these allow no meaningful comparisons to controls. The large reviews of the experience at major U.S. centers have not addressed this question directly, although information gathered on neurological function in the lower extremities may give some insight into the likelihood of bladder and bowel continence. Specifically, given no net improvement over controls in lower extremity function, it is quite unlikely that a significant salutary effect on continence should occur, but more complete estimates will have to await the results of the current trial. It is also important to consider that the procedure remains quite new, with the very first patients treated in 1997 and the majority only in the past few years. Accordingly, a substantial proportion of the patient population has not yet reached the age of usual development of continence and cannot yet be evaluated. Some effort, however, has been made to quantify urodynamic changes following fetal surgery for myelomeningocele. Video urodynamic testing has been carried out in 16 of the first 25 patients treated at a principal U.S. fetal surgery center, including cystometrography, fluoroscopic evaluation of filling and voiding, pelvic floor electromyography, and postvoid residual urine measurement (Holzbeierlein et al., 2000). In addition, this study included a retrospective review of renal sonograms, voiding cystourethrography, need for catheterization, number of urinary tract infections, and use of medications. Patients were assessed at a mean age of 6.5 months and compared to published rates from other studies. A slightly lower than expected incidence of urinary tract infection and reflux was felt to represent a bias of close urological follow-up rather than an improvement in neurological function. The urodynamic profile of infants in this group generally showed a small bladder capacity, decreased compliance, uninhibited detrusor contractions, and areflexia, consistent with that expected of a similar population of myelomeningocele patients treated conventionally.

Cognitive Function. Obtaining an estimation of the effect of in utero repair of myelomeningocele on cognitive function is, at present, even more problematic. Similar considerations apply, but no surrogate measure can be offered as with continence, and a still longer period will have to elapse before a substantial number of patients reaches an age that will allow either formal neuropsychological testing or assessment of school performance. Some preliminary evidence has been reported, in a cohort consisting of the first 29 cases treated at a major U.S. center (Bruner, 1999b). The developmental outcome of these 29 infants was evaluated at 2–18 months of age using the Bayley Scale of infant development. With a correction of age for prematurity, a mean score of 100 (range, 80–118) was obtained for the mental development index. No assessment of a comparison group was reported, suggesting no adverse effect of surgery. Nonetheless, the question remains important, and it seems reasonable to hold out hope that a positive effect may indeed be recognized in the future, since the procedure has a demonstrated and important impact on the incidence of hindbrain herniation and shunt-dependent hydrocephalus.

Fetal and Maternal Safety. While a number of encouraging results have been obtained in the early experience with fetal surgery for myelomeningocele in humans, enthusiasm for the potential benefits are necessarily tempered by consideration of the not insignificant risk of placental abruption, chorioamnionitis, premature labor, and fetal demise. A probably small, but nonetheless present, additional risk to the mother must also be carefully weighed. While necessarily fatal conditions present a relatively compelling indication to attempt a procedure regarded as risky even to the fetus, survival is the rule in the majority of patients with myelomeningocele, albeit with considerable morbidity. As in the early history of any form of surgical treatment, it is probably reasonable to expect at least a modest improvement in complication rates with developments in technique and greater experience of the operating surgeons. Nonetheless, reports to date have indicated a fetal loss rate of 4% (Tulipan et al., 2003), with 7 of 177 fetuses dying of complications directly attributable to the surgery: 5 due to prematurity, 1 intrauterine fetal demise, and 1 due to pulmonary hypoplasia. Overall, the risk of extreme prematurity (less than 30 weeks' gestational age) was 11%. Concerns that earlier surgery may lead to an increased risk of prematurity have not been borne out in observations to date. In a review of the first 95 patients treated at a principal U.S. fetal surgery center, fetuses were divided according to whether they had undergone early (mean, 23.6 weeks' gestational age) or late (mean, 26.3 weeks' gestational age) surgery (Hamdan et al., 2002). Gestational age at delivery was not found to be significantly different at 34.0 and 34.4 weeks, respectively. In the complete experience to date, no maternal deaths have been reported in association with any fetal surgery procedure, and future fertility appears to be unaffected (Farrell et al., 1999).

Risk/Benefit Analysis

These risks must be weighed carefully, not only with a global perspective by the treating physician team, but also on an individual basis by prospective parents, according to their individual wishes and values. While in utero repair of myelomeningocele has now been performed in over 300 fetuses, clear evidence of benefit has, to date, been lacking. The human cost of myelomeningocele is considerable, given its often significant associated disability; however, the malformation is not considered life-threatening in the majority of cases. Until evidence of efficacy and safety can be confirmed, fetal surgery for correction of any nonlethal condition must be considered experimental and is not indicated. Due to the enormous potential benefit but also the considerable risk to the fetus, as well as to the mother, the three U.S. centers with the most extensive experience with the procedure have undertaken to enroll all eligible patients in a National Institute of Child Health and Human Development–sponsored randomized clinical trial.

National Institute of Child Health and Human Development Trial: Management of Myelomeningocele Study

Three maternal-fetal surgery units in the United States—the University of California at San Francisco, the Children's Hospital of Philadelphia, and Vanderbilt University—have established an operative technique for the in utero repair of myelomeningocele. Since its inception in 1997 and over the past 5 years, a concerted effort has been made to compile and analyze data collected from the more than 180 fetuses undergoing this procedure. Unfortunately, these data are retrospective, and all comparisons were made with historical controls. Additionally, very little follow-up data were available from the children who underwent the surgery. Recognizing the need for more rigorous data to determine whether fetal repair of myelomeningocele, with its attendant maternal and neonatal morbidity, is warranted, the National Institute of Child Health and Human Development funded a multicenter randomized, controlled trial denoted the Management of Myelomeningocele Study (MOMS) (Fetal Surgery Units: MOMS, 2002)

Recruitment. The three participating centers listed above, in collaboration with George Washington University, are committed to testing the value of in utero surgery in the context of a randomized trial and have agreed not to offer myelomeningocele repair outside the trial until the end of recruitment, irrespective of whether a patient is eligible to participate in the trial. Other potential fetal therapy centers have also agreed that prenatal surgery for myelomeningocele repair will not be offered outside the trial.

Population. Two hundred pregnant women with a fetal diagnosis of myelomeningocele and in the second trimester of pregnancy will be randomized to either prenatal or postnatal repair at one of the three MOMS treatment centers, with follow-up to be conducted by an independent team of examiners.

Objectives. Two principal research questions will be addressed:

1. Does intrauterine repair of fetal myelomeningocele at 19 0/7–25 6/7 weeks' gestation using a standard multilayer closure improve the outcome compared with standard postnatal repair, as measured by death or the need for ventricular decompressive shunting by 1 year of life?
2. Does intrauterine repair of fetal myelomeningocele improve neurological function at 30 months' corrected age, as measured by a combined rank score on the Bayley Scales of Infant Development Mental Development Index and the difference between motor level and lesion level?

At the time of this writing, recruitment to the trial has begun.

FUTURE GOALS AND DIRECTIONS

Endoscopic Repair

Animal studies have suggested that the intrauterine environment causes secondary injury to the congenitally dysplastic spinal cord. This, in turn, suggests that early closure of the myelomeningocele sac might prevent secondary injury and therefore improve the neurological outcome. As a direct result of these studies, endoscopic intrauterine myelomeningocele repair was first attempted in the United States in 1994. At that time, a limited number of patients underwent repair using an endoscopic approach employing a maternal split-thickness skin graft to cover the myelomeningocele defect. The endoscopic approach held the promise of minimizing uterine trauma, thereby reducing the risk of preterm labor and delivery, a problem that had plagued previous attempts at fetal surgery.

Of the four operations performed, two resulted in fetal losses and a third infant was delivered prematurely at 28 weeks' gestation (Bruner et al., 1999a). One death occurred after the premature delivery of a fetus at 24 weeks and 4 days. The suspected cause of labor was chorioamnionitis. The second death was due to placental abruption at the time of surgery at 24 weeks and 3 days. In addition, the two survivors still required definitive closure of the myelomeningocele postnatally. The authors concluded that fetal morbidity and mortality related to the endoscopic procedure were disappointingly high and that myelomeningocele repair under direct vision through a 6- to 8-cm hysterotomy would be superior to repair performed endoscopically given the endoscopic technology available at that time (Bruner et al., 1999a, 2000).

Robot-Assisted Repair

Advances in technology have led to the development of robot-assisted surgical endoscopic devices such as the da Vinci system (Intuitive Surgical, Mountain View, CA), which overcome many of the deficiencies of conventional endoscopy. These devices translate the surgeon's hand movements at a remote console to robotically manipulated instruments in the operative field. The computer interface filters these motions to remove tremor and augment precision. The da Vinci system also incorporates specialized instruments with wrist-like ends that mimic the human hand and dual cameras that provide a three-dimensional view of the operative field. The introduction of such devices has allowed animal studies to be conducted to study the feasibility of performing in utero myelomeningocele repair using the da Vinci robot–assisted endoscopic system.

In a recently published study, investigators demonstrated that with the aid of the da Vinci system's advanced articulated instruments and three-dimensional optics, endoscopic intrauterine myelomeningocele repair is feasible (Aaronson et al., 2002). Six fetal lambs underwent intrauterine creation and repair of a full-thickness skin lesion using the da Vinci system. Four of the six survived until sacrifice. Two lambs died in the perioperative period, presumably due to impaired uteroplacental circulation. The da Vinci system and other advances in endoscopic technology have allowed a re-examination of endoscopic in utero myelomeningocele repair. The advantages of the endoscopic surgical approach include avoidance of a hysterotomy, which may preclude the need for cesarean delivery and lessen the risk of uterine rupture, as well as decrease the risk of preterm labor. What has been demonstrated as technically feasible now needs to be refined in a larger animal study using a suitable animal model of a myelomeningocele lesion.

Timing of Repair

As detailed above, recent large reviews of the experience with fetal surgery to date demonstrate an improvement in certain outcomes, notably shunt-dependent hydrocephalus, with earlier repair (Tulipan et al., 2003). The earliest repairs reported to date have been performed at 22–25 weeks' gestational age and demonstrate the greatest improvement in outcomes. This raises the conceptual question of whether still earlier repairs might theoretically lead to further improvements in outcomes. Answering this question, however, involves certain fundamental hurdles, as the technical difficulty of performing the repairs in still smaller patients, as well as the risk and especially the consequences of premature labor in younger fetuses, may prove prohibitive. Any efforts to push these boundaries will first have to await convincing documentation of the benefit of this treatment modality from the current clinical research effort, if such evidence is indeed what the near future holds.

REFERENCES

Aaronson OS, Tulipan NB, Cywes R, et al (2002). Robot-assisted endoscopic intrauterine myelomeningocele repair: a feasibility study. Pediatr Neurosurg 36(2):85–89.

Adzick NS, Harrison MR (1994). Fetal surgical therapy. Lancet 343(8902):897–902.

Adzick NS, Sutton LN, Crombleholme TM, Flake AW (1998). Successful fetal surgery for spina bifida. Lancet 352:1675–1676. Correspondence and reply in Lancet 1999;353:406–407.

Babcook CJ, Goldstein RB, Barth RA, et al (1994). Prevalence of ventriculomegaly in association with myelomeningocele: correlation with gestational age and severity of posterior fossa deformity. Radiology 190:703–707.

Bannister CM, Russell SA, Rimmer S (1998). Pre-natal brain development of fetuses with a myelomeningocele. Eur J Pediatr Surg 8(Suppl 1):15–17.

Bentley JR, Ferrini RL, Hill LL (1999). American College of Preventive Medicine public policy statement. Folic acid fortification of grain products in the U.S. to prevent neural tube defects. Am J Prev Med 16:264–267.

Bruner JP, Richards WO, Tulipan N, Arney TL (1999a). Endoscopic coverage of fetal myelomeningocele in utero. Am J Obstet Gynecol 180:153–158.

Bruner JP, Tulipan N, Davis GH (2001). Open fetal surgery for nonlethal malformations. Infert Reprod Med Clin North Am 12(4):829–849.

Bruner JP, Tulipan N, Paschall RL, et al (1999b). Fetal surgery for myelomeningocele and the incidence of shunt-dependent hydrocephalus. JAMA 282(19):1819–1825.

Bruner JP, Tulipan NB, Richards WO, et al (2000). In utero repair of myelomeningocele: a comparison of endoscopy and hysterotomy. Fetal Diagn Ther 15(2):83–88.

Crombleholme TM, Harrison MR, Langer JC, et al (1988). Early experiences with open fetal surgery for congenital hydronephrosis. J Pediatr Surg; 23:1114–1121.

Drewek MJ, Bruner JP, Whetsell WO, Tulipan N (1997). Quantitative analysis of the toxicity of human amniotic fluid to cultured rat spinal cord. Pediatr Neurosurg; 27:190–193.

Economic burden of spina bifida—United States, 1980–1990 (1989). MMWR 38:264–267.

Epstein F, Marlin A, Hochwald G, Ransohoff J (1976). Myelomeningocele: a progressive intra-uterine disease. Dev Med Child Neurol 18(Suppl 37):12–15.

Farrell JA, Albanese CT, Jennings RW, et al (1999). Maternal fertility is not affected by fetal surgery. Fetal Diagn Ther 14:190–192.

Fetal Surgery Units Network: Management of Myelomeningocele Study (MOMS) (2002). Available at http://www.spinabifidamoms.com/english/index.html. Elizabeth A Thom (Principal Investigator), George Washington University, Data and Study Coordinating Center. Contact information: MOMS@biostat.bsc.gwu.edu.

Hamdan AH, Walsh W, Heddings A, et al (2002). Gestational age at intrauterine myelomeningocele repair does not influence the risk of prematurity. Fetal Diagn Ther 17(2):66–68.

Harrison MR (2001). Historical perspective. In Harrison MR, Evans MI, Adzick NS, et al (eds): *The Unborn Patient: The Art and Science of Fetal Therapy,* 3rd ed. Philadelphia: WB Saunders, pp. 11–18.

Harrison MR, Adzick NS, Longaker MT, et al (1990). Successful repair in utero of a fetal diaphragmatic hernia after removal of herniated viscera from the left thorax. N Engl J Med 322:1582–1584.

Heffez DS, Aryanpur J, Cuello Rotellini NA, et al (1993). Intrauterine repair of experimental surgically created dysraphism. Neurosurgery 32(6):1005–1010.

Heffez DS, Aryanpur J, Hutchins GM, Freeman JM (1990). The paralysis associated with myelomeningocele: clinical and experimental data implicating a preventable spinal cord injury. Neurosurgery 26:987–992.

Holzbeierlein J, Pope JC, Adams MC, et al (2000). The urodynamic profile of myelodysplasia in childhood with spinal closure during gestation. J Urol 164(4):1336–1339.

Hunt GM (1990). Open spina bifida: outcome for a complete cohort treated unselectively and followed into adulthood. Dev Med Child Neurol 32:108–118.

Hunt GM (1997). The median survival time in open spina bifida. Dev Med Child Neurol 39:568.

Iams JD, Johnson FF, O'Shaughnessy RW, West LC (1988). A prospective random trial of home uterine activity monitoring in pregnancies at increased risk of preterm labor, II. Am J Obstet Gynecol 159:595–603.

Iskandar BJ, Tubbs S, Mapstone TB, et al (1998). Death in shunted hydrocephalic children in the 1990s. Pediatr Neurosurg 28:173–176.

Johnson MP, Sutton LN, Rintoul N, et al (2003). Fetal myelomeningocele repair: short-term clinical outcomes. Am J Obstet Gynecol 189:482–487.

Korenromp MJ, van Gool JD, Bruinese HW, Kriek R (1986). Early fetal leg movements in myelomeningocele. Lancet 1(8486):917–918.

Kuller JA, Katz VL, Wells SR, et al (1996). Cesarean delivery for fetal malformations. Obstet Gynecol Surv 51:371–375.

Langer JC, Harrison MR, Schmidt KG, et al (1989). Fetal hydrops and death from sacrococcygeal teratoma: rationale for fetal surgery. Am J Obstet Gynecol 160:1145–1150.

Lind T (1978). The biochemistry of amniotic fluid. In Fairweather DVI, Eskes TKAB (eds): *Amniotic Fluid: Research and Clinical Applications*. 2nd Edition Amsterdam: Exerpta Medica, pp. 59–80.

Luthy DA, Wardinsky T, Shutleff DB, et al (1991). Cesarean section before the onset of labor and subsequent motor function in infants with meningomyelocele diagnosed antenatally. N Engl J Med 324:662–666.

Mangels KJ, Tulipan N, Bruner JP, Nickolaus D (2000). Use of bipedicular advancement flaps for intrauterine closure of myeloschisis: technical report. Pediatr Neurosurg 32(1):52–56.

March of Dimes (2003). Quick Reference and Fact Sheets. Spina Bifida. Available at http://www.marchofdimes.com/professionals/681_1224.asp.

Mathews TJ, Honein MA, Erickson JD (2002). Spina bifida and anencephaly prevalence—United States, 1991–2001. MMWR 51(RR13):9–11.

McLone DG, Knepper PA (1989). The cause of the Chiari II malformation: a unified theory. Pediatr Neurosci 15:1–12.

Meuli M, Meuli-Simmen C, Hutchins GM, Freeman JM (1995a). In utero surgery rescues neurological function at birth in sheep with spina bifida. Nat Med 1:342–347.

Meuli M, Meuli-Simmen C, Hutchins GM, et al (1997). The spinal cord lesion in human fetuses with myelomeningocele: implications for fetal surgery. J Pediatr Surg. 32(3):448–452.

Meuli M, Meuli-Simmen C, Yingling CD, et al (1995b). Creation of myelomeningocele in utero: a model of functional damage from spinal cord exposure in fetal sheep. J Pediatr Surg 30(7):1028–1033.

Meuli M, Meuli-Simmen C, Yingling CD, et al (1996). In utero repair of experimental myelomeningocele saves neurological function at birth. J Pediatr Surg 31(3):397–402.

Meuli-Simmen C, Meuli M, Hutchins GM, et al (1995). Fetal reconstructive surgery: experimental use of the latissimus dorsi flap to correct myelomeningocele in utero. Plast Reconstr Surg 96:1007–1011.

Michejda M (1984). Intrauterine treatment of spina bifida: primate model. Z Kinderchir 39:259–261.

Osaka K, Tanimura T, Hirayama A, Matsumoto S (1978). Myelomeningocele before birth. J Neurosurg 49(5):711–724.

Paek BW, Farmer DL, Wilkinson CC, et al (2000). Hindbrain herniation develops in surgically created myelomeningocele but is absent after repair in fetal lambs. Am J Obstet Gynecol 183(5):1119–1123.

Quinn TM, Adzick NS (1997). Fetal surgery. Obstet Gynecol Clin North Am 24:143–157.

Rauzzino M, Oakes WJ (1995). Chiari II malformation and syringomyelia. Neurosurg Clin North Am 6:293–308.

Rintoul NE, Sutton LN, Hubbard AM, et al (2002). A new look at myelomeningoceles: functional level, vertebral level, shunting, and the implications for fetal intervention. Pediatrics 109:409–413.

Roberts HE, Moore CA, Cragan JD, et al (1995). Impact of prenatal diagnosis on the birth prevalence of neural tube defects, Atlanta 1990–1991. Pediatrics 96:880–883.

Ruge JR, Masciopinto J, Storrs BB, McLone DG (1992). Anatomical progression of the Chiari II malformation. Child Nerv Syst 8:86–91.

Shurtleff DV, Luthy DA, Nyberg DA, et al (1994). Meningomyelocele: management in utero and post natum. Ciba Foundation Symp 181:270–286.

Steinbok P, Irvine B, Cochrane DD, Irwin BJ (1992). Long-term outcome and complications of children born with meningomyelocele. Child's Nerv Syst 8:92–96.

Sutton LN, Adzick NS, Bilaniuk LT, et al (1999). Improvement in hindbrain herniation demonstrated by serial magnetic resonance imaging following fetal surgery for myelomeningocele. JAMA 282(19):1826–1831.

Tubbs RS, Chambers MR, Smyth MD, et al (2003). Late gestational intrauterine myelomeningocele repair does not improve lower extremity function. Pediatr Neurosurg 38(3):128–132.

Tulipan N, Bruner JP, Hernanz-Schulman M, et al (1999a). The effect of intrauterine myelomeningocele repair on central nervous system structure and neurologic function. Pediatr Neurosurg 31:183–188.

Tulipan N, Hernanz-Schulman M, Bruner JP (1998). Reduced hindbrain herniation after intrauterine myelomeningocele repair: a report of four cases. Pediatr Neurosurg 29:274–278.

Tulipan N, Hernanz-Schulman M, Lowe LH, Bruner JP (1999b). Intrauterine myelomeningocele repair reverses preexisting hindbrain herniation. Pediatr Neurosurg 31(3):137–142.

Tulipan N, Sutton LN, Bruner JP, et al (2003). The effect of intrauterine myelomeningocele repair on the incidence of shunt-dependent hydrocephalus. Pediatr Neurosurg 38(1):27–33.

Van den Hof MC, Nicolaides KH, Campbell J, Campbell S (1990). Evaluation of the lemon and banana signs in one hundred thirty fetuses with open spina bifida. Am J Obstet Gynecol 162:322–327.

Velie EM, Shaw GM (1996). Impact of prenatal diagnosis and elective termination on prevalence and risk estimates of neural tube defects in California, 1989–1991. Am J Epidemiol 144:473–479.

Worley G, Schuster JM, Oakes WJ (1996). Survival at 5 years of a cohort of newborn infants with myelomeningocele. Dev Med Child Neurol 38(9):816–822.

19

Postnatal Surgery for Myelomeningocele

JONATHAN P. MILLER
ALAN R. COHEN

Myelomeningocele, the most serious form of spina bifida, affects 2500 to 6000 newborns per year in the United States (McLone, 1998). For neonates born with this condition, the initial management has a profound impact on their survival and the disabilities they may have to cope with throughout their lives. Postnatal surgical treatment for myelomeningocele has been well established for many years. The surgeon must first replace the neural tissues within the spinal canal and then reconstruct the thecal sac and close the back. Large areas may be difficult to close and sometimes require innovative techniques, particularly if there is an associated kyphotic deformity. Associated abnormalities including hydrocephalus and the Chiari II malformation must also be addressed by the neurosurgeon.

HISTORY OF SURGICAL TREATMENT

Spina bifida has been recognized since ancient times. The first detailed description of a child with spina bifida was published in 1587 by Peter van Forrest (Forestus, 1587), who also was the first to attempt surgical repair by ligating the myelomeningocele sac in 1610 (Forestus, 1610). The first anatomical illustration of a myelomeningocele was produced in 1641 (Tulpius, 1641). In 1761, the Italian anatomist Giovanni Baptiste Morgagni became the first to associate the clinical changes observed in spina bifida patients with the spinal cord defect, but he himself did not believe that surgery should play a role in the treatment of these patients (Morgagni, 1761). By 1881, Lebedeff had determined that spina bifida was due to a failure of the neural tube to close (Lebedeff, 1881), and 5 years later, Friedrich von Recklinghausen was able to classify the several types of spina bifida and review the surgical therapies attempted thus far (von Recklinghausen, 1886).

The first large surgical series of patients with spina bifida was reported by Sir John Fraser, who in 1929 reported his experience with 191 spina bifida patients treated at the Royal Hospital for sick children, Edinburgh, between 1898 and 1923 (Fraser, 1929). Of the 131 patients surgically treated, only 82 survived until discharge from the hospital, and among 46 of these traced at follow-up, 30 were still alive. Even among the survivors, the associated clinical conditions (especially hydrocephalus) were severe. Fraser wrote: "I wish I could say the results were good—in a few cases, they might be so described—but the greater proportion were evidently crippled in body or in mind or both, and, as the records were gone through, one was inclined to say: 'Cui bono?' " (Fraser, 1929) Such complications led many in the 1930s and 1940s to delay surgery to allow for full epithelialization of the placode (Ingraham and Swan, 1943).

Surgical treatment of spina bifida became much more aggressive in the early 1950s, largely due to the development of the ventriculoperitoneal shunt, which made it possible to avoid many of the devastating consequences of hydrocephalus. Even so, many physicians argued that surgical treatment was not warranted in severely affected infants since the prognosis was so poor that to prolong such a life through surgery would be cruel. One prominent advocate of this nonsurgical approach was English physician John Lorber, who enumerated four criteria that should exclude affected children from treatment: advanced hydrocephalus, total paraplegia, scoliosis/kyphosis, or other gross congenital abnormalities (Lorber, 1971). Lorber based his recommendation on two assumptions: that the mortality due to severe spina bifida is unacceptably high and that the quality of life of survivors is unacceptably low. Both of these assumptions have been challenged in recent years. Lorber believed that severe spina bifida is a uniformly fatal disease and surgery will only delay the inevitable (Lorber and Salfield, 1981). However, several large trials have shown that aggressive surgical management of patients with spina bifida dramatically improves survival to more than 80% (Ames and Schut, 1972; McLone, 1983). Lorber's second assertion, that life with severe spina bifida is not worth living, has also been challenged. He wrote that "the prospects for open employment, marriage, or anything approaching a normal life are poor, and the cost to the community is immense" (Lorber and Salfield, 1981). However, when parents of children with spina bifida were surveyed to determine how in hindsight they felt about their decision regarding whether to treat their infant, the vast majority reported they were satisfied with their decision to treat aggressively. Among the 274 sets of parents surveyed, only 5% reported regretting the decision they made. Furthermore, all nine sets of parents who elected to delay treatment later regretted their decision not to treat the child more aggressively (McLone, 1998). In one study of aggressively treated patients, many were able to achieve ambulation, social continence, and IQs in the normal range (McLone, 1983). In essence, Lorber's criteria allow a number of reasonably functional children to die to avoid the societal burden of the severely disabled. At present, almost all children with myelomeningocele are treated aggressively, regardless of the severity of the neurological dysfunction, provided that cranial and renal ultrasonography and cardiac echocardiography do not indicate an abnormality incompatible with life.

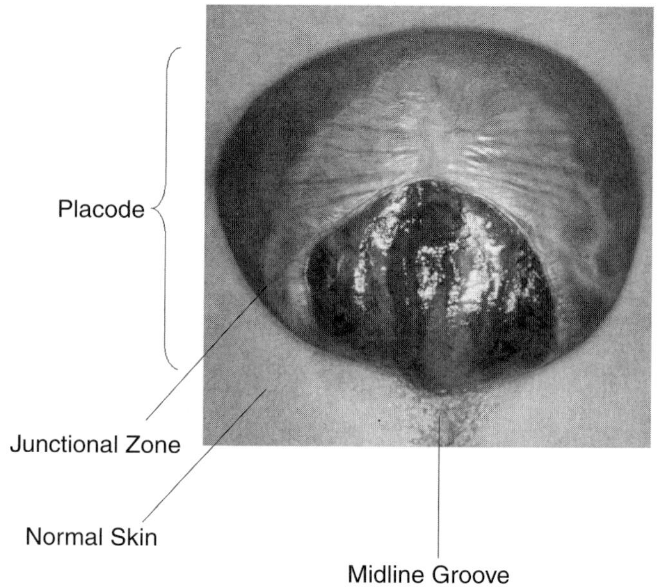

FIGURE 19.1. Photograph of a typical myelomeningocele. The exposed surface represents the inside of what should have been a closed tube and is covered with ependyma. Note the midline groove, which is continuous with the central canal of the spinal cord above the exposed placode. The junctional zone and surrounding normal skin are easily visible. Deep to the myelomeningocele are the pia and arachnoid enclosing an enlarged subarachnoid space and nerve roots.

SURGICAL ANATOMY

Myelomeningocele represents failure of the spinal cord to curl properly around the central canal and fuse in the dorsal midline during development (days 18 to 27 of human embryogenesis), resulting in an open book configuration at some level in the spinal canal (Fig. 19.1; see also Fig. 19.2*A*). Most (85%) are in the lumbar or sacral spine, 10% are in the thorax, and 5% are cervical (Dias and Walker, 1992). The structures normally derived from the neural tube are nearly always present but are open dorsally and everted from the midline. The exposed superficial (dorsal) surface represents the everted interior of the neural tube and is thus covered with ependyma. A narrow groove is usually visible along the midline, which represents the primitive neural groove and which is continuous with the central canal of the spinal cord above (and occasionally below) the exposed placode. A small pit at the rostral end of the groove opens into the central canal and discharges cerebrospinal fluid (CSF) from the proximal cord. The deep (ventral) surface underneath the placode represents the entire outside of what should have been a closed neural tube, and is covered with pia and arachnoid that enclose an intact subarachnoid space. Motor roots exit from the ventral surface on either side of the midline, and sensory roots enter the ventral surface lateral to the motor roots at the periphery of the placode like a book that has been opened (see Fig. 19.2*A*). Both root systems pass through the subarachnoid space to their respective root sleeves. The CSF in the subarachnoid space deep to the placode pushes the placode dorsally. Deep to the subarachnoid space is an open basin lined by dura with underlying epidural fat. Lateral to the placode is a junctional (intermediate) zone of thin epithelium fused with dystrophic skin. The vertebral bodies are flattened and widened, with pedicles everted nearly horizontal in the coronal plane, a widened interpedicular distance, a shortened pedical height, bifid or hypoplastic laminae, large transverse processes that extend laterally, and absent spinous processes. Thoracic lesions frequently cause severe kyphosis. Paraspinal muscles are present but everted and displaced anteriorly, often acting as spine flexors rather than extensors and sometimes markedly attenuated due to the lack of innervation. Above the placode the spinal cord may be normal, although there is an increased frequency of associated abnormalities such as split cord malformation, arteriovenous malformations, lipomas, dermoids, neuroenteric cysts, myelomeningocele manqué (dorsal roots exiting from the cord or neural placode and aberrantly entering the dura), or split notocord syndrome (Dias and Walker, 1992; McLone, 1998).

OTHER SURGICAL CONSIDERATIONS: HYDROCEPHALUS AND CHIARI II MALFORMATION

Hydrocephalus refers to enlargement of the cerebral ventricles due to obstruction of ventricular outflow (noncommunicating) or disruption of reaborption at the arachnoid granulations (communicating). The majority (80% to 90%) of patients with myelomeningocele have hydrocephalus that requires treatment. The etiology of hydrocephalus in spina bifida is not known with certainty, although there are several theories. Aqueductal stenosis or fourth ventricular outflow obstruction may cause a noncommunicating hydrocephalus or underdevelopment of the arachnoid granulations may result in a communicating hydrocephalus. Hydrocephalus among patients with spina bifida is most likely multifactorial in origin. If symptomatic, it always requires surgical treatment, usually with a ventriculoperitoneal shunt that allows drainage of CSF through a tunneled catheter from the cerebral ventricles into the peritoneal space.

The Chiari II malformation is defined as displacement of the cerebellar vermis through the foramen magnum into the upper cervical spinal canal. The malformation is associated with a number of abnormalities that affect the entire brain. Infratentorial abnormalities include kinking of the medulla, cephalad angling of the cervical nerve roots, low-lying torcular Herophili and tentorium, small posterior fossa, enlarged foramen magnum, tectal beaking, and changes in brainstem nuclei (Gilbert et al., 1986). Abnormalities above the tentorium include dysgenesis of the corpus callosum, large massa intermedia, gray matter heterotopias, and polymicrogyria (small, disorganized gyri) in the medial occipital lobes. Chiari II malformation has been associated with a higher incidence of lobar agenesis, holoprosencephaly, schizencephaly, septum pellucidum cysts, arachnoid cysts and midline lipomas. Nearly all patients with myelomeningocele have an associated Chiari II malformation, and although only a relatively small fraction become symptomatic, this condition is the overall leading cause of death in patients with myelomeningocele. Therefore, the presence of brainstem symptoms should prompt surgical treatment with a ventriculoperitoneal shunt and/or decompression of the posterior cranial fossa.

PREOPERATIVE MANAGEMENT

Prenatal Management: Labor and Delivery

Since a multidisciplinary approach by a team of specialists familiar with spina bifida is needed to adequately treat a newborn with a myelomeningocele, parents of an affected fetus should be referred to a tertiary care center that has a neonatal intensive care unit and a pediatric neurosurgery service. It is not clear whether labor or vaginal delivery versus cesarean section affects the outcome of infants born with myelomeningocele. One nonrandomized prospective study of 200 singleton pregnancies implied that labor increases the risk of neurological injury and is associated with a higher level of motor dysfunction, presumably due to trauma to the placode during labor (Luthy et al., 1991). However, several retrospective studies have failed to show any difference between vaginal and cesarean delivery, with or without labor. For example, one retrospective study found that infants born by vaginal delivery and those born by cesarean section had comparable spinal defect levels, comparable incidences of hydrocephalus, mortality at birth, development at 1 year, and incidence of neonatal meningitis (Bensen et al., 1988). Another retrospective study of 208 patients also found no difference in motor and sensory function among infants born by vaginal delivery and those born by cesarean section before labor (Cochrane et al., 1991). Since vaginal delivery is statistically safer than cesarean section, and since it is not clear that labor is definitely associated with a worse outcome for infants with spina bifida, it may be appropriate to deliver these infants vaginally even if the diagnosis is made before birth. Gibbus formation, spinal cord hypoplasia, and breech presentation are not indications for cesarean section (Shurtleff and Lemire, 1995).

Perinatal Management

Initial management focuses on stabilizing the infant and preparing for surgical repair of the myelomeningocele, which ideally occurs within 48 hours of birth. The myelomeningocele should not be allowed to dry; it should be immediately covered with a sterile saline-moistened gauze dressing and the entire trunk wrapped circumferentially with plastic wrapping. Subsequently, the infant is positioned prone or on the side to avoid mechanical trauma to the neural placode. The infant must be kept normothermic and euvolemic, and latex precautions are used from birth to minimize exposure of the infant to the latex allergen. To minimize the risk of meningitis, no oral feedings should be administered prior to the operation so that there will be no fecal contamination of the open myelomeningocele. If contamination does occur, no chemical antimicrobial solutions should be used on the exposed neural tissue. Prophylactic antibiotics are frequently used, although it has not been shown conclusively that these provide any additional benefit over perioperative antibiotics. After initial stabilization, the neonate is carefully examined to determine whether there are any additional malformations that may delay or obviate the need for myelomeningocele repair, which occur in about 1% of infants with myelomeningocele.

The Initial Neurological Evaluation

The initial neurological examination is performed to document the level of the spinal defect and assess for the presence and severity of hydrocephalus. To test for sensory level, a painful stimulus is applied to the lower extremities from distal to proximal until the infant grimaces. To test for motor level, a painful stimulus is applied above the sensory level of the lesion and the most distal voluntary motion is noted. A level at T12 or above is associated with complete lower extremity paralysis. With a lesion between L1 and L3, the infant will demonstrate hip flexion. A level between L2 and L4 will also produce intact hip adduction, hip flexion, and inverted feet. If the level is between L5 and S2, there will be knee flexion as well. Infants with a sacral level may appear intact except for plantar flexion and rockerbottom feet (since the intrinsic muscles of the foot are innervated by S3). There may be some degree of spinal shock. Care must be exercised in interpreting abnormal reflexes, since they may not reflect voluntary function. For example, stimulation of the perineum may cause contraction and spread of a response that should not be mistaken for voluntary anal contraction. The infant typically has an incomplete functional transection of the spinal cord and therefore may show signs of myelopathy, including hyperreflexia and clonus (Stark, 1971). Upper motor neuron signs have been reported in approximately two-thirds of the infants. A flaccid pelvic floor and patulous anus are often present, but the presence of an anal wink or sphincter tone does not accurately predict anal sphincter function in the future (Hahn, 1995). Signs are generally symmetric bilaterally, and any asymmetry should prompt investigation for an additional lesion such as diastematomyelia or hemimyelocele (McLone, 1998).

The size and extent of the defect and associated abnormalities that may influence the repair are determined. Although 15% of patients have kyphosis at birth, kyphectomy is rarely needed at the time of initial repair. Kyphoscoliosis or significant asymmetry between the lower extremities at birth may indicate an underlying split cord malformation (Stark, 1971). The entire spine should be examined closely for stigmata of occult spina bifida including hypertrichosis, hemangioma, or hyperpigmented areas, which may indicate a tandem lesion.

The cranial nerve examination can provide evidence for increased intracranial pressure or the Chiari II malformation. Other signs of intracranial hypertension include increased head circumference, fullness of the anterior fontanelle, and separation of cranial sutures. Cranial ultrasonography is useful to characterize the degree of hydrocephalus, although the ventricles may not enlarge until after the spinal defect is closed. More definitive imaging with computed tomography is sometimes helpful. Magnetic resonance imaging is usually not necessary in the perinatal period, but should be performed later in infancy to evaluate the hindbrain malformation. If severe kyphosis is present, plain radiographs of the spine should be obtained. Signs of the Chiari II hindbrain malformation include central or obstructive apnea, stridor, and opisthotonus. The presence of stridor should prompt inspection of the vocal cords by direct laryngoscopy to document their function.

OPERATIVE REPAIR

Preoperative Preparation

Once considered a surgical emergency, myelomeningocele repair can be performed safely up to 72 hours after birth. Any further delay markedly increases the chance of meningitis or ventriculitis (Charney et al., 1985), which can have a significant impact on intellectual development (Wills et al., 1990). Delayed closure has been associated with a 37% incidence of ventriculitis compared with 7% with early closure (McLone, 1998). If it is absolutely necessary to delay the repair beyond 72 hours after birth, cultures from the lesion should be obtained and confirmed to have no growth before proceeding with surgery. If cultures are positive, the operation should be postponed and the patient should be treated with antibiotics until the infection clears.

To protect the myelomeningocele during intubation, the infant is positioned supine on a donut. Subsequently, the patient is positioned prone with all pressure points well padded. The table is set in a slight Trendelenburg position to minimize drainage of CSF from the spinal defect. The entire back is prepared and draped to allow for a more extensive closure technique if it becomes necessary. The scrub solution should not come in contact with the neural placode.

Operative Technique

The primary objectives of myelomeningocele closure are to isolate the neural tissue and CSF from the external environment, avoid meningitis, and protect the functional tissue in the neural placode. Consideration must also be given to minimizing the chance of retethering of the spinal cord and limiting disruption of the thoracolumbar musculature. The procedure described below and outlined in Figure 19.2 allows reconstruction both of the spinal cord central canal and of the pia-arachnoid-lined subarachnoid space, allowing the spinal cord to float freely in a CSF compartment. Since the exposed neural tissue is likely to be viable, restoration of the natural anatomy will produce an environment that will likely lead to recovery of neural function. Throughout the operation, the dissection may be facilitated by magnification with loupes, and only bipolar cautery should be used near the neural elements (McLone, 1998).

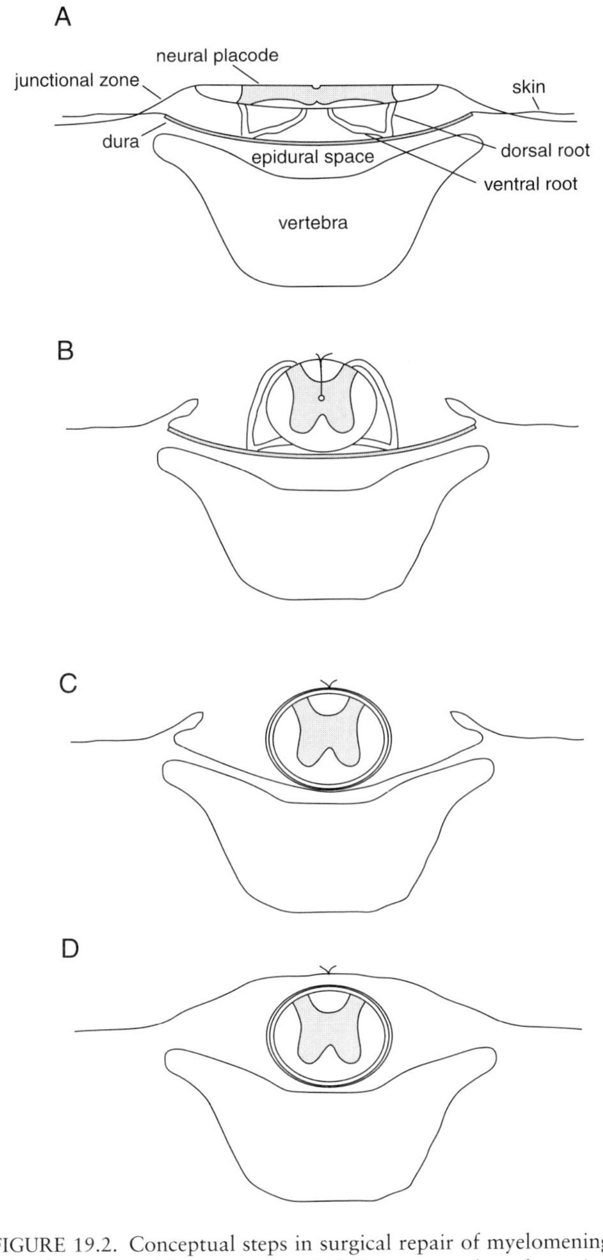

FIGURE 19.2. Conceptual steps in surgical repair of myelomeningocele, shown in axial cross section. (*A*) The untreated myelomeningocele. Note the "open book" appearance, with ventral and dorsal roots exiting from the ventral surface, lying medially and laterally, respectively. (*B*) Reconstruction of the neural tube. The placode is dissected from surrounding tissue by incision through the junctional zone, using caution to exclude dermal elements. The pia is closed in the midline. (*C*) Reconstitution of the thecal sac. The dura is dissected free from the fascia and skin to produce a watertight midline closure. (*D*) Midline closure of fascia and skin to cover the defect.

The initial incision is made at the junctional zone, which is the margin between the arachnoid of the neural placode and the dystrophic epidermis (Fig. 19.2*A*). The neural plaque is freed from the surrounding junctional zone circumferentially, using great care because any residual skin elements may grow to form inclusive epidermoid or dermoid tumors, which are responsible for 15% of cases of later symptomatic cord tethering (Scott et al., 1986). Because some neural elements may be functional, every effort is made to preserve them. Large vessels are sometimes intermingled with nerve roots that exit anteriorly from the placode and should be carefully preserved. Arachnoid adhesions between the placode and the underlying dura are lysed. If a thickened filum is identified, it should be transected distal to the last nerve root (McLone, 1998). At this point, the neural tissue will be floating free on a sac of CSF. Any associated malformations should be repaired before continuing.

The neural placode is then reconstructed into a tube (Fig. 19.2*B*). It is thought that closure of the neural tube decreases the incidence of retethering, presumably by minimizing the area of adherent neural elements that may result in scarring and later tethering. Additionally, reconstruction of the neural tube makes the detethering procedure easier if it is required later. To reconstruct the central canal, the pia-arachnoid junctions on either side are approximated using 7-0 to 10-0 nonabsorbable sutures, beginning at the cephalic end and progressing caudally. It is sometimes necessary to mobilize the dura prior to closure of the pia. In cases in which the placode is very wide or the defect in the canal is shallow, it may not be possible to reconstruct the tube without jeopardizing perfusion of the tissue.

The next step is to identify the intact dura at the rostral end of the defect, just below the last intact lamina. The dura is dissected free from the surrounding tissue by developing a plane in the epidural space that is extended from rostral to caudal on both sides. The dura should be freed medially only as much as is necessary to approximate the lateral edges in the midline. The dura is then closed in the midline to reconstruct the thecal sac using nonabsorbable 5-0 suture, producing a watertight closure whenever possible (Fig. 19.2*C*). However, to prevent ischemia and optimize potential recovery, it is extremely important that the dural closure not compress the underlying tissues; if the defect is large, the dura may be patched using thoracolumbar fascia or bovine pericardium. If possible, the thoracolumbar fascia is mobilized and closed over the dura in the midline. The skin is mobilized by blunt dissection through the subcutaneous tissue, and absorbable sutures are then used to close the subcutaneous tissue in the midline. Lastly, the skin is closed with nonabsorbable sutures that are left in place for 2 weeks (Fig. 19.2*D*). To facilitate future orthopedic procedures, closure should take place in the midsagittal plane whenever possible.

Closure of Large Defects

There is some controversy about the repair of large defects where inadequate tissue is available for the standard closure. Neural tissue should be preserved whenever possible; if the mass of tissue exceeds the volume of spinal canal, it may be necessary to construct a protruding sac. If the defect is moderately wide, longitudinal relaxing incisions in the fascia lateral to the defect that are subsequently grafted may be all that is required to obtain a tension-free closure. A large number of both cutaneous and musculocutaneous flaps have been described for very large defects, but none have been successful enough to be used in common practice (Reigel and McLone, 1987). Some surgeons suggest that extensive reconstruction with flaps is unnecessary. One series found that extensive flap reconstruction was not needed in any of 358 consecutive patients. Others assert that as many as one-quarter of all myelomeningocele defects are too large for standard midline closure (Ramasastry and Cohen, 1995). The consequences of a large reconstructive procedure must be carefully considered. Using muscles of the upper torso to cover the defect can be counterproductive, since wheelchair or crutch-dependent patients depend on these muscles for locomotion. Disruption of these muscles can also lead to progression of scoliosis or kyphosis later in childhood. Deep dissection near the latissimus dorsi must be done with great care to prevent injury to retroperitoneal structures or the development of pneumothorax. Skin flaps also have drawbacks: approximately 20% of rotatory skin flaps have necrosis of the tips of the tissue, and they often fail due to ischemia.

Kyphosis

Kyphosis, or excessive flexion of the spine, affects approximately 15% of spina bifida patients at birth. Patients with thoracic lesions are most likely to suffer from kyphosis, usually because of a wedge-shaped vertebra at the level of the defect that causes dorsal buckling of the spine. If possible, definitive spinal reconstruction for kyphosis should be delayed until the infant is older, but sometimes kyphectomy is necessary to complete the initial myelomeningocele repair successfully (Reigel, 1979). If kyphectomy is to be performed, care must be taken during anterior dissection since epidural bleeding can be extensive. If kyphectomy has been performed, the infant requires an orthosis from 3 months to 2 years of age (Pang, 1995).

Hydrocephalus

Approximately 15% of patients with a myelomeningocele are born with severe hydrocephalus and require immediate shunt placement, which can be performed in the same operative setting as the repair. Since the increased CSF pressure associated with hydrocephalus increases the chance of wound dehiscence and CSF leakage from the myelomeningocele dural closure, it is usually preferable to implant a ventroperitoneal shunt prior to myelomeningocele closure in any patient who has evidence of hydrocephalus. To insert a shunt at the same time as the myelomeningocele repair, the patient is positioned supine and the myelomeningocele is protected in a donut-shaped sponge support. A standard frontal ventriculoperitoneal shunt is inserted, and the patient is subsequently repositioned prone for the myelomeningocele repair during the same anesthesia.

It is possible to place the shunt and perform the repair without repeating the preparation and draping (Hubballah and Hoffman, 1987; Chadduck and Reding, 1988). For this combined procedure, the patient is placed in a park-bench position and the skin in the right occipital area, posterior neck, entire back including the myelomeningocele defect, and the right flank and abdomen are prepared; then the entire area is draped into the surgical field. A towel is placed over the myelomeningocele to drape it out of the field. A right occipital shunt is then inserted, and the distal tubing is passed over the back to enter the peritoneum at the right lateral abdominal wall. This approach simplifies draping during the initial procedure, but may complicate the care of the infant later if a shunt revision or Chiari decompression is required.

The risk of shunt infection appears to be the same whether the shunt and myelomeningocele repair take place in one or two steps. One retrospective study found infection rates of 29% and 21%, respectively, a difference that was not statistically significant (Gamache, 1995). However, the risk of shunt infection is significantly increased if shunt placement and myelomeningocele repair are delayed for more than 2 days after birth. In one study, three-fourths of the patients undergoing shunt insertion and closure more than 2 days after birth developed shunt infections, and 13% of these patients died as a result (Gamache, 1995).

Latex Allergy

Latex hypersensitivity can be a significant problem for spina bifida patients. Studies have shown that 36% to 51% of these patients develop latex allergy (Nieto et al.,

1996; Cremer, 1997). Patients who have undergone more operations (especially shunt operations) are at higher risk (Nieto et al., 1996); therefore, the allergy may result from frequent exposure to the allergen due to multiple surgeries early in life. It is also possible that spina bifida involves a genetic predisposition to latex allergy. Anaphylaxis is often the initial presentation (Mazagri and Ventureyra, 1999); among patients with latex allergy, as many as 26% had an anaphylactic reaction in the operating room (Holzman, 1997). Intraoperative latex anaphylaxis is a serious complication, carrying a mortality of 3.4% (Mazagri and Ventureyra, 1999). During spina bifida surgery only latex-free supplies should be used, and patients should receive additional prophylaxis with hydrocortisone and diphenhydramine. Although anaphylaxis can still occur with premedication, appropriate precautions can reduce the incidence of latex reactions to less than 0.3 % (Holzman, 1997).

POSTOPERATIVE MANAGEMENT

General Postoperative Care

To avoid CSF leakage, the myelomeningocele site should be kept above the level of the head for at least the first 3 days after repair. The infant may be laid supine, prone, or on the side and may be held upright for oral feedings. To prevent infection, antibiotics are usually given for 24 hours and a plastic drape is placed between the wound and the anus to prevent fecal contamination of the wound. The infant should be monitored closely for any sign of brainstem dysfunction, such as apnea, that may indicate a symptomatic Chiari II malformation. Sometimes the infant shows an improved motor level of function within the first few days after the operation. Some infants require clean intermittent catheterization, a bowel regimen, and physical therapy. The spina bifida patient should be transferred to the regular patient floor as soon as enteral feedings are tolerated so that the parents can have a better bonding experience and become comfortable caring for the infant. It is important that the infant receive adequate nutrition to allow healing and recovery from the stress of surgery, and supplemental nutrition should be administered if necessary. The initial hospital stay is usually about 5 days if there are no complications (McLone, 1998).

Early Complications

Operative mortality in myelomeningocele repair is near zero, but morbidity from postoperative complications can be significant. The most common complication is superficial wound dehiscence (Pang, 1995). The wound should be followed closely for separation of the skin edges or CSF leakage, particularly if the infant does not have a shunt. One sign of leakage is a previously full fontanelle that becomes soft as CSF decompresses through the repair site. The risk of leakage is greater in larger wounds. If an infant develops a leak prior to shunt insertion, an external ventricular drain should be placed until the CSF is sterilized.

Because of the potential for fecal contamination of the repaired myelomeningocele defect, there is a high risk of contamination by enteric bacteria. Local wound infections, which usually occur 5 to 7 days after the myelomeningocele repair, have been reported to have an incidence of 1% to 1.5% (Pang, 1995). Signs of local infection include induration and purulent drainage from the surgical site, often accompanied by ileus, mild hypothermia, and mild leukocytosis. Treatment includes sterile dressing changes and intravenous antibiotics.

Meningitis poses a more significant threat to the neonate and can be associated with significant cognitive morbidity. Signs of infection include poor feeding, temperature instability, skin that is mottled or ashen and blotchy (livido reticularis), and leukopenia (less than 4000 cells/mm^3) with bandemia. Seizures may also occur. Magnetic resonance imaging is helpful in identifying intradural abscess at the site of repair. A ventricular tap may be necessary to obtain CSF if a ventriculoperitoneal shunt is not in place. Treatment includes broad-spectrum intravenous antibiotics with effective penetration into the CSF and externalization of the shunt (Pang, 1995).

Spina bifida is associated with an increased risk of necrotizing enterocolitis. Since patients with thoracic lesions may not have the characteristic abdominal findings of necrotizing enterocolitis, the diagnosis may be less clear in these patients.

Hydrocephalus

Even though a ventriculoperitoneal shunt is required at the time of the initial repair in only 15% of patients, up to 80% of the total will ultimately require a shunt. During the first few days after repair, the infant should be closely monitored for signs of increased intracranial pressure. Because of the relative compliance of the immature white matter, an increase in head circumference and splitting of sutures are relatively late changes and should not be relied on exclusively. Other signs of increased intracranial pressure include irritability, lethargy, emesis, bulging of the anterior fontanelle, distention of the myelomeningocele repair, or distended scalp veins. There may also be worsening of brainstem signs from a symptomatic Chiari II malformation. At the first sign of increased intracranial pressure, a ventriculoperitoneal shunt should be inserted. If a shunt is not required prior to discharge, the parents should be instructed to observe the infant for the symptoms listed above.

Complications related to the shunt are frequent problems for children with spina bifida, especially those with high lesions or severe ventriculomegaly. Overall, about half of all spina bifida patients with a shunt require at least one shunt revision during the first year (Caldarelli et al., 1996), and 20% to 40% require multiple revisions (Steinbok et al., 1992). Only 10% require shunt revision beyond 2 years of age (Steinbok et al., 1992). Shunt malfunctions are due either to mechanical problems (75%) or to infection (25%). Timing of shunt placement seems to be significant, as shunts placed prior to the myelomeningocele repair have an 83% change of becoming infected, compared with an infection rate of 23% for simultaneous placement and 7.3% for shunt placement after the repair. Elevated CSF protein at the time of shunt placement has been associated with a 91% chance of shunt infection (Caldarelli et al., 1996).

Endoscopic third ventriculostomy is an alternative to ventriculoperitoneal shunting that has been used successfully to treat various types of noncommunicating hydrocephalus (Cohen, 1998). This procedure involves the creation of an opening in the floor of the third ventricle under endoscopic guidance that allows CSF to communicate directly between the third ventricle and the subarachnoid space rather than through the cerebral aqueduct and fourth ventricle, which may be obstructed. The outcome for endoscopic third ventriculostomy is generally poor in infants with spina bifida, but the procedure may be helpful if a child presents with a shunt malfunction later in life. Since the anatomy of the third ventricle is frequently abnormal in patients with spina bifida, with a thickened floor and enlarged massa intermedia, a midsagittal magnetic resonance image should be carefully reviewed prior to the procedure. If ventricular anatomy is appropriate, a majority of spina bifida patients with shunt malfunction can be successfully treated with endoscopic third ventriculostomy (Cohen, 1998).

Chiari II Malformation

Almost all patients with myelomeningocele have an associated Chiari II malformation, and even though the malformation becomes symptomatic in only about 10% of all infants with myelomeningocele (Pollack et al., 1996), it remains the leading cause of death for all patients with spina bifida, accounting for 79% of all deaths in one series (McLone, 1983). The symptoms and signs most commonly associated with neonatal Chiari II malformation are swallowing difficulties (69%), intermittent obstructive or central apnea (58%), stridor (56%), aspiration (40%), arm weakness (27%), and opisthotonus (18%) (Park et al., 1983). Other signs include cyanosis, bradycardia, nystagmus, vocal cord paralysis, torticollis, hypotonia, and spasticity. Brainstem auditory evoked potentials are consistently abnormal in patients with symptomatic Chiari II malformations, with a positive predictive value of 88% (Taylor et al., 1996). While 59% to 71% of children with myelomeningocele without Chiari II malformation have some degree of swallowing dysfunction, difficulty swallowing thin liquids tends to occur only in the setting of the Chiari II malformation and is the most common presenting symptom. Among all infants with Chiari II malformation, only 23% eventually become symptomatic (Worley et al., 1996), and the severity of brainstem symptoms does not correlate well with the degree of caudal herniation (Pang, 1995). However, most (75%) of those who do develop symptoms eventually require surgical decompression (at an average age of 14 months), 23% require tracheostomy, and 34% to 38% do not survive (Park et al., 1983; Worley et al., 1996). Predictors of a poor outcome include respiratory arrest, vocal cord paralysis, and arm weakness; in one study, 71% of infants having at least one of these symptoms died. Central apnea is associated with a 56% mortality rate (Cochrane et al., 1991). With rapid diagnosis and decompression, 69% of the infants have resolution of their symptoms within 48 hours (Pollack et al., 1996).

The treatment for symptomatic Chiari II malformation is placement of a ventriculoperitoneal shunt; if a shunt is already in place, it is necessary to rule out shunt malfunction. If symptoms occur after a functional shunt has been in place for at least 48 hours, the next step is hindbrain decompression, which should be performed early to minimize symptom progression (Pang, 1995). Magnetic resonance imaging of the craniovertebral junction and cervical spine is helpful to plan the procedure. After exposure of the posterior craniovertebral elements, a small portion of the occipital bone and the cervical lamina that overlie the cerebellar peg are removed. The laminectomy is kept narrow to minimize the risk of cervical kyphosis later in life. There is frequently a band of dura contributing to brainstem compression that must be released. Since spina bifida is often associated with a low-lying tentorium and torcular Herophili, and since the occipital sinus may be a venous lake, opening of the dura can cause significant bleeding, which usually can be controlled with vascular clamps. However, to avoid this potential complication, it is sometimes sufficient to selectively section the outer restrictive bands without cutting through the entire thickness of the dura. This usually allows sufficient dural expansion to provide decompression. Intraoperative ultrasonography is used to confirm decompression of the brainstem extending below the most inferior portion of the tonsils. The ultrasound scan should demonstrate CSF circulating around the cerebellum and in the cervical canal.

Since the Chiari II malformation may continue to pose a threat even after repair, it is essential to monitor patients for symptoms and signs of brainstem dysfunction throughout childhood. The most common (and often missed) symptom of recurrent Chiari II malformation is moderate to severe sleep-disordered breathing, consisting of obstructive apnea, central apnea, or central hypoventilation (Kirk et al., 1999).

CONCLUSIONS

Postnatal surgical treatment for myelomeningocele can have a profound impact on survival and functionality for patients with this condition. Repair of the defect involves reconstruction of the neural tube and closure of the skin over the abnormal tissue. Large defects and kyphosis may require innovative techniques, and associated abnormalities such as hydrocephalus and the Chiari II malformation must also be addressed by the neurosurgeon.

REFERENCES

Ames MD, Schut L (1972). Results of treatment of 171 consecutive myelomeningoceles—1963 to 1968. Pediatrics 50:466–470.

Bensen JT, Dillard RG, Burton BK (1988). Open spina bifida: does cesarean section delivery improve prognosis? Obstet Gynecol 71:532–534.

Caldarelli M, DiRocco C, LaMarca F (1996). Shunt complications in the first postoperative year in children with meningomyelocele. Childs Nerv Syst 12:748–754.

Chadduck WM, Reding DL (1988). Experience with simultaneous ventriculoperitoneal shunt placement and myelomeningocele repair. J Pediatr Surg 23:913–916.

Charney EB, Weller SC, Sutton LN, Bruce DA, Schut LB (1985). Management of the newborn with myelomeningocele: time for a decision-making process. Pediatrics 75:58–64.

Cochrane D, Aronyk K, Sawatzky B, Wilson D, Steinbok P (1991). The effects of labor and delivery on spinal cord function and ambulation in patients with meningomyelocele. Childs Nerv Syst 7:312–315.

Cohen A (1998). Endoscopy and the management of third ventricular lesions. In Apuzzo M (ed): *Surgery of the Third Ventricle*, 2nd ed. Baltimore: Williams & Wilkins, pp. 889–936.

Cremer R (1997). The role of shunted hydrocephalus in the development of allergy to latex in patients with spina bifida (letter to the editor). J Allergy Clin Immunol 100:719.

Dias MS, Walker ML (1992). The embryogenesis of complex dysraphic malformations: a disorder of gastrulation? Pediatr Neurosurg. 18:229–253.

Forestus P (1587). *De Capitis et Cerebre Morbis ac Symptomatis. Observationum Medicinalium*, libri III. Leiden: Ex Off Plantiniana.

Forestus P (1610). *Observationum et Curationum Chirurgicarum*, libri V, lib III, obs VII. Lugduni: Raphelengium.

Fraser J (1929). Spina bifida. Edinburgh Med J 36:284.

Gamache FW Jr. (1995). Treatment of hydrocephalus in patients with meningomyelocele or encephalocele: a recent series. Childs Nerv Syst 11:487–488.

Gilbert JN, Jones KL, Rorke LB, Chernoff GF, James HE (1986). Central nervous system anomalies associated with meningomyelocele, hydrocephalus, and the Arnold-Chiari malformation: reappraisal of theories regarding the pathogenesis of posterior neural tube closure defects. Neurosurgery 18:559–564.

Hahn YS (1995). Open myelomeningocele. Neurosurg Clin North Am 6:231–241.

Holzman RS (1997). Clinical management of latex-allergic children. Anesth Analg 85:529–533.

Hubballah MY, Hoffman HJ (1987). Early repair of myelomeningocele and simultaneous insertion of ventriculoperitoneal shunt: techniques and results. Neurosurgery 20:21–23.

Ingraham FD, Swan H (1943). Spina bifida and cranium. I. A survey of five hundred forty-six cases. N Engl J Med 228:559.

Kirk VG, Morielli A, Brouillette RT (1999). Sleep-disordered breathing in patients with myelomeningocele: the missed diagnosis. Dev Med Child Neurol 41:40–43.

Lebedeff A (1881). Uber die Enstehurg der Anencephalie und Spina Bifida dei Vogelin und Menschen. Virchows Arch Pathol Anat Physiol 86:263.

Lorber J (1971). Results of treatment of myelomeningocele. An analysis of 524 unselected cases with special references to possible selection of treatment. Dev Med Child Neurol 13:279–303.

Lorber J, Salfield SA (1981). Results of selective treatment of spina bifida cystica. Arch Dis Child 56:822–830.

Luthy DA, Wardinsky T, Shurtleff DB, Hollenbach KA, Hickok DE, Nyberg DA, et al (1991). Cesarean section before the onset of labor and subsequent motor function in infants with meningomyelocele diagnosed antenatally. N Engl J Med 324:662–666.

Mazagri R, Ventureyra EC (1999). Latex allergy in neurosurgical practice. Childs Nerv System 15:404–407.

McLone DG (1983). Results of treatment of children born with a myelomeningocele. Clin Neurosurg 30:407–412.

McLone DG (1998). Care of the neonate with a myelomeningocele. Neurosurg Clin North Am 9:111–120.

Morgagani JB (1761). *De Sedubis et Causis Morborum per Anatomen Indigatis,* libri V. Venice.

Nieto A, Estomell F, Mazon A, Reig C, Nieto A, Garcia-Ibarra F (1996). Allergy to latex in spina bifida: a multivariate study of associated risk factors in 100 consecutive patients. J Allergy Clin Immunol 98:501–507.

Pang D (1995). Surgical complications of open spinal dysraphism. Neurosurg Clin North Am 6:243–257.

Park TS, Hoffman HJ, Hendrick EB, Humphreys RP (1983). Experience with surgical decompression of the Arnold-Chiari malformation in young infants with myelomeningocele. Neurosurgery 13:147–152.

Pollack IF, Kinnunen D, Albright AL (1996). The effect of early craniocervical decompression on functional outcome in neonates and young infants with myelodysplasia and symptomatic Chiari II malformations: Results from a prospective series. Neurosurgery 38:703–710.

Ramasastry SS, Cohen M (1995). Soft tissue closure and plastic surgical aspects of large open myelomeningoceles. Neurosurg Clin North Am 6:279–291.

Reigel D (1979). Kyphectomy and myelomeningocele repair. In Ransohoff J (ed): *Modem Techniques in Surgery: Neurosurgery.* Mount Kisco, NY: Futura, pp. 1–9.

Reigel DH, McLone DG (1987). *Myelomeningocele. Operative Treatment and Results.* Basel: Karger.

Scott RM, Wolpert SM, Bartoshesky LE, Zimbler S, Klauber GT (1986). Dermoid tumors occurring at the site of previous myelomeningocele repair. J Neurosurg 65:779–783.

Shurtleff DB, Lemire RJ (1995). Epidemiology, etiologic factors, and prenatal diagnosis of open spinal dysraphism. Neurosurg Clin North Am 6:183–193.

Stark GD (1971). Neonatal assessment of the child with a myelomeningocele. Arch Dis Child 46:539–548.

Steinbok P, Irvine B, Cochrane DD, Irwin BJ (1992). Long-term outcome and complications of children born with meningomyelocele. Childs Nerv Syst 8:92–96.

Taylor MJ, Boor R, Keenan NK, Rutka JT, Drake JM (1996). Brain stem auditory and visual evoked potentials in infants with myelomeningocele. Brain Dev 18:99–104.

Tulpius N (1641). *Cum Atieis Figuris*. Amsterdam: Apud Ludovican Elzevirium.

von Recklinghausen F (1886). Untersuchungen uber che Spina Bifida. Arch Pathol Anat 105:243.

Wills KE, Holmbeck GN, Dillon K, McLone DG (1990). Intelligence and achievement in children with myelomeningocele. J Pediatr Psychol. 15:161–176.

Worley G, Schuster JM, Oakes WJ (1996). Survival at 5 years of a cohort of newborn infants with myelomeningocele. Dev Med Child Neurol 38:816–822.

20

Neurosurgical Management of Adults with Spina Bifida

HAROLD L. REKATE

Accurate epidemiologic information before the development of valve-regulated shunts is unavailable. Nonetheless, during that time, few infants born with spina bifida and hydrocephalus survived the newborn period. The first reports of concepts for managing these children derived from treatments used in the 1960s and published in the early 1970s. The first generation of these survivors are now reaching middle age. Based on decades of careful study in multidisciplinary clinics, an increasing number of publications deal with the management of infants and children born with this complex congenital anomaly. However, there is little if any published information available from which to derive treatment protocols for adults with this condition. This problem primarily reflects the newness of this population of patients, who previously rarely survived infancy. An important secondary explanation is related to the settings in which care is delivered to these patients.

Especially in the United States and Great Britain, it was recognized early that these patients had extremely complex conditions and would benefit from coordinated multidisciplinary care. A number of academic centers committed resources to providing coordinated care for these infants and children, and spina bifida became the paradigm of the value of coordinated care in the management of children with complicated multisystemic birth defects. Coordinated care was usually based in academic medical centers and usually occurred in children's hospitals. In the United States, the primary payer for the treatment of many of these children became individual programs in each state designed to take care of children with birth defects. They usually had names such as *Crippled Children's Program.*

This system grew as the number of these children who survived increased after contemporary concepts of treatment were introduced. Changes in the mechanisms and levels of funding have placed significant strains on the systems providing care. Some clinics have had to close, creating challenges in providing care to these complicated patients. Justification for these clinics has rarely been challenged, but comparisons of outcomes in such patients treated in multidisciplinary clinics and in those receiving services from individual providers are unavailable. Probably the best information derives from a study of patients who were first managed in a multidisciplinary setting and then offered noncoordinated care by the same physicians after the clinic itself closed (Kaufman et al., 1994). Initially, the medical care costs dropped dramatically after the clinic closed. There were fewer patient contacts, and fewer surgical procedures were performed. After 3 years, however, the costs of caring for these children rose dramatically because the incidence of decubitus ulcers, urinary tract infections, renal failure, and insidious shunt failure increased. The initial cost savings were soon overwhelmed by medical problems that might have been prevented or ameliorated if earlier care had been provided (Kaufman et al., 1994). These patients and their families were overwhelmed by assuming the responsibility of coordinating care for themselves or their own children, respectively.

At the Arizona Children's Rehabilitation Services' Multidisciplinary Spina Bifida Clinic in Phoenix, overseen by the Children's Health Center at St. Joseph's Hospital and Medical Center, we had a brief opportunity to view this problem from another perspective. Because our clinic is overseen by the Arizona State Department of Health

Services, care is discontinued at age 21. Our clinic coordinator had maintained contact with most of the adults who had "graduated" from the clinic during the previous decade. Many of these patients were covered under a single health maintenance organization Medicaid provider of care. Needed care was ordered by the specialist and approved by the patient's primary care provider, who served as a gatekeeper. Little resistance was encountered in obtaining approval for surgical procedures or diagnostic tests. Patients did not receive medical care—not because it was unavailable, but because they did not seek it. There was no coordination of care, and they had difficulty recognizing the early signs of deterioration. Traveling to appointments with a multitude of specialists became frightening, and, for some, physically impossible. Most had not had an imaging study since leaving the clinic. Few had undergone urinalysis, and then only as a result of overtly febrile urinary tract infections. Many community ambulators had reverted to wheelchairs, and decubitus ulcers were common.

We petitioned for and obtained clearance to establish an adult spina bifida clinic with the intention of offering adults care similar to that received by children with this condition. A pilot program with 10 patients was to be the start of the adult program. The physicians involved donated their time for outpatient care, and the hospital supplied the other clinicians needed to make the clinic a success, including physical and occupational therapists and psychologists. Imaging studies and surgical procedures that were ordered were reviewed by the patient's gatekeepers, and all were approved as necessary. Only 3 of the 10 patients were living independently and employed. Almost all required surgical procedures such as shunt revision, spinal cord detethering, aggressive management of decubitus ulcers, bladder augmentation, or contracture releases. The cost of medical care for these patients was extremely high, and the experimental program was abandoned after its first year as being too expensive. Coordinated care is effective in preventing many of the long-term complications of spina bifida in adults as well as in children, but economic considerations usually preclude this "luxury." Patients are left to be responsible for coordinating their own care.

Finally, finding specialists in neurosurgery, urology, and orthopedics who are trained to manage the late complications of spina bifida in adults and who are interested in seeing this type of patient is extremely difficult. In childhood and adolescence, these patients usually are cared for by physicians practicing in children's hospitals. Typically at the age of 18 or 21, the patients are no longer considered appropriate to be treated in a children's hospital and are instructed to find adult neurosurgeons, urologists, and orthopedists to assume responsibility for their care. At best, this is a frightening and dangerous time for these patients. The physicians who have provided care to them for many years and who understand the subtle nuances of their complex difficulties are replaced with physicians who want to provide excellent care but have not previously seen what works and what does not in each particular case. At worse, adult practitioners are unwilling to see patients with complex conditions who require considerable time and many visits that are often emergencies. Frequently, these patients receive much of their care in the emergency room.

This chapter describes the complex nature of the neurosurgical problems confronting adults with the congenital abnormality of spina bifida and how they should be managed, and defines the role of the neurosurgeon in caring for these patients.

HYDROCEPHALUS IN ADULTS WITH SPINA BIFIDA

When adults develop hydrocephalus, the number of underlying causes such as infection, tumor, or hemorrhage is relatively small. The cerebral ventricles enlarge because of an obstruction along the pathway of cerebrospinal fluid (CSF) flow from the ventricles to the arachnoid villi. The latter are specialized pouches of arachnoid invaginated into the dural venous sinuses. These organelles allow CSF to flow into the venous system. In young adults, the signs and symptoms of hydrocephalus and shunt failure are straightforward and include severe headache, nausea, vomiting, irritability progressing to somnolence, and eventually coma if untreated. Unless the patient is elderly or the condition has been present for a very long time, the size of the ventricles decreases substantially when treated with ventriculoperitoneal (VP) shunting. The diagnosis of hydrocephalus is not difficult, and the ventricles expand at the time of shunt failure. Many of these patients have single, defined points of obstruction and may be managed with endoscopic third ventriculostomy (ETV). Infants, however, tend to be much more complicated to manage. Their initial causes of hydrocephalus are more diverse, and shunt failure is much more difficult to diagnose (Rekate, 2002), especially in the context of hydrocephalus associated with spina bifida. All patients born with spina bifida aperta have a Chiari II malformation, although it is subtle in some infants. The malformation is the cause of the hydrocephalus that so often accompanies this condition. Ventriculomegaly occurs in about 90% of babies born with spina bifida. At least 70% of these babies receive VP shunts.

What causes hydrocephalus in the context of the Chiari II malformation? There are four potential sites of obstruction within the CSF pathway affected by the abnormalities present in a Chiari II malformation (Fig. 20.1) (Rekate, 2001). An individual patient may have one or all

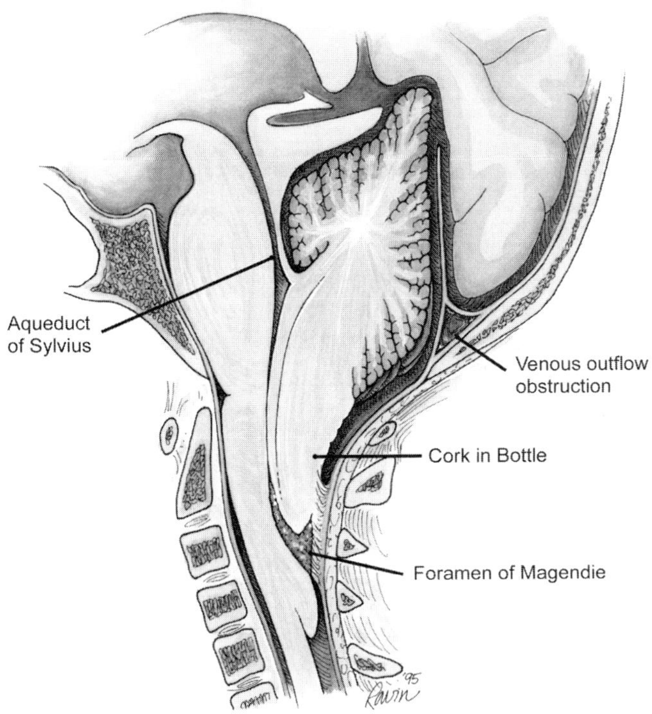

FIGURE 20.1. Illustration of a Chiari II malformation showing the four potential sites of obstruction of the cerebrospinal fluid pathways causing hydrocephalus in the context of spina bifida. *Source:* With permission from the Barrow Neurological Institute.

of these points of obstruction. In infancy, it may not be possible to define the actual site of CSF obstruction, and probably it is unnecessary unless the possibility of treating the hydrocephalus with ETV is entertained. Each of these four sites is associated with a characteristic syndrome of presentation at the time of shunt failure. The symptoms of presentation for each patient are likely to continue into adulthood and to form an important part of the information needed to treat adults with hydrocephalus and spina bifida. Each of the four potential sites of obstruction to flow is associated with a different clinical picture at the time of shunt failure, and each is described separately. It should be recognized that more than one site may be obstructed in a single patient (Rekate, 2002).

Aqueductal Stenosis

The posterior fossa is smaller than normal in the context of a Chiari II malformation, and the tentorium is oriented vertically. These features lead to an incompetent tentorial notch. The superior aspect of the cerebellum often rises well above the tentorial notch. This feature can lead to anterior and superior distortion of the tectum of the midbrain (*tectal beaking*) and secondarily to obstruction of the aqueduct of Sylvius. These children are usually diagnosed in utero with marked enlargement of the ventricles and a very large head that makes it difficult or impossible to deliver the baby except by cesarean section. At shunt failure, the closed aqueduct means that the total volume of CSF is quite small. Small additions of CSF by production of CSF that cannot be removed rapidly increase intracranial pressure (ICP) and the size of the ventricles. These patients become symptomatic at all ages, with overt and classic signs of shunt failure: rapid deterioration, severe headaches, vomiting, and lethargy. Several authors have reported excellent results from treating children and adults with ETV (Jones et al., 1996; Teo and Jones, 1996). Our own experience has been somewhat less positive (Baskin et al., 1998).

Obstruction of the Outlet Foramina of the Fourth Ventricle

The degree of hindbrain herniation in the context of a Chiari II malformation can be extreme. Occasionally, the medullary kink is found as low as C5. In this situation the foramen of Luschka is within the spinal canal. The chronic mixing of amniotic fluid and CSF in utero leads to chronic arachnoidal scarring (Duru and Rekate, 1997). This scarring, combined with the characteristic eversion of the fourth ventricular choroid plexus into the subarachnoid space outside the fourth ventricle, leads to occlusion of the foramen of Magendie in almost all cases of Chiari II malformation. The second site of obstruction to the flow of CSF is therefore the outlet foramina of the fourth ventricle. Hall and colleagues recognized the relationship between scoliosis and shunt failure (Batnitzky et al., 1976; Hall, et al., 1979). In spina bifida patients with obstruction of the outlet foramina of the fourth ventricle, shunt failure leads to what Oi and colleagues describe as hydromyelic hydrocephalus and what most authors describe as syringomyelia (Batnitzky et al., 1976; Hall et al., 1979; Oi et al., 1991).

Syringomyelia can lead to weakness and sensory loss in the upper extremities and to scoliosis with or without headache or other signs of shunt failure or hydrocephalus. These same symptoms would be expected from a symptomatic Chiari II malformation. Magnetic resonance imaging of the brain and spine shows some increase in ventricular size, including the third ventricle, and syringomyelia. Repairing the shunt usually resolves the problems caused by this subtle form of shunt failure. Hydromyelic hydrocephalus from obstruction of the outlet foramina of the fourth ventricle also occurs later in life but is extremely rare. The cause of this condition as an acquired phenomenon in patients who do not have spina bifida is meningitis, usually a chronic granulomatous form such as tuberculosis, fungal meningitis, or carcinomatous meningitis.

The "Cork in the Bottle"

In the normal pattern of CSF flow, the ventricular and spinal fluids mix in the cisterna magna and then flow over the convexity of the brain to the cortical subarachnoid space. Patients with a Chiari II malformation do not have a cisterna magna because the brain and spinal cord are crowded within the upper cervical canal. This crowding can lead to obstruction of CSF flow between the spinal and cortical subarachnoid spaces. Imaging studies show ventricular dilatation. This condition is known as *communicating hydrocephalus* according to the Dandy classification or as *extraventricular obstructive hydrocephalus* according to the later Ransohoff classification (Ransohoff et al., 1960). In this context, shunt failure is often subtle and can mimic many other conditions.

There is little evidence that most patients with hydrocephalus and shunts require routine imaging studies. If their shunt fails, either they will be overtly symptomatic or they will develop a state of shunt-independent arrest of hydrocephalus (Rekate et al., 1982). In contrast, in patients with hydrocephalus related to a Chiari II malformation, insidious deterioration may be the rule rather than the exception (Fig. 20.2).

Subtle deterioration is a common and somewhat frightening aspect of the management of hydrocephalus in the context of adult spina bifida. One of the most common subtle signs of shunt malfunction in this group is the onset of "staring spells" similar to *absence* epilepsy. Electroencephalography in these patients is either normal or shows intermittent slowing. There are no guidelines for how frequently imaging studies should be obtained in older children and adults with shunted hydrocephalus and spina bifida, but such routine studies are warranted (Rekate, 2001). Because coordinated care is lacking in adults with this condition and because at least some patients are living independently, they are at risk for subtle deterioration that goes unnoticed by their family. Fur-

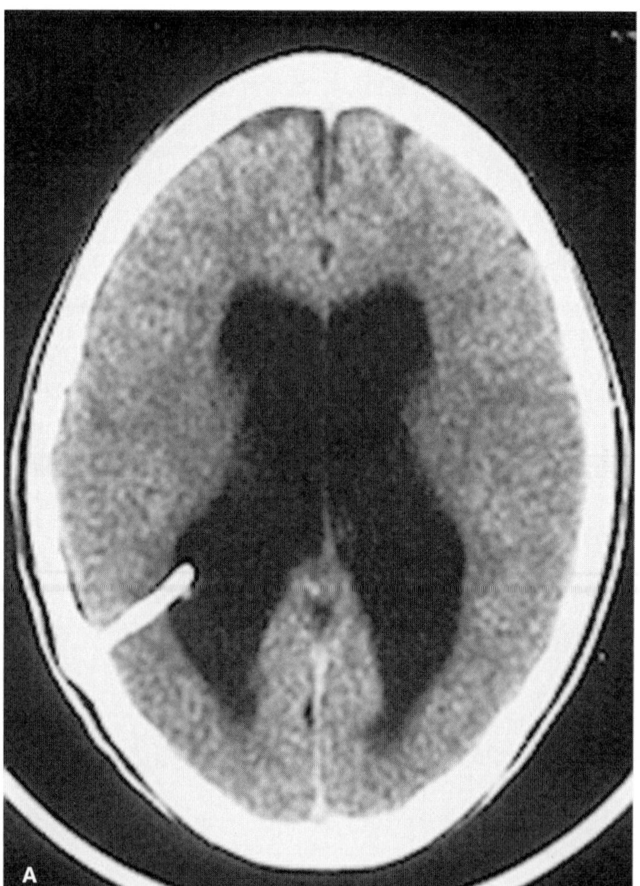

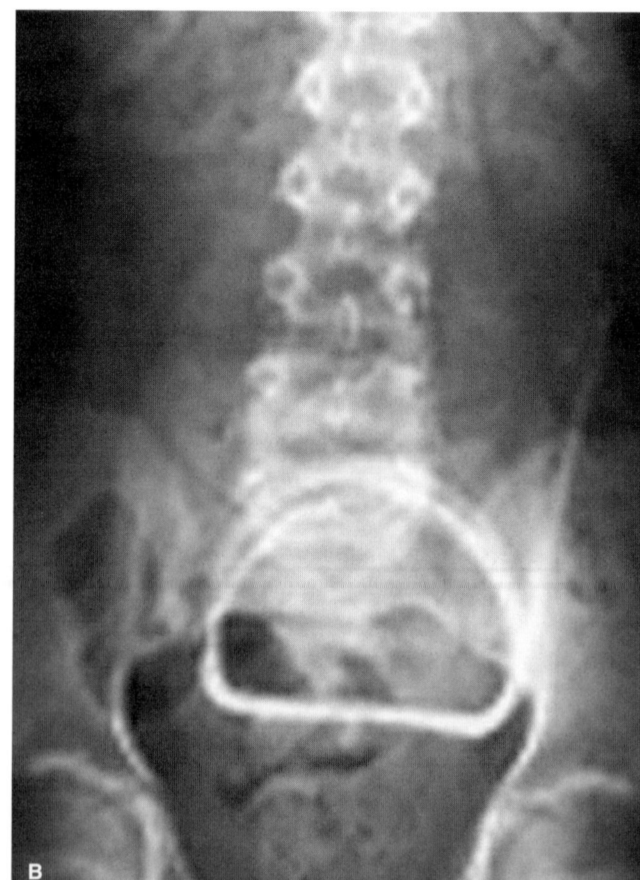

FIGURE 20.2. (*A*) Computed tomographic scan of a 15-year-old girl obtained for routine surveillance at an annual multidisciplinary spina bifida clinic showing enlargement of the lateral ventricles without overt signs of increased intracranial pressure. (*B*) Abdominal film of the same patient showing unrecognized disconnection of the shunt system. The distal end was in the peritoneal cavity. When questioned, this girl, who had been earning straight A's in all classes, was now failing several. She was surly toward her family. Psychological assessment showed that her IQ, previously tested at 120, now tested at 65. She underwent shunt revision, and 4 months later had resumed her previous successful academic career and regained her positive attitude.

thermore, these studies may not be ordered because the patients no longer receive routine care from neurosurgeons familiar with these problems.

Hydrocephalus Related to Venous Obstruction

In patients with a Chiari II malformation, the posterior fossa is quite small and the tentorium is oriented vertically, as discussed earlier. Frequently, this configuration leads to downward displacement of the dural venous sinuses with the torcular Herophili lying at the level of the foramen magnum, where it can be compressed by crowding of all of the structures that occupy the space. This crowding can lead to a significant increase in dural venous sinus pressure. In infants with distensible skulls, CSF cannot be absorbed due to the increased sagittal sinus pressure. In response, the size of the cortical subarachnoid spaces and ventricles increases, leading to hydrocephalus. After a shunt is inserted, the skull fuses. At the time of shunt failure, ICP may increase rapidly to very high levels with little or no increase in ventricular size. This syndrome has been termed *normal volume hydrocephalus* (Engel et al., 1979). In this condition, closure of the sutures has been converted to pseudotumor cerebri. Almost all of these patients are sent home from emergency rooms with the reassurance that imaging has shown that their shunt is working well (Rekate, 2001, 2002).

These patients frequently develop a severe form of slit-ventricle syndrome with intermittent proximal shunt failure, with or without spontaneous resolution. The distal obstruction of the natural CSF pathways leads to an accumulation of CSF in the cortical subarachnoid space that pushes the brain inward. As the brain is distorted around the holes in the ventricular catheter, the ventricular catheter becomes permanently or temporarily obstructed. In patients without spina bifida, this serious problem would best be handled by lumboperitoneal shunting (Rekate and Wallace, 2003). The presence of a dysraphic state and spinal cord tethering makes lumboperitoneal shunting difficult, if not impossible. It is, however, still necessary to access the cortical subarachnoid space when planning shunt placement in these complicated patients.

In this difficult situation, decompressing a Chiari II malformation and creating a new cisterna magna using a patch of the upper cervical dura has worked well. A piece of lumboperitoneal shunt catheter is placed into the newly created cisterna magna and brought up to the foramen magnum. This flimsy tubing is spliced to a standard piece of peritoneal shunt using a stepdown connector. The new shunt tubing is spliced into the existing VP shunt proximal to the valve. This construct, which has been recommended by Egnor (M. Egnor, personal communication, 2002), leads to mixing of ventricular and subarachnoid CSF, preventing the likelihood of ventricular catheter obstruction. Drainage (decompression) of the cortical subarachnoid space may actually increase the volume of the ventricular system.

Multiple sites of obstruction to the flow of CSF often make the management of older children and adults with shunt failure difficult both diagnostically and therapeutically. This is the condition most likely associated with subtle deterioration without overt signs of increased ICP. Education and screening imaging studies are uniquely indicated for these patients. Adults are no longer under the direct observation of anxious parents and face considerable challenges in obtaining screening medical care. Few of these patients are employed or financially and socially independent. They are no longer served by coordinators of multidisciplinary clinics. The universal goal of independence for adults requires more thought, planning, and creative strategies than is needed for individuals with most other survivable birth defects.

SYMPTOMS RELATIVE TO THE CHIARI II MALFORMATION

The Chiari II malformation is a universal part of the complex central nervous system (CNS) malformations in patients born with open neural tube defects. McLone and Knepper (1989) have shown that the Chiari II malformation is caused by leakage of CSF in utero. This leakage leads to microcephaly as the brain grows and to herniation of the posterior fossa contents into the upper cervical canal. Three distinct syndromes are associated with the Chiari II malformation, and to some extent their symptoms depend on the age at which the patient becomes symptomatic. In the perinatal form, newborns cannot breath spontaneously and must be resuscitated in the delivery room. These children have a poor prognosis and usually require permanent ventilator assistance or they die in early infancy. Postmortem studies in these unfortunate babies show disorganization of the brainstem and no identifiable 9th and 10th cranial nerve nuclei.

The infantile form tends to manifest later, usually between the ages of 6 weeks to 6 months. The children become symptomatic with stridor; have difficulty swallowing, as shown by drooling; retropulsion of the neck; irritability; and poor upper extremity tone. Unlike children with the perinatal form, these children often benefit from decompression of the brainstem in the cervical spinal canal. Vocal cord function and the ability to swallow and protect the airway recover. This condition should be considered somewhat of an emergency because of the inability to protect the airway. Furthermore, the earlier in the course of the process the decompression is performed, the more likely the child is to recover.

It is the late adolescent or adult form of spina bifida that concerns us. These patients have done well in infancy and childhood. From adolescence through adulthood, they develop a characteristic syndrome of suboccipital headaches, numbness in the upper extremities, and finally, increasing weakness and coordination difficulties in the hands. In contrast to the first two forms, this particular condition does not appear to be caused by compression of the neural elements. Instead, it appears that the brainstem and spinal cord are attached to the dorsal surface of the craniocervical dura (Fig. 20.3). In this context, brainstem dysfunction can result from multiple factors that can be treated in different ways. The most important diagnostic test is to ascertain that the shunt is working. As discussed above, 20% of older patients with spina bifida do not develop ventriculomegaly at the time of shunt failure, and many of these patients respond to shunt revision. In these situations, a manometric test of shunt function or a radionuclide shunt study is necessary to exclude the possibility that the symptoms are caused by shunt failure rather than by a symptomatic Chiari II malformation.

The second problem that is easy to confuse with a symptomatic Chiari II malformation is symptomatic tethering of the distal spinal cord. In this situation, the abnormalities of neurological structure interact throughout the neuraxis. Attachment of the spinal cord at its distal terminus affects the entire CNS. Detethering the distal spinal cord leads to ascension of the brainstem in the cervical canal and to symptomatic improvement of the condition (L. Harris, personal communication, 1990).

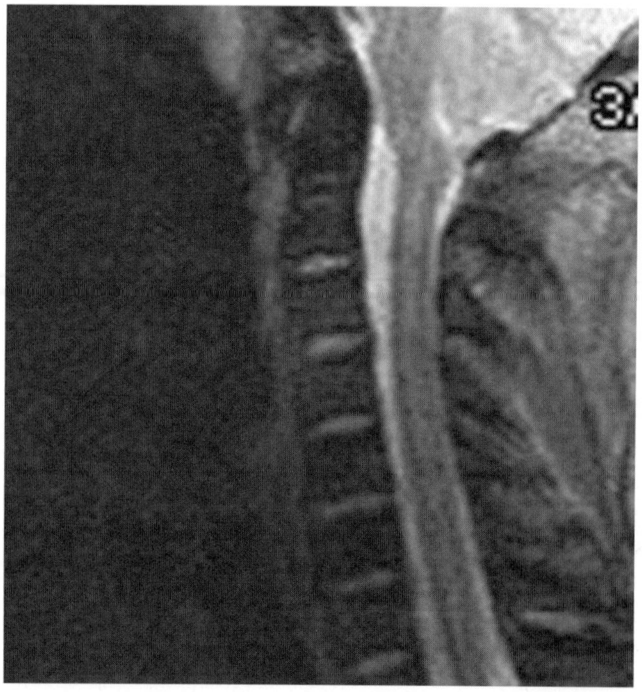

FIGURE 20.3. Midline sagittal magnetic resonance image shows adherence of the herniated brainstem to the posterior cervical spinal dura.

If the patient has symptoms suggestive of both hindbrain dysfunction and a tethered spina cord, detethering the spinal cord is likely to improve the symptoms. If the patient is asymptomatic at the level of the distal spinal cord (Fig. 20.4), it is usually best to address the Chiari II malformation. The risks of intervention are substantially lower, and subsequent surgeries may thereby be avoided.

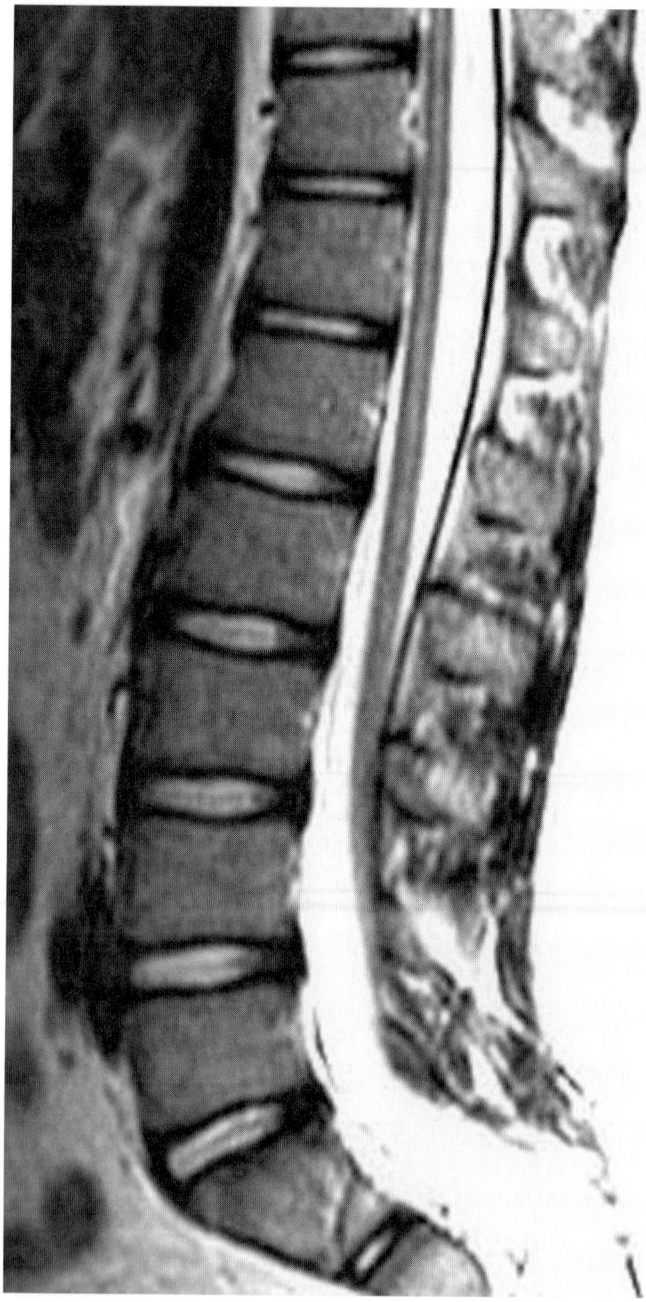

FIGURE 20.4. Sagittal magnetic resonance image of the lumbar spine in a spina bifida patient with no overt signs or symptoms of spinal cord tethering.

If surgery is performed for symptoms relative to the brainstem, the operation is distinct from the operation that would be performed in patients with a Chiari I malformation. It is rarely if ever necessary to remove bone from the foramen magnum. This structure is usually large in the presence of a Chiari II malformation. The posterior fossa is small and the tentorium is oriented vertically. This relationship often places the torcula at the level of the foramen magnum. In this context, bone removal of the posterior fossa is unnecessary and often even dangerous. Occasionally, the early results of decompressing Chiari II malformations were devastating due to excessive blood loss.

The surgical procedure involves a midline laminectomy without extension into the facets. The laminectomy is extended far enough inferiorly to be certain that the brainstem is free of overlying laminae. C3 is usually included but has been found to extend well below that level. When the dura is opened, strands of arachnoidal scar are found tenting the brainstem back to the opened dura posteriorly. Under microscopic magnification, these strands are cut. The brainstem can be seen to fall into the bottom of the cervical canal. In these situations, my preference is to identify the choroid plexus everted into the subarachnoid space. The choroid plexus is followed into the fourth ventricle opening, and the foramen of Magendie is opened to ensure the free flow of CSF.

Once the brainstem has been detethered, a decision is made about how much room is present in the resultant cervical spinal cord. A patch is seldom required. Occasionally, however, there is too little room and a patch is necessary, depending on the surgeon's preference.

The outcome of this type of decompression in properly selected individuals with a Chiari II malformation has been excellent. Most patients are free of headaches after the surgical pain has eased. Almost all experience significant improvement in arm strength and function. The surgical procedure is a midline operation, and the opening need not be extended far laterally. We have had only one patient who developed a spinal deformity after this procedure—an infant with a very large head operated on within the first few weeks of life. The only other complication we have encountered has been the development of a pseudomeningocele, which was probably related to an unrecognized subsequent shunt failure.

SYMPTOMATIC TETHERED CORD IN ADULTS WITH SPINA BIFIDA

The risk of developing symptoms of tethered cord syndrome does not end when growth ceases. Although tethered cord syndrome results from the failure of the spinal cord to ascend as the patient grows, the inciting event results from the movement of the distal end of the spinal cord during motion. Yamada et al. (1981) suggest that with movement, oxidative metabolism of the spinal cord fails, leading to neurological deterioration. Release of the tethered cord leads to documentable improvement in oxidative metabolism. Younger children and adolescents exhibit three syndromes relative to a symptomatic tethered cord that lead to detethering surgery. For a long time, the most common indication for detethering was failure of continence on intermittent catheterization. This indication is now less likely to lead to tethered cord syndrome because urological management of this problem has improved. Treatment of progressive scoliosis is a controversial indication for detethering. Spinal straightening can result from detethering, but recurrence is common and may be related to anatomical retethering. It is unlikely that scoliosis would be used as an indication for detethering in adults.

The third indication for tethered cord release in children and adolescents is likely to be the only indication for detethering the spinal cord in adults. This condition is associated with a combination of severe back and leg pain, often in the distribution of several nerve roots, and loss of motor and sensory function. The problem often begins with a mild traumatic event. These events tend to be the result of axial-loading injuries such as falls but have also been reported in other conditions, such as riding in a car with no shock absorbers. Patients with low lumbar lesions are the most difficult to treat when this problem occurs. A minimal increase in neurological deficits can change an adult with spina bifida from a community ambulator to a home ambulator who needs an assistive device or a wheelchair to get around in the community.

The major difficulty that neurosurgeons and their adult patients confront is that surgery in this situation may or may not lead to neurological recovery, while neurological function is clearly at further risk from the procedure. Unlike in children, the back and leg pain in adults caused by a tethered cord does not resolve quickly after detethering. It may take a month or more, and complete resolution of the pain cannot be guaranteed. Symptoms often recur months or years after detethering in adults. In my experience, however, the neuropathic pain associated with recurrent tethered cord syndrome in these patients is unresponsive to all treatment but surgery. The risk–benefit analysis is not straightforward. However, surgery should not be considered until conservative measures have failed, and no outcome can be guaranteed.

Another important aspect of surgical decision making relates to diagnosis. No radiographic procedure can determine that a patient's symptoms are caused by tethered cord syndrome and not by other causes. Arthritic changes in the lower spine related to chronic abnormal neurological intervention and mobility may lead to severe pain with mobility as well as to chronic subluxation of the hips in patients with weak hip extensors and accentuated lumbar lordosis. These patients should be managed with a period of immobility. They will respond if the problem is mechanical and will not respond if it is caused by the tethered cord syndrome.

REPRODUCTION

Successful independence in adulthood includes reproductive functions. Although the number of spina bifida patients reaching adulthood and even middle age is increasing, little is known about their reproductive capacity. Although the actual percentage is unknown, a significant minority of males with spina bifida are potent. In surveys on education in sexuality among patients with spina bifida, expectations of intimacy are almost universal and about 25% of patients have had intimate relationships not otherwise described. This is four times more likely among women than men. Using many key words and combinations of words, I have been unable to find a reference that indicates whether males with spina bifida can successfully father a child.

Most discussions regarding reproduction in the context of spina bifida are limited to conception, pregnancy, and delivery of babies. The first aspect of this discussion relates to the risk of a woman with spina bifida conceiving a fetus. Before the folic acid campaign, the rate of this birth defect in the general population varied widely but was accepted to range between 1 and 3 per 1000 births. The published risk for a woman with spina bifida conceiving a fetus with the same anomaly is about 4% (Rietberg and Lindhout, 1993). For patients with seizures on anticonvulsants, especially carbamazepine, this percentage increases and may double (Frey and Hauser, 2003).

The prophylactic use of folic acid before conception decreases the incidence of spina bifida conceptions perhaps more than 50%. The current recommendation is that normal women who may become pregnant should consume at least 0.4 mg folic acid per day. High-risk women such as those with a seizure disorder on anticonvulsants and women with spina bifida should take 4 mg/day (Erickson, 2002).

How to ensure compliance with this recommendation is a subject for a major public health debate. In a very well controlled study from Nova Scotia, a major public health initiative in the mid-1990s to convince women to take supplemental folate did not influence the incidence of neural tube defects in the region (2.5–2.6 per 1000 births). After folate was added to wheat products sold to the populace, however, the incidence decreased more than 50% (McLone and Knepper, 1989).

The obstetrical issues related to the delivery of children of mothers with spina bifida are of significant concern. Most of these mothers have shunts. Will their shunts continue to work during pregnancy, and does that consideration affect the method of delivery? The body of information on pregnancy and hydrocephalus is growing. One study (Wisoff et al., 1991) found a high incidence of shunt failure in the third trimester when intra-abdominal pressure increased dramatically, resulting in an increase in ICP. Most of these patients became asymptomatic after delivery, although some needed pre- or postnatal shunt revision. The authors recommended early delivery in symptomatic patients when the problem is likely related to an increase in intra-abdominal pressure. The authors also accepted vaginal delivery, but their threshold for performing cesarean section in patients who develop signs of increased ICP during delivery (Wisoff et al., 1991) was relatively low. This study involved patients seen by a neurosurgeon during their pregnancy. A larger study (Liakos et al., 2000) that involved giving a questionnaire to women with shunts showed a very low baseline level of shunt-related complications during pregnancy and delivery. This study recommended that decisions regarding the method of delivery be made on obstetrical rather than neurosurgical grounds.

The primary concern associated with delivering babies in patients with spina bifida is the possible exacerbation of symptoms of tethered cord in the mother. As stated, the most common presentation of adult tethered cord syndrome is severe back pain and radicular pain, with a decrease in neurological findings usually associated with a traumatic event. The delivery of a baby in the lithotomy position could be such a traumatic event. In one study of 11 women who became symptomatic from a tethered cord, 5 became symptomatic when they delivered their baby (Huttmann et al., 2001). A general review of the issues related to pregnancy and delivery indicates that a decision to perform a cesarean section should be made on obstetrical grounds. However, significant challenges related to pelvic anatomy and to the shunting issues already discussed could impact the decision (Rietberg and Lindhout, 1993). Data collection and reporting of outcomes and decision making in this new population are needed to formulate intelligent recommendations on this difficult subject. For now, each decision should be made on an individual basis, with full eduction of the mother before the onset of labor.

CONCLUSION

Adults with spina bifida remain at risk for all of the complications suffered by children with this complicated birth defect. The rate of development of these complications is unknown because no long-term follow-up information is available from adults with spina bifida. As these patients become subject to the normal problems of aging but at an accelerated rate, their management becomes increasingly difficult. Problems include arthritic changes of the upper extremities (especially the shoulders), arthritic changes in the hips and knees, an increased incidence of bowel and bladder cancer, and especially deterioration related to severe obesity. The medical care system, payers, and the patients themselves must work together to develop a system that will improve these patients' chances of leading an independent life.

REFERENCES

Baskin JJ, Vishteh AG, Wesche DE, Rekate HL, Carrion CA (1998). Ventriculoperitoneal shunt failure as a complication of laparoscopic surgery. JSLS 2:177–180.

Batnitzky S, Hall PV, Lindseth RE, Wellman HN (1976). Meningomyelocele and syringohydromyelia. Some radiological aspects. Radiology 120, 351–357.

Duru S, Rekate HL (1997). Is prenatal repair of myelomeningocele feasible? Crit Rev Neurosurg 7:129–138.

Engel M, Carmel PW, Chutorian AM (1979). Increased intraventricular pressure without ventriculomegaly in children with shunts: "normal volume" hydrocephalus. Neurosurgery 5:549–552.

Erickson JD (2002). Folic acid and prevention of spina bifida and anencephaly. 10 years after the U.S. Public Health Service recommendation. MMWR Recomm Rep 51:1–3.

Frey L, Hauser WA (2003). Epidemiology of neural tube defects. Epilepsia 44(Suppl 3):4–13.

Hall P, Lindseth R, Campbell R, Kalsbeck JE, Desousa A (1979). Scoliosis and hydrocephalus in myelocele patients. The effects of ventricular shunting. J Neurosurg 50:174–178.

Huttmann S, Krauss J, Collmann H, Sorensen N, Roosen K (2001). Surgical management of tethered spinal cord in adults: report of 54 cases. J Neurosurg 95:173–178.

Jones RF, Kwok BC, Stening WA, Vonau M (1996). Third ventriculostomy for hydrocephalus associated with spinal dysraphism: indications and contraindications. Eur J Pediatr Surg 6(Suppl 1):5–6.

Kaufman BA, Terbrock A, Winters N, Ito J, Klosterman A, Park TS (1994). Disbanding a multidisciplinary clinic: effects on the health care of myelomeningocele patients. Pediatr Neurosurg 21:36–44.

Liakos AM, Bradley NK, Magram G, Muszynski C (2000). Hydrocephalus and the reproductive health of women: the medical implications of maternal shunt dependency in 70 women and 138 pregnancies. Neurol Res 22:69–88.

McLone DG, Knepper PA (1989). The cause of Chiari II malformation: a unified theory. Pediatr Neurosci 15:1–12.

Oi S, Kudo H, Yamada H, Kim S, Hamano S, Urui S, et al (1991). Hydromyelic hydrocephalus. Correlation of hydromyelia with various stages of hydrocephalus in postshunt isolated compartments. J Neurosurg 74:371–379.

Ransohoff J, Shulman K, Fishman RA (1960). Hydrocephalus: a review of etiology and treatment. J Pediatr 56:399–411.

Rekate HL (2001). Pathophysiology and management of hydrocephalus in spina bifida. In Sarwark JF, Lubicky JP (eds): Caring for the Child with Spina Bifida. Rosemont, IL: American Academy of Orthopedic Surgeons, pp. 395–408.

Rekate HL (2002). Adults with hydrocephalus treated in infancy and childhood. Semin Neurosurg 13:19–28.

Rekate HL, Nulsen FE, Mack H, et al (1982). Establishing the diagnosis of shunt independence. Monogr Neural Sci 8:223–226.

Rekate HL, Wallace D (2003). Lumboperitoneal shunts in children. Pediatr Neurosurg 38:41–46.

Rietberg CC, Lindhout D (1993). Adult patients with spina bifida cystica: genetic counselling, pregnancy and delivery. Eur J Obstet Gynecol Reprod Biol 52:63–70.

Teo C, Jones R (1996). Management of hydrocephalus by endoscopic third ventriculostomy in patients with myelomeningocele. Pediatr Neurosurg 25:57–63.

Wisoff JH, Kratzert KJ, Handwerker SM, Young BK, Epstein F (1991). Pregnancy in patients with cerebrospinal fluid shunts: report of a series and review of the literature. Neurosurgery 29:827–831.

Yamada S, Zinke DE, Sanders D (1981). Pathophysiology of "tethered cord syndrome." J Neurosurg 54:494–503.

21

Orthopedic Surgery

LUCIANO DIAS

The overall management of the child with spina bifida has evolved significantly in the past 30 years. The orthopedic management has also evolved. With better knowledge of the orthopedic pathology, new surgical techniques have been developed to improve function.

The goal of orthopedic treatment is to make the musculoskeletal system as functional as possible. Ambulation is not the goal for every child.

For the ambulatory child, with the advent of gait analysis, we can better understand the most important orthopedic deformities that are interfering with gait, and in so doing, we can perform more effective procedures for improvement in function. Throughout this chapter, we will be discussing *functional orthopedic procedures,* which will vary according to the child's functional level of ambulation.

It goes without saying that orthopedic management is part of a team approach. There is need for a well-trained group of paramedical personnel consisting of a pediatric orthopedic nurse, physical therapists, and orthotists. Close communication between the orthopedic surgeon and the neurosurgeon is important. Emphasis on the intellectual and personality development of children with spina bifida, including wheelchair mobility and wheelchair sports programs, is an important part of overall care.

CLASSIFICATION

A practical classification of spina bifida, based on the neurological level of the lesion, is as follows:

Group I

Thoracic or high lumbar level lesion
No quadriceps function
Usually a household ambulator up to the age of 13 years, with the use of an hip-knee-ankle-foot-orthosis or reciprocating gait orthosis
95%–99% are wheelchair users as adults, although exceptions are seen

Group II

Low lumbar level lesion
Quadriceps and medial hamstring function
No gluteus medius/maximus function
Ambulation requires ankle-foot orthoses (AFO) and crutches
79% retain community ambulation as adults
Most use wheelchairs for long-distance mobility
Significant difference in ability to walk between children with L4 and L3 level lesions (Asher and Olson, 1983)
Medial hamstring function is needed for community ambulation

Group III

Sacral level lesion
High sacral—no gastrocsoleus strength; walks with and without support but uses AFO braces; has characteristic gluteus lurch with excessive pelvic obliquity and rotation during gait
Low sacral—good gastrocnemius/soleus strength and normal gluteus medius and maximus function; walks without the need for AFOs; gait is close to normal.

The use of this classification is important when planning orthopedic surgery, since different techniques and postoperative care change according to the functional level.

ORTHOPEDIC EXAMINATION

For the ambulatory child, two examinations should be performed: horizontal and vertical.

Horizontal Evaluation

With the child on the examining table, the clinician should evaluate the following: (*1*) *Sitting balance*. The ability to sit without hand support is a good indication of nearly normal central nervous system function. For the high-level child, if one- or two-handed support is required for sitting, walking ability with an orthosis and external support is likely to be severely impaired. (*2*) *Upper extremity function*. Decreased grip strength and atrophy of the thenar musculature are reliable signs of hydromyelia. Spasticity involving the elbow, forearm, or hand musculature can interfere with the child's ability to use a walker or crutches or even to use a manual wheelchair. (*3*) *Spine alignment*. With the child in a sitting position, it is important to evaluate the presence of abnormal spine curvatures such as scoliosis or kyphosis. It is also important to evaluate the presence or absence of pelvic obliquity—suprapelvic, related to spinal curvature, or infrapelvic, related to contractures at the hip such as adduction or abduction contractures. Scoliosis is quite common in the high-level child. Annual spinal radiographs are indicated to assess this functional level. Kyphosis is also common and is usually congenital. The incidence of scoliosis is quite low in the child with a low lumbar or sacral level lesion. Any abnormal spinal curvature in children with lesions at these two levels is highly suggestive of tethering of the spinal cord (Gabrieli et al., 2003). (*4*) *Hip*. Secondary to muscle paralysis, spasticity, and abnormal posture habitually assumed after birth, contractures at the hip are quite common in children with high-level and low lumbar level lesions. Flexion contractures, detected by the Thomas test, can have a significant effect on the low lumbar level child's gait. The severe anterior pelvic tilt is compensated for by a significant lumbar lordosis, and gait is more difficult with a slow velocity (Lourenco et al., 2001). Frequently, hip flexion contractures are associated with knee flexion contractures. Abduction or adduction contractures can also cause significant gait problems leading to abnormal pelvic obliquity and causing abnormal curvatures of the spine. Hip flexion and adduction contractures are frequently associated with and secondary to asymmetrical gait in the low lumbar level child. Internal hip rotation deformity, especially when associated with an external tibial torsion, is a frequent source of increased valgus stress at the knee joint. (*5*) *Knee*. Knee flexion contractures are common in high-level and low lumbar level children. When this deformity exceeds 20°, it can lead to problems with bracing and to a significantly crouched gait. (*6*) *Rotational deformities of the tibia*. Precise measurement of the tibial torsion is often a challenge. The bimalleolar axis technique should not be used since the fibula is always posterior in these children. The thigh-foot angle (TFA) technique is more reliable. The child should be prone; with the knee flexed to 90°, the foot is brought to a neutral position and the TFA is measured. Internal tibial torsion (ITT) is always congenital and frequently associated with a clubfoot deformity. On the other hand, abnormal external tibial torsion (over 10°) is an acquired deformity that may not be present in the earlier years. Excessive external tibial torsion (ETT) of over 20° in the sacral level child can cause an abnormal valgus stress at the knee joint (Lim et al., 1998). (*7*) *Ankle*. An abnormal valgus malalignment of the ankle joint is common secondary to an abnormal shortening of the fibula and can interfere with orthotic wear, leading to increased pressure at the medial malleolus (Dias, 1978) (*8*) *Foot*. Approximately 90% of patients with spina bifida have some type of foot deformity. Some deformities, such as clubfoot, are present at birth. Others, such as a calcaneus foot, result from muscle imbalance, and still others, such as an equinus deformity, are caused by a tendon contracture. The possibility of a tethered cord should be considered in children with spasticity. The goal of orthopedic management of foot deformities is to obtain a supple, plantigrade, braceable foot.

Vertical Evaluation

Visual Gait Analysis and Computerized Gait Analysis. When computerized gait analysis is not available, visual gait analysis using a digital video camera is highly recommended.

Clinical application. Much attention has been devoted to the application of clinical gait analysis in the treatment of children with cerebral palsy. Gait analysis also has proved to be helpful in two main groups of patients with spina bifida: (*1*) the low lumbar level child who walks with a below-knee orthosis and external support and (*2*) the sacral level child who walks with an ankle-foot orthosis and no support. The average walking velocity for the child with a low lumbar level lesion is about 60% of normal. The child with a high sacral level lesion walks with a velocity of about 75% of normal (Vankoski et al., 1997).

Kinetic-kinematic patterns. Because of gluteus medius and maximus weakness, compensatory movements occur at the pelvis and hip to facilitate forward progression and maintain independent ambulation. Such characteristics include increased active pelvic rotation and stance phase hip abduction. The lower the motor level, the less pronounced these movements are. All children with low lumbar level lesions show an increased anterior pelvic tilt (Gabrieli et al., 2003). Gait analysis has also shown the benefit and influence of forearm crutches on pelvic and hip kinematics in children with spina bifida. The use of crutches enables the patient to transfer some weight-bearing to the upper extremity, decreasing the demand on weak lower extremity musculature. This allows the patient to maintain functional ambulation with a closer to normal gait pattern. Pelvic rotation, which is quite high with no crutch-walking, decreases considerably with crutch walking (Vankoski et al., 1997).

Gait analysis, in our experience, has been helpful in the decision-making process for the treatment of orthopedic deformities such as hip flexion-adduction contractures, unilateral dislocation or subluxation of the hip in the child with a low lumbar level lesion, and unilateral dislocation of the hip in a child with a sacral level lesion. Gait analysis has been found to be particularly helpful in the treatment of rotational malalignments of the lower extremity, especially external tibial torsion, which leads to significantly increased valgus stress at the knee joint. The use of gait analysis in the patient with a low lumbar and sacral level spina bifida has the same value as the use of gait analysis in the patient with spastic cerebral palsy. Understanding the effect of the hip deformities on walking leads to intervention at an early stage. Further understanding of the quality of gait in the crutch-walking child has led to a more conservative approach to hip subluxation and dislocation. The high valgus stress at the knee joint found with gait analysis has led to correction of rotational malalignment.

PRINCIPLES OF ORTHOPEDIC MANAGEMENT

Orthopedic procedures and postoperative care in spina bifida are different from those in other neuromuscular pathologies such as cerebral palsy. For instance, in spina bifida, tendon releases (tenotomies) are much more common than the tendon lengthenings frequently used in cerebral palsy. Tendon transfers are rare; however, they are occasionally done in the low sacral level child with a foot deformity. Rarely, if ever, is an arthrodesis at the foot performed since foot rigidity is highly correlated with pressure sores (Burke et al., 1991). Hip dislocation is always treated in the ablebodied child and is untreated in the child with a high or low lumbar level spina bifida (Gabrieli et al., 2003). Surgical treatment of the contractures affecting gait are more important than surgical relocation of the hip.

Since prolonged immobilization leads to significant osteopenia and enhances the risk of postoperative fractures in spina bifida, postoperatively we try to avoid casting and aim to start motion and ambulation after a short period of rest (1 week).

Orthopedic deformities in children with spina bifida are caused by (*1*) muscle imbalance as a result of the neurological abnormality; (*2*) a habitually assumed posture after birth (seen in the high-level child); and (*3*) associated congenital deformities such as clubfoot. The goal of treatment of children with spina bifida is to establish a pattern of development that is as close to normal as the level of paraplegia and central nervous system involvement permits. Orthopedic management should be tailored to meet specific goals during childhood, taking into account the expected adult function.

In spite of the best medical and surgical care, about 50% of children with spina bifida, as they reach adulthood, are nonambulators. Thus, care must be taken to prevent pelvic obliquity and correct spine deformities. In the high-level child hip and knee contractures do not require surgical treatment since they do not interfere with the sitting position. Orthopedic treatment should be directed at establishing a stable sitting posture for these patients.

Walking requires the spine to be balanced over the pelvis, allowing only small degrees of hip flexion contractures and knee contractures, and mandates a plantigrade, supple, braceable foot. Effective community ambulation, with low-energy consumption and minimal bracing with AFOs, is possible in about 50% of adult patients. In the low lumbar and sacral level child, the orthopedic surgeon should strive for functional mobility by any efficient and effective means that allows the patient to go easily from place to place, to explore the environment, and to grow and develop.

Surgical procedures to improve mobility should also take into account the child's age. For instance, a 3-year-old high-level child with good sitting balance but with a knee and hip flexion contracture that prevents the use of a brace (reciprocating gait orthosis [RGO]) should have these deformities corrected by surgery since this child has the potential to walk for at least another 10 years. The same child at the age of 10 with the same deformities should be left alone since most high level children will cease ambulation by age 12–13.

The functional level is an important factor in determining how aggressive orthopedic procedures are done to correct deformities that are not compatible with good function.

Treatment of Hip Contractures

Flexion. A flexion contracture of the hip is more frequently seen in children with high lumbar and thoracic lesions and is caused by the unopposed action of the hip flexors (iliopsoas, sartorius, rectus, and tensor fascia latae), by long periods of lying supine/sitting, or by spasticity of the hip flexors, commonly seen in patients with tethered cord, especially those with high-level lesions. Flexion, abduction, and external rotation contractures are also frequently present in the high-level child.

Hip flexion contracture is measured using the Thomas test. In the first 2 years of life the deformity gradually decreases. For this reason, a hip flexion deformity rarely requires surgical treatment in patients younger than 24 months of age. Furthermore, the treatment of a hip flexion contracture varies with the child's functional level. In the high-level child, a flexion contracture of up to 30°–40° may be accepted if it does not interfere with the child's bracing and walking. Frequently, when the flexion contracture is greater than 30°–40° in a child walking with an RGO, it will result in very short stride length and increased lumbar lordosis. In such situations, hip flexor release is indicated; however, for the child with a low lumbar level lesion, a flexion deformity of as little as 20° can result in a major impairment in walking ability and velocity. In these cases, a hip flexor lengthening is indicated.

The hip flexor release is performed through an anterior approach and involves the release of the tensor fascia latae, sartorius, rectus, and iliopsoas. In the low lumbar level child, preservation of some hip flexor power is important. In this patient, the tensor fascia latae is released and the sartorius is detached from the anterior-superior iliac spine and reattached to the antero-inferior iliac spine. The rectus is released proximally, and the iliopsoas is lengthened inside the pelvis (above the brim lengthening). After surgery a hip splint should be used, maintaining the hip in extension for the first 7 days, followed by early immobilization and use of the splint at night for a prolonged period of time.

Adduction Contracture. Not uncommonly, a hip flexion contracture is also associated with an adduction contracture. In the low lumbar level child it can cause gait asymmetry, which can be well documented with the use of gait analysis, and subsequent surgical treatment is advised. An adduction deformity is treated by an adductor myotomy and includes the adductor longus, the gracilis, and, if necessary, the adductor brevis. In more severe cases, it may be necessary to add a subtrochanteric valgus osteotomy of the proximal femur to achieve enough abduction to correct the pelvic obliquity (S. Montgomery, personal communication). Internal fixation with a plate is indicated to avoid cast immobilization. Similar to the protocol for a hip flexor release, a hip splint is used full-time for the first 7 days and thereafter only at night.

Abduction Contracture. This deformity is generally caused by contracture of the tensor fascia latae but is frequently associated with some degree of flexion contracture. It occurs often in children with high-level lesions and can be prevented by early splinting and physical therapy. Surgery is indicated when the abduction contracture causes pelvic obliquity and scoliosis and interferes with function. Mild to moderature contractures are corrected by a proximal release of the tensor fascia latae (Ober procedure). In the more severe deformity, it is not uncommon to also perform a distal release of the tensor fascia latae (Yount procedure). Postoperatively, a hip splint is made with the operated hip in neutral abduction and rotation and the opposite hip in 20° of abduction. The splint is used full-time for 1 week and thereafter only at night.

In the sacral level child, hip contractures are rarely seen. The presence of strong, active gluteus musculature prevents the development of these deformities. If a contracture is present, one must suspect a tethered cord.

Hip Internal Rotation Deformity. With the advent of gait analysis in spina bifida, it was found that abnormal hip internal rotation can cause increased valgus stress at the knee joint, especially if external tibial torsion is present. This valgus stress at the knee is a common cause of knee pain in adult life (Selber and Dias, 1998; Williams et al., 1993).

When the valgus stress is significant, as documented by gait analysis, an external derotation osteotomy of the femur is indicated. The derotation is done proximally with a right-angle AO plate fixation. With the rigid fixation no cast is necessary. A hip splint is used full-time for 1 week, after which early motion is instituted. Weight-bearing must wait until solid bone healing has occurred (4–6 weeks).

Excessive hip external rotation is rare but can cause awkward gait. In these patients, an internal derotation osteotomy of the femur proximally is indicated. Here too AO plate fixation is used to avoid cast immobilization.

Rotational osteotomies are usually done after the age of 6 years. In the young patient, to temporarily improve the gait, Becker twister cables attached to the AFO are indicated.

Hip Subluxation and Dislocation. Nearly half of the children with spina bifida show some degree of hip instability during the first 10 years of life. Muscle imbalance between the hip flexors and extensors and between the hip abductors and adductors accounts for this tendency. Lack of muscle force is also a main cause of hip instability.

Congenital hip dislocation is rare and may occur in children with sacral level lesions without muscle imbalance. It should be treated conservatively by standard methods of treatment for congenital hip dislocation (Pavlik harness, closed or open reduction, and spica cast immobilization). Teratological dislocations usually occur in children with high-level lesions. Initial roentgenograms show a severely dysplastic acetabulum with the head of the femur displaced proximally. Teratological dislocation should not be treated.

The approach to hip problems in children with spina bifida has evolved over the past 30 years. Treatment has shifted from benign neglect to extensive surgical reconstruction. This has occurred without clear indications, consistent patient selection criteria, or standardized evaluation or outcome measures. Although most reconstructions in the past were offered to ambulatory patients, nonambulators have also had hip reconstruction that offered little benefit and frequently led to stiff hips that often remained dislocated. Treatment decisions were, and often still are, based mainly on the radiographic picture rather than on the functional consequence of the unstable hip. There is general agreement, however, that ambulatory ability per se is not predicated on reducing stable hips. A functional group classification can be used to guide treatment of the unstable hip.

In the high-level child, hip dislocation occurs in 50%–70% of the time because of imbalance between the abduction and adduction forces. The dislocation occurs most frequently during the first 3 years of life. The dislocations in older children usually are caused by contractures or spasticity of the unopposed adductors and hip flexors associated with tethered cord syndrome.

Unilateral or bilateral hip dislocation in high-level lesions does not interfere with walking ability. Surgical reduction is not indicated, and treatment should be directed to associated contractures that may interfere with bracing. Such treatment allows for proper sitting posture, facilitates perineal care, and provides normalized alignment for the application of orthoses. There appears to be no convincing evidence to support hip reduction in this group.

For the low lumbar level child, reduction of unilateral subluxed or dislocated hips remains controversial. In 1975, Barden et al. noted no correlation between the status of the hip and the ability to walk in children followed up for 20 years. Feiwell (1980) reported that reducing the hip in the acetabulum did not improve hip range of motion or reduce the amount of bracing needed, and stated that a few children had increased hip stiffness after surgery. He stressed that maintaining a level pelvis and flexible hips was more important than reduction of the hips. In the past, hip reconstruction, with or without muscle transfers, produced inconsistent results.

Modern gait analysis has shown that the gait of children in this group (walking with crutches and AFOs) can be improved without hip reduction by simply repositioning the leg with soft tissue releases, with or without realignment osteotomies to normalize the functional range of motion (Gabrieli et al., 2003).

Sacral-level children typically have gluteus medius and maximus function, and the degree of excessive pelvic obliquity and rotation is related to the strength of the gluteus musculature. Because these children place a strong demands on the hip, the hip instability should be approached aggressively to achieve concentric reduction, adequate acetabular coverage, and supplementary muscle augmentation, if necessary. In the sacral-level child, for successful treatment of dislocated and subluxed hips, the following guidelines should be followed: (*1*) correct any capsular laxity by capsular plication; (*2*) correct any soft tissue contractures by release of the adductors and intrapelvic lengthening of the iliopsoas; (*3*) correct any malalignment of the proximal femur (femoral antetorsion/coxa valga) by varus derotation osteotomy. The surgeon should avoid excessive varus because these patients require good hip abduction function for stance stability and to improve their foot clearance during the swing phase; (*4*) correct any acetabular dysplasia. Most of these patients will do well with a Dega or Pemberton pelvic osteotomy. If the degree of acetabular dysplasia is severe, a Chiari pelvic osteotomy or a shelf procedure, as described by Staheli (1992), is indicated.

The Sharrard iliopsoas transfer should be avoided since this procedure will eliminate the iliopsoas, a major power-generating force (Sharrard, 1970). If tendon transfers are needed for augmentation of the hip abductor power, the external oblique transfer is the procedure of choice (Litner and Lindseth, 1994). It is important to remember that the incidence of hip dislocation in the sacral-level child is not common. The fact that the gluteus medius and maximus are present to a certain degree will ensure a higher surgical success rate.

Proximal Femoral Resection with Interposition Arthroplasty. One of the most serious problems in hip surgery in spina bifida is severe stiffness of the joint. If the hip is stiff in extension, the child cannot sit; if it is stiff in flexion, the child cannot stand. If it is stiff in between, the child can neither sit nor stand. Very little has been written about the management of this complication, but resection of the femoral head and neck is not effective. The proximal femoral resection and interposition arthroplasty (Castle and Schneider, 1978) can be used for this extremely serious complication in patients with spina bifida.

Knee. The two most common deformities are (*1*) knee flexion contracture and (*2*) knee extension contracture. Two other less common deformities are valgus or varus deformity.

Flexion contracture. Knee flexion contractures are the most common. They are seen in the high-level and low lumbar level child. They are rarely seen in the sacral-level child and, when present, are mild (less than 10°). The factors that lead to a fixed knee flexion contracture are (*1*) the typical position assumed in the supine position, with hips in abduction, flexion and external rotation, knees in flexion, and feet in the equinus position. The early use of night splints, such as the total body splint, can prevent these deformities; (*2*) a gradual contracture of the hamstrings and biceps, also with contracture of the posterior knee capsule secondary to quadriceps weakness and prolonged sitting; (*3*) spasticity and contracture of the hamstrings as a result of tethered cord syndrome; (*4*) quadriceps weakness and paralysis of the gastrocnemius, soleus, gluteus medius, and maximus.

In children with low lumbar level lesions, the flexion deformity usually occurs later. With an increase in height and weight, even the use of an orthosis to block ankle dorsiflexion does not prevent the gradual development of a knee flexion deformity. There is no obvious contracture of the hamstrings, but there is contracture of the posterior knee capsule (Dias, 1982).

A crouched gait has a high energy cost. Studies have shown that if there is an increased knee flexion of more than 40° during gait, the energy cost of walking is increased. Recent studies have shown that in children with external tibial torsion of more than 20°, despite the absence of a fixed knee flexion contracture, a crouched gait is present because of the inability of the AFO brace to improve extension of the knee during the stance phase (Lim et al., 1998). In this situation, correction of the external tibial torsion by an internal rotation osteotomy will improve knee extension during the stance phase. Recent gait analysis studies at our Motion Analysis Center have also shown, for instance, that a patient with a knee flexion contracture of 15° on the examining table will show a flexed position of 30° during gait. The flexion of the knee during gait is usually double the knee flexion contracture. Because of the increased energy use with a crouched gait, correction of a knee flexion contracture of 20° or more is indicated in the low lumbar and sacral level child. For the high-level child who is using an RGO, we can sometimes accept a higher degree of contracture. The brace needs to be adjusted to accommodate the flexion deformity of the knee.

A radical flexor release is indicated for the child with a high-level lesion. A transverse incision is used, extending from medial to lateral, approximately 1 cm above the flexor crease. All of the medial and lateral hamstring tendons are divided and resected. Next, the origin of the gastrocnemius is freed from the medial and lateral femoral condyles, exposing the posterior knee capsule, and an extensive capsulectomy is performed. The posterior cruciate ligament should be left intact. It should be possible to achieve either full extension of the knee joint at the end of the surgery or –10° of full extension.

For the low lumbar and sacral level lesion, knee flexor lengthening is indicated. In these children, the hamstring tendons are lengthened to preserve some flexor power. The hamstrings are helpful in achieving extension of the hip joint. Postoperatively, a long-leg cast is applied for 3 weeks, followed by a long-leg splint or a total body splint. During the same surgical procedure, it is important to correct any hip flexion contracture, if present. In the low lumbar and sacral level child, it is also important, after cast removal, to have an intensive physical therapy program for strengthening of the quadriceps mechanism.

A supracondylar extension osteotomy of the femur is rarely indicated. It is used primarily in older community ambulators with a fixed knee flexion deformity of more than 20° in whom a radical knee flexor release was unsuccessful. In the older child who is not a community ambulator, no surgical treatment is indicated because the knee flexion contracture does not interfere with mobility. This supracondylar extension osteotomy can be performed through a multiple drill hole technique and a Greenstick-type extension without the need for rigid fixation. Recently, it was suggested (Kramer and Stevens, 2001) that for flexion deformities of 20° or less, anterior stapling of the distal femoral physis should be used in a growing child, leading to gradual correction of the flexion deformity.

Extension contracture. Extension contracture of the knee is much less common than flexion deformity. It is usually congenital, frequently associated with other congenital anomalies such as ipsilateral hip dislocation and equinovarus deformity of the foot. Knee extension contractures can decrease ambulation, making wheelchair sitting and transfers and getting into and out of a motor vehicle very difficult. Treatment with serial casting, attempting to achieve at least 90° of knee flexion, is successful in most patients. If nonsurgical treatment does not correct the deformity, lengthening of the quadriceps mechanism is indicated. The use of the VY quadriceps lengthening procedure is favored (Curtis and Fisher, 1969). Ninety degrees of knee flexion should be obtained at the time of surgery. After surgery, the knee is immobilized in a cast at 45°–60° of flexion for approximately 2–3 weeks. After cast removal, active and passive range-of-motion exercises are started.

A knee extension contracture can also be acquired. It is seen after immobilization for a femur or supracondylar fracture. If conservative treatment fails to improve the motion, surgical treatment, as described above, is indicated.

Knee varus-valgus deformity. This condition is seen after supracondylar fractures of the femur or proximal metaphyseal fractures of the tibia. No treatment is indicated if the deformity is mild and does not interfere with the child's gait or bracing; otherwise, in the growing child, the hemiepiphysiodesis stapling technique (Stevens and Toomey, 1988) should be used. If growth is already completed, osteotomies of the distal femur or proximal tibia are indicated.

External-internal tibial torsion. The susceptibility of paralyzed limbs to angular deformities is well known. Rotational deformities of the paralyzed limbs in spina bifida, however, have received scant attention until recently

(Lim et al., 1988; Vankoski et al., 1997; Dias, 2003; Dunteman et al., 2000). In the adult sacral level population, it has been reported (Selber et al; Williams et al., 1993) that a 24% incidence of late knee pain secondary to rotational malalignments and knee deformities is seen. Most often, this appearance of the knee valgus results from a combination of lateral pelvic and hip internal rotation, external tibial torsion, and stance phase knee flexion (Lim et al., 1988). Over time, the constant proximal swivel movement of the pelvis and hip over the planted, stanced foot induces rotational deformities and external tibial torsion.

The possible sources of a high incidence of knee pain were demonstrated by motion analysis showing an excessively high internal knee varus moment related to the magnitude of external tibial torsion in association with increased pelvic rotation and lateral trunk sway. It was concluded that increased external tibial torsion is likely to result in an abnormal varus knee stress, a thigh-foot angle (TFA) of greater than 20° appears to increase this stress significantly, and knee flexion is an important related parameter. This abnormal stress predisposes the knee to late arthrosis, and an internal derotation osteotomy of the tibia to normalize the TFA improves the long-term outcome. The decrease of this abnormal internal varus moment after internal rotation osteotomy of the tibia has been documented with pre- and postoperative motion analysis. An improvement in knee extension during the stance phase was found after correction of this rotational malalignment.

The other components of this abnormal stress at the knee can be recognized through gait analysis. It is not uncommon for an increased internal rotation of the hip to be associated with excessive external tibial torsion. In these patients, usually high sacral level patients, correction of the excessive hip internal rotation by an intertrochanteric external rotation osteotomy of the femur and correction of the abnormal external tibial torsion by a supramalleolar internal rotation osteotomy are indicated. Improving external tibial torsion will improve the effectiveness of the AFO brace and achieve better extension of the knee during the stance phase. The excessive pelvic rotation, which is also one of the components of the abnormal knee stress, can be decreased only by the use of external support, crutches.

Because of the known high rate of delayed union, osteotomies of the tibia should be performed above the distal tibial physis. An osteotomy of the distal fibula is performed through a separate incision. It is important to avoid the use of a power saw when performing the tibial osteotomy. Multiple drill holes and a corticotomy with an osteotome are indicated. An AO plate is preferred for internal fixation. A short-leg cast is applied after surgery, and no weight-bearing is allowed for at least the first 3 weeks. After that time, the patient is allowed to achieve partial weight-bearing with crutches or a walker until the osteotomy is well healed.

Internal tibial torsion. Internal tibial torsion is not an acquired deformity. It is present from birth and usually is associated with patients who were born with a talipes equinovarus. Internal tibial torsion can result in quite significant in-toeing, with the patient tripping and falling. This is usually seen in low lumbar and sacral level children. The initial treatment in the first 5–6 years involves twister cables attached to the AFO brace; however, if the problem is significant after 5 years of age, an external rotation osteotomy of the tibia should be performed distally, as was described for external tibial torsion. Recent gait analyses performed at our Motion Analysis Center have shown that internal tibial torsion does not lead to an abnormal internal valgus or varus moment of the knee joint. It is important to recognize at the time of surgery that if there is any muscle imbalance, such as an active or spastic anterior tib tendon, associated with the tibial torsion, a tenotomy with tendon excision should be performed simultaneously with the osteotomy. It is also not uncommon that an adduction deformity of the forefoot may be present. In these patients a cuboid closing wedge osteotomy, sometimes in association with an opening wedge osteotomy of the medial cuneiform, is also performed simultaneously with the osteotomy of the tibia.

Foot. Approximately 80%–90% of children with spina bifida have deformities of the foot secondary to muscle imbalance. These deformities are either present at birth, such as talipes equinovarus or vertical talus, or are acquired, a classic example being the calcaneus deformity. Only patients with a very low sacral level lesion, with no muscle imbalance, will have no foot deformity. Even these children can have some intrinsic muscle paralysis and with time may develop a cavus deformity. Since the great majority of children with spina bifida will require the use of braces, a plantigrade, supple, braceable foot is the final treatment goal. Surgical treatment is frequently necessary for correction of foot deformities.

The following principles apply to surgery: (*1*) tendon excisions are more reliable than tendon transfer or tendon lengthenings; (*2*) arthrodesis should be avoided whenever possible because of the stiffness that results. Correction of bony deformities can be obtained by appropriate osteotomies that preserve joint motion. A mobile, flail foot is easier to brace than a rigid foot. Studies have shown that arthritic changes in the ankle joint frequently develop after a subtalar fusion. Pressure sores and ulcerations have been reported to be more frequent after triple arthrodesis than after soft tissue procedures and osteotomies (Burke et al., 1991). Deformities resulting from muscle imbalance are gradually progressive. If they are not treated early, bony deformities will occur, which require osteotomies to achieve full correction. Even subtle muscle imbalances can lead to more significant deformities. Recognition of these muscle imbalances by serial muscle testing, coupled with early intervention, may prevent fixed bony deformities. After surgery and cast removal, it is also important to maintain the correction and prevent recurrence with the use of well-molded AFO braces and splints.

Clubfoot. Approximately 30% of children with spina bifida have a clubfoot at birth. There is a marked difference between the idiopathic clubfoot and the equinovarus deformity in children with spina bifida; the latter resembles the deformity seen in arthrogryposis multiplex congenita. In spina bifida, the clubfoot deformity is characterized by a severely rigid foot. Frequently, a supination deformity caused by the unopposed action of an active anterior tibial muscle is also present. Rotational malalignment of the calcaneus and talus, as well as calcaneocuboid and talonavicular subluxation, is always present, and a cavus component may occur. In many patients there is also a severe internal tibial torsion associated with the equinovarus deformity.

Correction rarely, if ever, is achieved by conservative management. Serial casting most likely will reduce the deformity, but surgical treatment is indicated in most patients. Serial casting should be used initially to achieve partial correction, especially of the forefoot deformity. It also will help to stretch the soft tissue and the skin, permitting better closure of the incision at the time of surgery. The best time for surgical treatment of clubfoot is approximately 10–12 months of age. The surgical treatment consists of a radial posteromedial-lateral release. A Cincinnati transverse incision, with wide exposure of all anatomical structures medial, posterior, and lateral, is preferred. At surgery, all tendons are excised rather than lengthened. A tenotomy of the anterior tibial tendon with excision should always be performed to correct the supination deformity and prevent its recurrence. The subtalar joint, including the interosseous ligament, is released completely. Correction of the rotational malalignment of the talus and os calcis is very important. Postoperatively, a long-leg splint is used, with the foot in mild equinus to decrease any irritation at the suture line for the first 2 weeks. The cast is then changed for a long-leg cast applied with the foot in the corrected position for another 6 weeks. At the time of final cast removal, the Kirschner wires (K-wires) are also removed and an AFO splint is fitted for night use for an indefinite period, as well as an AFO brace for daytime use. A higher percentage of poor results is seen in the high-level child (Neto et al., 1996). The explanation for this difference is that in the low-level child, weight-bearing is achieved earlier, and therefore, standing and walking are more frequent, contributing to maintenance of a good foot position. In the high-level child, for whom standing and walking are limited and who spends more time in a wheelchair, despite the use of AFO braces, there is a higher incidence of recurrence of the deformity. There is no question that the incidence of poor and fair results is higher in spina bifida clubfoot compared to the surgical results in idiopathic clubfoot. We emphasize that at the time of cast removal, every child with spina bifida should be using a standing A-frame for at least 3 hours a day.

A second type of acquired equinovarus deformity can also be seen in spina bifida. This is usually secondary to tethering of the spinal cord. If the foot is supple, then a simple tendon excision will achieve correction. If the foot is rigid, then a similar radical posteromedial-lateral release is indicated.

The most common residual deformity after clubfoot surgery is an adduction deformity of the forefoot, which is frequently secondary to growth imbalance between the lateral and medial columns. Bracing is the first line of treatment, but if the adduction deformity is rigid and interferes with brace wear, then surgical correction can be achieved by a closing wedge osteotomy of the cuboid and, if needed, an opening wedge osteotomy of the medial cuneiform. The surgery should be performed after the medial cuneiform is well ossified, which is usually when the child is 5 years of age or older (Lourenco et al., 2001).

If after clubfoot surgery the deformity recurs, a second posteromedial-lateral release may be quite difficult in view of the extensive scar tissue following surgery. The best procedure for achieving a plantigrade foot in these patients is a talectomy (Dias and Stern, 1987). The talus excision is accomplished through an oblique anterolateral incision. Generally, the talus can be removed in one piece, but the dissection can be especially difficult at the talonavicular, talocalcaneal, and tibiotalar joints because these joints are nearly obliterated by the scar tissue. It is important not to leave any talus fragment behind because such a remnant can cause a recurrence of the deformity. Recognizing that the residual adduction deformity of the forefoot is common after talectomy and knowing that the talus is part of the medial column of the foot, a closing wedge osteotomy of the cuboid, balancing the medial and lateral columns, should be performed. At the end of the procedure, the os calcis is thrust posteriorly and held in position by a K-wire wire that is passed through the os calcis and ankle mortis. Postoperatively, a short-leg cast is applied with the foot in the corrected position, and the immobilization is continued for 6 weeks, at which time the K-wire is removed and a well-molded below-knee AFO splint is fabricated for night use. An AFO brace should be used during the day. After several years of follow-up, the development of Charcot joints has not been seen after talectomy (Dias and Stern, 1987). There is no doubt that the need for talectomy is decreasing due to our improved technique for surgical correction of clubfoot. The extensive radical posteromedial-lateral release with tendon excision and casulectomy, together with correction of the talus and os calcis rotational malalignment, has remarkably improved the result of clubfoot surgery in spina bifida.

Equinus deformity. An equinus deformity occurs more frequently in high-level children. It is usually an acquired deformity that can be prevented by bracing and splinting (AFO); however, when it does occur, it requires surgical treatment to achieve a plantigrade, braceable foot. If the deformity is mild, a simple tendo-achilles excision can be performed. This is an outpatient procedure. A short-leg cast is applied with the foot in a neutral position and is worn for about 7 days; then an AFO brace and a night splint are used. For the more severe equinus deformity, where there is a contracture of the posterior tibiotalar and talocalcaneal joints, a radical posterior release is necessary. A limited Cincinnati transverse incision, where all tendons are excised, and an extensive capsulectomy of the ankle and subtalar joint are performed. It is very important to divide the calcaneofibular ligament to achieve full correction. A short-leg cast is used for at least 6 weeks, followed by an AFO splint at night and a brace during the day. If the equinus deformity is very severe, there may be problems with skin closure using the Cincinnati incision. In such cases, a longitudinal incision can be performed medial to the tendo-achilles, but a short posterolateral incision may also be required for complete access and release of the calcaneofibular ligament.

Vertical talus. Approximately 10% of children with spina bifida have a vertical talus deformity at birth that is characterized by malalignment of the hindfoot and midfoot. The talus is in an almost vertical position, the calcaneus is in equinus and valgus, the navicular is dislocated dorsally and laterally from the talus, and, at times, the cuboid may be dorsally subluxed in relation to the calcaneus. Bone and joint deformities result from the soft tissue contracture. These cause remodeling of bone and cartilage to adapt to the abnormal forces (hypoplasia of the middle facet). The most common type of vertical talus is present at birth. A second developmental type can also be seen (Kodros and Dias, 1999). Neither type can be corrected by conservative means. In congenital vertical talus, manipulation and serial casting may partially correct the soft tissue contractures in preparation for a complete posteromedial-lateral release, which should be performed when the child is about 10–12 months of age. The procedure is somewhat similar to clubfoot surgery in which an extensive posteromedial-lateral release is performed. The single-stage surgical correction is done with the patient in the prone position using the standard transvere Cincinnati incision. As realignment of the talus, calcaneus, navicular, and cuboid is achieved, K-wires are used for internal fixation. Postoperatively, a long-leg splint is used for the first 2 weeks and then a long-leg cast for another 6 weeks. At cast removal, the K-wires are also removed and the patient is fitted with an AFO orthosis for day use as well as an AFO brace for nighttime.

Calcaneus and calcaneovalgus deformity. Calcaneus deformity occurs in approximately 30% of children with spina bifida, most often in the low lumbar and sacral levels with active dorsiflexors and weak plantar flexors. It can also be seen in the high-level child, in which case there is spasticity of the ankle dorsiflexors and evertors with paralyzed plantar flexors. The calcaneovalgus deformity is more common and is caused by the imbalance between the active anterior compartment muscles and inactive muscles in the posterior compartment. The valgus deformity is caused by the muscle imbalance between the evertors, which can be either active or spastic, and the invertors, which are paralyzed. This valgus deformity may be either at the subtalar joint alone or associated with a valgus deformity at the ankle joint. When the deformity is present at birth, the foot appears to be in acute dorsiflexion because of the active dorsiflexors. Usually the deformity is not rigid and the foot can be brought to a neutral position by splinting. If the deformity is rigid, then serial casting is indicated followed by an AFO splint. Most commonly, the calcaneus deformity is not present at birth, but will develop gradually secondary to the persistent muscle imbalance. If untreated, the calcaneus deformity produces a bulky, prominent heel that is prone to pressure sores and can make bracing and shoe wear difficult. To prevent bony deformities, early correction of the muscle imbalance is indicated. As stated before, a tendon release is more effective than tendon transfers. An anterolateral release by simple tenotomy of all ankle dorsiflexors and a tenotomy of the peroneus brevis and longus can achieve a braceable, supple, plantigrade foot. The anterolateral release is a more simple procedure than the anterior tibial transfer to the os calcis. The anterior or anterolateral release can be performed on an outpatient basis, requires a very short time in a cast (1 week), and can be done as early as 18 months of age. In the older child in whom there is a significant bony deformity with the os calcis in a vertical position, surgical correction is directed toward the os calcis deformity. A closing wedge osteotomy of the os calcis in association with a plantar release can improve the alignment of the os calcis and hindfoot, allowing more effective bracing and avoiding the development of pressure sores on the heel area. It is important to proceed at the same time with a release of all the extensor tendons, and if the peroneus longus and brevis are also active or spastic, their release and resection is indicated.

In summary, early intervention for the calcaneovalgus deformity, before the vertical position of the os calcis is well established, is recommended. Then, through a simple anterolateral release, it is possible to achieve a very braceable foot that will not have problems with pressure sores later on in life.

Supination deformity. A supination deformity may be associated with an adduction deformity of the forefoot. It is produced by the unopposed action of the tibialis anterior when the peroneus brevis and longus are paralyzed. The deformity occurs more often in children with a low lumbar or sacral level lesion. It can also be seen after clubfoot surgery in which the anterior tibial tendon was not excised. If the muscle imbalance persists, the supination deformity can become fixed. If the foot is supple, a simple tenotomy of the anterior tibial tendon is indicated. In certain patients, especially those with lesions at a very low level (low sacral) who have gastrocsoleus strength and the ability to walk with no orthosis, the anterior tibial tendon can be transferred to the midfoot (lateral cuneiform) in line with the third metatarsal. In spina bifida we do not recommend split transfer of the anterior tibial tendon. When the deformity is fixed, in addition to the tenotomy of the anterior tibial tendon transfer, it is necessary to proceed with a plantar closing wedge osteotomy of the medial cuneiform. This will enable plantar flexion of the first ray and realignment of the forefoot. In the more severe supination deformity, including the entire forefoot, a more extensive metatarsal osteotomy is required. If a simple tenotomy is performed, a short-leg cast is used for 1 week, followed by an AFO brace and a splint. If bony procedures are performed, a short-leg cast is used for 6 weeks, followed by the AFO brace and splint.

Varus and cavovarus deformity. A cavovarus deformity occurs mainly in children with a sacral-level lesion. It is also quite common in the child with intraspinal lipoma. Cavus is the primary deformity, and the varus is secondary to it. The degree of rigidity of the varus deformity determines the treatment. If the varus is supple, a plantar release should be performed without hindfoot surgery. If the varus is rigid, then after plantar release, with or without midtarsal or first metatarsal osteotomy, the varus deformity of the hindfoot should be corrected by a closing wedge osteotomy of the calcaneus (Dwyer, 1959). Any muscle imbalance must be corrected at the same time. For either the plantar release or the plantar release in association with the os calcis osteotomy, a short-leg cast is used for 6 weeks, followed by an AFO brace and a splint. A triple arthrodesis is rarely performed in patients with spina bifida and is indicated only as a salvage procedure.

Hindfoot-ankle valgus. A progressive valgus deformity may occur at the ankle or in combination with hindfoot valgus. This deformity is most common in children with low lumbar lesions and high sacral lesions. A severe valgus deformity can cause significant problems with brace fitting. The medial malleolus is bulky, the head of the talus is shifted medially, and pressure ulceration of these areas is frequent. Clinically, a calcaneus foot is obvious, and often external tibial torsion is also present. Gastrocsoleus muscle strength is decreased or absent. Excessive laxity of the tendo-achilles is characterized by marked passive ankle dorsiflexion. The calcaneovalgus deformity appears quite early, but problems with orthotic fitting usually do not arise until after the age of 6 years. Fibular shortening is common in children with low lumbar and high sacral lesions. In the paralytic limb, abnormal shortening of the fibula and lateral malleolus results in a valgus tilt of the talus, with subsequent valgus deformity at the ankle. With abnormal shortening of the fibula, normal distribution of forces in the distal tibial articular surface is altered, causing increased compression forces on the lateral portion of the tibial epiphysis, inhibiting growth, and decreasing compression on the medial portion of the tibial epiphysis, accelerating growth. Such imbalance causes the lateral wedging that leads to a valgus inclination of the talus. The degree of lateral wedging of the tibial epiphysis correlates well with the degree of fibular shortening. Surgical treatment of the ankle valgus deformity is indicated when the deformity causes problems with orthotic fitting and cannot be alleviated with orthoses. Three different methods of surgical treatment have been described. The Achilles tendon tenodesis to the fibular has shown unpredictable results. This treatment is presently not advised. A hemiepiphysiodesis is indicated for mild-moderate deformities (Stevens and Toomey, 1988). Experience with this technique using a cannulated AO screw has been quite rewarding. It is important to place the screw in a most medial position and quite vertical. This procedure can be performed on an outpatient basis. To avoid permanent closure of the physis, the screw should be removed within 2 years of its insertion. With the temporary growth arrest of the medial aspect of the physis and continued growth of the lateral aspect, there is a gradual correction of the lateral wedging of the tibial epiphysis that corrects the valgus tilt. If overcorrection occurs or if there is permanent arrest of the medial part of the physis, the epiphysiodesis should be completed laterally. In the more severe ankle valgus deformity in the older child with no remaining growth potential, a supramalleolar varus internal rotation osteotomy is indicated (Lubicky and Altiok, 2001). Osteotomies of the distal tibia have a high incidence of complications, such as delayed union, nonunion, wound infection, wound dehiscence, and loss of correction. To prevent some of these complications, multiple holes should be drilled and the osteotomy should be completed with an osteotome rather than with power instruments. If external tibial torsion is present, internal rotation of the distal fragment should be performed concurrently.

It is also important, when analyzing the valgus deformity, to recognize that frequently there may be an associated valgus of the hindfoot. One should not attempt to correct the severe hindfoot valgus with an extra subtalar arthrodesis (Grice procedure). Even when the deformity is corrected, the rigid foot may be vulnerable to ulceration. The medial sliding osteotomy of the os calcis is indicated (Torosian and Dias, 2000). The amount of displacement of the distal fragment is generally 50% of the width of the fragment. A threaded K-wire is used for internal fixation. After surgery, a well-padded short-leg non-weight-bearing cast is applied. The K-wire is removed at 2 weeks and a short-leg walking cast is applied for another 4 weeks. The results of this procedure are quite rewarding.

CONCLUSIONS

The orthopedic care of the child with spina bifida has changed significantly in the past 30 years. The main goal is to achieve and improve mobility in the environment using functional surgical procedures when needed, state-of-the-art orthotics, and a sound physical therapy program.

Surgical procedures that were used quite frequently in the past, such as iliopsoas transfer, are no longer needed. The knowledge that motion of the hip joint is more important than a reduced hip is now well accepted.

With the knowledge obtained from motion analysis, we have been able to look at and understand better the deformities of the lower extremity that interfere with gait and allow for a better selection of functional procedures. A knowledgeable and experienced physical therapist and orthotist are also very important for successful orthopedic care. Constant communication between the orthopedic surgeon, neurosurgeon, and urologist is imperative for the early diagnosis and treatment of tethered cord syndrome.

REFERENCES

Asher M, Olson J (1983). Factors affecting the ambulatory status of patients with spina bifida cystica. J Bone Joint Surg 65A:350.

Barden GA, Meyer LC, Stelling FH III (1975). Myelodysplastics: fate of those followed for 20 years or more. J Bone Joint Surg 57A:643.

Burke SW, Weiner LS, Maynard MJ (1991). Neuropathic foot ulcers in myelodysplasia. Orthop Trans 15:102.

Castle ME, Schneider C (1978). Proximal femoral resection interposition arthroplasty. J Bone Joint Surg 60A:1051.

Curtis PE, Fisher RL (1969). Congenital hyperextension with anterior subluxation of the knee. J Bone Joint Surg 51A:255–269.

Dias LS (1978). Ankle valgus in children with myelomeningocele. Dev Med Child Neurol 20:627–633.

Dias LS (1982). Surgical management of knee contractures in myelomeningocele. J Pediatr Orthop 1:127–131.

Dias LS (2003). Foot deformities in myelomeningocele. In DuParc J (ed) *Surgical Techniques in Orthopaedics and Traumatology Volume 8 Lower Leg Ankle and Foot.* Paris: Elsevier, pp. 55-670-A-10–55-670-B-10.

Dias LS, Stern LS (1987). Talectomy in the treatment of resistant talipes equinovarus deformity in myelomeningocele and arthrogryposis. J Pediatr Orthop 7:39–41.

Dunteman RC, Vankoski SJ, Dias LS (2000). Internal derotation osteotomy of the tibia: pre- and postoperative gait analysis in persons with high sacral myelomeningocele. J Pediatr Orthop 20:623–628.

Dwyer FC (1959). Osteotomy of the calcaneum for pes cavus. J Bone Joint Surg Br 41-B:80–86.

Feiwell E (1980). Surgery of the hip in myelomeningocele as related to adult goals. Clin Orthop 148:87.

Fraser RK, Hoffman EB, Sparks LT, Buccimazza SS (1992). The unstable hip and mid-lumbar Myelomeningocele. J Bone Joint Surg Br 74:143–146.

Gabrieli APT, Vankoski SJ, Dias LS, Milani C, Lourenco A, Filho JL, Novak R (2003). Gait analysis in low lumbar myelomeningocele patients with unilateral hip dislocation or subluxation. J Pediatr Orthop 23:330–334.

Kodros SA, Dias LS (1999). Single-stage surgical correction of congenital vertical talus. J Pediatr Orthop 19:42–48.

Kramer A, Stevens PM (2001). Anterior femoral stapling. J Pediatr Orthop 21:804–807.

Lim R, Dias L, Vankoski S, Moore C, Marinello M, Sarwark J (1998). Valgus knee stress in lumbosacral myelomeningocele: a gait analysis evaluation. J Pediatr Orthop 18:428–433.

Lourenco AF, Dias LS, Zoellick DM, Sodre H (2001). Treatment of residual adduction deformity in clubfoot: the double osteotomy. J Pediatr Orthop 21:718–718.

Lubicky J, Altiok H (2001). Transphyseal osteotomy of the distal tibia for correction of valgus/varus deformities of the ankle. J Pediatr Orthop 21:80–88.

Neto JC, Dias LS, Gabrieli AP (1996). Congenital talipes equinovarus in spina bifida: treatment and results. J Pediatr Orthop 16:782–785.

Selber P, Dias L (1998). Sacral level myelomeningocele: long-term outcome in adults. J Pediatr Orthop 18:423–427.

Sharrard WJW (1970). Long-term follow-up of posterior transplant for paralytic dislocation of the hip. J Bone Joint Surg 52B:779.

Staheli LT (1992). Slotted acetabular augmentation in childhood and adolescence. J Pediatr Orthop 12:569.

Stevens PM, Toomey E (1988). Fibular-achilles tenodesis for paralytic ankle valgus. J Pediatr Orthop 8:169.

Torosian CM, Dias LS (2000). Surgical treatment of severe hindfoot valgus by medial displacement osteotomy of the os calcis in children with myelomeningocele: J Pediatr Orthop 20:226–229.

Vankoski S, Moore C, Statler KD, Sarwark JF, Dias L (1997). The influence of forearm crutches on pelvic and hip kinematics in children with myelomeningocele: don't throw away the crutches. Dev Med Child Neurol 39:614–619.

Williams JJ, Graham GP, Dunne KB, Menelaus MB (1993). Late knee problems in myelomeningocele. J Pediatr Orthop 13:701–703.

22

Urological Care and Management of Patients with Neural Tube Defects

DAVID B. JOSEPH

The goals of urological care and management of a child with spina bifida center on maintaining normal renal function, gaining urinary continence, and making the eventual transition of personal care to gain independence. The significant achievements in other specialties, particularly neurosurgery, have unmasked the importance of maintaining normal renal function and a healthy bladder environment for urinary storage and elimination. Over 90% of children with spina bifida have a normal upper urinary tract (kidney and ureter) at the time of birth (Bauer and Joseph, 1990). Without follow-up, 50% of the children will suffer considerable upper urinary tract (kidney and ureter) damage due to lower urinary tract (bladder and urethra) hostility (Bauer and Joseph, 1990). (Fig. 22.1). With appropriate urological management, children at risk for renal damage can be identified early, and intervention can be initiated to prevent long-term compromise of kidney function. During the first several years of life, the urological focus on a child's health is based on maintaining normal kidney function. As the child begins to approach school age, interest is directed gaining urinary continence. There are overlapping factors that affect both kidney function and urinary control.

Several principles must be appreciated that are not unique to urology or to children with spina bifida. The most important is that no two children are alike. From a medical point of view, we are unable to simply look at a child's back and determine what type of bladder or kidney function the child has and what the future holds. For that reason, children with spina bifida undergo very close urological observation.

The following description of urological care is based on a protocol used at our Children's Hospital. It works well for our children because of our particular resources. Institutions create protocols based on their program's philosophy and resources. The philosophy presented here can be carried out elsewhere. However, there are multiple approaches for any particular problem, and children can be successfully managed with a different approach. With any approach, it is critical to have consistent urological follow-up and active participation by the family in the urological management of their child.

Children are managed based on the philosophy of their institution. Two general management philosophies prevail; proactive (attempting to identify children at risk for upper urinary tract deterioration and treat them before a problem occurs) and retrospective (following a child closely and beginning management at the first sign of any adverse change) (Bauer et al., 1984; Edelstein et al., 1995; Hopps and Kropp, 2003) Institutions favoring a retrospective approach rely on close evaluation of the upper urinary tract and documentation of urinary infections. It is felt that adverse upper urinary tract changes can be detected early with minimally invasive assessment using ultrasonograph. The adverse changes can then be reversed with medical, pharmacological, and operative management. Treating children as needed allows precise selection of the children requiring therapy, limiting the stress and potential side effects of invasive procedures, medications, catheterization, and surgery. Proactive advocates favor early identification of upper tract damage in at-risk children, assessing bladder function and managing hostile bladder parameters in an attempt to preserve normal renal function and prevent exposure to upper tract deterioration. Pediatric urologists have had good results treating children both ways. The protocol presented here is based on a proactive philosophy.

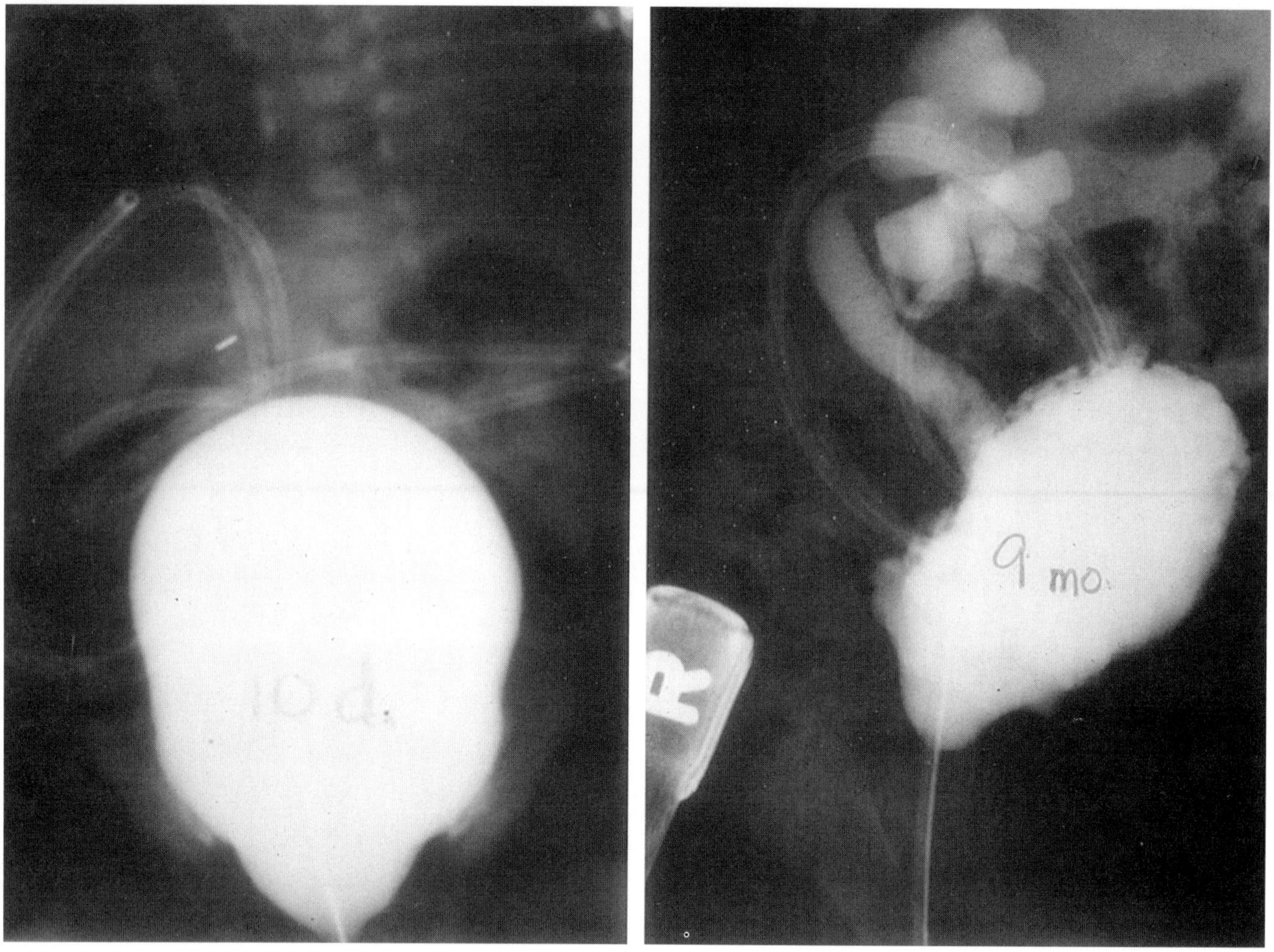

FIGURE 22.1. *Left:* A 6-week-old male. The bladder has a smooth bladder wall, there is no vesicoureteral reflux (VUR), and the bladder neck is open. *Right:* A 9-month-old male. The bladder is trabeculated, there is left grade III/V VUR, and the bladder neck is open. This is the same child, which indicates how quickly significant deterioration of the upper urinary tract can occur.

NEWBORN PROTOCOL

The infant bladder functions as a reservoir for urinary storage and as a muscle when voiding. Babies with normal bladder function void by reflex, when the bladder is full, and when stimulated by touch or temperature. The fact that a baby with spina bifida has a wet diaper does not equate with normal synergistic voiding. Studies must be performed to determine if the bladder is functioning appropriately or if there is evidence of bladder hostility that is detrimental to the upper urinary tract (Bauer and Joseph, 1990). *Bladder hostility* refers to characteristics of the bladder that directly result in damage to the kidneys. This includes excessive filling and storage pressure, repeated high-pressure bladder contractions, and high-pressure voiding or urinary leaking. Therefore, it is helpful to know the resting bladder pressure during storage, the pressure generated during elimination of urine, whether unusual bladder contractions occur, and if the external urinary sphincter (muscle) is relaxing appropriately when the bladder contracts (bladder-sphincter synergy). When the external urinary sphincter contracts at the same time that the bladder contracts, abnormally high voiding pressure occurs, a condition called *bladder-sphincter dyssynergy.* A wet diaper can also be caused by overflow incontinence due to decreased outlet resistance, a poorly compliant bladder, or a combination of both. If the denervated external sphincter is thick and fibrotic, detrimental elevated leak pressure can be present. Bladder storage pressure may also be compromised and elevated due to thickened, fibrotic changes from a denervated neurogenic bladder. To determine an infant's bladder dynamics, special bladder (urodynamic) studies are required. These studies are undertaken approximately 6 weeks after the back has been closed or the spinal cord released. Waiting for this period of time decreases the potential risk of obtaining transient data due to spinal "shock" from surgery rather than from the true underlying condition. Baseline assessment of the kidneys should be established with a renal sonogram. Blood work (serum creatinine testing) is performed to assess kidney function, particularly in children with abnormal kidney changes.

Intermittent Catheterization

We begin intermittent urethral catheterization on all newborns with spina bifida (Bauer et al., 1984; Sidi et al., 1986; Joseph et al., 1989). An 8 Fr feeding tube is used in full-term boys and girls. On occasion, a small urethra in boys may require the use of a 5 Fr feeding tube. Rarely will a smaller catheter be needed. Catheterization is initiated every 4 hours and tapered based on the amount of urine obtained, decreasing the frequency of catheterization when catheterized urine volumes consistently remain less than 30 cc. Catheterization is resumed in any neonate who undergoes neurosurgical intervention such as back closure or shunt placement. In our experience and that of others, urethral trauma secondary to catheterization has not been encountered (Joseph et al., 1989). Approximately 25% of our newborns will be discharged, with the family preforming intermittent catheterization (unpublished data). This will be continued at least through the first urodynamic study. We have found it beneficial to begin catheterization in the neonate to identify the small group of children who have difficulty voiding and have significant residual urine. In addition, all families become familiar with the technique of catheterization, which can be very helpful if this treatment is recommended at a later date.

Urodynamics

To determine whether a child is at risk for upper urinary tract deterioration, bladder function must be assessed. This can be achieved with urodynamic testing (Blaivas et al., 1977), which determines the bladder's ability to store and eliminate urine. The urodynamic study is complicated and uncomfortable, particularly when the child has normal sensation. The test can be combined with contrast imaging of the bladder to evaluate the presence of vesicoureteral reflux (urine backing up into the kidneys) and structural bladder changes caused by abnormal innervation. Urodynamic testing assesses multiple variables, which include bladder resting pressure, leak pressure, uninhibited bladder contractions, bladder areflexia, and bladder sphincter synergy or dyssynergy. The Credé, anal, and bulbar cavernosa reflexes can also be checked. Urodynamic testing is invasive and requires placement of a rectal catheter, a urethral catheter and electromyographic (EMG) electrodes. The procedure can become technically demanding and presents with several artifacts. However, when it is performed in a consistent manner, controlling for multiple variables, the urodynamic result is reproducible and can be used objectively. Factors that play an important role in the reliability of the results, particularly in the newborn, include the rate of infusion of the testing medium and the temperature of the infused medium (Joseph, 1992, 1993).

A low dose of a prophylactic antibiotic is started at birth and continued at least until the first urodynamic study is done. The infant is maintained on prophylactic antibiotics when vesicoureteral reflux or hostile bladder changes are encountered.

The results of the urodynamic study will help direct the required follow-up. When the urodynamic study is normal or shows favorable bladder function, the child will be scheduled for a return visit in appropriately 6 months to reassess kidney growth with a sonogram. The urodynamic study will be repeated yearly at least through the age of 3–4 years to identify bladder changes that cannot be recognized by observing the baby's daily voiding routine. Dynamic bladder changes noted on successive urodynamic studies may reflect the effects of a chronic urinary infection, progressive nerve damage, or the onset of a tethered spinal cord. Often the first indication of spinal cord tethering is manifested by changes in bladder and bowel function. During infancy, it is difficult to determine if any adverse changes have occurred unless urodynamic analysis has been performed early, establishing a baseline for later comparison.

TREATMENT OF HOSTILE CHANGES

When a hostile bladder environment is noted on urodynamic testing, treatment will be recommended based on the specific abnormality. All therapy follows progressive steps, beginning with the easiest to perform and the least invasive.

Following the first urodynamic study, intermittent catheterization will be continued, stopped, or renewed. Intermittent catheterization is recognized as one of the most important urological advances over the past 30 years in the treatment of the neurogenic bladder (Lapides et al., 1972). Intermittent catheterization successfully eliminates urine from the bladder, mimicking normal voiding. This can decrease symptomatic urinary infections and reduce the effects of hostile bladder pressure on the kidneys. Since intermittent catheterization is performed in a clean but not sterile fashion, most children will become colonized with bacteria. Asymptomatic bacteriuria does not need to be treated routinely. Approximately 50% of children with bacteriuria will have symptoms resulting in a clinical urinary tract infection. Symptomatic infections are usually easily controlled with low-dose prophylactic antibiotics. Nitrofurantoin macrocrystals,

1–2 mg/kg/dose, can be used effectively in infants older than 3 months of age. This medication is rapidly absorbed from the small intestine and concentrated in urine, but it has little effect on vaginal and perineal flora. These factors decrease the risk of developing resistance to it.

Intermittent Catheterization

All of our families are exposed to the technique of intermittent catheterization during the newborn hospitalization period. This decreases apprehension if catheterization is renewed in the future. Depending on the child's problem, catheterization may be required every 4 hours. An 8 Fr catheter is standard for full-term boys and girls. Boys do not need to be circumcised in order to proceed with catheterization. Catheterization is continued as a clean technique. For most children, there is no significant difference between reusing a catheter with a clean technique or using a new catheter with a sterile technique. Various options are available for cleaning catheters in order to reuse them. Techniques vary from simple cleansing with soap and water to boiling in water or treating in a microwave oven. They are equally effective. We recommend using a different catheter (not necessarily a new one) for each catheterization during the day. Once a day, the catheters are washed in soapy water, rinsed, and placed on a paper towel positioned over a plate. A microwavable cup filled with water is put in the center of the plate. The plate, cup, and catheters are then microwaved for approximately 10 minutes. The steam from the boiling water will further cleanse the catheters. The power of the microwave will affect the life of a catheter. Eventually, the catheters will become brittle or flimsy and need to be replaced.

Credé Maneuver

Some children have a large amount of residual of urine that can be eliminated by the Credé maneuver (pushing on the bladder with the fingertips above the pubis). This technique is very helpful when there is minimal bladder outlet resistance. However, it is not appropriate for all children, particularly if there is concurrent vesicoureteral reflux, if the child has been shown to have a Credé reflex (contraction of the external urinary sphincter with compression of the bladder), or if there is elevated outlet resistance due to external sphincter fibrosis. Performing the Credé maneuver when these conditions are present can result in elevated upper urinary tract pressure, which over a long period of time is detrimental to the kidneys.

Pharmaceuticals

Medication will be started when excessive, uncontrolled bladder contractions (hyperreflexia) are present. Commonly used medications are oxybutynin (Ditropan), tolterodine (Detrol), hyoscyamine (Levsin), and propantheline (Table 22.1).

Most medications used to control bladder contractions have anticholinergic activity. Multiple medications are available, indicating that no one particular medication has a clear advantage over the others. Anticholinergic side effects vary from one child to another and among medications. These include flushing of the face and neck, occasional problems with overheating (particularly in the summer months), gastrointestinal (GI) upset, dry mouth, dry eyes, change in visual accommodation, and moodiness. Any or all of these side effects may occur. Traditionally, medications have been given two or three times a day; however, new forms of some of the medications allow for single daily dosing (Table 22.1). Single-dose therapy may decrease some of the more common side effects and improve compliance. Some children cannot tolerate any side effect when the medication is taken by mouth. If these children are on a catheterization protocol, they can be given crushed, intravesical oxybutynin, resulting in similar therapeutic benefits, but with decreased systemic absorption and fewer side effects (Amark et al., 1998).

Vesicostomy

There is a small group of infants with significant bladder hostility who do not respond well to medication and/or catheterization. When this occurs, a vesicostomy is beneficial to allow continuous low-pressure elimination of urine. This will help decrease bladder pressure and preserve normal kidney function (Cohen et al., 1978; Snyder et al., 1983; Hutcheson et al., 2001). A vesicostomy is created by making a small opening in the dome of the bladder and attaching the bladder to the abdominal wall. The open bladder is positioned between the pubic bone and the umbilicus. This will allow for normal diaper usage. A vesicostomy is well tolerated and reversible. It is common for the infant to develop a rash around the opening because of continuous urine dribbling. This will improve with time but may initially require topical treatment using a protective barrier of zinc oxide or an antifungal agent. When a rash persists, we use a "custom paste" combining zinc oxide, an antifungal agent, and a stoma adhesive. Occasionally oral Diflucan will be required. Bathing is not restricted with a vesicostomy. Any water entering the vesicostomy will drain out. The vesicostomy provides excellent bladder decompression and decreases the pressure on the kidneys due to poor bladder compliance during storage and high-pressure voiding.

When a vesicostomy is not appropriate, formal bladder reconstruction with augmentation cystoplasty may be required (Adams and Joseph, 2002).

TABLE 22.1. *Medications Used in the Urological Care of Patients with Neural Tube Defects*

Type (Brand Name)	Minimal Dosage	Maximal Dosage	Long-Acting Dosage
Cholinergic			
Bethanechol (Urecholine)	0.7 mg/kg/d bid	0.8 mg/kg/d qid	
Anticholinergic			
Oxybutynin (Ditropan)	0.2 mg/kg bid	0.2 mg/kg qid	XL 5–15 mg qd
Hyoscyamine (Levsin)	0.03 mg/kg bid	0.1 mg/kg qid	Time cap 1–2 bid
Tolterodine (Detrol)	1 mg bid	2 mg bid	LA 2–4 mg kd
α-Adrenergic Agonist			
Phenylephrine (Entex)	0.5 mg/kg	1.0 mg/kg tid	LA 1 tab bid
Pseudoephedrine (Sudafed)	30 mg qid (6–12 yr)	60 mg qid (>12 yr)	
Ephedrine	1 mg/kg/d qid	3 mg/kg/d qid	
α-Adrenergic Antagonist			
Doxazosin mesylate (Cardura)	0.5 mg qhs	8 mg qhs	
Prazosin (Minipress)	0.05 mg/kg bid	0.1 mg/kg tid	
Terazosin (Hytrin)	0.5 mg qhs	10 mg qhs	
Phenoxybenzamine	0.3 mg/kg bid	0.5 mg/kg tid	
Smooth Muscle Relaxant			
Dicyclomine (Bentyl)	0.1 mg/kg bid	0.3 mg/kg tid	
Flavoxate (Urispas)	3 mg/kg bid	3 mg/kg tid	
Tricyclic			
Imipramine (Tofranil)	25 mg/qhs	75 mg/qhs	

URINARY CONTINENCE

As the child ages, the upper urinary tract should remain normal and interest can be shifted to focus on gaining urinary continence. The age at which a child begins to address urinary continence is individualized based on his or her physical capabilities and social situation. It is practical to consider urinary continence when a child enters school. While this is a realistic goal, it may not be appropriate for all children. To gain urinary continence, adherence to a consistent voiding program is necessary. This program may include medications, intermittent catheterization, and possibly operative reconstruction. When a urinary continence program is initiated, it should be continued even while the child is in school.

Some children with spina bifida can void and achieve normal urinary continence. The majority of children, however, require a combination of treatment measures similar to the methods described above for reducing bladder hostility. Urodynamic bladder testing will help assist the pediatric urologist in developing a continence program that is specific for the child's problem and needs. Most often, conservative reversible treatment regimens using medications and catheterization are initiated first. When this management has been maximized and incontinence persists, operative intervention will be recommended.

To achieve urinary continence, three important factors of bladder function need to be assessed: the ability of the bladder to store an adequate volume of urine at low pressure; the ability of the bladder neck and/or external urinary sphincter to remain closed when the child is not voiding; and the ability of the bladder to contract and eliminate urine. Any one or all three of these factors may be dysfunctional. Treatment will depend on the specific abnormality.

When the bladder capacity is small, resting bladder pressure is elevated, or abnormal contractions occur, anticholinergic medications can be tried to expand the capacity, decrease the pressure, and reduce the contractions. Catheterization is often required to eliminate urine when bladder contractions are poorly coordinated, weak, or nonexistent. When medications and catheterization have been maximized and the child has not gained continence, the bladder may need to be enlarged through augmentation and the bladder neck may need to be strengthened. All GI segments, from the stomach to the colon, have been used to augment the bladder (Lockhart and Politano, 1986; Sidi and Gonzalez, 1986; Bogaert et al., 1995; Adams and Joseph, 2002). Most often, the small or large bowel is selected. There are advantages and disadvantages in using any segment of bowel. The large bowel is in close proximity to the bladder, and its large diameter results in a smaller segment that needs to be harvested. It should be noted, however, that using the large bowel may result in a greater discharge of mucus, and a change in bowel continence can occur in some children. For those reasons, the small bowel (ileum) is the most common choice. All bowel segments are reconfigured into a cup like patch that is added to the bladder. Reconfiguring the tubular bowel segment into a cup creates a spherical shape when the bowel is placed on the bladder, maximizing the surface area and creating a reservoir with the greatest capacity (Hinman, 1988). Detubularizing the bowel segment also decreases elevated pressure that can occur when the bowel segment contracts due to peristalsis.

A limited number of children benefit from use of the stomach, particularly if they have renal insufficiency or a short gut due to other abnormalities. The stomach does not result in mucus secretion, and there are fewer problems with bacteriuria and stone formation. But a stomach patch will secrete acid, which can be a source of discomfort and minor bleeding (Bogaert et al., 1995; Rink and Adams, 1995; Shelton et al., 1995; Leonard and Wiliot, 2000).

Complications

All bowel segments secret mucus, an excellent culture medium for bacteria and a nidus for stone formation. The large bowel tends to secret more mucus than the small bowel, but there is no significant difference regarding segment of choice and stone formation (Palmer et al., 1993; Rink and Adams, 1995; Khoury et al., 1997). The secreted mucus needs to be irrigated intermittently from the child's bladder or the reconstructed reservoir (Adams and Joseph, 2002). Failure to do so will result in excessive accumulation of mucus, poor urinary drainage, and an increased risk of urinary infections, odor, and the formation of bladder calculi. Draining the bladder completely and irrigating it routinely helps diminish these problems.

All GI segments have the potential for causing various metabolic abnormalities due to the reabsorption and loss of electrolytes, bicarbonate, and acid. Routine monitoring of the child's electrolyte balance is required. Nutritional supplementation may be necessary for some children.

Bladder ruptures have been reported and can be life-threatening (Sheiner and Kaplan, 1988; Rink and Adams, 1995). Immediate drainage of the bladder and repair of a significant rupture are mandatory to diminish the morbidity associated with this problem (Slaton, 1994). The etiology of a bladder rupture is unknown, but it is likely multifactorial and influenced by lack of compliance with catheterization, chronic inflammation, and focal areas of ischemia (Crane et al., 1991).

Superficial bladder tumors are rare but have been described 10–15 years after augmentation cystoplasty (Barrington et al., 1997; Soergel et al., 2004). The tumors are usually small, confined within the bladder, and easily treated with cystoscopic resection. Individuals who have undergone reconstruction with bowel benefit from yearly cystoscopic surveillance of the bladder or reservoir after 10 years.

A low lifelong risk of bowel obstruction results following augmentation. However, this is not a significant increase in children who have already had other intra-abdominal operative procedures.

Augmenting the bladder with a portion of bowel usually commits the child to intermittent catheterization. Therefore, it is essential that all children and their caretakers feel comfortable with catheterization and become proficient in using the technique several weeks prior to reconstructive surgery. After the augmentation, it is essential that catheterization is continued on a very strict schedule. Often when children are responsible for self-catheterization, poor technique will lead to either incomplete emptying or excessive stretching of the bladder and the augmented segment. If this is not corrected, a life-threatening bladder rupture can occur. Teenagers often become complacent regarding the importance of maintaining a strict catheterization schedule and need to be supervised when they are managing their own care.

While augmentation enterocystoplasty is the current state of the art, its potential risks and side effects have prompted investigation of other methods of bladder rehabilitation. Electrical bladder stimulation has been attempted and may show some promise with improving compliance, but overall the results of treatment have not been clinically significant. Augmenting the bladder with engineered tissue has the potential of revolutionalizing bladder reconstruction and dramatically decreasing the morbidity seen with the use of bowel (Lai et al., 2002; Zhang et al., 2000).

Bladder Neck Incompetence

When urinary incontinence exists due to bladder neck or sphincter incompetence, medications can be tried but are rarely successful (Bugg and Joseph, 2003). Operative intervention is usually required to tighten each area. Multiple procedures have been described, indicating that no technique is effective for all of the different types of outlet abnormalities. (Kryger and Barthold, 2000). Some operative techniques use natural bladder tissue fashioned into a one-way "valve" (Kropp, 1986; Pippi Salle et al., 1997; Snodgrass, 1997). This valve prevents urine from leaking and requires a catheter to be passed for drainage of urine. Another technique uses a strip of fascia (the strong tissue that surrounds a muscle) that is placed around the bladder neck and tightened like a belt (Bugg and Joseph, 2003). Regardless of the technique, most bladder neck repairs rely on the child's need to catheterize in order to eliminate urine.

The artificial urinary sphincter is a mechanical device with three components: a cuff positioned around the bladder neck, a pump placed either in the labia or the scrotum, and a pressurized balloon reservoir located beneath the rectus muscle (Kryger and Gonzalez, 2001; Herndon et al., 2003). At rest, the sphincter is activated, the cuff pressurized, and the bladder neck or proximal urethra closed. When the child wants to void or catheterize, the pump is compressed, which forces fluid from the cuff into the reservoir. This opens the cuff, and urine is eliminated with a natural contraction, with straining, or via intermittent catheterization. Over the next several minutes, the cuff will gradually fill and close the bladder neck. Improvements over the past several years with the artificial urinary sphincter have eliminated many of the initial mechanical problems. However, it must be recognized that the sphincter is a mechanical device, and when it is placed in a young child, some form of malfunction during the child's life requiring repair is expected (Herndon et al., 2003). Many problems can be repaired with simple replacement of one of the components. Infection of the prosthesis is the most serious problem and substantially increases the risk for urethral erosion. When an infection occurs, removal of the sphincter will likely be required (Herndon et al., 2003).

The goal of any bladder neck reconstruction is to increase outlet resistance. An increase in resistance can change the bladder dynamics and unmask potential bladder hostility not previously recognized (Bauer et al., 1986). For that reason, all children undergoing bladder neck reconstruction must be followed closely for changes in bladder dynamics. Periodic reassessment with urodynamic testing may be required. This becomes particularly important in children who are noted to show a new onset of hydronephrosis and signs of upper urinary tract deterioration.

Continent Catheterizable Channel

It should be appreciated that intermittent catheterization is a common method of maintaining normal kidney function and urinary continence. Most often, catheterization is performed through the normally positioned urethra. As the child begins to mature, this may become difficult. In boys this is due to virilization of the posterior urethra and prostate. In addition, some children who use a wheelchair have difficulty reaching the genital area for self-catheterization. When catheterization of the native urethra is difficult, it is possible to place a small catheterizable channel between the bladder and the body wall. The stoma (opening) of the channel can be hidden within the umbilicus or placed very low on the abdominal wall. (Fig. 22.2) Various tissues have been used to create a catheterizable channel, including the appendix, ureter, fallopian tube, and small bowel (Liard et al., 2001). The appendix (Mitrofanoff) is particularly appealing because of its small tubular caliber, long length, and close proximity to the bladder (Cendron, 1991). The appendix is typically the first choice for a catheterizable channel (Fig. 22.3). Another source of tissue will be required in children who have had an appendectomy or whose appendix will be used for the antegrade colonic enema (Yerkes et al., 2003). Most often, this is fashioned from a very small, tubularized segment of the ileum (Monti/Yang), particularly when augmentation cystoplasty is required (Monti et al., 1997; Perez et al., 2001).

Bowel Control

It is practical to consider bowel continence at the same time that a child is working toward urinary continence. It is essential for the child to maintain an appropriate stool consistency, which can be achieved by a diet that includes

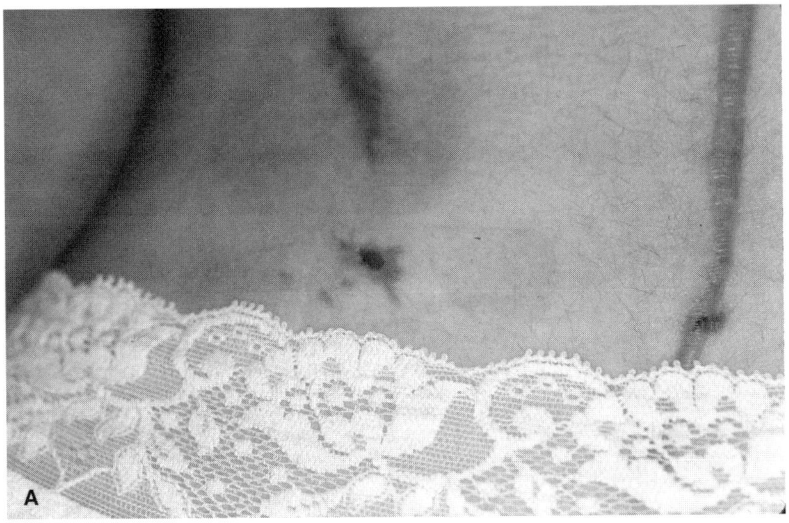

FIGURE 22.2 (*A*) Catheterizable stomal site in the right lower quadrant. This child has undergone continent undiversion of a previous ileal conduit.

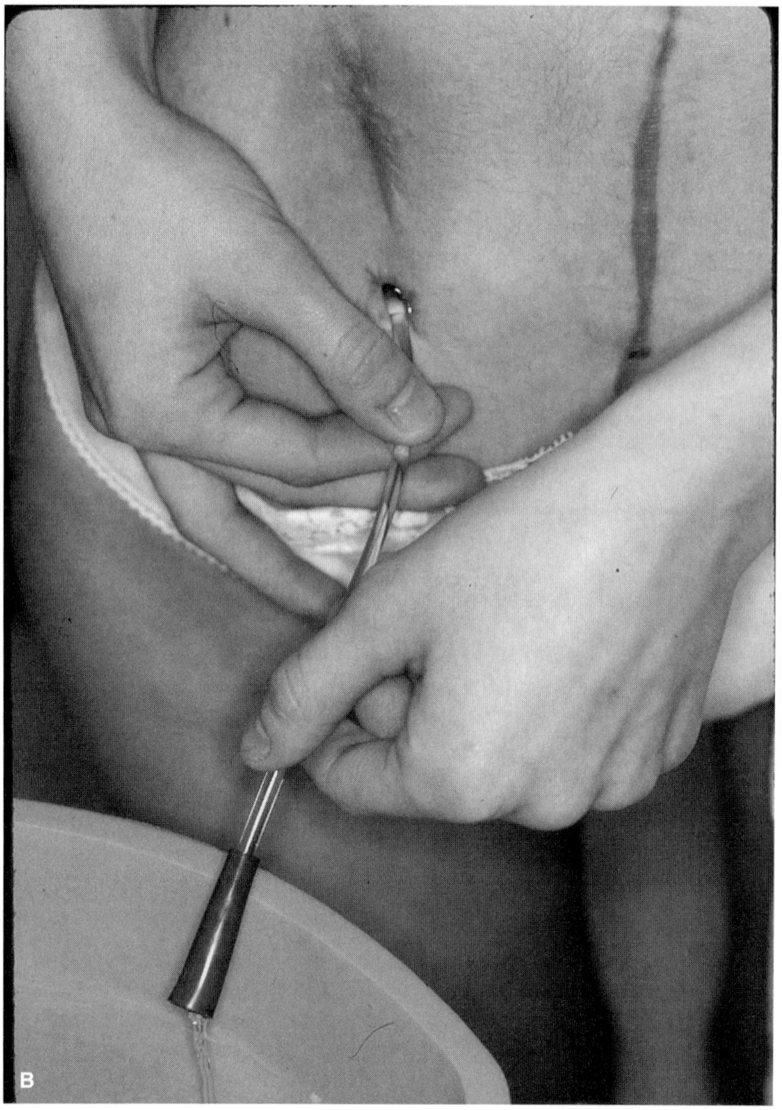

FIGURE 22.2 (*continued*). (*B*) Catheterization and drainage of Mitrofanoff.

plenty of fluid and fiber. Some children benefit from fiber supplementation. Even when the stool is of normal consistency, some children need assistance with eliminating the stool from their rectum and colon. There are various recommended techniques, including digital manipulation, rectal suppositories, and enemas. When rectal enemas are employed, only the terminal portion of the colon is "washed" free of the stool, leaving the bulk of the stool in the remainder of the colon. When the above techniques do not achieve bowel continence, irrigation of the entire colon beginning at its origin (the cecum) can be effective. This antegrade colonic enema requires a catheter to be passed into the cecum (Perez et al., 2001; Yerkes et al., 2003). A conduit for the catheter can be created by reinforcing the appendix within the cecum and opening the distal end of the appendix as a small stoma either in the right lower quadrant or the umbilicus. When the appendix is not available, alternatives such as a cecal button (similar to a gastrostomy button) can be inserted, a secondary tubularized segment of ileum can be tunneled into the cecum, or a cecal flap can be created (Perez et al., 2001). Colonic irrigation may take anywhere from 30 to 90 minutes. The child remains in the bathroom while the colon is irrigated, at which time the child can read or proceed with the daily homework assignment.

Transitional Years

Urological care should slowly transition from the parent or caretaker to the teen. This transition can be difficult for both parties. Teenagers should be educated about their anatomy, any dysfunction, and the reasons they need to perform certain activities or take medication. It is important that the adult allow the teenager to assume responsi-

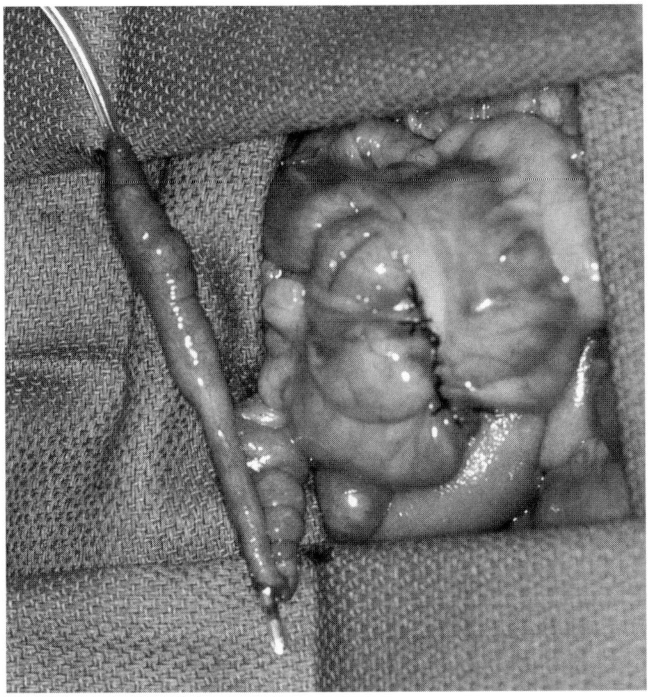

FIGURE 22.3 Mobilization of the appendix to be used as a continent catheterizable channel (Mitrofanoff). When the appendix is left intact with the cecum, it can be used to irrigate the colon (antegrade colonic enema procedure) for bowel continence.

bility for bladder and bowel needs. While the parent provides independence, it is necessary to continue close monitoring to ensure that the teenager is accomplishing the goals of the treatment program.

Direct communication with the teenager is required to reinforce the importance of catheterization, particularly if the teenager has undergone reconstruction. To determine whether catheterization is being accomplished, a parent can monitor the use of supplies. When medications are self-administered, the parent should periodically document the number of pills or capsules remaining in the monthly supply.

The teenage years are a struggle for children with spina bifida, just as they are for other children. However, the medical consequences resulting from lack of attention to specific personal needs are much greater. Parents may need to refocus their child on what is required to maintain healthy kidneys and urinary continence.

Follow-up

Long-term follow-up is essential to monitor renal status and general health. Most individuals who intermittently catheterize or who have undergone urinary reconstruction will likely have chronic bacteriuria. Overtreatment of bacteriuria can be problematic and is best reserved for symptomatic events. Both the upper and lower urinary tracts need to be monitored for urolithiasis on a yearly basis (Palmer et al., 1993). Yearly cystoscopy 10 years after augmentation cystoplasty can be beneficial.

CONCLUSION

With appropriate urological care, most children with spina bifida will transition through life with normal renal function. Gaining urinary and bowel continence is a practical goal and can be achieved with a combination of medical and surgical intervention. Achieving continence while maintaining normal renal function allows for an improved self-image and independence.

REFERENCES

Adams MC, Joseph DB (2002). Urinary tract reconstruction in children. In Walsh PC, Vaughan ED, Wein AJ. Philadelphia: WB Saunders, 3, 2508–2563.

Amark P, Eksborg S, Juneskans O, Bussman G, Palm C (1998). Pharmacokinetics and effects of intravesical oxybutynin on the paediatric neurogenic bladder. Br J Urol 82:859–864.

Barrington JW, Fulford S, Griffiths D, Stephenson TP (1997). Tumors in bladder remnant after augmentation enterocystoplasty. J Urol 157:482.

Bauer SB, Reda EF, Colodny AH, Retick AB (1986). Detrusor instbility: A delayed complication in association with the artificial sphincter. J Urol 135:1212–1215.

Bauer SB, Joseph DB (1990). Management of the obstructed urinary tract associated with neurogenic bladder dysfunction. Urol Clin North Am 17(2):395–406.

Bauer SB, Hallett M, Khoshbin S, Lebowitz RL, Winston KR, Gibson S, Colodny AH, Retik AB (1984). Predictive value of urodynamic evaluation in newborns with myelodysplasia. JAMA 252:650–652.

Blaivas JG, Labib KL, Bauer SB, Retik AB (1977). Changing concepts in the urodynamic evaluation of children. J Urol 117:778–781.

Bogaert GA, Mevorach RA, Kim J, Kogan BA (1995). The physiology of gastrocystoplasty: once a stomach always a stomach. J Urol 153:1977.

Bugg CE Jr., Joseph DB (2003). Bladder neck cinch of pediatric neurogenic outlet deficiency. J Urol 170:1501–1503.

Cendron M, GJ (1991). The Mitrofanoff principle: technique and application in continent urinary diversion. Urol Clin North Am 18:615–621.

Cohen JS, Harbach LB, Kaplan GW (1978). Cutaneous vesicostomy for temporary urinary diversion in infants with neurogenic bladder dysfunction. J Urol 119(1):120–121.

Crane JM, SH, Billman GF, Kaplan GW (1991). Ischemic necrosis: hypothosis to explain the pathogenesis of spontaneously ruptured enterocystoplasty. J Urol 146:141.

Edelstein RA, Bauer SB, Kelly MD, Darbey MM, Peters CA, Atala A, Mandell J, Colodny AH, Retik AB (1995). The long-term urological response of neonates with myelodysplasia treated proactively with intermittent catheterization and anticholinergic therapy. J Urol 154:1500–1504.

Sheiner JR, Kaplan GW (1988). Spontaneous bladder rupture following enterocystoplasty. J Urol 140:1157.

Herndon CDA, Rink RC, Shaw MB, Simmons GR, Cain MP, Kaefer M, Casale AJ (2003). The Indiana experience with artificial urinary sphincters in children and young adults. J Urol 169:650–654.

Hinman F (1988). Selection of intestinal segments for bladder substitution: physical and physiological characteristics. J Urol 139:519.

Hopps CV, Kropp KA (2003). Preservation of renal function in children with myelomeningocele managed with basic newborn evaluation and close followup. J Urol 169:305–308.

Hutcheson JC, Cooper CS, Canning DA, Zderic SA, Snyder HM III (2001). The use of vesicostomy as permanent urinary diversion in the child with myelomeningocele. J Urol 166(6):2351.

Joseph DB (1992). The effect of medium-fill and slow-fill saline cystometry on detrusor pressure in infants and children with myelodysplasia. J Urol 147(2):444–446.

Joseph DB (1993). The use of iothalamate meglumine 17.2% as an effective testing medium in lower urinary tract urodynamic assessment of children. J Urol 149(1):92–93.

Joseph DB, Bauer SB, et al (1989). Clean, intermittent catheterization of infants with neurogenic bladder. Pediatrics 84(1):78–82.

Khoury AE, Salomon M, Doche R, Sobou F, Ackerley C, Jayanthir, et al (1997). Stone formation after augmentation cystoplasty: the role of intestinal mucus. J Urol 158:1133.

Kropp KA, Angwafo FF (1986). Urethral lengthening and reimplantation for neurogenic incontinence in children. J Urol 135:533–536.

Kryger JV, Gonzalez R, Barthold JS (2000). Surgical management of urinary incontinence in children with neurogenic sphincteric incompetence. J Urol 163:256–263.

Kryger JV, Leverson G, Gonzalez R (2001). Long-term results of artificial sphincters in children are independent of age at implantation. J Urol 165:2377–2379.

Lai JY, Yoon CY, Yoo JJ, Wulf T, Atala A (2002). Phenotypic and functional characterization of in vivo tissue engineered smooth muscle from normal and pathological bladders. J Urol 168(4 Pt 2):1853–1857; discussion 1858.

Lapides J, Diokno AC, Silbert SJ, Lowe BS (1972). Clean intermittent self-catheterization in the treatment of urinary tract disease. J Urol 107:458.

Leonard MP, Dharamsi N, Williot PE (2000). Outcome of gastrocystoplasty in tertiary pediatric urology practice. J Urol 164:947.

Liard A, S-LE, Mathiot A, Mitrofanoff P (2001). The Mitrofanoff procedure: 20 years later. J Urol 165:2394.

Lockhart JL, Bejany D, Politano VA (1986). Augmentation cystoplasty and the management of neurogenic bladder disease and urinary incontinence. J Urol 135:969.

Monti PR, Lara RC, Dutra MA, De Carvalho JR (1997). New techniques for construction of efferent conduits based on the Mitrofanoff principle. J Urol 49:112–115.

Palmer LS, Kogan SJ, Franco I, Reda E, Gill B, Levitt SB (1993). Urolithiasis in children following augmentation cystoplasty. J Urol 150:726.

Perez M, Lemelle JL, Barthelme H, Marquand D, Schmitt M (2001). Bowel management with antegrade colonic enema using a Malone or a Monti conduit—clinical results. Eur J Pediatr Surg 11(5):315–318.

Pippi Salle JL, McLorie GA, Bagli DJ, Khoury AE (1997). Urethral lengthening with anterior bladder wall flap (Pippi Salle procedure): modifications and extended indications of the technique. J Urol 158:585–590.

Rink RC, Hollensbe DW, Adams MC (1995). Complications of bladder augmentation in children: a comparison of gastrointestinal segments. (Am Urol Assoc) UPDATE Series 14 Vol. 122.

Shelton CA, GA, Wacksman J, Lewis AG (1995). Gastrocystoplasty: technical and metabolic characteristics of the most versatile childhood bladder augmentation modality. J Pediatr Surg 30:283.

Sidi AA, Dykstra DD, Gonzalez R (1986). The value of urodynamic testing in the management of neonates with myelodysplasia: a prospective study. J Urol 135:90–93.

Sidi AA, Reinberg Y, Gonzalez R (1986). Influence of intestinal segment and configuration on the outcome of augmentation enterocystoplasty. J Urol 136:1201.

Slaton JW, Kropp KA (1994). Conservative management of suspected bladder rupture after augmentation cystoplasty. J Urol 152:713.

Snodgrass W (1997). A simplified Kropp procedure for incontinence. J Urol 158:1049–1052.

Snyder HM III, Kalichman MA, Charney E, Duckett JW (1983) Vesicostomy for neurogenic bladder with spina bifida: followup. J Urol 130(4):724–726.

Soergel TM, Cain MP, Misseri R, Gardner TA, Koch MO, Rink RC (2004). Transitional cell carcinoma of the bladder following augmentation cystoplasty for the neuropathic bladder. J Urol 172:1649–1651.

Yerkes EB, Cain MP, King S, Brei T, Kaefer M, Casale AJ, Rink RC (2003). The Malone antegrade continence enema procedure: quality of life and family perspective. J Urol 169(1):320–323.

Zhang, Y, Kropp BP, Moore P, Cowan R, Furness PD 3rd, Kolligian ME, Frey P, Cheng EY (2000). Coculture of bladder urothelial and smooth muscle cells on small intestinal submucosa: potential applications for tissue engineering technology. J Urol 164 (3 Pt 2):936–941.

23

Cognition, Education, and Learning Disorders

GREGORY S. LIPTAK

ABNORMALITIES OF THE BRAIN

Although the terms *spina bifida* and *meningomyelocele,* which will be used synonymously in this chapter, refer to the back and spinal cord, the neurological abnormalities of this condition involve the entire neural axis (Bannister et al., 1998). Gilbert et al. (1986) reported that 92% of children with meningomyelocele who had died had abnormal migration of cortical neurons, 72% had cerebellar dysplasia, 20% had hypoplasia or aplasia of cranial nerve nuclei, 16% had fusion of the thalami, and 12% had agenesis of the corpus callosum. These findings have been confirmed with cranial magnetic resonance imaging (MRI). For instance, Kawamura et al. (2001, 2002) have found partial agenesis of the corpus callosum, hypoplasia of the cerebral hemispheres, polymicrogyria, and heterotopic gray matter, as well as the expected cervicomedullary anomalies, such as herniation of the cerebellar tonsils through the foramen magnum. Individuals with the cerebral anomalies were more likely to have cognitive impairment.

Between 70% and 80% of children with meningomyelocele develop hydrocephalus (McLone, 1992). Hydrocephalus and its treatment also appear to disrupt the development of white matter tracts and myelination, as well as the development of cortical neurons (del Bigio, 1993; Erickson et al., 2001).

For years, the co-occurrence of cerebellar disorders with the Chiari II malformation, which is found in three-fourths or more of children with meningomyelocele, has been acknowledged. Historically, cerebellar abnormalities have been associated with motor performance and motor learning (Van Mier and Petersen, 2002). Yet, only recently has the role of the cerebellum in cognition been recognized. For example, Gao et al. (1996) showed that the cerebellum is engaged during the acquisition and discrimination of sensory information, while Gebhart et al. (2002) have shown that the right posterolateral cerebellar hemisphere assists the left cerebral hemisphere in generating specific types of spoken word associations. Individuals who have had resection of part of the cerebellum secondary to brain tumors have been identified as having a unique syndrome called *cerebellar cognitive affective syndrome* (Levisohn et al., 2000). This is characterized by impairments in executive function (including planning and sequencing), visual-spatial function, expressive language, verbal memory, and modulation of affect. Thus, given the cerebral and cerebellar abnormalities found in individuals who have meningomyelocele, the occurrence of cognitive deficits should be no surprise.

COGNITIVE ABILITIES

Most children who have meningomyelocele with shunted hydrocephalus have been reported to have intelligence in the low average range, while children with meningomyelocele without shunted hydrocephalus have cognition typical of children who are not disabled (Yeates et al., 1995; Bier et al., 1997). Children with meningomyelocele who have had an episode of shunt infection (ventriculitis) have significantly lower scores of intelligence, often in the range of mental retardation, more seizures, higher future risks of shunt infection and malfunction, and worse school performance (McLone, 1992; Kanev and Sheehan, 2003). Some studies have found that frequent shunt revisions have a negative effect on IQ (Mazur et al., 1988; Holler et al., 1995; Hunt et al., 1999; Dennis and

Barnes, 2002), although others have not replicated this finding (Ralph et al., 2000).

Abnormalities of the corpus callosum and the presence of epilepsy also are negatively related to intelligence (Barf et al., 2003). The corpus callosum provides an important pathway for communication across different parts of the brain. However, it also contributes to the development of cerebral specialization of language and other cognitive skills (Hannay et al., 1999). Impairment of the corpus callosum early in development also may interfere with the plasticity of the brain (functional substitution). Children with meningomyelocele who have abnormalities of the corpus callosum are more likely to have impaired nonverbal skills (Hannay et al., 1999).

Children born prior to routine ventricular shunt insertion who had severe hydrocephalus with large heads often were described as having the "cocktail party syndrome" (Tew, 1979; Tew and Laurence, 1979, Hurley et al., 1990). This refers to the tendency of these children to chatter on about topics that are not always meaningful or appropriate to the situation; they may use and repeat memorized common phrases like "Hello, how are you today?" or "What's up?" They may be able to repeat parts of a story that they have heard without really understanding what the story means. Typically, the content of these verbal expressions is often absent or trivial at best. Thus, these children, as well as those who are less affected by hydrocephalus, have difficulty deriving meaning from context (Barnes and Dennis, 1998).

When administered tests of intelligence, children with meningomyelocele and shunted hydrocephalus typically perform worse on performance than on verbal scales (Hurley et al., 1983; Wills et al., 1990; Brookshire et al., 1995; Casari and Fantino, 1998), with gaps of 20 or more points not uncommon. Most studies of cognition in children with meningomyelocele have involved school-age children. Therefore, the nature of cognition in preschool children and the long-term outcomes in adults are not as well understood. Some studies of young adults have shown the same pattern of higher verbal than performance scores on intelligence tests (Hommet et al., 1999; Dennis and Barnes, 2002).

Studies of school-age children with meningomyelocele have shown that they use and understand single words; however, they have difficulty using language in a flexible and adaptive manner (Dennis and Barnes, 1993; Dennis et al., 1994; Fletcher et al., 2002) and have difficulty with reading comprehension (Barnes and Dennis, 1992). In school, math comprehension is commonly impaired (Friedrich et al., 1991), and writing problems are frequent (Barnes et al., 2002; Dennis and Barnes, 2002). These students may have problems with short-term memory, especially list learning (Cull and Wyke, 1984; Yeates et al., 1995; Scott et al., 2003). Many children with meningomyelocele have problems with construction of meaning and pragmatic communication. As children age and impairments in more complex language and executive functioning become apparent, the verbal disorders become more obvious.

Impairments in executive functioning also have been found (Fletcher et al., 1996; Dise and Lohr, 1998; Brewer et al., 2001; Mahone et al., 2002). Metacognitve skills (e.g., mental flexibility, mental efficiency, learning from experience, and conceptual sophistication) generally are more affected than behavioral inhibition (Mahone et al., 2002). As mentioned above, associations between cognition and MRI findings have been documented. For instance, Fletcher et al. (1996) found that children with hydrocephalus who had proportionately greater posterior than anterior cerebrospinal fluid percentages had significantly poorer visuomotor dexterity and visuospatial skills than those who had normal percentages of cerebrospinal fluid.

LEARNING DISORDERS

Learning disabilities can be defined as low academic achievement that is unexpected based on the child's overall cognitive abilities. Children who have meningomyelocele often fall into this category, although some clearly have lower IQs commensurate with their achievement. However, it is important to realize that learning disabilities also may be manifest as achievement that is sustainable only by extremely high levels of effort and support—as if the child were running hard just to stay in place. Especially in the early grades (fourth grade and below), children with meningomyelocele may be able to keep up but may be expending a great deal of energy—much more than their peers—to do so. This may not be recognized as a problem by school personnel.

Myklebust (1975) and Rourke (1989) evolved the concept of nonverbal learning disorders. Verbal learning disorders are more common in the general school-age population and have been attributed to problems in the left cerebral hemisphere, while nonverbal disabilities, which are less common, have been attributed to the right side. This is an oversimplification of neuroanatomical correlations; most people believe that both types of learning disabilities involve multiple areas of the brain, including the centers that provide integration and interhemispheric transfer of information (Klaas et al., 1999); yet, the category of nonverbal learning disorder holds heuristic value. Children with the syndrome of nonverbal learning disabilities (NVLD) have multiple deficits—in tactile perception, in visual perception, in complex psychomotor skills, and in dealing with novel circumstances (Rourke et al., 2002). Children who demonstrate this pattern typically have strengths in verbal and auditory abilities but weaknesses in nonverbal areas; this pattern is found in some children with meningomyelocele.

Rote verbal memory is a strength in children who have NVLD. They are better auditory than visual learners, and oral production is better than language comprehension (though problems with oral expression may also be seen (Dennis and Barnes, 1993). Table 23.1 outlines some of the difficulties they experience as well as the corresponding manifestations.

Children with NVLD experience difficulty with visual attention and visual-spatial perception, flexibility, abstract thinking, executive function and organizational skills, the pragmatics of language (Fletcher et al., 2002), generalizing information (e.g., you send a child to buy a quart of milk; however, the store only has pints and half-gallons, so the child does not buy any milk), and motor coordination. Executive function skills include planning future activities, organizing, inhibiting competing (inappropriate) responses, self-regulation, remembering rules (like carrying or borrowing during addition and subtraction), initiating tasks (like contacting another teen for companionship), and remembering to remember an activity (like clean intermittent catheterization). Children with NVLD may have strategic and metacognitive deficits (Mahone et al., 2002). They do better thinking in a linear fashion rather than in gestalt terms, and they have difficulty with context (e.g., if the student misses a few words of a sentence of a story, or of a lecture, he or she will get lost; or a child with spina bifida cannot read a map but can follow a sequence of words to find a location). Children with NVLD have difficulty learning new concepts, especially in novel situations; they rely extensively on previously learned rote information; they have difficulty adapting to new situations, which affects their ability to learn; and their information processing tends to be unimodal rather than intermodal (Rourke et al., 2002).

The pattern of NVLD, which is caused by differences in the structure of the nervous system, is not unique to children who have meningomyelocele, but appears more commonly in children who have sustained traumatic injuries to the right side of their brain and in children with conditions affecting white matter such as Williams syndrome, Asperger disorder, velocardiofacial syndrome, and Klinefelter syndrome (McDonald, 2002). Some children with meningomyelocele may have mild difficulties with only a few of the features of NVLD, while others have severe difficulties with all of them.

Yeates et al. (2003) found that about half of children with meningomyelocele have characteristics of NVLD, yet they display significantly more variability in their patterns of assets and deficits than their sibling controls. Significant variability occurs among children with meningomyelocele and may be related to genetic as well as medical factors, including the number of shunt revisions, the severity of the hydrocephalus, and the severity of cerebellar lesions. In addition, as children age, the difference between verbal and nonverbal abilities may change. This makes generalizing about all children with meningomyelocele a risky business. Since most children with meningomyelocele also exhibit some difficulty with verbal memory, oral expression, language comprehension, narrative discourse, and reading comprehension, the cognitive profile in most children with meningomyelocele typically is not one of pure NVLD.

TABLE 23.1. *Areas of Difficulty Seen in Nonverbal Learning Disabilities with Corresponding Manifestations*

Areas of Difficulty	Manifestations
Visual-spatial perception	Difficulty tying shoes* Poor handwriting*
Visual attention	Difficulty reading people's intent in social situations
Adaptation or flexibility with new environments	Resistance to new situations; anxiety due to breaking routines
Abstract thinking	Trouble with many high school subjects
Executive function and organization	Disorganized desk; incomplete assignments
Language pragmatics	Trouble reading between the lines, especially in social situations
Seeing the whole picture	Unable to understand context; cannot break down assignments into manageable parts
Generalizing information	Cannot go from one task to a similar (but not identical) task

*These activities require motor programming and the ability to learn procedures as well as visual spatial abilities.

ATTENTION DEFICIT HYPERACTIVITY DISORDER

Some children with meningomyelocele have classic attention deficit hyperactivity disorder (ADHD). For example, Davidovitch et al. (1999) reported that one-third of children with meningomyelocele have ADHD and about 30% of these children respond to methylphenidate. Their poorly modulated attention may affect higher-order integration skills. Other children may be inattentive and have poor organizational skills but not true ADHD (Shaffer et al., 1985), and it may be difficult to differentiate primary ADHD from attention deficits that are secondary to other neurological impairments, such as problems with alertness and arousal (Brewer et al., 2001). Their inability to integrate, organize, and interpret information can impair their attention, especially when they try to accomplish unfamiliar tasks; as a result, they may be diagnosed as having attention deficit disorder without regard paid to executive functioning.

EFFECTS ON ACADEMIC ABILITIES AND SCHOOL PERFORMANCE

Preschool children with meningomyelocele may appear precocious at an early age because of their strong verbal skills; however, by the time they are 3 years of age, they typically demonstrate weak number skills that persist into adulthood (Wills et al., 1990; Dennis and Barnes, 2002). They score lower on standardized math tests than do children without spina bifida. Handwriting may be taxing (Pearson et al., 1988). These children may have difficulty using scissors, tying shoelaces, and buttoning buttons. They may have difficulty holding a pencil.

In the past, children with meningomyelocele were placed in schools specifically designed for children with disabilities (Kirk et al., 2002). Now they generally are mainstreamed in normal classes (Carr et al., 1983; Dodd, 1984). Problems with both types of placement have been observed (Wasson et al., 1992). Even today some children may experience restricted or delayed school attendance due to inaccessible school facilities or lack of facilities for toileting.

Several studies have shown that children and adolescents with meningomyelocele do worse than their typically developing peers on measures of intelligence and/or achievement, and are more likely to receive special services or repeat a grade (Tew and Laurence, 1984; Fowler et al., 1985; Friedrich et al., 1991; Appleton et al., 1994; Jacobs et al., 2001). Scores in mathematics are consistently lower, and those in other academic areas (i.e., reading, spelling) are inconsistently lower. In addition, students attending regular schools demonstrate better outcomes on IQ tests and on skills tests in reading and arithmetic than children in special schools (Carr et al., 1983; Wasson et al., 1992). The presence of a shunt has been associated with lower IQ scores and lower mathematics scores in some studies (Kalucy et al., 1996).

Children with meningomyelocele are less likely to advance to postsecondary education than children without meningomyelocele. In one study, 34% of children with meningomyelocele were involved in postsecondary education compared to 47% of the general population. Youth with meningomyelocele were 1 to 2 years delayed in educational attainment compared to age-matched peers (Bomalaski et al., 1995). In a follow-up of 48 adults who had attended a specialty clinic, 7 were attending college. Achievement and IQ scores, as well as measures of language and visual-spatial ability, differentiated those who attended college from those who did not (Hurley and Bell, 1994). Although survival into adulthood has improved for individuals with meningomyelocele, the rate of employability has not and remains around 30% (Tew et al., 1990).

Meningomyelocele may affect children's ability to learn in several ways. First, it has an obvious direct effect on cognition. Second, it is associated with increased absences from school (Weitzman et al., 1986). These may be from acute illnesses, visits to health professionals, inappropriate health beliefs and perceptions of vulnerability, worsening of chronic symptoms, or hospitalizations. In addition to absence from school, children with meningomyelocele may be absent from academic classes because they are pulled out for therapy services (e.g., physical and occupational therapy) or catheterization and other medical procedures. Third, the inability to understand academic subjects, diminished expectations and lower self-esteem, fatigue, pain, and preoccupation with symptoms that often accompany spina bifida may be associated with a decreased sense of self-efficacy (Mobley et al., 1996). Children in fact, may develop *learned helplessness*, believing that their efforts to change the environment are ineffective, and will stop trying academically or reaching out socially. Because social skills and athletic abilities, as well as many aspects of academic learning, are impaired in children with meningomyelocele (Humphries et al., 1996; Hommeyer et al., 1999), it is difficult for school-age children with meningomyelocele to develop a sense of industry (Erikson, 1959).

Academic demands change as children grow older. In elementary school, the curriculum is highly structured, with an emphasis on rote learning. Pragmatic learning is emphasized, and analyses are simple. Redundancy is built into the curriculum. However, in later grades, demands for speed, efficiency, organizational ability, and automaticity increase. Concepts become increasingly abstract and require mental flexibility. Information processing becomes less linear and more simultaneous. Children who have meningomyelocele have emerging learning difficulties that may not be apparent in the earlier grades (Rowley-Kelly and Reigel, 1993).

Numerical literacy, or the ability to do mathematics, is adversely affected in children who have nonverbal learning disorder, including children who have meningomyelocele. Visual-spatial difficulties can make learning certain types of mathematics, such as geometry, a major challenge. Similarly, problems with estimation and the ability to solve word problems are associated with problems with visual-spatial integration (Barnes et al., 2002). Children with meningomyelocele also have worse procedural skills that persist to adulthood (Dennis and Barnes, 2002). They also have diminished speed of retrieval (efficiency). Even as early as 36 months of age, they may demonstrate delays in the ability to count or seriate.

As children grow older, expectations in school change. The inability of children with NVLD to keep up with their peers becomes more noticeable. For example, at around the time of third grade, "learning to read" becomes "reading to learn," which is more difficult for children with NVLD (useful resources in this topic are available at http://ericec.org/readlist.html "learning to read, reading to learn"). Word recognition and sight reading are strong, but overall reading comprehension is weak. Math skills such as telling time and counting money tend to be difficult. Children with NVLD may have difficulty separating relevant from less relevant material and may fail to understand the meaning, function, and purpose of writing. They have difficulty getting the main idea from a story or a movie and get caught up in the details. Other changing demands in school include the increasing complexity of tasks, increasing abstraction, increased demand for written output, and increasing need for analytical abilities. Because these children have difficulty generalizing, they have problems going from one example of an academic activity (like division with integers) to another related activity (like division with fractions) (Marlowe, 2000). Or they seem to repeat the same mistakes.

In middle school, a whole sequence of events needs to be organized to do an assignment. Remembering, planning, and organizing these sequences are difficult for these children because they lack the executive ability to bring skills together effortlessly and use them for more integrated learning. At the same time, increasing physical demands occur, such as moving from class to class between periods in a limited amount of time and carrying books while in a wheelchair or using braces. This may lead to fatigue, which further decreases academic performance. Thus, children with spina bifida often demonstrate increasing deficits as they go from elementary to middle to high school.

Children may demonstrate a decline in school function for several medical reasons. These include ventricular shunt malfunction, which may present with subtle symptoms including worsening academic performance. Anticonvulsants and anticholinergics (used to help manage bladder function) may lead to lethargy and affect school performance. Children with meningomyelocele are at increased risk for depression and/or anxiety (Appleton et al., 1997), which can affect functioning in school.

EFFECTS ON SOCIAL ABILITIES

Children with spina bifida have been found to be socially immature and passive, more isolated, more dependent on adults, and less likely to make independent decisions (Blum et al., 1991; Holmbeck et al., 2003). Successful social interactions require learning empathy, an ability to understand how others see themselves, reciprocity, image building, greeting skills, and social attributions (Levine, 1980). Children need to learn to match affect, pace interactions, and sustain relationships over time. This requires abilities in verbal pragmatics, social problem-solving skills, and social memory, as well as the ability to predict consequences.

Nonverbal learning disorder affects communication in a number of ways. These include an impaired ability to interpret visual social cues such as body language, gestures, and facial expressions. In addition, NVLD impairs the understanding of tone of voice, mood, and emotional cues. It affects comprehension not immediately contained in words, such as humor, nuances, and sarcasm, and affects the pragmatics of language, such as what to say when. For an individual with an NVLD, the interpretation of social cues such as facial expressions and body language can become a major problem, and can lead to confusion and social rejection. Table 23.2 lists the social interactions and changes that occur as a child progresses through school.

Because children with NVLD have difficulty with novel and complex situations, they may be reluctant to try new activities, such as a new game or going to summer camp. A great deal of meaning in relationships is communicated nonverbally. Because children with NVLD have difficulty with visual attention and understanding nonverbal cues, they have problems interpreting behavior. Although these children may be talkative, they often interrupt and have difficulty entering conversations correctly. They may have difficulty understanding jokes because they do not understand how things normally fit together, interact, or intersect.

As children become teens, social demands increase and the ability to read cues like body language and tone of voice becomes more critical. Anyone who has observed a group of teenage girls in a mall witnesses remarkable shifts of mood, topic, and feeling. Like a flock of birds in flight, they change direction in unison with great precision. Individuals with NVLD may have difficulty interpreting intention, humor, and abstractions, and cannot follow transitions or the subtle social rules and conventions. Social interactions require different linguistic sets, such as conversations with parents versus those with friends. Children with NVLD may not be able to discriminate between these situations and therefore act inappropriately, leading to social rejection.

TABLE 23.2. *Social Interactions and Changes Throughout School*

Time	Social Interactions
Kindergarten	Play reciprocally
	Share and resolve conflicts
Lower grades	Appreciate the perspectives of others
Middle grades	Develop close relationships and friendships
	Develop a reputation
	Learn to conform
	Learn to match affect with others
Upper grades	Develop membership in subgroups
	Increase tolerance for diversity
	Interact with peers of the opposite sex

Source: Levine (1980).

FAILURE TO RECOGNIZE NONVERBAL LEARNING DISORDER

Because children with NVLD have good verbal skills, teachers in the early grades may overestimate their overall abilities. Because these children fail to meet expectations in other areas or have inconsistent performance, they often are viewed as being lazy, unmotivated, or having a poor attitude. They may be incorrectly diagnosed as having ADHD (though some may have ADHD as a separate entity). Because these children do not interpret social situations well and commit many faux pas, they may be viewed as being insensitive. They may be rejected by peers, teased, and ridiculed, which leads to social isolation. Repeated failures in school and with peers may lead to anxiety, depression, or acting-out, oppositional behaviors; students may decide that success is impossible, learn to be helpless, and lose all desire (learned helplessness) (Bandura, 1977). They may be victimized by their peers or adults (Little, 2001, 2002).

ASSESSMENT OF CHILDREN WITH MENINGOMYELOCELE

Preschool children with meningomyelocele should have formal evaluations of their cognitive abilities if they have developmental delay on screening tests. All children with meningomyelocele with shunted hydrocephalus should have a formal evaluation before they enter kindergarten or first grade. Parents, school personnel, and clinicians should work together in the process of evaluation. Parts of the assessment may include (*1*) direct observation of the child's interactions with parents, teachers, and peers; (*2*) interviews of the student, family, teachers, and therapists; (*3*) examination of school records and past evaluations; (*4*) use of formal checklists completed by parents, teachers, or the student; and (*5*) formal psychoeducational testing. Formal neuropsychological testing of the child is often helpful. Table 23.3 lists the evaluations performed in a typical neuropsychological evaluation. Assessment is best approached by a multidisciplinary team using standardized neurodevelopmental and educational tests (rather than an isolated IQ test) to evaluate the child's strengths and weaknesses, neurological status, academic skills, and emotional concerns. The resulting description is more valuable in helping to develop a plan of intervention than a mere list of test scores or a label such as ADHD. Assessment should be ongoing and include classroom observations as well as informal assessments, including samples of classwork and teacher-made tests. Because a child's ability to perform will change as academic demands increase, monitoring over time is critical to understanding the child's abilities and needs.

TABLE 23.3. *Components (Domains) of a Comprehensive Neuropsychological Examination*

Sensory perceptual examination
Visual
Auditory
Somatosensory
Psychomotor abilities (motor performance)
Visuospatial functions
Calculation
Constructional abilities
Mood and temperament
Language
Oral expressive
Aural receptive
Written narrative
Attention and processing speed
Working memory
Memory and learning
Complex problem solving, judgment, and executive functioning
Abstract thinking
Intelligence
Academic skills
Adaptive behavior

INTERVENTIONS TO MAXIMIZE LEARNING

General Issues

Children require a safe environment, as well as access to the school and all of its activities. School personnel may not be knowledgeable about the child's condition or how to manage acute exacerbations and may be extremely anxious about having the child in school (Hunt, 1981). A formal process of entry into school may be helpful. This includes early notification of the school by the parents and health-care providers regarding the child's desire to attend the program, as well as a discussion of the child's condition and needs. The family, providers and school develop a formal health-care plan. Training of school personnel may be helpful. Table 23.4 lists the components of a school-based health-care plan for a child who has meningomyelocele. Since frequent absences from school can adversely affect a child's ability to learn (Fowler et al., 1985), keeping the child healthy can directly increase the child's ability to function academically.

The next step is to delineate the child's academic strengths and weaknesses in order to provide insight to the child, family, and school personnel. Expectations of the school should be congruent with the child's abilities, motivation, and temperament. Failure to understand the child's condition and individual characteristics can lead to expectations that are unreasonably high or detrimentally low.

TABLE 23.4. *Components of a School-Based Health-care Plan for a Child with Meningomyelocele*

1. Universal precautions
2. Preparation for entry
   a. Initial evaluation
   b. Medical evaluation (bladder and bowel programs, hydrocephalus, medications, latex allergies, diet, and skin care)
   c. Medical history
   d. Meetings to develop plan
   e. Related services (physical, occupational, and speech/language therapies, classroom aide, scribe, catheterization, adaptive physical education)
      Training of school staff
3. Physician's orders
4. Emergency plan
   a. Names, addresses, and phone numbers of family and caretakers
   b. Emergency phone numbers
      Ambulance, primary care physician, specialists, therapists, home care company, utility companies, hospital, emergency department
   c. Child-specific emergency plan
   d. Other school personnel to contact
5. Child-specific guidelines
   a. Background information
      Conditions, medical history, special health-care needs, baseline status, medications, diet, assistive technological aids, transportation needs
   b. Procedures required, including mobility and accessibility
   c. Equipment
   d. Child-specific techniques
   e. Special considerations and precautions (e.g., latex allergy)
   f. List of possible problems—observation, reason, action
6. Parental authorization for specialized health care
7. Follow-up and modification of the plan

Source: Haynie et al. (1989).

Next, the child's academic and other needs are prioritized, followed by designing specific strategies to improve various aspects of the child's life including classroom, homework, social skills, and activities of daily living (including self-help skills such as catheterization and taking medications). Providing the child's environment with as much predictability as possible, planning for transitions, allowing plenty of time for tasks, and providing structure (organization) to the environment are strategies that can be helpful in any setting. Based on these, recommendations regarding the program, placement, and staffing are made.

Several laws have been enacted to ensure that children have access to education in the least restrictive environment. The Individuals with Disabilities Education Act (IDEA), Public Law 102-119, which incorporates other earlier legislative efforts, provides children with meningomyelocele with improved access to educational services. This law entitles children with disabilities ages 3–21 to a free, appropriate education. It provides funds to states to develop and support special education programs. It guarantees children an education in the least restrictive environment and inclusion in educational and social programs. Related services must be paid for by the school. A related service is any additional service that is needed to allow the child to benefit from instruction. These services include transportation, audiology, recreation, school health services, psychological services, physical therapy, occupational therapy, speech and language therapy, catheterization, assistive technology, and social work services. Every child has a written plan (Individualized Education Plan [IEP]), and parents have the right to question placement decisions and the right to due process to settle differences. Two criteria have to be met for a child to qualify under IDEA: (*1*) the child must have a disability, and (*2*) special education services are necessary to address the disability. Children who have meningomyelocele can be classified as having a disability under IDEA in several different ways, including the categories "learning disabled," "orthopedically impaired," or "other health impaired." The second criterion can be met if any aspect of the disability has a negative impact on any aspect of participation in the general curriculum—including academic, behavior, communication, vocational skills, basic life skills, social skills, and physical needs.

If for some reason the child does not qualify under IDEA, Section 504 of the Rehabilitation Act of 1973 provides access to services. This law states that no qualified person with a handicap shall be excluded from participation in any program or activity that receives benefits from federal financial assistance. Under this legislation, a child does not have to be enrolled in special education or eligible under IDEA in order to receive related services from a school. However, parents have fewer rights and children receive fewer services under Section 504.

Loomis et al. (1997) found that family encouragement of independence and achievement was linked with good outcomes in young adults with meningomyelocele. McKernon et al. (2001) found that the quality of parenting and the family environment were associated with children's problem-focused coping behaviors. Therefore, one of the most important interventions is encouraging parents to have high expectations for their child with meningomyelocele. For example, children with meningomyelocele should be encouraged to do chores and follow the rules of the house. Educational materials are available to help parents understand their child's cognitive abilities and advocate for them with schools (e.g., Thompson 1997; Tanguay, 2001; NLD on the Web, 2003; SANDI, 2004). Health-related care by a multidisciplinary team that is knowledgeable about spina bifida and regular therapeutic interventions may maximize health and well-being (Kinsman et al., 2000; Rendeli et al., 2002). Parents should be encouraged to stay involved since they will have to advocate for the child repeatedly. They also should be aware of the rules and regulations concerning special education and other interventions at their child's school.

Specific Interventions

Interventions to optimize educational and social skills need to use the child's strengths, which usually are based on verbal rote repetitions. Interventions need to be ongoing, and are both remedial and compensatory. Remedial techniques are designed to strengthen a certain area of weakness, such as, teaching memory techniques or mnemonics. Compensatory strategies are designed to offset or provide an alternative strategy, such as, providing checklists or assistive technology devices (Russel, 2004).

Because they have difficulty with gestalt, children with meningomyelocele should be provided with a context. Activities need to be modeled. Providing lists and planners can help them organize materials. Classroom changes can include accommodations such as minimizing paper-and-pencil tasks because of poor finger dexterity and visual-spatial problems, modifications such as placement in an environment that has a well-established routine, and strategies such as grouping the child with good role models or having teachers "think out loud" during tasks in order to give them a verbal perspective on their internal thinking. Using assistive technology, like a computer for word processing in place of writing, should be encouraged (Tanguay, 2002).

Increasing skills related to "learning to learn" and "remembering to remember" can help executive control processes. Repetition to overlearn an activity, which leads to automaticity, can increase the child's ability to do that task independently. Helping the child to make lists (scripts) for everyday activities like "(*1*) take shower, (*2*) take medications, (*3*) catheterize, (*4*) get dressed, (*5*) brush my teeth" and giving the child sufficient time can help with sequential activities (Lutkenhoff and Oppenheimer, 1997). Providing similar lists in a written and pictorial display can give insights into why certain procedures are done, such as, (*1*) catheter in bladder → (*2*) empty bladder → (*3*) no infection and no reflux → (*4*) kidneys stay healthy, and may promote adherence to regimens of care.

Some children benefit from medications to increase attention, or to decrease anxiety or depression. Teaching a child with learning disorders can be exhausting because it requires constant work; having support from parents, colleagues, and friends is critical to the success of the endeavor. Table 23.5 lists some strategies for providing educational instructions to children who have meningomyelocele. However, very little evidence has been published demonstrating that these techniques work (or do not work).

A special area of intervention is that of improving social skills, which are as important for well-being as academic and other skills. Table 23.6 lists certain strategies that have been used, some of which have been shown in case series to be effective (Minskoff, 1980a, 1980b; Loomis et al., 1994; King, 1997; Barnhill, 2002). Accurately perceiving social cues and responding appropriately are skills that can be taught, especially by focusing

TABLE 23.5. *Strategies for Providing Educational Instructions to Children Who Have Meningomyelocele*

Strategy	Examples
Use rote verbal repetition	Ask for verbal feedback Repeat instructions Describe social situations verbally Develop verbal coping strategies
Use assistive devices and organizers to compensate for deficitsin executive function and visual spatial problems	Planners Calendars Word processors Watches with alarms Calculators
Use linear sequences to explain concepts	Written chains instead of maps Generate outline before writing Put things in a list and number them Use sequential linguistic instruction, not whole language
Preview, plan, and prepare students for novel situations or transitions	Explain new concepts and situations verbally ahead of time
Do not assume knowledge about context	Be explicit about schedules and feelings
Organize materials visually	Use graph paper to line up numbers

TABLE 23.6. *Examples of Interventions to Improve Social Skills*

Interventions for parents
Social skills curriculum
Peer mentorship (circle of friends)
In vivo coaching
Social stories (comic strip conversations)
Didactic teaching about social skills and emotions
Group-based interventions

Source: Loomis et al. (1994).

on concrete rote behaviors. In these programs, children are placed in highly structured environments where they receive support and many opportunities for practice. Collaborations occur between home and school (Duke et al., 1996), and children are given assignments for practice.

In one method, the *circle of friends,* children are put in a structured peer network with scheduled time and shared activities. There they can practice various activities together, such as observing a soap opera on television with the sound muted while trying to determine what emotions the actors are portraying. They then practice showing those emotions. They can also play games like liar's bluff, act out specific characters, and practice telling jokes. These complex social interactions can be broken down into more discrete activities like eye contact, tone of voice, body language, choice of words, turn-taking, transitions from subject to subject, and so on. Children receive formal instruction in the social interactions shown in Table 23.2.

As with educational interventions, providing and rehearsing numbered lists may help with social behavior. For example, decision making consists of the following: (*1*) define the problem and the facts; (*2*) define options; (*3*) weigh the options; (*4*) pick an option; (*5*) carry out your plan; and (*6*) evaluate your choice. Problem solving includes the following: (*1*) what went right and wrong?; (*2*) what could you do differently?; and (*3*) what other options are available?

SUMMARY

Figure 23.1 illustrates the World Health Organization model as applied to some aspects of learning in children with meningomyelocele (Simeonsson et al., 2002). Children who have meningomyelocele with shunted hydrocephalus typically have anomalies of the central nervous system that are associated with learning disorders. Although their IQ scores are in the low-normal range, they often score worse on performance than on verbal measures. Many can be described as having characteristics of NVLD. In school they tend to have more problems with mathematics than with other subjects. They exhibit impaired social skills and demonstrate problems attributable to poor executive functioning, including failure in planning to plan. Their main strength lies in aural rote repetition. As the academic challenges of higher grade levels increase, their learning disorders become more evident.

Strategies to address these disorders include remediation and compensation. Building on their strengths can help develop new skills and strategies. Extensive planning and cooperation with school personnel are required. In order to be effective advocates for their child, parents need to stay involved and be knowledgeable about the rules and regulations that govern special education. In addition to addressing academic subjects, interventions that address social interactions are critical to optimize the potential of children who have meningomyelocele.

REFERENCES

Appleton PL, Ellis NC, Minchom PE, Lawson V, Boll V, Jones P (1997). Depressive symptoms and self-concept in young people with spina bifida. J Pediatr Psychol 22:707–722.

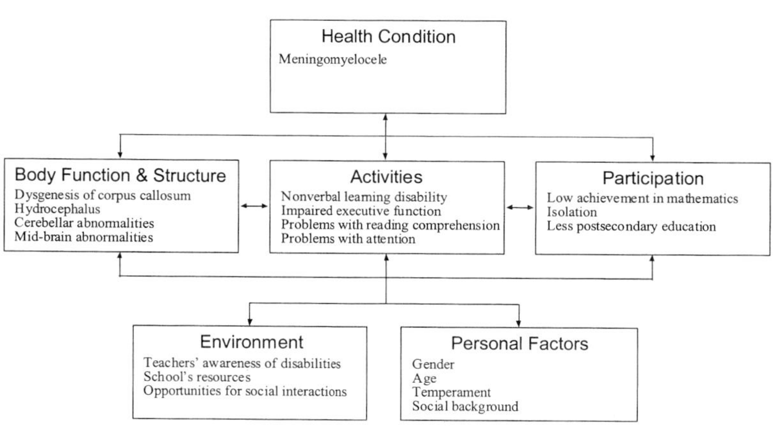

FIGURE 23.1. World Health Organization International Classification of Function (ICF) model applied to one aspect of functioning in children with meningomyelocele.

Appleton PL, Minchom PE, Ellis NC, Elliott CE, Boll V, Jones P (1994). The self-concept of young people with spina bifida: a population-based study. Dev Med Child Neurol 36:198–215.

Bandura A (1977). Self-efficacy: towards a unifying theory of behavioral change. Psychol Rev 84:191–215.

Bannister CM, Russell SA, Rimmer S (1998). Pre-natal brain development of fetuses with a myelomeningocele. Eur J Pediatr Surg 8(Suppl 1):15–17.

Barf HA, Verhoef M, Jennekens-Schinkel A, Post MW, Gooskens RH, Prevo AJ (2003). Cognitive status of young adults with spina bifida. Dev Med Child Neurol 45:813–820.

Barnes MA, Dennis M (1992). Reading in children and adolescents after early onset hydrocephalus and in normally developing age peers: phonological analysis, word recognition, word comprehension, and passage comprehension skills. J Pediatr Psychol 17:445–465.

Barnes MA, Dennis M (1998). Discourse after early-onset hydrocephalus: core deficits in children of average intelligence. Brain Lang 61:309–334.

Barnes M, Pengelly S, Dennis M, Wilkinson M, Rogers T, Faulkner H (2002). Mathematics skills in good readers with hydrocephalus. J Int Neuropsychol Soc 8:72–82.

Barnhill GP (2002). The effectiveness of social skills intervention targeting nonverbal communication for adolescents with Asperger syndrome and related pervasive developmental delays. Focus Autism Other Dev Disabil 17:112–118.

Bier JA, Morales Y, Liebling J, Geddes L, Kim E (1997). Medical and social factors associated with cognitive outcome in individuals with myelomeningocele. Dev Med Child Neurol 39:263–266.

Blum RW, Resnick MD, Nelson R, St Germaine A (1991). Family and peer issues among adolescents with spina bifida and cerebral palsy. Pediatrics 88:280–285.

Bomalaski MD, Teague JL, Brooks B (1995). The long-term impact of urological management on the quality of life of children with spina bifida. Urol 154:778–781.

Brewer VR, Fletcher JM, Hiscock M, Davidson KC (2001). Attention processes in children with shunted hydrocephalus versus attention deficit-hyperactivity disorder. Neuropsychology 15:185–198.

Brookshire BL, Fletcher JM, Bohan TP, Landry SH, Davidson KC, Francis DJ (1995). Verbal and nonverbal skill discrepancies in children with hydrocephalus: a five-year longitudinal follow-up. J Pediatr Psychol 20:785–800.

Carr J, Halliwell MD, Pearson AM (1983). Educational attainments of spina bifida children attending ordinary or special schools. Spec Educ Forward Trends 10:22–24.

Casari EF, Fantino AG (1998). A longitudinal study of cognitive abilities and achievement status of children with myelomeningocele and their relationship with clinical types. Eur J Pediatr Surg 8(Suppl 1):52–54.

Cull C, Wyke MA (1984). Memory function of children with spina bifida and shunted hydrocephalus. Dev Med Child Neurol 26:177–183.

Davidovitch M, Manning-Courtney P, Hartmann LA, Watson J, Lutkenhoff M, Oppenheimer S (1999). The prevalence of attentional problems and the effect of methylphenidate in children with myelomenigocele. Pediatr Rehabil 3:29–35.

delBigio MR (1993). Neuropathological changes caused by hydrocephalus. Acta Neuropathol 85:573–585.

Dennis M, Barnes M (1993). Oral discourse skills in children and adolescents after early-onset hydrocephalus: linguistic ambiguity, figurative language, speech acts, and script-based inferences. J Pediatr Psychol 18:639–652.

Dennis M, Barnes M (2002). Math and numeracy in young adults with spina bifida and hydrocephalus. Dev Neuropsychol 21:141–155.

Dennis M, Jacennik B, Barnes M (1994). The content of narrative discourse in children and adolescents after early-onset hydrocephalus and in normally-developing age peers. Brain Lang 46:129–165.

Dise JE, Lohr ME (1998). Examination of deficits in conceptual reasoning abilities associated with spina bifida. Am J Phys Med Rehabil 77:247–251.

Dodd KD (1984). Where should spina bifida children go to school? Z Kinderchir 39(Suppl 2):129–131.

Duke MP, Martin EA, Nowicki S Jr (1996). *Teaching Your Child the Language of Social Success.* Atlanta: Peachtree.

Erickson K, Baron IS, Fantie BD (2001). Neuropsychological functioning in early hydrocephalus: review from a developmental perspective. Child Neuropsychol 7:199–229.

Erikson E (1959). Identity and the life cycle. Psychol Issues 1:1–171.

Fletcher JM, Barnes M, Dennis M (2002). Language development in children with spina bifida. Semin Pediatr Neurol 9:201–208.

Fletcher JM, McCauley SR, Brandt ME, Bohan TP, Kramer LA, Francis DJ, Thorstad K, et al (1996). Regional brain tissue composition in children with hydrocephalus. Relationships with cognitive development. Arch Neurol 53:549–557.

Fowler MG, Johnson MP, Atkinson SS (1985). School achievement and absence in children with chronic health conditions. J Pediatr 106:683–687.

Friedrich WN, Lovejoy MC, Shaffer J, Shurtleff DB, Beilke RL (1991). Cognitive abilities and achievement status of children with myelomeningocele: a contemporary sample. J Pediatr Psychol 16(4):423–428.

Gao JH, Parsons LM, Bower JM, Xiong J, Li J, Fox PT (1996). Cerebellum implicated in sensory acquisition and discrimination rather than motor control. Science 272:545–547.

Gebhart AL, Petersen SE, Thach WT (2002). Role of the posterolateral cerebellum in language. Ann NY Acad Sci 978:318–333.

Gilbert JN, Jones KL, Rorke LB, Chernoff GF, James HE (1986). Central nervous system anomalies associated with meningomyelocele, hydrocephalus, and the Arnold-Chiari malformation: reappraisal of theories regarding the pathogenesis of posterior neural tube closure defects. Neurosurgery 18:559–564.

Hannay HJ, Fletcher JM, Brandt M (1999). Role of the corpus callosum in the cognitive development of children with congenital brain malformations. In Broman SH, Fletcher JM (eds): *The Changing Nervous System: Neurobehavioral Consequences of Early brain Disorders.* New York: Oxford University Press. pp. 149–171.

Haynie M, Porter SM, Palfrey JS (1989). Children assisted by medical technology in educational settings. Boston: Project School Care, The Children's Hospital.

Holler KA, Fennell EB, Crosson B, Boggs SR, Mickle JP (1995) Neuropsychological and adaptive functioning in younger versus older children shunted for early hydrocephalus. Child Neuropsychol 1:63–73.

Holmbeck GN, Westhoven VC, Phillips WS, Bowers R, Gruse C, Nikolopoulos T, Totura CM, Davison K (2003). A multimethod, multi-informant, and multidimensional perspective on psychosocial adjustment in preadolescents with spina bifida. J Consult Clin Psychol 71:782–796.

Hommet C, Billiard C, Gillet P, Barthez M, Lourmiere J, Santini JJ, de Toffol B, Corcia P, Autret A (1999). Neuropsychologic and adaptive functioning in adolescents and young adults shunted for congenital hydrocephalus. J Child Neurol 14:144–150.

Hommeyer JS, Holmbeck GN, Wills KE, Coers S (1999). Condition severity and psychosocial functioning in pre-adolescents with spina bifida: disentangling proximal functional status and distal adjustment outcomes. J Pediatr Psychol 24:499–509.

Humphries T, Krekewich K, Snider L (1996). Evidence of nonverbal learning disability among learning disabled boys with sensory integrative dysfunction. Percept Mot Skills 82:979–987.

Hunt GM (1981). Spina bifida: implications for 100 children at school. Dev Med Child Neurol 23:160–172.

Hunt GM, Oakeshott P, Kerry S (1999). Link between the CSF shunt and achievement in adults with spina bifida. J Neurol Neurosurg Psychiatry 67:591–595.

Hurley AD, Bell S (1994). Educational and vocational outcome of adults with spina bifida in relationship to neuropsychological testing. Eur J Pediatr Surg 4(Suppl 1):17–18.

Hurley AD, Dorman C, Laatsch L, Bell S, D'Avignon J (1990). Cognitive functioning in patients with spina bifida, hydrocephalus, and the "Cocktail Party" syndrome. Dev Neuropsychol 6:151–172.

Hurley AD, Laatsch LK, Dorman C (1983). Comparison of spina bifida, hydrocephalic patients and matched controls on neuropsychological tests. Z Kinderchir 38(Suppl 2):116–118.

Jacobs R, Northam E, Anderson V (2001). Cognitive outcome in children with myelomeningocele and perinatal hydrocephalus: a longitudinal perspective. Dev Phys Disabil 13:389–405.

Kalucy M, Bower C, Stanley F (1996). School-aged children with spina bifida in western Australia: parental perspectives on functional outcome. Dev Med Child Neurol 38:325–334.

Kanev PM, Sheehan JM (2003). Reflections on shunt infection. Pediatr Neurosurg 39(6):285–290.

Kawamura T, Morioka T, Nishio S, Mihara F, Fukui M (2001). Cerebral abnormalities in lumbosacral neural tube closure defect: MR imaging evaluation. Childs Nerv Syst 17(7):405–410.

Kawamura T, Nishio S, Morioka T, Fukui K (2002). Callosal anomalies in patients with spinal dysraphism: correlation of clinical and neuroimaging features with hemispheric abnormalities. Neurol Res 24(5):463–467.

King GA (1997). Social skills training for withdrawn unpopular children with physical disabilities: a preliminary evaluation. Rehabil Psychol 42(1):47–60.

Kinsman SL, Levey E, Ruffing V, Stone J, Warren L (2000). Beyond multidisciplinary care: a new conceptual model for spina bifida services. Eur J Pediatr Surg 10(Suppl 1):35–38.

Kirk S, Gallagher J, Anastasiow N (2002). *Educating Exceptional Children,* 10th ed. Boston: Houghton Mifflin.

Klaas PA, Hannay JH, Caroselli JS, Fletcher JM (1999). Interhemispheric transfer of visual, auditory, tactile, and visuomotor information in children with hydrocephalus and partial agenesis of the corpus callosum. J Clin Exp Neuropsychol 21(6):837–850.

Levine MD (1980). *A Pediatric Approach to Learning Disorders.* New York: Wiley.

Levisohn L, Cronin-Golomb A, Schmahmann JD (2000). Neuropsychological consequences of cerebellar tumour resection in children: cerebellar cognitive affective syndrome in a paediatric population. Brain 123(Pt 5):1041–1050.

Little L (2001). Peer victimization of children with Asperger spectrum disorders. J Am Acad Child Adolesc Psychiatry 40(9):995–996.

Little L (2002). Middle-class mothers' perceptions of peer and sibling victimization among children with Asperger's syndrome and nonverbal learning disorders. Issues Compr Pediatr Nurs 25(1):43–57.

Loomis JW, Javornisky JG, Monahan JJ, Burke G, Lindsay A (1997). Relations between family environment and adjustment outcomes in young adults with spina bifida. Dev Med Child Neurol 39(9):620–627.

Loomis JW, Lindsey A, Javornisky JG, Monahan JJ (1994). Measures of cognition and adaptive behavior as predictors of adjustment outcomes in young adults with spina bifida. Eur J Pediatr Surg 4(Suppl 1):35–36.

Lutkenhoff M, Oppenheimer SG (eds) (1997). *Spinabilities: A Young Person's Guide to Spina Bifida.* Bethesda, MD: Woodbine House.

Mahone EM, Zabel TA, Levey E, Verda M, Kinsman S (2002). Parent and self-report rating of executive function in adolescents with myelomeningocele and hydrocephalus. Child Neuropsychol 8:258–270.

Marlowe WB (2000). An intervention for children with disorders of executive functions. Dev Neuropsychol 18:445–454.

Mazur JM, Aylward GP, Colliver J, Stacey J, Menelaus M (1988). Impaired mental capabilities and hand function in myelomeningocele patients. Z Kinderchir 43(Suppl 2):24–27.

McDonald BC (2002). Recent developments in the application of the nonverbal learning disabilities model. Curr Psychiatry Rep 4(5):323–330.

McKernon WL, Holmbeck GN, Colder CR, Hommeyer JS, Shapera W, Westhoven V (2001). Longitudinal study of observed and perceived family influences on problem-focused coping behaviors of preadolescents with spina bifida. J Pediatr Psychol 26(1):41–54.

McLone DG (1992). Continuing concepts in the management of spina bifida. Pediatr Neurosurg 18(5–6):254–256.

Minskoff E (1980a). Teaching approach for developing nonverbal communication skills in students with social perception deficits, Part 1: the basic approach and body language cues. J Learning Disabil 13:118–124.

Minskoff E (1980b). Teaching approach for developing nonverbal communication skills in students with social perception deficits, Part 2: proxemic, vocalic, and artifactual cues. J Learning Disabil 13(4):203–208.

Mobley CE, Harless LS, Miller KL (1996). Self-perceptions of preschool children with spina bifida. J Pediatr Nurs 11:217–224.

Myklebust HR (1975). Nonverbal learning disabilities: assessment and intervention. In Myklebust HR (ed): *Progress in Learning Disabilities.* New York: Grune & Stratton, pp. 85–121.

NLD on the Web (2003). Nonverbal Learning Disorder on the Web! Available at www.nldontheweb.org.

Pearson AM, Carr J, Hallwell MD (1988). The handwriting of children with spina bifida. Z Kinderchir 43(Suppl 2):40–42.

Ralph K, Moylan P, Canady A, Simmons S (2000). The effects of multiple shunt revisions on neuropsychological functioning and memory. Neurol Res 22:131–136.

Rendeli C, Salvaggio E, Sciascia CG, Bianchi E, Caldarelli M, Guzzetta F (2002). Does locomotion improve the cognitive profile of children with meningomyelocele? Childs Nerv Syst 18(5):231–234.

Rourke BP (1989). *Nonverbal Learning Disabilities: The Syndrome and the Model.* New York: Guilford Press.

Rourke BP, Ahmad SA, Collins DW, Hayman-Abello BA, Hayman-Abello SE, Warriner EM (2002). Child clinical/pediatric neuro psychology: some recent advances. Annu Rev Psychol 53:309–339.

Rowley-Kelly FL, Reigel DH (eds) (1993). *Teaching the Student with Spina Bifida.* Baltimore; Paul H Brookes.

Russel CL (2004). Understanding nonverbal learning disorders in children with spina bifida. Teach Except Child 36(4):8–13.

SANDI (2004). The SANDI project: the Spina Bifida Assessment of Neurobehavioral Development, International. http://ped1.med.uth.tmc.edu/spinabifida. Accessed March 23, 2004.

Scott MA, Fletcher JM, Brookshire BL, Davidson KC, Landry SH, Bohan TC, Kramer LA, et al (2003). Memory functions in children with early hydrocephalus. Neuropsychology 4:578–589.

Shaffer J, Friedrich WN, Shurtleff DB, Wolf L (1985). Cognitive and achievement status of children with myelomeningocele. J Pediatr Psychol 10(3):325–336.

Simeonsson RJ, McMillen JS, Huntington GS (2002). Secondary conditions in children with disabilities: spina bifida as a case example. Ment Retard Dev Disabil Res Rev 8(3):198–205.

Tanguay P (2001). *Nonverbal Learning Disabilities at Home: A Parent's Guide.* Philadelphia: Jessica Kingsley.

Tanguay P (2002). *Nonverbal Learning Disabilities at School: Educating Students with NLD, Asperger Syndrome, and Related Conditions.* Philadelphia: Jessica Kingsley.

Tew B (1979). The "cocktail party syndrome" in children with hydrocephalus and spina bifida. Br J Disord Commun 14(2):89–101.

Tew B, Laurence KM (1979). The clinical and psychological characteristics of children with the "cocktail party" syndrome. Z Kinderchir Grenzgeb 28(4):360–367.

Tew B, Laurence KM (1984). The relationship between intelligence and academic achievements in spina bifida adolescents. Z Kinderchir 39(Suppl 2):122–124.

Tew B, Laurence KM, Jenkins V (1990). Factors affecting employability among young adults with spina bifida and hydrocephalus. Z Kinderchir 45(Suppl 1):34–36.

Thompson S (1997). *The Source for Nonverbal Learning Disorders.* East Moline, IL: LinguiSystems.

Van Mier HI, Petersen SE (2002). Role of the cerebellum in motor cognition. Ann NY Acad Sci 978:334–353.

Wasson CM, Bannister CM, Ward GS (1992). Factors affecting the school placement of children with spina bifida. Eur J Pediatr Surg 2(Suppl 1):29–34.

Weitzman M, Alpert JJ, Klerman LV, Kayne H, Lamb GA, Geromini KR, Kane KT, Rose L (1986). High risk youth and health: the case of excessive school absence. Pediatrics 78:313–322.

Wills KE, Holmbeck GN, Dillon K, McLone DG (1990). Intelligence and achievement in children with myelomeningocele. J Pediatr Psychol 15(2):161–176.

Yeates KO, Enrile BG, Loss N, Blumenstein E, Delis DC (1995). Verbal learning and memory in children with myelomeningocele. J Pediatr Psychol 20(6):801–815.

Yeates KO, Loss N, Colvin AN, Enrile BG (2003). Do children with myelomeningocele and hydrocephalus display nonverbal learning disabilities? An empirical approach to classification. J Int Neuropsychol Soc 9(4):653–662.

24

Transition to Adulthood

GREGORY S. LIPTAK

As medical care has improved, more children who have spina bifida are surviving to adulthood. Findings from one study indicate that at least 75% of children born with meningomyelocele can be expected to reach their early adult years (Bowman et al., 2001). The World Health Organization (WHO, 2002) and governments around the world have emphasized the goals of improving social integration and decreasing secondary conditions for adults who have disabilities. In the United States, federal legislation, such as the Americans with Disabilities Act (ADA), mandates equal access to facilities such as public transportation, state and local government services including state universities, stores and recreational facilities, independent living within the community, and employment for individuals who have disabilities.

Unfortunately, individuals who have spina bifida often fail to participate fully in society once they become young adults (Date et al., 1993; Dillon et al., 2000). They frequently do not finish high school. Of those who do, fewer go on to postsecondary education. Many fail to live independently of their parents, even though they want to. They may not obtain any work (Lonton et al., 1984), or if they do, the jobs may not be meaningful; earnings typically are lower than for those who do not have disabilities.

For example, in a study of 53 young adults who had spina bifida and lived in Kentucky, 86% completed at least 12 years of school, but 80% earned less than $10,000 per year, and 82% had received Supplemental Security Income for an average of 9 years. Ninety-three percent had never been married; 24% were currently sexually active; only 30% were employed; and 23% were driving. They spent an average of 29 hours per week watching television (their prime activity) and 6 hours talking on the telephone. Only 16% made all their monetary decisions on their own; 66% were using intermittent catheterization for bladder continence; only 51% were using a bowel program, and only 41% were continent of stool (Mier et al., 2003). In a study from Ireland, McDonnell and McCann (2000) found that only 36% of adults with spina bifida were employed, 33% were regular drivers, 17% were married or engaged, and 8% were parents. Secondary medical conditions that interfere with functioning occur commonly. For example, a group of 98 adults with spina bifida accounted for 353 admissions to Johns Hopkins Medical Center during the study period; 166 (47.0%) of the admissions were due to potentially preventable secondary conditions such as serious urological infections, renal calculi, pressure ulcers, and osteomyelitis (Kinsman and Doehring, 1996). A higher rate of depression (Appleton et al., 1997), as well as poor health-care outcomes (Newachek, 1989; Oi et al., 1996), have been reported for many youth and adults with spina bifida. Thus, young adults with spina bifida have more medical complications and do not achieve the same levels of integration or success as those who are not disabled.

TRANSITION

Transition for adolescents is defined as the movement from child-centered to adult-oriented activities. Important transitions for adolescents with spina bifida include the transition from child-centered pediatric to adult-oriented health care, the transition from school to work, and the transition from home to community (Table 24.1). When a child with spina bifida receives primary health care from a family physician or general practitioner, transfer to a new adult-oriented primary care provider, such as an internist, is not necessary. However, the individual providing adult-oriented care should be interested in and knowledgeable about spina bifida. Even when a capable primary care physician is identified, transfer of

TABLE 24.1. *Topics That Need to Be Considered During the Transition from Childhood to Adulthood*

Domain	Examples
Health care	Transition from child-oriented to adult-oriented providers Optimal self-care Nutrition support services Care coordination
Advocacy/legal services	Support in obtaining needed services in the community Creation of a trust fund or will
Education	Finding appropriate educational resources Financial aid
Employment	Career counseling Supported employment programs
Independent living skills	Cooking and housekeeping Money management
Financial assistance	Social Security Administration, such as Supplemental Security Income (SSI) Obtaining healthcare insurance
Housing	Adaptive equipment, such as ramps or lifts Homemaker services
Socialization and recreation	Identifying friends and peers Finding accessible community leisure programs Exercise programs
Transportation	Driver education Training to find and use accessible public transportation

specialty care (e.g., orthopedics, neurosurgery, urology) from child-centered to adult-centered care is necessary. Most children with spina bifida receive comprehensive care from a multidisciplinary program. Few of these programs, however, are available to adults with spina bifida. If a comprehensive team is not available, the complexity of spina bifida may require the specialized services of someone trained in physical medicine and rehabilitation or in neurology. Adequate communication among the individuals providing care to the adult (one aspect of care coordination) needs to be insured.

Health care is a necessary but not a sufficient goal of transition. Poor health can destroy the opportunity for adequate functioning. Also, if optimal health care can keep adults with spina bifida well, it increases opportunities for the other transitions, allowing them to live their lives the way they choose. Realistic goals for adolescents and young adults with spina bifida include gradual separation and individuation from parents, establishment of relationships outside the family unit, acceptance of responsibility for decisions as well as behavior and its consequences, and maturation of vocational choices and development of a career identity. The goal of transition is an adult who enjoys the best health possible, has a sense of well-being, and is integrated into the community (Anderson and Vogel, 2002; Anderson et al., 2003). Transition has been described as a process, not an event, and time lines are available to assist with children who have developmental disabilities and chronic conditions (CHDD, 2003a).

In a survey of adolescents with spina bifida (Buran et al., 2004), only a few were engaging in the full range of adolescent activities such as decision making, friendship activities, and household responsibilities; nor did they achieve positive outcomes, like self-management and employment. Without a solid basis of achievements in adolescence, the transition to adulthood will be difficult at best. The Maternal and Child Health Bureau has stated as one of its goals that "All youth with special needs will receive services needed to support the transition to adulthood" (MCHB, 2003). This means that teenagers will receive guidance and support during the transition to adult health care as well as vocational and career training to prepare for adult jobs. However, in a recent national survey of individuals with special health-care needs, only 6% of teenagers met that goal (Newacheck and Kim, 2005).

Because very few studies have been published that examine the transition process in individuals who have spina bifida, it is difficult to make many evidence-based recommendations or even to know how much concern individuals might have regarding the process of transition. For example, in a study of youth with cystic fibrosis, Anderson et al. (2002) noted that "Most importantly, the patients reported their level of concern about transfer as minimal, far less than what CF physicians had perceived." Therefore, it is important for health-care providers and educators to address issues related to transition not only with the family but with the child too.

THEORETICAL BASES FOR TRANSITION

Knowledge of several theories is useful to understand and optimize the process of transition. These include Erikson's (1959) psychosocial developmental theory, Rutter's (1989) chains of adversity, Bandura's (1977) social learning theory with emphasis on self-efficacy, and Piaget's theory of cognitive development (Elkind, 1981). Other models that are helpful include the chronic illness care model developed by Wagner (1998) and structural family therapy (Rolland, 1994).

Erikson (1959) defined *identity versus role diffusion* as the psychosocial crisis that has to be met during adolescence. To achieve a sense of personal identity, adolescents use role models and peer groups to experiment with different identities and roles. Unfortunately, youths with spina bifida have fewer positive role models in popular culture such as the movies, television, and periodicals. Because youths who have spina bifida often appear different (e.g., using a wheelchair or braces) and may know only a few individuals who also have similar disabilities, peer identification is more difficult. For example, mainstreaming individuals who have spina bifida in school means that very few other children in their grade will have similar disabilities.

Moreover, physical or cognitive impairments in children with spina bifida may lead to limited success in meeting earlier psychosocial developmental challenges, upon which developing a sense of identity is based. For example, Erikson (1959) posited that the sense of autonomy is enhanced by muscular maturation as toddlers learn to walk, climb, hop, and jump to explore their environment. Children who have spina bifida often have limited ability to perform these activities. Thus, developing a sense of autonomy, which affects the ability to develop a sense of identity, is especially difficult for many adolescents who have spina bifida. Likewise, developing a sense of identity (vs. inferiority), which is the task of school-age children, may be impaired in children with spina bifida by their learning disabilities as well as their physical impairments, which affect participation in sports.

Erikson (1959) also included gaining independence from the family as important in developing identity; yet, individuals who have disabilities may have to live with their families longer than others due to restricted finances, poor independent skills (e.g., inability to shop independently), and limited transportation. Families also may have difficulty "letting go" of the adolescent/young adult, since for years they were responsible for maintaining this person's care (Sawin et al., 2003).

Immediately after adolescence, young people face the psychosocial challenge of *intimacy versus isolation*. Most individuals who have spina bifida, even those with significant cognitive limitations, have many strengths and hope to achieve typical adult interpersonal relationships. If these individuals cannot develop a sense of identity, cannot achieve independence from their families of origin, and have difficulty finding a peer group, their sense of isolation may be deepened. Developing a sense of intimacy with another individual may, therefore, be more difficult. Moreover, nonverbal learning disabilities, which occur commonly in children with spina bifida (Fletcher et al., 2002), affect social interaction and may be a further barrier to developing meaningful relationships with others.

Conditions that impair physical sexual functioning, such as severe mobility impairments or loss of innervation to the sexual organs (erectile dysfunction and retrograde ejaculation in the male, decreased lubrication in the female, and decreased sensation in both males and females), can also impair the development of intimacy. Because cultural norms of beauty often do not include individuals with disabilities, these adolescents may have more difficulty identifying someone who recognizes their intrinsic worth and who desires an intimate relationship with them.

The chains of adversity framework developed by Rutter (1989) also provides insight into the process of transition faced by adolescents who have spina bifida. The chain of adversity in someone with spina bifida occurs when the individual's physical impairments initiate a sequence of outcomes that are disadvantageous. For example, an individual with spina bifida is likely to have learning disabilities as well as worse school attendance because of health-related problems. This results in less school success and may lead to early departure from school. The adolescent thus may lack scholastic qualifications for optimal employment, leading to unemployment or underemployment in unskilled work. The result is a poor employment record, which adversely affects the individual's ability to fulfill typical adult roles such as independent provider, spouse, or parent. Interventions that break the chain of adversity promote more positive outcomes.

Bandura (1977) postulated that self-efficacy is the belief in one's capacity to organize and execute the actions required to manage prospective situations. The opposite of self-efficacy is learned helplessness. In this state, individuals believe that unpleasant or aversive stimuli cannot be controlled, and they cease trying to remedy an aversive circumstance even if they can exert some influence. Self-efficacy affects the choices that children make, the effort they put forth, how long they persist when they confront obstacles or failures, and how they feel. The most effective way of creating a strong sense of efficacy is through mastery experiences. Successes build the belief in one's personal efficacy, while failures undermine it. For example, if a child who has spina bifida with learning disorders fails repeatedly in a classroom because he or she does not understand the material, that child eventually will stop trying. Self-efficacy also can be boosted by vicarious experiences provided by social models. However, as mentioned above, children with spina bifida have few role models they can observe or emulate. The third way to enhance self-efficacy is through social persuasion, and the fourth way is through mood. Positive mood enhances perceived self-efficacy, while despondent mood diminishes it. Learned helplessness has been linked to depression and to learning disabilities (Matek and Wierzbicki, 1998; Dunn et al., 1999). As mentioned above, learning disabilities clearly are more common in individuals with spina bifida, and depression is also probably more common.

Piaget (Elkind, 1981) hypothesized that the *formal operational* stage is one in which adolescents develop the capacity for abstract, thinking. Consequences of this include argumentativeness, self-consciousness and self-focus, idealism, planning, and decision making. Another consequence of this is the sense of permanence. Thus, adolescents with spina bifida may realize for the first time in their lives that their condition is permanent. This may contribute to the occurrence of depression. Also, if the young person with spina bifida has learning disabilities and problems with executive functioning, the ability to plan and make decisions may be impaired, yet expectations from the environment may be the same as they are for youth who do not have these disabilities. Children with spina bifida and nonverbal learning disabilities typically have problems with executive function (Mahone et al., 2002). They do better thinking in linear fashion rather than in gestalt terms and have difficulty with context. Impairments in executive function may impair activities of self-care, such as remembering the sequences of self-care tasks, the importance of catheterizing on time and understanding realistic consequences if this is not done, and the importance of checking for and preventing pressure sores (Russel, 2004).

Another useful theoretical model is that of family structure (Minuchin, 1974; Rolland, 1994). A chronic condition like spina bifida affects the entire family system, leaving no one untouched. The teenager's attitudes toward spina bifida, adaptive strategies, ability to achieve self-help, and adherence to treatment regimens (compliance) all depend on the family. Family relationships and expectations are a principal source of good mental health (or psychopathology) for individuals. Also, prescribed treatments may help the patient but harm the family unit. Thus, families should be considered to be a health-related family system rather than just the patient and his or her family.

Family problems may be the result of boundaries that are too porous (enmeshed) or too rigid (disengaged). With enmeshment, family members are overinvolved and overresponsive—such as, the mother who goes to the college dormitory to disimpact her 20-year-old son of stool. With overprotection, excessive nurturing and restricted autonomy occur; the child disappears behind the illness and is less likely to be able to achieve independent skills. Rigid families maintain fixed patterns of behavior, even if they no longer are functional, and with *triangulation,* the focus on the condition detours conflict, preventing adequate resolution of crises. Both individual and family needs must be met in order for the family to develop healthy psychosocial adaptation to crises. Successful transition requires a balance between connection and individuation, and family adaptability and cohesion are core traits that prevent family dysfunction and optimize transition. Thus, paying critical attention to families by identifying family patterns of interaction, expectations, and belief systems can be crucial to optimizing transition for individuals who have spina bifida.

FACILITATORS AND BARRIERS

Several investigations of adolescents with other chronic conditions and risk factors suggest a number of characteristics that may enhance the likelihood of successful transition for adolescents who have disabilities (Hirst, 1989; Kokkonen et al., 1991; Nasr et al., 1992; Wysocki et al., 1992; Loomis et al., 1997; Werner, 1997; Flouri and Buchanan, 2002; Anderson et al., 2003). These include internal and external factors. Internal factors include higher functional level, better health, positive social orientation (temperament), commitment to learning, social competencies, locus of control, and more formal education. External factors include higher income, a close bond with a caregiver, support including an array of alternative caretakers—grandparents, siblings, neighbors—who step in when parents are not present, boundaries and expectations at home such as chores, and active engagement in acts of required helpfulness in middle childhood and adolescence.

Potential barriers to transition, shown in Table 24.2, can be divided into three categories: the child and the condition, the family, and the community (Viner, 2000, 2001; Lewis-Gary, 2001; Fox, 2002). Barriers related to the child and the condition include lack of developmental readiness (e.g., nonverbal learning disabilities), lack of social skills (e.g., social anxiety), impairments that affect communication or interactions (e.g., urinary incontinence), and the presence of learned helplessness or depression. Factors related to the family include the desire to protect the child, including the vulnerable child syndrome, difficulty letting go or *eternal vigilance* (Holmbeck et al., 2002), unrealistic expectations, and lack of economic means. For example, activities such as catheterizing the child, ensuring that medications are taken in a timely fashion, and ensuring that numerous visits to health-care providers occur, create dependency relationships between parents and their children not typically found with children who are not disabled. Thus, parents of teenagers who have disabilities may have more difficulty letting go (Strax, 1991). Or they may not be able to let go because the teenager does not have the capacity to be independent.

TABLE 24.2. *Barriers to Effective Transition*

Category	Examples
Child and condition	Lack of developmental readiness Lack of social skills Impairments that affect communication or interactions Learned helplessness Depression
Family	Inability to let go of the child Unrealistic expectations Lack of economic means
Community	Lack of knowledgeable, available, adult-oriented healthcare providers Poor reimbursement for care Decreased access to other resources, such as accessible housing

Factors related to the community include lack of knowledgeable, available, adult-oriented health-care providers and lack of reimbursement for care. The health care of adults with spina bifida requires increased time both during and in between visits; insurance may not provide adequate coverage due to the presence of a pre-existing conditions clause, and many insurance policies provide limited coverage for therapy. In addition, very few studies have examined spina bifida and the aging process, thus limiting the body of knowledge available to providers. Children who have spina bifida routinely encounter low performance expectations from health-care providers and other professionals. For example, pediatricians often continue talking with parents rather than with children, even when the children are more than 10 years of age and able to take increasing responsibility for their health care. Decreased access to other resources, such as recreation, accessible housing and jobs, supportive social networks, and employment training, also acts as a barrier to transitions.

PROMOTING TRANSITIONS

Chronic Illness Model

Wagner (1998) developed a model that can be useful in promoting health-related transitions. This model, shown in Fig. 24.1, has been evaluated in chronic conditions in adults as well as asthma in children and found to be related to outcomes of care (Bodenheimer et al., 2002a, 2002b). Attaining the goals of optimal functional and clinical outcomes in the individual who has spina bifida requires productive interactions between the patient (and family) and the healthcare providers. The patient should be *informed* and *activated,* that is, willing to monitor his or her status and perform procedures, like catheterization, that are necessary to maximize health. The providers should be *prepared* (including being knowledgeable about spina bifida) and *proactive,* that is, attentive to preventive measures and anticipatory guidance, and not passively awaiting the family to bring complaints to them. For instance, adults with shunted hydrocephalus may develop subtle signs and symptoms of shunt failure. Periodic monitoring can help assess this problem and lead to more timely intervention. For these interactions to happen, support from the health-care system and from the larger community is required.

Self-management support refers to the assistance that healthcare providers give to families and individuals to make them as self-reliant as possible. This means ensuring that individuals are knowledgeable about spina bifida. Table 24.3 lists criteria required for a minimal level of knowledge regarding spina bifida. Universal checklists are available to determine levels of knowledge regarding activities required to become independent (CHDD, 2003b).

Self-management support also means giving patients a central role in determining their care. Providers and patients work together to define problems, set priorities, establish goals, create treatment plans, and solve problems along the way. Group visits and telephone follow-up, as well as one-to-one interactions, can make communication between patients and providers more efficient and more useful to the patient and his or her family.

If an individual with spina bifida has learning disabilities, it may be difficult for that individual to become activated and informed. A decision needs to be made about whether the individual would benefit from *remediation*—that is, additional instructional time or different instructional approaches—or *compensation*—that is, recognizing that remediation has failed or needs to be supplemented and that compensatory approaches (e.g., a written schedule or an electronic reminder system) are

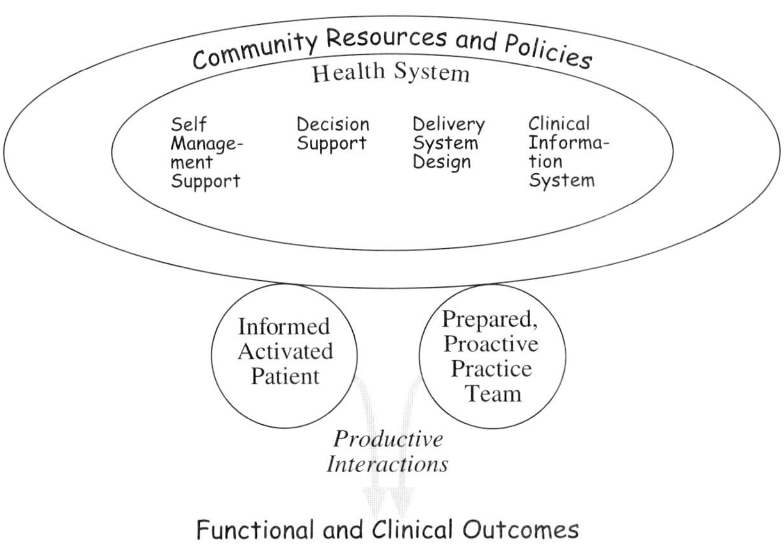

FIGURE 24.1. Care model for child health. *Source:* Ed Wagner.

TABLE 24.3. *Minimal Level of Knowledge Regarding the Medical Condition*

1. Can describe spina bifida and its implications for daily life
2. Knows names of medications, dosages, effects, and potential ad effects
3. Remembers to take medications
4. Knows assistive technology (e.g., orthotics) and procedures (e.g., catheterization)
5. Can access past medical history, and is aware of allergies and other special needs
6. Can order/renew prescriptions and medical supplies
7. Knows providers; can make appointments with them and prepare questions for visits
8. Knows who to contact in an emergency and how to contact them
9. Has some knowledge of health insurance coverage

needed to produce the desired level of performance. In this instance, self-management support needs to provide remediation (e.g., additional instruction) or compensation (e.g., family, friends, computers, personal aides, mentors—who can assist the individual to identify and perform activities that he or she may not be able to perform), or both.

Delivery system design refers to the process of care. For example, traditionally, primary care offices have been oriented to provide acute care. Visits are scheduled every 15–20 minutes and providers take a passive role, waiting for families to call them if a problem occurs. However, for optimal care that keeps the person as healthy as possible, changes in the design of the delivery system need to be made. Visits should be longer and adequately reimbursed. Providers should address prevention of secondary conditions. In addition to determining what care is needed, specific roles and tasks need to be elucidated. For transitions to be successful, health-care providers from both the pediatric and adult side need to be knowledgeable about the patient's condition, treatments and needs, and guidelines for care, and should address transition issues prior to the transfer of care.

Decision support refers to giving health care (and related) providers the most recent evidence-based information on spina bifida so that they can provide the best care possible. Practitioners should be knowledgeable about the resources available in the community to help individuals with spina bifida with their transitions. Technical systems such as computer-based prescription-writing programs that can check dosages and identify potential drug interactions before they occur also are part of decision support.

Clinical information systems refer to the components that track individuals as well as populations of patients. The transfer of accurate medical information from the pediatric to the adult-oriented health-care system is a critical part of successful transition. Because spina bifida is so complex, individuals who have this condition should have access to their medical records so that if they are out of town and become ill, the treating physician can access this information. An effective clinical information system also allows proactive actions to be taken. For example, individuals who have spina bifida and respiratory problems, such as from Chiari II malformations, can be contacted in the fall and reminded about taking the influenza vaccine. Individuals who take anticholinergic medications like oxybutynin (Ditropan) can receive warnings regarding their increased risk for hyperthermia in warmer weather.

Spina bifida has been described as the most complex medical condition compatible with life. Table 24.4 lists some of the impairments and disabilities found in adolescents and adults with this condition. This long list of possible (and likely) complications means that individuals and their health-care providers need extensive knowl-

TABLE 24.4. *Impairments and Disabilities Found in Adolescents and Adults with Spina Bifida*

- I. Spinal Cord and Spine
  - A. Primary abnormalities of the cord
    - 1. Syrinx
  - B. Tethering
  - C. Motor impairment
    - 1. Neurogenic bowel
      - a. Incontinence
      - b. Constipation
    - 2. Male sexual dysfunction
    - 3. Weakness and paralysis
      - a. Orthopedic contractures
      - b. Joint pain and deterioration
      - c. Diminished mobility
    - 4. Neurogenic bladder
      - a. Urinary tract infections
      - b. Reflux
      - c. Incontinence
      - d. Hypertension
      - e. Renal failure
  - D. Sensory impairment
    - 1. Decubitus ulcers
- II. Brain
  - A. Hydrocephalus
    - 1. Ventricular shunt dysfunction
  - B. Chiari II malformation
    - 1. Respiratory impairment, including apnea
  - C. Learning disabilities
    - 1. Poor social skills
  - D. Epilepsy
- III. Other
  - A. Obesity
  - B. Poor nutrition

edge to identify and manage complications, secondary conditions, and co-morbidities.

Characteristics of the Health-Care System

The following characteristics of the health-care system may facilitate the transition of youth who have spina bifida (Reiss and Gibson, 2002): (*1*) a policy on the timing of transfer; (*2*) needs-based training to enable the young person to learn the items shown in Table 24.2; (*3*) a coordinated transfer process, including a written plan, and a pretransfer visit with an adult provider and his or her staff; (*4*) an interested and capable adult service that is equivalent in quality to the pediatric program; (*5*) administrative support; and (*6*) primary care involvement. Bonomi et al. (2002) have developed an instrument, the Assessment of Chronic Illness Care (ACIC), that allows evaluation of the systems of care available for individuals who have spina bifida or other chronic conditions. The Cystic Fibrosis (CF) Foundation of the United States requires CF centers to have adult programs in order to receive accreditation (Schidlow, 2002). The impact of this policy is not certain for CF, nor is it clear what effect a similar policy would have on programs that care for children who have spina bifida.

Assessment

Specific steps that may optimize transitions include (*1*) assessment of the individual, family, and community; (*2*) development of a transition plan; and (*3*) implementation of the plan (Sawyer et al., 1998; Lewis-Gary, 2001). Evaluating the adolescent's ability to negotiate the transitions from adolescence to adulthood includes assessing the child and his or her family, as well as the larger environment, in terms of potential barriers and facilitators for the transition. The first step in this phase is to evaluate the child's developmental readiness. Questionnaires and checklists are available to evaluate the readiness of adolescents with chronic conditions for transition to adulthood (CHDD, 2003b). The items listed in Table 24.2 should be included in that assessment.

The second step is to evaluate the youth's and family's functioning, social supports, and goals. Information obtained from the family on daily activities, relationships, rights, and responsibilities can help define current family functioning. The importance of social supports has been underscored by the work of Werner (1997), who found that in a population of adults with chronic conditions, successful adult functioning at age 33 years was correlated with having had a relationship with a supportive adult as a young person. Identifying both the adolescent's and the family's goals for future independent living, work, and health care will help determine how much consideration they have given to the issue of transition and how realistic the goals are.

The third step is to evaluate the environment outside the family. The best planning for transition should begin long before the child becomes an adolescent, and certainly before he or she leaves school. Because children gain not only knowledge but also social prowess and skills in problem solving and decision making while in school, the school is one of the most critical environments to evaluate. All students in the United States who have disabilities are protected under the Individuals with Disabilities Education Act (IDEA) or Section 504 of the Rehabilitation Act of 1973 (PL 93-112), which prohibits discrimination on the basis of disability in federally funded or assisted education and employment programs. These children have the right to receive education with reasonable accommodations, including specialized education and related aids and services (Committee on Children with Disabilities, 2000). Every school should have a Section 504 plan for that school that outlines the procedures for developing an accommodation plan and providing necessary services for such students. Under IDEA, the individual education program for children who have cognitive disabilities must include plans for transition by the time the child is 14 years old. Some states mandate a transition plan even before this age.

Other aspects of the environment that need to be evaluated include the availability of programs that can assist individuals with finding affordable and accessible housing and suitable employment. Information about model programs and technical assistance for those interested in helping youths with these issues are available through the National Information Center for Children and Youth with Disabilities (NICHCY, 2003).

Adolescents with disabilities and their families need to address questions such as: How will the youth gain income (e.g., through employment, public assistance, or reliance on family or friends)? What kind of continuing education will be pursued after high school, if any? Where will the youth live, and what types of supports will be needed for optimal independence, autonomy, safety, and privacy? How will these supports (such as a personal care aide or homemaker services) be obtained? How will continuing health-care needs be met and paid for? Can the youth drive or use public transportation? If not, how will transportation needs be met? Does the youth have strong peer supports and good mental health, or will special supports be needed in this area? Can he or she make appropriate judgments and choices, or is help with advocacy needed? How will long-term future needs be met?

Planning

Interventions to help with transitions must be planned carefully to meet several goals: (*1*) to maximize the person's developmental potential; (*2*) to optimize the person's health; (*3*) to promote relief from stress and positive coping patterns in the adolescent and the family; (*4*) to promote positive family functioning in support of the adolescent's increasing independence; and (5) to support development of self-efficacy in the adolescent. A planning process that provides self-management means that the individual with spina bifida plays a central role in determining his or her care and develops a sense of responsibility for personal health and well-being. This may require remediation or compensation and should be monitored by the transition team. Providers and patients work together collaboratively to define problems, set priorities, establish goals, create specific plans, and follow up with each other on a regular basis.

Implementation

All of the following activities are designed to increase independence and self-efficacy for the adolescent during the process of transition (AAP, 2002).

1. Identify a transition coordinator, often an advanced practice nurse (nurse practitioner or nurse specialist), who has responsibility for transition arrangements. The role of the coordinator is to assess the needs of the adolescent and family, plan comprehensive care, and facilitate, coordinate, and monitor care to ensure that all needed services are being received. Being a coordinator means being knowledgeable about the adolescent and family, as well as about community resources available to meet the individual's needs. In some cases, the adolescent, with appropriate assistance from parents or another adult, will be able to assume this role. This is the ideal situation for promoting future independence, but it may not be feasible for adolescents or families with barriers such as cognitive limitations or very high levels of stress and chaos in daily life.

   Coordination services may be difficult to obtain because the current health-care financing system includes limited opportunity for providers to be appropriately paid for time spent in these indirect care activities. In this case, the primary care physician or nurse practitioner may assume this role and absorb the cost, or the parents and adolescent may become the coordinators by default instead of by choice, and will need assistance to accomplish this task.
2. Provide health maintenance and preventive care with emphasis on nutrition, physical fitness, sexuality, substance abuse prevention, personal safety, and emotional health. Unlike the care of younger children, with its strong focus on health promotion and anticipatory guidance, adolescent health-care visits often occur in conjunction with health crises. These crises are more frequent among youths who have spina bifida, diverting attention from health promotion and prevention to medical problems that are often managed in the specialist's office. Therefore, emphasizing health maintenance and preventive issues is even more important in the person with spina bifida (Raddish et al., 1993).
3. Teach self-care in order to prevent secondary conditions. For example, youths with spina bifida need to learn how to prevent skin breakdown, obesity, chronic constipation, and joint contractures. They need to recognize the signs and symptoms of ventricular shunt dysfunction, urinary tract infection, tethered spinal cord, and Chiari II malformation. All these youths need to learn how to stay fit physically and to attend to their emotional health. During routine health-care visits, the health-care provider can perform an interpretive interview and a teaching physical examination (Johnson, 1995). During the interview, the concerns of the family and adolescent are addressed, and they are provided with relevant information for each concern. Medical and rehabilitative interventions are discussed, and plans for future care can be developed. Assistive technologies, such as computer-based instructional programs, may help individuals with learning disabilities compensate, thus optimizing their ability for self-care.

   During the teaching physical examination, the youth's abilities and disabilities are reviewed system by system. After the examination, more specific health education can be provided, in writing or as a resource on the Internet, either by the primary health-care provider or by a health education specialist. Reinforcing this teaching at home and at school will assist the youth to feel more competent and enhance self-efficacy, and may help break adverse chains such as the school failure chain described earlier.
4. Support the establishment of a trusting relationship with new providers when the adolescent is ready to change to adult care providers. If feasible, a period of joint visits including the old pediatric and new adult providers of care may be beneficial (Schidlow and Fiel, 1990; Strax, 1991; Boyle et al., 2001).
5. Develop an up-to-date medical summary that is portable and accessible. This document should inform the new care providers about the adolescent's condition, current management of the condition, and the client's strengths, needs, and goals. This information should be provided to the adolescent. Some health-care providers help adolescents to create their own personal medical summary—basically a condensed version of the medical record compiled by the client. Such a summary provides emergency information, lists of medical problems, long-term medications, service providers, daily routines and equipment such as adaptive devices, information on positioning, therapeutic goals, toileting, meals, and communication mechanisms, and brief summaries of health-care visits and laboratory tests and X-rays. This document is intended to improve communication with health-care providers as well as to encourage the individual with disabilities to be more aware of his or her care. Developing this document over time, in collaboration with

the adolescent, enhances its effectiveness and may enhance self-efficacy. An example of a summary data set that is accessible and portable is the Emergency Information Form for Children with Special Health Needs (AAP, 2003) developed by the American Academy of Pediatrics and the American College of Emergency Physicians.

6. Provide preservice and continuing education for ily medicine or physicians who completed a medical-pediatrics residency, who see both children and adults, may help to bridge the gaps between the two cultures of pediatric and adult medical care (Rosen, 1995). Community resources that can assist with adult services also should be identified for the new caregivers, since adult providers may not have used these agencies previously.
7. Ensure future financing for health-care needs. For example, assist the youth in obtaining all assistance for which she or he may be entitled, such as Social Security Disability Income, and in obtaining employment that offers comprehensive health insurance as a benefit option.
8. Provide access to programs such as driver education, employment training, sex education, and social skills training.
9. Evaluate the outcomes of interventions by (*a*) measuring whether or not the intended interventions are actually taking place, (*b*) determining the level of satisfaction of the adolescent and his or her family with the interventions, and (*c*) and monitoring the process and progress toward objectives. When variances from the planned course of action are identified or objectives are not being met, analysis is needed to determine whether the variance is related to provider, system or patient-related factors. The plan then can be modified accordingly, thus increasing the probability of its success.

CONCLUSION

More individuals with spina bifida are surviving to adulthood. However, little is known about their quality of life and health or about the process of transition from adolescence to adulthood. Based on studies primarily involving individuals who have other chronic conditions, the process of transition for youth with spina bifida should include collaboration between child-centered and adult-oriented providers. Use of the chronic illness model can help identify the areas that need to be addressed on both individual and systemwide levels related to issues of health. Effectively assisting individual adolescents to become healthy, competent, contributing adults is important. It is equally important, however, that we advocate for changes in systems and policies that will lead to the development of a society where all people are fully valued and supported.

REFERENCES

AAP (2002). A consensus statement on health care transitions for young adults with special health care needs. Pediatrics 110:1304–1306.

AAP (2003). Emergency information for children with special needs. Available at http://www.aap.org/advocacy/blankform.pdf.

Anderson CJ, Krajci KA, Vogel LC (2003). Community integration among adults with spinal cord injuries sustained as children or adolescents. Dev Med Child Neurol 45:129–134.

Anderson CJ, Vogel LC (2002). Employment outcomes of adults who sustained spinal cord injuries as children or adolescents. Arch Phys Med Rehabil 83:791–801.

Anderson DL, Flume PA, Hardy KK, Gray S (2002). Transition programs in cystic fibrosis centers: perceptions of patients. Pediatr Pulmonol 33:327–331.

Appleton PL, Ellis NC, Minchom PE, Lawson V, Boll V, Jones P (1997). Depressive symptoms and self-concept in young people with spina bifida. J Pediatr Psychol 22:707–722.

Bandura A (1977). Self-efficacy: towards a unifying theory of behavioral change. Psychol Rev 84:191–215.

Bodenheimer T, Wagner EH, Grumbach K (2002a). Improving primary care for patients with chronic illness. JAMA 288:1775–1779.

Bodenheimer T, Wagner EH, Grumbach K (2002b). Improving primary care for patients with chronic illness: the chronic care model, Part 2. JAMA 288:1909–1914.

Bonomi AE, Wagner EH, Glasgow RE, VonKorff M (2002). Assessment of chronic illness care (ACIC): a practical tool to measure quality improvement. Health Serv Res 37:791–820.

Bowman RM, McLone DG, Grant JA, Tomita T, Ito JA (2001). Spina bifida outcome: a 25-year prospective. Pediatr Neurosurg 34:114–120.

Boyle MP, Farukhi Z, Nosky ML (2001). Strategies for improving transition to adult cystic fibrosis care, based on patient and parent views. Pediatr Pulmonol 32:428–436.

Buran CF, Sawin KJ, Brei TJ, Fastenau PS (2004). Adolescents with myelomeningocele: activities, beliefs, expectations, and perceptions. Dev Med Child Neurol 46:244–252.

Center on Human Development and Disability (CHDD), University of Washington (2003a). Transition timeline. Introduction and contents. Available at Seattle http://depts.washington.edu/healthtr/Timeline/timeline.htm.

Center on Human Development and Disability (CHDD), University of Washington (2003b). Adolescent autonomy checklists. Introduction and contents. Available at http://depts.washington.edu/healthtr/Checklists/intro.htm.

Committee on Children with Disabilities (2000). Provision of educationally-related services for children and adolescents with chronic diseases and disabling conditions. Pediatrics 105:448–451.

Date I, Yagyu Y, Asari S, Ohmoto T (1993). Long-term outcome in surgically treated spina bifida cystica. Surg Neurol 40:471–475.

Dillon CM, Davis BE, Duguay S, Seidel KD, Shurtleff DB (2000). Longevity of patients born with myelomeningocele. Eur J Pediatr Surg 10(Suppl 1):33–34.

Dunn DW, Austin JK, Huster GA (1999). Symptoms of depression in adolescents with epilepsy. J Am Acad Child Adolesc Psychiatry 38:1132–1138.

Elkind D (1981). *Children and Adolescents: Interpretive Essays on Jean Piaget,* 3rd ed. New York: Oxford University Press.

Erikson E (1959). Identity and the life cycle. Psychol Issues 1:1–171.

Fletcher JM, Barnes M, Dennis M (2002). Language development in children with spina bifida. Semin Pediatr Neurol 9:201–208.

Flouri E, Buchanan A (2002). What predicts good relationships with parents in adolescence and partners in adult life: findings from the 1958 British birth cohort. J Fam Psychol 16:186–198.

Fox A (2002). Physicians as barriers to successful transitional care. Int J Adolesc Med Health 14:3–7.

Hirst M (1989). Patterns of impairment and disability related to social handicap in young people with cerebral palsy and spina bifida. J Biosoc Sci 21:1–12.

Holmbeck GN, Johnson SZ, Wills KE, McKernon W, Rose B, Erklin S, Kemper T (2002). Observed and perceived parental overprotection in relation to psychosocial adjustment in preadolescents with a physical disability: the mediational role of behavioral autonomy. J Consult Clin Psychol 70:96–110.

Johnson CP (1995). Transition into adulthood. Pediatr Ann 24:268–273.

Kinsman SL, Doehring MC (1996). The cost of preventable conditions in adults with spina bifida. Eur J Pediatr Surg 6(Suppl 1):17–20.

Kokkonen J, Saukkonen AL, Timonen E, Serlo W, Kinnunen P (1991). Social outcome of handicapped children as adults. Dev Med Child Neurol 33:1095–1100.

Lewis-Gary MD (2001). Transitioning to adult health care facilities for young adults with a chronic condition. Pediatr Nurs 27:521–524.

Lonton AP, Loughlin AM, O'Sullivan AM (1984). The employment of adults with spina bifida. Z Kinderchir 39(Suppl 2):132–134.

Loomis JW, Javornisky JG, Monahan JJ, Burke G, Lindsay A (1997). Relations between family environment and adjustment outcomes in young adults with spina bifida. Dev Med Child Neurol 39:620–627.

Mahone EM, Zabel TA, Levey E, Verda M, Kinsman S (2002). Parent and self-report rating of executive function in adolescents with myelomeningocele and hydrocephalus. Child Neuropsychology 8:258–270.

Mattek PW, Wierzbicki M (1998). Cognitive and behavioral correlates of depression in learning-disabled and nonlearning-disabled adult students. J Clin Psychol 54:831–837.

Maternal and Child Health Bureau (MCHB) (2003). Achieving and measuring success: A national agenda for children with special health care needs. Available at http://www.mchb.hrsa.gov/programs/specialneeds/measuresuccess.htm.

McDonnell GV, McCann JP (2000). Link between the CSF shunt and achievement in adults with spina bifida. J Neurol Neurosurg Psychiatry 68:800.

Mier R, Holcomb LA, Minter C (2003). Community functioning among adult spina bifida patients (abstract). Dev Med Child Neurol 45:29.

Minuchin S (1974). *Families and Family Therapy*. Cambridge, MA: Harvard University Press.

Nasr SZ, Campbell C, Howatt W (1992). Transition program from pediatric to adult care for cystic fibrosis patients. J Adolesc Health 13:682–685.

Newacheck PW (1989). Adolescents with special health needs: prevalence, severity, and access to health services. Pediatrics 84:872–881.

Newacheck PW, Kim SE (2005). A national profile of health care utilization and expenditures for children with special health care needs. Arch Pediatr Adolesc Med 159:10–17.

NICHCY (2003). *National Dissemination Center for Children with Disabilities*. Available at http://www.nichcy.org

Oi S, Sato O, Matsumoto S (1996). Neurological and medico-social problems of spina bifida patients in adolescence and adulthood. Childs Nerv Syst 12:181–187.

Raddish M, Goldmann DA, Kaplan LC, Perrin JM (1993). The immunization status of children with spina bifida. Am J Dis Child 147:849–853.

Reiss J, Gibson R (2002). Health care transition: destinations unknown. Pediatrics 110:1307–1314.

Rolland JS (1994). *Families, Illness, and Disability. An Integrative Treatment Model*. New York: Basic Books.

Rosen D (1995). Between two worlds: bridging the cultures of child health and adult medicine. J Adolesc Health 17:10–16.

Russel CL (2004). Understanding nonverbal learning disorders in children with spina bifida. Teaching Except Child 36:8–13.

Rutter M (1989). Pathways from childhood to adult life. J Child Psychol Psychiatry 30:23–51.

Sawin KJ, Bellin MH, Roux G, Buran C, Brei TJ, Fastenau PS (2003). The experience of parenting an adolescent with spina bifida. Rehabil Nurs 28(6):173–185.

Sawyer SM, Collins N, Bryan D, Brown D, Hope MA, Bowes G (1998). Young people with spina bifida: transfer from paediatric to adult health care. J Paediatr Child Health 34:414–417.

Schidlow DV (2002). Transition in cystic fibrosis: much ado about nothing? A pediatrician's view. Pediatr Pulmonol 33:325–326.

Schidlow DV, Fiel SB (1990). Life beyond pediatrics. Transition of chronically ill adolescents from pediatric to adult health care systems. Med Clin North Am 74:1113–1120.

Strax TE (1991). Psychological issues faced by adolescents and young adults with disabilities. Pediatr Ann 20:507–511.

Viner R (2000). Effective transition from paediatric to adult services. Hosp Med 61:341–343.

Viner R (2001). Barriers and good practice in transition from paediatric to adult care. J R Soc Med 94:2–4.

Wagner EH (1998). Chronic disease management: what will it take to improve care for chronic illness? Eff Clin Pract 1:2–4.

Werner EE (1992). The children of Kauai: resiliency and recovery in adolescence and adulthood. J Adolesc Health 13:262–268.

Werner EE (1997). Vulnerable but invincible: high-risk children from birth to adulthood. Acta Paediatr (Suppl)422:103–105.

World Health Organization (2002). *The World Health Report 2002. Reducing Risks, Promoting Healthy Life*. Geneva: WHO.

Wysocki T, Hough BS, Ward KM, Green LB (1992). Diabetes mellitus in the transition to adulthood: adjustment, self-care, and health status. J Dev Behav Pediatr 13:194–201

25

Transition/Separation, Toilet Training, and Sexuality

DAVID B. SHURTLEFF
CAROLE A. SOBKOWIAK
WILLIAM WALKER

This chapter will discuss general concepts of child emotional and behavioral development in the areas of toilet training, separation/transition, and sexuality, comparing children with and without disabilities. Myelomeningocele, the most severe form of neural tube defects associated with survival, will serve as an example of the spectrum of neural tube defects. The first section will deal with general concepts that every care provider should consider reviewing with patients and families. There are many reasons that make this general review necessary, including recent developments in the diagnosis, prevention, management, and outcomes for these complex patients. The first and most important reason is the authors' experience with parents who have complained about not having all the possible complications outlined for them from the beginning. All care providers for patients with myelomeningocele, and similarly affected patients, should consider providing their own specialty opinions about the management of these children, integrating their advice with the possible alternatives offered by others in their own field and by the patient's care providers from other specialties.

Professionals, care providers, and parents of children with any disability should recognize that the transition from childhood to adulthood requires an infant or child to progress though stages of development, and to learn age appropriate skills of independence, self-care, and social interactions to achieve autonomy (Brazelton, 1992). Brazelton provided a comprehensive description of early emotional and behavioral development for infants and children without disabilities. Families teach some of these skills, and children learn others without being formally taught. Anyone caring for a child, including one with a disability, should consider reviewing and understanding each developmental *touchpoint*.

Erikson (1950) and Piaget (1929) described the need for appropriate early infancy and childhood learning within a social context in order to develop an intact, functional personality later in life. To become a competent adult, they state, a child must understand society's emphasis on attainable goals (Erikson, 1950; Brazelton, 1992). This emphasis is not just theoretical. While the four domains in the title of this chapter (urine and stool toilet training, transition/separation, and sexuality) are critically important to the proper development of a child's psyche, they are also topics that are either avoided in social discourse or not fully understood. No literature known to us addresses these concepts in children born with neural tube defects. This chapter will discuss the skills that infants and children should master in order to develop into competent teenagers and adults. In each subsection we will suggest, in our opinion, how rearing a child with an impairment can be modified, facilitating acquisition of the requisite skills at approximately the same age as children without disabilities.

The reader is cautioned that the language in this chapter is for professionals and other adults. Terms used to teach a child or a person with a developmental delay should be adjusted to a language level appropriate for their intellectual level. For example, feces or stool can be described during toilet training as *poop* or *number two* and urination as *pee* or *number one*. Only a rare infant or child understands terms such as *defecation, feces, stool, urination,* or *passage of urine*. Parents should consider not only learning these terms, but also teaching their children to communicate with professionals using alternative terms and to talk to other persons in public.

INITIAL CONTACT AND COUNSELING

When counseling parents of a patient with spina bifida, we believe it is important to provide them with as accurate information as possible. Prognosis varies with the type of spina bifida and the extent of nervous, musculoskeletal, genitourinary, and gastrointestinal system involvement; specifics can be gleaned from the other chapters in this text and from references at the end of this chapter.

The type of spina bifida, the degree of impairment, and possible malformations of other organ systems can be determined by prenatal testing or intrauterine, newborn, or postnatal examination, as discussed in this book and elsewhere (Matsumoto and Sato, 1999; Sarwark and Lubicky, 2001). Children can be assessed at birth or later; more specific information can be provided to parents and, if old enough, to the patient. The prognosis may change, becoming more specific and accurate as the child with disabilities develops. This evolution allows the current health professional to explain the differences in the predictions by prior providers due to the current assessment.

Parents are particularly interested in their child's potential to grow up into a socially functional adult. Professionals should remind parents that, raised properly, the majority of children born with any one of the varieties of spina bifida can become socially well-adjusted adults.

Forty years ago, one of us (DBS) learned an important lesson in the development of a child with a disability: 6- to 9-year-old patients with myelomeningocele did not know whether they were boys or girls. A subsequent study demonstrated that parents were embarrassed to ask whether their infant or young child could become a competent reproductive human being! This lack of information is in stark contrast to what is actually known. Adult patients with myelomeningocele are able to reproduce (Carter and Evans, 1973; Laurence and Beresford, 1975; Shurtleff et al., 1975; Dunne and Shurtleff, 1986; Arata et al., 2000; Blackburn, 2002). Discussing a patient's potential sexuality remains the same whenever the patient and family enter a practice. For the parents of a fetus or newborn, these concepts can be discussed in a straightforward manner. For parents of children initially treated elsewhere, their understanding of a particular concept should be clarified prior to any further discussion. If their understanding is correct, the issue will not require further discussion unless their knowledge is out-of-date. Therefore, we discuss with new families, regardless of age, the parents' knowledge of their fetus's or child's sexuality and reproductive potential.

Females with the various forms of spina bifida and normal reproductive organs will usually experience orgasm, and are usually fertile and capable of bearing children (Shurtleff et al., 1975; Comarr, 1976; Shurtleff and Sousa, 1977). Exceptions to this general statement are children with exstrophy of the cloaca and the rare patient with additional malformations of the reproductive organs. Males have a much more complex genitourinary system that depends on an intact autonomic nervous system, as described in Chapter 22. Males can have erections that are due to urinary bladder base stimulation, erotic thoughts, or noxious stimulation of the thigh, perineum, pubic area, or penis (Comarr, 1976). They can be fertile if their prostate, epididymus, and at least one testicle are not malformed and have not been destroyed by infection. Ejaculation may be retrograde, forward, or nonexistent; ejaculation is not necessary for fertility. Some males will ooze prostatic fluid containing sperm during the sex act, successfully impregnating their partner without ejaculation. Retrograde ejaculation can be reversed either by adding an artificial sphincter proximal to the prostate (Jumper et al., 1990) or by closing the urinary bladder neck and adding a catheterizable stoma. For the 75% to 80% of males with infertility, there is a 75% to 80% probability that needle aspiration of the testes can recover sperm or the DNA of its precursor cells. These cells or DNA can be used to fertilize the partner's egg via intracytoplasmic sperm injection (Cass et al., 1986; Vroege et al., 1998; Hultling et al., 2000; Pasqualotto et al., 2002). The fourth and last portion of the male sex act is *potency*. This term is used to include the ability to satisfy a sex partner, not just satisfactorily performing sexual intercourse. There are many ways to achieve orgasm (Comarr, 1976). Parents are unlikely to either understand or divulge such information, and peers cannot be relied upon. Males and females with any type of spina bifida need to learn from movies, television, a sexual counselor, or sexually explicit literature how to use these techniques to satisfy their sexual partner (Blackburn, 2002).

The last aspect of reproduction discussed with both sexes is their ability to lower the recurrence of spina bifida in relatives, their parents, and the affected child's children, as discussed in the chapters on etiology, pathoembryology, and prevention in this book. The only studies known to us about the recurrence rate in first-degree family members (mother's and father's brothers and sisters and the affected child's siblings) suggest that the recurrence rate in first-degree relatives is approximately 1 in 30. For second-degree relatives (mother's, sister's, or brother's children) the rate is approximately 1 in 220. However, the accurate recurrence risk data for family members are not well known (Toriello and Higgins,

1983). Others report a recurrence risk among mothers or an affected child's first-degree relatives as high as 1 in 70 to 1 in 140 in first-degree relatives of the mother (Timson, 1972; Chatkupt et al., 1994). McManus (1987) reports recurrence rates in second- and third-degree relatives of 1 in 90 and 1 in 40 for sisters of the mother of an affected child and for the offspring of those sisters. She reported mother's brothers and father's sisters and brothers to have lower recurrence risks of 1 in 140–190. Arata et al. (2000) reported that affected mothers appear to have only a 0.5% to 1% chance of having a child with a neural tube defect.

The Medical Research Council (MRC Vitamin Research Group, 1991) first conclusively proved that when women with a prior child with a neural tube defect took 4 mg folic acid daily beginning 3 months prior to conception, there was a 70% reduction of recurrence in subsequent offspring. Wald et al. (2001) have recommended 5 mg daily. Because of the higher occurrence in first- and second-degree relatives, we recommend 4 mg daily beginning 3 months prior to a planned conception. We suggest that the effect in the United States may be closer to a 40%–50% reduction for two reasons. First, Berry et al. (1999) demonstrated a 79% reduction in occurrence in high-incidence north China but only 40% in south China when women took 0.4 mg of folic acid periconceptionally. The incidence of neural tube defects in the United States is closer to that of southern rather than northern China. Second, recent data from Canada and Mexico are the first to indicate that lower-incidence communities on the North American continent can achieve a 45%–55% reduction in occurrence with a regimen of 5 mg folic acid per week (De Villarreal et al., 2002), 0.4 mg daily (Gucciardi et al., 2002), and supplementation added to dietary fortification (Persad et al., 2002).

A discussion of etiology, genetics, and prevention is also important to help parents learn about causation and to decrease any remaining guilt associated with the diagnosis of a fetus or infant with a congenital anomaly. Guilt-ridden parents have greater difficulty helping their child develop an intact personality (Brazelton, 1992). Frequently, the parents' imagined causes for their child's neural tube defect occurred long after the closure of the neural tube at 27 days' gestation; the parents can be firmly reassured that their guilt is misplaced.

INFANCY AND TODDLERHOOD

Transition/Separation for Infants and Toddlers without Disabilities

Brazelton (1992) in his book *Touchpoints: Your Child's Emotional and Behavioral Development: Birth–3: The Essential Reference for the Early Years,* describes the emotional and behavioral development of children without disabilities. Readers are encouraged to review this text, adapting Brazelton's recommendations to their patients with disabilities. The remainder of this chapter will discuss salient aspects of Brazelton's (1992) and Erikson's (1950) books as they may relate to children with myelomeningocele.

Transition and the development of autonomy begin as an infant with the ability to move away from the mother (Miezio, 1983; Brazelton, 1992; Peterson et al., 1994). The infant creeps or crawls out of sight of the mother but returns quickly for assurance that she is still there. If the primary caretaker tries to leave the child, vocalizations are used to resist and prevent it. The duration of these child-initiated periods of exploration gradually grows longer, particularly when the child begins to walk. The distances also become longer, gradually progressing from rooms in the house to the play yard (garden in England), from the garden to day care, church school, preschool, school, and the homes and gardens of peers. Separating from a parent and substituting other care providers also occurs naturally for longer periods of time and greater distances. These child-initiated separations help build the child's concept of autonomy (Brazelton, 1992).

Toilet Training for the Child without a Disability in General

The timing of toileting skill acquisition in children with myelomeningocele should approximate the age of other children in the family and should consider the individual child's development. The typical method used to teach toilet training to a child without a disability involves a positive reward system for getting rid of excreta in the toilet. This process should not cause guilt in the child; it may last until 6 to 8 years of age for both day and night control (Brazelton, 1992). This recommended process, according to Brazelton, does not imply that stool or urine is bad. However, in most societies, a negative attitude toward excreta is introduced by discouraging children from having toileting accidents (Piaget, 1929; Erikson, 1950). A second critical skill that evolves during this same developmental period is the acquisition of language. The young child learns socially acceptable words for urine and stool and to not repeat vulgar or obscene words for these same entities. Examples of words that children overhear and repeat until admonished by their parents are well known Anglo-Saxon vulgarities.

Each culture has its own methods for teaching the child to conform to attainable goals, including toilet training (Piaget, 1929; Erikson, 1950). Toddlers without disabilities begin developing their toilet training skills when they are in a stage of denial (Brazelton, 1992). A 2- or 3-year-old frequently uses the word *no* as one of the first experiments in learning autonomy and testing limits (Brazelton,

1992). Therefore, we need to review how each of us learned or were taught socially appropriate toileting hygiene and how to discuss it.

Dependence on the sense of smell as a backup warning for stool or urine leakage is not completely reliable in either the child or the adult with or without a disability. "A man who smells bad is the last to smell himself" (an old Yankee saying based on a well-known phenomenon, habituation). Toileting accidents for the child with spina bifida of any degree with perineal nerve involvement usually occur with small leaks, initially generating little odor. The odor gradually increases, becoming more pungent as the child becomes involved in other activities and does not recognize the slowly increasing malodor. The initial odor also dulls later recognition of the noxious odor, a phenomenon known to anyone who has entered an area downwind from the original source of a foul odor. After a relatively brief time, the bad odor is no longer detectable (habituation). Children, therefore, frequently and truthfully deny that they have a bad odor because their noses have lost the ability to sense their own malodor.

Toilet Training for the Child without a Disability—Stool

Children without a disability and their parents usually learn toilet training before developing sufficient vocabulary or understanding to remember how it was learned. They learn on their own, by trial and error, and from caretaker cues. We all experience this same sequence of events but have not verbalized it because we were too young to understand cause and effect. Adult teachers, therefore, cannot verbalize the interpretation of the defecation sensations and requisite muscle control from their own experience. Stool toilet training requires that the child comprehend the predefecation urge and the subsequent events. Peristalsis can only be vaguely localized through the small and large bowels; the person without a disability definitely recognizes and localizes a peristaltic wave entering the rectum. Reflex opening of the proximal anal sphincter almost immediately follows this predefecation sensation. This allows the contents of the rectum to touch the mucous membrane of the anal canal. Sensory nerve endings that previously touched only the mucous membrane of the anal canal now detect a delicate soft sensation, which we interpret as gas. If we feel a rough substance, it is stool. The third sensation is a soft, hot substance that signals diarrhea. The only way to prevent the immediate passage of rectal contents, after analyzing these signals from the anal canal sensory nerves, is by contracting the voluntary anal sphincter. Failure to effectively close the anus is confirmed by the sensation of these same elements touching the skin of the perineum, buttocks, or thigh.

Toilet Training for the Child without a Disability—Urination

Toilet training for urine control is similar to stool control, though there are some differences. The vague feeling of a full urinary bladder or preurination urge is equivalent to the predefecation urge and is also carried to the brain by the autonomic nervous system. Painful stretching of the bladder is sensed via somatic nerves in the covering peritoneum that are mediated via the 12th vertebral roots. The simultaneous contraction of the urinary bladder detrusor and opening of the urinary bladder neck initiates the flow of urine into the proximal urethra. This is sensed via the fourth and fifth sacral somatic nerves. The external, voluntary urethral sphincter is also contracted via the fifth sacral somatic nerves. The sensory and motor components of urine control are similar to, but less complicated than, those of stool control and present their own problems for the child. The need to pass urine more frequently throughout the day and the difficulty in preventing urinary leakage pose greater social problems for a child than stool control. Blackburn (2002) reports that odor secondary to urine incontinence interferes with social adaptation in 60% of adults, while only 17% complained of stool odor. Eight of 12 adults with myelomeningocele and failure to adapt socially identified either incontinence of urine or its effect on psychosexual maladjustment as the reason; none mentioned stool accidents (Shurtleff et al., 1975). The other aspects of stool control noted above also apply to urine control.

Sexuality Training for and Learning by the Child without a Disability

An important but frequently overlooked aspect of transition and a necessary precursor for independent toilet training is the child's ability to undress and dress. These two skills are learned gradually during late infancy and early childhood. The removal of clothing also encourages autonomy. However, unless undressing occurs in the proper social circumstances, it leads to condemnation rather than approval. Parents teach their young children not to expose their perineum—frequently called their *private parts*—in public, particularly in the presence of the opposite sex. During this developmental period, infants and children fondle their genitalia and parents tell them that this should not be done (Erikson, 1950; Brazelton, 1992); at least, the child soon learns not to do so in the presence of others. Masturbation is a normal aspect of development (Brazelton, 1992). The social disapproval of masturbation should be explained in terms appropriate for the child's age but should not include threats of bodily harm. The child of 3 to 4 years of age may also ask where babies come from; their interest is usually brief and superficial. Simple explanations will both correctly inform the child and end their questioning (Brazelton, 1992). They observe that their mother develops a large abdomen, comes home from the hospital, or comes out of a home birthing room with a great reduction in her abdominal girth and a baby. Stories such as a stork delivering the baby are not appropriate.

Children at this age also notice differences between boys and girls, men and women. Some will satisfy this natural curiosity by comparing their private parts to those of other children of both sexes. Children with disabilities are no different in their curiosity or methods of exploration. One mother related the following story about three children who were 4 and 5 years of age. The children came in from playing outdoors to urinate. They all entered the bathroom together. The first, a boy, stated, "This is how I pee." A prolonged tinkle ensued. The second, a girl, said the same. Her shorter but louder stream of urine could then be heard splashing in the toilet bowl. The third, the woman's son, stated, "I don't have to take my pants down, and I pee quicker." He then flipped his urostomy bag over the top of his pants and pulled the plug. The subsequent swoosh was indeed quicker. Then two awed little voices exclaimed together, "Wow, are you lucky!"

INFANCY AND TODDLERHOOD FOR THE CHILD WITH SPINA BIFIDA

Transition/Separation for the Infant or Toddler with Spina Bifida

Lower extremity paralysis impairs mobility and interferes with the developmental process of separation/transition. Less well recognized, however, are the poor general tone and decreased motor abilities in the body and upper extremities of children with myelomeningocele and their effect on these same processes, regardless of the level of paralysis (Fay et al., 1986; Shurtleff, 1986; Wolf and McLaughlin, 1992; Hurley, 1993; Norrlin et al., 2003). Professionals and parents of small children with spina bifida should consider introducing their affected child to multiple methods of alternative mobility, such as wheeled toys, for two reasons (Miezio, 1983; Norrlin et al., 2003).

First, several authors have noted that children with higher-level myelomeningocele do not maintain biped ambulation beyond middle or late childhood (De Souza and Carroll, 1976; Samuelsson and Skoog, 1988; Bartonek et al., 1999; Iborra et al., 1999; Williams et al., 1999; Dias, 2001). The earliest age for cessation of walking in children with myelomeningocele enrolled in an active walking program was 7 years, 6 months for thoracic level patients; 6 years, 11 months for high lumbar level patients; and 9 years, 1 month in patients with low-level lesions (Williams et al., 1999). At a mean age of 14 years, 10 months, Samuelsson and Skoog (1988) reported 0% of ambulatory patients among those with thoracic or high lumbar (L1–L2) level lesions, 54% of ambulatory patients with L3 level lesions, 67% of ambulatory patients with L4 level lesions, 80% of ambulatory patients with L5 level lesions, and 100% of ambulatory patients with sacral level lesions. De Souza and Carroll (1976) reported that in the second and third decades of life, all thoracic level, 90% of high lumbar level, 66% of low lumbar level, and 50% of sacral level lesion patients with myelomeningocele were not able to ambulate in the community and required a wheelchair for extended mobility. Dias (2001) reported that only 1 of 32 patients with a thoracic-high lumbar level lesion and weak (three/five or fewer) quadriceps muscles ambulated as adults despite being enrolled in a vigorous biped ambulatory program as children. Iborra et al. (1999) reported that at a mean follow-up age of 15.9 years, the median age for beginning to walk was 37.1 months, while the median age at cessation of walking was 128 months; 74.8% of their patients were still walking at the time of follow-up. Bartonek et al. (1999) studied ambulation over a 12-year period in 60 patients with a mean age of 22 years (range, 12–54 years). Nineteen (32%) demonstrated a loss of ambulatory ability over time. With such a large proportion of children with myelomeningocele becoming wheelchair-dependent, it would seem at least partially appropriate to consider teaching methods of wheeled mobility early in life and to avoid the concept *of retreating to a wheelchair.* This retreat must be a depressing event for children brought up to believe that ambulation is an important goal to achieve and keep.

Secondly, with these mobility devices, children can be as mobile as they desire and can explore their environment. They can participate in floor-level activities and, later in childhood, can actively participate in wheelchair activities inaccessible to children solely dependent on crutch and braces, such as basketball, bowling, archery, and racing. McDonald (2001) discusses mobility devices. He recommends the Caster cart; we suggest that the "Alligator" can precede the use of the Caster cart. The Alligator is simply a flat, wheeled device similar to those used by mechanics to slide under automobiles. We recommend having a protective layer of covered foam on the top to protect against pressure decubitus formation. The undersurface of the plywood frame has either four small swivel caster wheels, two at each end, or two casters at one end and two regular wheels at the other (Fig. 25.1).

Other options for early mobility include hand-propelled devices into which the infant or young child can crawl. Handles allow the child to move forward and backward and pivot. One example is shown in Figure 25.2. There are many other devices available locally or on the Internet (Miezio, 1983).

Infants and toddlers should be allowed to be on the floor and encouraged to move about by rolling, scooting,

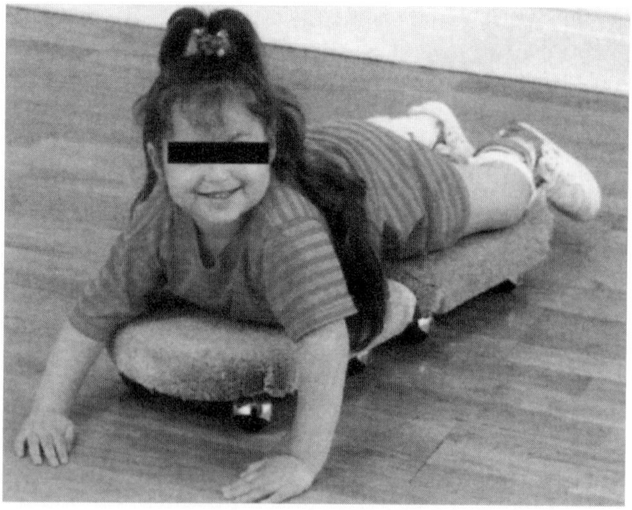

FIGURE 25.1. This mobility device and others can be obtained from Sammons Preston Roylan at WWW.sammonspreston.com or 1-800-323-5547 or built from the instructions in the text. It allows infants with disabilities to learn separation from their care providers and begin the process of autonomy.

combat crawling, and propelling themselves on a wheeled device (Miezio, 1983). Butler et al. (1984) have demonstrated that children as young as 18 months can learn to manipulate a motorized wheelchair, augmenting the typical stages of physical separation of toddlers from their primary caretakers. We recommend that these devices be close to the floor, allowing the infant or early toddler to crawl or scoot onto and off them.

We have learned that cumbersome devices designed to aid walking may actually impair the small child's mobility. We recommend that braces that might encumber mobility be used only during walking exercises and during naps or at bedtime to maintain joints free of contracture. When out of their braces, children should be dressed in pants and footwear made of material that will slide easily over rugs and rough surfaces in order to make mobility convenient and to protect their skin from friction burns.

From the very first, it is necessary to encourage self-accomplishment by the infant and young child (Brazelton, 1992). A study of our patient population revealed that a maternal belief in independence was a common psychosocial contributor to independence in self-care skills, achievement in school, and high self esteem (Goodwyn, 1990). During this early developmental period, play activities with same-age peers at the floor level should be encouraged. Adults should also consider engaging the infant in interactive floor-level play (Brazelton, 1992). The child's toys can be kept in a place where they can be reached from the floor or a wheeled device. We recommend that caretakers actively encourage children with a disability to explore their environment and allow them to fetch their own toys or other desired articles. Caretakers should discourage others from automatically responding to the child's request to have toys or other desired objects brought to her. Carefully encourage the child's drive for self-achievement while minimizing the child's frustration (Miezio, 1983). Allowing the child to use only verbal commands to demand action by others on his behalf may lead to learned helplessness and a poorly adjusted child (Fay et al., 1986; Hurley, 1993; Rowley-Kelly, 1993).

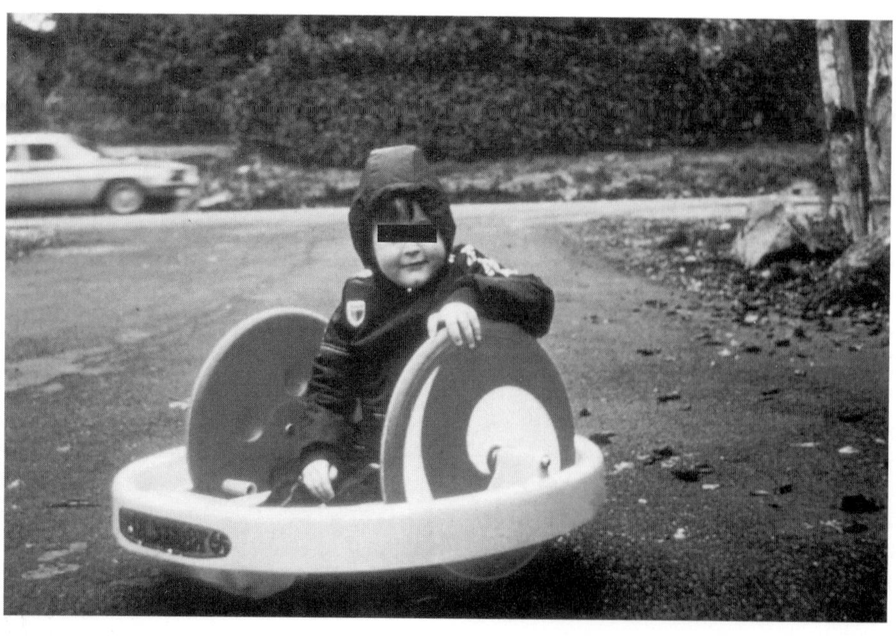

FIGURE 25.2. This mobility device is an example of a toy sold at stores for children without disabilities in the United States. For children with disabilities, it has a low profile that allows entry and exit by combat crawling and wheels that allow forward, reverse, and spinning movements similar to those of standard wheelchairs. Such a device is useful for training children with disabilities to negotiate rapidly in space by their own choice with less effort than with the use of braces and crutches.

Initial Ambulation for the Infant or Toddler with Spina Bifida

The natural development of upright posture in the infant without a disability occurs at 8 to 18 months of age, starting with a crouched-knee position. When their balance fails, they drop softly onto their buttocks (Brazelton, 1992). We have learned from our children and adults with spina bifida that in braces, they double their height in relation to sitting. As they attempt to stand with rigidly constrained ankles, knees, and sometime hips, they will fall to the ground much like a felled tree. No wonder they are terrified.

Forty years ago, we published advice derived from an incomplete study, recommending upright posture and simulation of "normal" ambulation (Shurtleff, 1966). Our colleagues in our multiple disciplinary clinics also reported on a standing frame, the Verlo, which could be used for standing and ambulation, much like the Parapodium of today (Taylor and Pemberton, 1972). This intervention proved to be of no benefit and, indeed, caused decubiti and fractures for the patients and frustration for their caregivers. One of the authors (DBS) now suggests to our skeptical physical therapists that they build a pair of stilts that will double children's height above the ground (their usual perception of their body in space). With these stilts strapped to their legs, they should prop themselves against a wall and take off, walking with or without appropriate supportive devices such as a parallel bar, walker, or crutches. It can be done—circus clowns do it all the time without assistive arm support. But can the average person or child? This difficulty is amplified by the considerable impairment of motor coordination and, to a lesser extent, by the visual perception exhibited by most infants born with myelomeningocele (Shaffer et al., 1985; Fay et al., 1986; Wolf and McLaughlin, 1992; Hurley, 1993; Hinderer et al., 1994; Lutkenhoff, 1999; McDonald, 2001).

Whether these suggestions and modifications to promote a child's mobility will enable them to develop appropriate autonomy is currently unknown. There are nine reported benefits of an upright standing or walking program: (*1*) improved urinary tract and bowel function; (*2*) improved cardiopulmonary function; (*3*) decreased osteoporosis; (*4*) decreased lower extremity fractures; (*5*) decreased lower extremity joint contractures; (*6*) reduced obesity; (*7*) decreased skin breakdown; (*8*) reduced degenerative joint disease; and (*9*) improved hand-eye-motor coordination function. None have been proven (Shurtleff, 1986). A study by Liptak et al. (1992) suggested that age- and disability-matched pairs in a parapodium program were more obese, watched more television, and were less mobile over rough surfaces than children with myelomeningocele brought up to use multiple methods of alternative mobility. The study by Liptak et al. demonstrated no significant differences in performance of activities of daily living between a group of similarly affected patients. In another study, patients with spina bifida enrolled in a program of early upright ambulation were found to have better independent skills of daily living compared to those involved in a program that emphasized the use of multiple methods of alternative mobility devices (Mazur et al., 1989). The patients in the biped ambulatory program used an A frame and had daily physiotherapy throughout their enrollment in residential schools; the patients in the multiple methods of alternative mobility program did not. Few of the patients in the multiple methods of alternative mobility group used standing or biped ambulatory devices and, if at all, only for a brief time. Since long-term ambulation is not a realistic goal for most high level lesion patients, its effect on development is the remaining indication for expensive and time-consuming ambulation programs in childhood. Whether a child's intensive drive toward upright ambulation and autonomy described by Brazelton (1992) is best served by intensive biped ambulatory training or by being able to explore the environment with the least restrictive bracing and multiple methods of alternative mobility, or a combination of these two approaches, has yet to be determined by accepted evidence-based criteria.

Toilet Training for the Infant or Toddler with Spina Bifida

There are many publications describing special methods to assist children with spina bifida to learn independent toilet training (Hill et al., 1969; Carr, 1981; Miezio, 1983; Okamoto et al., 1984; Kimura et al., 1986; Jumper, et al., 1990; Rowley-Kelly and Reigel, 1993; Lutenhoff, 1999; Elmark and Adams, 2000; Searles et al., 2000; Sarwark and Lubicky, 2001; Aslan and Kogan, 2002; Buyse et al., 2002). The reader is referred to these works for specific techniques and their rationale. This chapter will concentrate on toilet training as it relates to emotional and behavioral development.

Brazelton (1992) recommends toilet training for the child without disabilities after the age of 2 years or when the child (*1*) has developed sufficient language to understand the parents' chosen words to describe urine and stool; (*2*) is able to sit for at least 5 minutes independently, with or without a distracting activity; (*3*) is able to undress and dress the lower body; and (*4*) has expressed an interest.

How different the situation is for children born with spina bifida, with their delayed motor development, some with an inability to sit independently, and their sphincter motor impairment, lacking sensation in the anal canal and urethra. This problem is compounded by complex toileting procedures while encased in cumbersome braces and protective garments to guard against toilet accidents.

Toileting that depends on the immediate presence of the mother or another caretaker impairs the child's development of autonomy and delays the transition/separation process. For parents to effectively teach toileting skills to their child with sphincter impairment, they need to understand toilet training for the child without disability, the impact of their child's specific impairment, and how their child best learns. The child with fourth and fifth sacral nerve impairment lacks the ability to distinguish among stool, gas, and diarrheal fluid. Nor can the child contract the voluntary anal sphincters. Children with no function in the fourth and fifth sacral dermatomes have no sensation in either the anal canal or the skin of the perineal area, but many can identify a predefecation urge when peristalsis pushes bulky stool into the rectum. Learning disabilities are a common accompanying problem for these infants and children with spina bifida both with and without hydrocephalus (Chapter 23; Shaffer et al., 1985; Fay et al., 1986; Wolf and McLaughlin, 1992; Hurley, 1993; Hinderer et al., 1994; Lutkenhoff, 1999; McDonald, 2001).

Infants and toddlers without sensation in their legs and perineum, and swaddled in stool- and urine-collecting clothing, do not have the opportunities to become appropriately aware of their lower body and lower extremities. We believe that teaching the infant or toddler with any form of spina bifida to recognize that the lower part of their body and legs are part of them is an important objective at this age. Playing before a mirror with children nude can help them understand that the lower portion of their body and their legs are indeed a part of them. These paralyzed and senseless parts of their body should be incorporated into their concept of self. Modifying their clothing can improve their physical ability to don and doff their clothes and braces. Velcro fasteners are important facilitators. These two concepts may help the older child to become interested in his or her bodily functions and learn how to control them. We recommend a cool, uninterested attitude toward the older child when the diaper is soiled. As Brazelton (1992) and Erikson (1950) explain, even infants and toddlers understand their caretaker's communications through attitude and facial expression. Toddlerhood is the time to begin using nonverbal interactions to communicate that stool and urine are not pleasant. Whenever the diaper is found to be clean and dry, the caretaker should consider spending a short, pleasant time with the child. Continuing diaper cleanup as a pleasant experience into childhood conveys the wrong message to the child. At our suggestion, one of our students followed this approach with his 10-year-old daughter, who had developmental delay and incontinence but intact fourth and fifth sacral nerves. Impressed with the achievement of his nonverbal child, he applied the same positive attitude toward clean diapers and a cool attitude toward soiled diapers to a population of profoundly mentally retarded, nonverbal adults in an institution. When the attendants found clean diapers, they spent a few minutes providing a pleasant interaction. When soiled diapers were found, they changed the patients with no interaction. Within a few months, the number of soiled diapers markedly decreased.

Rutter (1980) described young children, deprived of learning interpersonal relationships and cognitive abilities, learning appropriate social behavior as older children and adjusting to be as functional as their peers. Brazelton (1992) indicates that some normal children are not fully toilet trained for 24 hours until 6 to 8 years of age; they do well unless they are made to feel guilty (see above). Hence, we believe that the actual techniques and timing of toilet training of children with sphincter impairment can be delayed until they understand and are physically able to perform the necessary and complex procedures without impairing their emotional adjustment. We recommend explaining to children with sphincter impairment that while they cannot prevent accidents, they should strive to keep themselves odor free.

Sexuality Training for the Infant or Early Toddler with Spina Bifida

When normal early childhood genital exploration among peers is postponed to later childhood, there can be severe social consequences. We know of three late childhood and early teenage boys convicted of and incarcerated for sexual molestation after engaging in curiosity-driven comparison of their genitalia with younger children, despite our testimony. A fourth was successfully exonerated after embarrassing social criminal investigations. A female with spina bifida was reportedly accused of indecent exposure for demonstrating her clean intermittent catheterization technique to some boys.

Playing nude in front of a mirror is effective in teaching the difference between boys and girls. Infants and young children enjoy learning about themselves from a mirror and exploring their body parts (Brazelton, 1992). We recommend that caretakers of the child with spina bifida consider directing the child's attention to the genitalia seen in the mirror, explaining the difference between girls and boys.

PRESCHOOL AND EARLY SCHOOL YEARS

Preschool and Early School Years for the Child without a Disability

The toddler progresses to the next stage of development having learned trust and mistrust from mother or primary caretakers. Shame, part of Erikson's (1950) first stage of development of man, is replaced by autonomy (Piaget, 1929; Brazelton, 1992). Autonomy, Erikson's (1950) second stage of development, is practiced through interaction with parents, caretakers, and family members. The young child may first identify with one parent and then the other, excluding the opposite parent during each time period (Brazelton, 1992). Close contacts experience the young child's frustration, anger, hostility, and aggression. Limit setting by these adults also helps the child to learn self-control (Erikson, 1950; Brazelton, 1992). Brazelton states that a sense of discipline is a parent's second most important gift to a child next to love. He also notes that setting limits in a consistent, effective manner is one of the most difficult tasks for parents. Limit setting is essential. It enables the child to learn self-control before interacting with peers. The young child benefits from social interaction with peers in five major ways (Erikson, 1950; Brazelton, 1992). During these interactions, they learn (*1*) the need for self-toileting as they tease one another about wearing diapers; (*2*) the difference between boys and girls; (*3*) the limits on exposing their perineum; (*4*) the limits on their anger and aggression toward others, Erikson's (1950) third stage of development; and (*5*) to accomplish joint tasks or develop industry as opposed to inferiority, Erikson's (1950) fourth stage of development. The young child begins to accomplish these developmental tasks by separating from family through attendance at church, school, neighbors' gardens (yards), play school, day care, and, by age 3 years, preschool. Initially, these activities are closely supervised and attended by the parents or caregiver. The time away from parents and caregiver gradually lengthens, becoming more frequent and less supervised. Children's absences from parents and caregiver provide opportunities to learn about themselves. They become more mobile and liberated, learning to use their wheeled vehicles—first the tricycle and then the bicycle. The reasons for and the importance of acquiring these independence skills and autonomy have been previously elaborated in this chapter.

Transition/Separation in the Preschool and Early School Years for the Child with Spina Bifida

Too often, the young child with spina bifida is separated from parents by hospitalization, an emotionally and physically traumatic experience for any child. At this age, children believe that the creation of all objects and order in their lives is under the control of their parents (Piaget, 1929). Hospitalizations, therefore, require explanation and support from the parents or primary caregiver, as described by Brazelton (1992). His studies indicate that preparation for hospital admission should include clear reasons and objectives and a full explanation of the sequence of events. The parent or primary caregiver should be with the child during admission, bloodletting and other painful procedures, preoperatively, and during recovery from anesthesia.

Separation for social reasons such as day care, parents' absences, preschool attendance, and so on should be associated with clear limits, the exact time of return, and assurances that the parent will return, helping the child overcome any anxiety about abandonment (Piaget, 1929; Erikson, 1950; Brazelton, 1992). Absences by a child from parents to be with same-age peers and to develop autonomy should be encouraged. Parents of children with spina bifida tend to avoid, rather than encourage, such separations because of the child's limited mobility, incontinence, and previous traumatic hospital separations. What children with spina bifida learn during separations from their parents are the same five concepts and skills noted above for children without a disability.

Erikson (1950) describes child play as an opportunity to learn self-control with other children, to develop new mastery skills over fantasy, and to develop give-and-take with peers through experimenting and experience. Brazelton (1992) and Piaget (1929) concur. Parents should be encouraged to involve their children with spina bifida in social activities with family and friends and in group activities such as music, arts and crafts, gardening, caring for pets or farm animals, church, school, preschool, swimming, rowing, sailing, bowling, childhood social groups such as Boy Scouts and Girl Scouts, Camp Fire Girls, Indian Guides, Brownies, Cub Scouts, and, of course, fishing. The main objective of these activities is to place the child in frequent situations to interact and play with other children, both similarly disabled and able-bodied, in order to learn autonomy.

Ambulation in the Preschool and Early School Years for the Child with Spina Bifida

The mobility needs discussed above for infants and toddlers become more important for the preschool- and early-school-age child. Floor-level play, unencumbered by heavy bracing, should be considered to provide opportunities to explore and learn autonomy. Caretakers should consider restricting brace- and crutch-assisted ambulation to exercise periods, teaching the child without producing frustration and intolerance or interfering with the child's opportunity to explore and be with same-age peers. We believe that the availability of mobility devices mentioned above and in Chapter 24 for the more severely motor-impaired and wheelchairs should be provided to brace- and crutch-assisted walkers in order to teach them how to compete in wheelchair activities and experience extended trips. As noted above, a number of authors note that many biped ambulatory children with spina bifida prefer wheelchair use as adults, at least part-time. Many of the activities suggested for increasing a child's social interactions, such as basketball, bowling, archery, and fishing, noted above, can be performed more easily with the assistance of a wheelchair. They cannot be performed when the children's arms are holding crutches. At this age, parents and caretakers should encourage multiple methods of alternative mobility and participation in, rather than observation of, other children's games and activities.

Toilet Training in the Preschool and Early School Years for the Child with Spina Bifida

The discussions about toilet training in this chapter do not provide the details of the many methods available to parents and caretakers. The reader is referred to other publications for that information (Hill et al., 1969; Carr, 1981; Sousa et al., 1983; Okamoto et al., 1984; Sulliva-Bolyai et al., 1984; Fay et al., 1986; Kimura et al., 1986; Shurtleff and Mayo, 1986; Wicks and Shurtleff, 1986; Lutkenhoff, 1999; Ekmark and Adams, 2000; Searles et al., 2000; Aslan and Kogan, 2002; Buyse et al., 2002; Wright, 2002). No single process will work for all children; no single process will be effective across the lifetime of a child. Therefore, ongoing consultation with specialists in toilet training a child with impaired sphincters is often needed. We suggest that the interested person contact a nurse coordinator of the local multidisciplinary spina bifida clinic for advice, references, and ongoing consultations appropriate for the child in question. We will discuss the need for participation by the child in whatever procedure is being used to help establish and support the child's autonomy and sense of self-worth.

Incontinence hampers participation in peer interactions and social activities. Medical and surgical management techniques are very good at preserving health. However, in our experience, they successfully establish continence in less than half of the children with spina bifida at this age. Attitudes toward soiled and clean diapers described above for the infant and toddler should continue. Caretakers should consider explaining to children that while they cannot prevent accidents because of their paralysis, odor-free cleanliness is achievable and necessary for social acceptance. This objective and others can be explained without embarrassing or humiliating the child. There are four additional objectives for a child of this age: (*1*) learn to dress and undress; (*2*) assist in preparing for toileting procedures; (*3*) learn that the nose may not detect the odor of urine or stool (habituation); and (*4*) cooperate with caregivers during toileting procedures until the child is completely independent. Learning to dress can be taught in the morning, at naptime, on awakening, before and after toileting, and while undressing at nighttime for bed. In a similar manner, learning to assist with toileting procedures should begin and be advanced in small increments as the child incorporates each step into the daily regimen. Learning may initially be slow and take extra time because of learning difficulties discussed in Chapter 23. It is essential to teach these skills to the child; otherwise, learned helplessness will result. Creating a detailed list of the steps required for successful toileting and posting them in the child's toileting area will help the child learn the entire process (see Chapter 23; Carr, 1981; Fay et al., 1986; Rowley-Kelly and Reigel, 1993).

That their child's nose does not detect foul odors needs to be acknowledged by parents and primary caretakers. Frequently, the odor increases slowly or develops when the child is concentrating on play. If children do not understand this process of habituation, they will deny that they smell bad. To teach them that their soiled clothing has a bad odor, the children can clean themselves with as little help as necessary. The soiled clothes should then be placed in an open container in a small room or closet. After a half hour or so, the children should be led to the space with the soiled clothing and asked if they now detect the odor. This exercise, repeated if necessary, can teach the children that their noses are unreliable and defuse their tendency to argue with caretakers who state that they have a bad odor and suggest the need to clean themselves.

Learning to cooperate with parents and caretakers in the toileting process requires teaching the child the following five concepts: (*1*) At this age, children are interested in their bodies' anatomy and function and how they differ from or are similar to others. The anecdote related above about the two boys, one with a urostomy bag, and a girl passing urine illustrate this phenomenon. (*2*) They are old enough to begin to understand how their sphincter mechanisms should, but do not, work. (*3*) They can be assured that their particular manner of toileting can be private, and neither revealed to nor discussed with others. Federal laws in the United States and the United Kingdom require that schools offer private toileting places for children with impaired sphincters (IDEA) (Blackburn, 2002). Children at this age begin to understand the need for privacy for their genitals. Like-sex caretakers should perform and teach them about clean intermittent catheterization and various anally introduced medications for stool elimination. They should also be taught to report to their like-sex parent any touching of their genitals by anyone other than their like-sex caretakers. Girls with spina bifida are at risk for seduction or rape if they lack understanding of sexuality. (*4*) Many persons with spina bifida can feel urinary bladder fullness and the predefecation urge. Some believe that children at this age can be taught these sensations during urodynamic studies and biofeedback sessions (Aslan and Kogan, 2002). (*5*) There is a need for odor-free cleanliness. Children with uncontrolled incontinence should be taught to examine themselves on a routine basis, both before and after physical activities that involve the Valsalva maneuver. They also need to learn to inspect and clean themselves when parents, friends, teachers, and others who are aware of their sphincter impairment suggest that they have a foul odor. Obviously, this goal can be achieved only if primary caretakers share knowledge of the impaired sphincters with individuals who come in close contact with the sphincter-impaired child. Subtle nonverbal communications should be used to prevent embarrassing the child.

Sexuality Training in the Preschool and Early School Years for the Child with Spina Bifida

The suggestions in the section on sexuality training for infants and early toddlers with spina bifida also apply to children in the preschool and early school years. At these ages, parents and caregivers can more easily explain sex differences and appropriate behaviors using language that the child can understand. Children at these ages are more likely to ask questions about sex and childbirth. For younger children, the explanations should be accurate but superficial (Brazelton, 1992). Explanations for older children should also inform them about their future sexual potential, particularly the risk of their birth defect in their own children (Blackburn, 2002). The subjects of privacy and protection of their genitals have been covered in the previous section on toileting.

LATE CHILDHOOD AND PREADOLESCENCE

Late Childhood and Preadolescence for the Child without Disability

This period of growth and development includes the second phase of conflict between the child and authority figures. Children of this age are entering into the last of the four stages of the development of man described by Erikson (1950): (*1*) learning limits on self-identity, compared to role diffusion, including physical genital maturity; the child must learn to distinguish between self-centered existence and participation in the world of peers; (*2*) learning intimacy, compared to isolation, centering on close personal relationships; the child must learn the difference between close, friendly relationships and intimate relationships with a personal partner; (*3*) learning generativity, compared to stagnation; deciding if they will become productive, contributing members of society or withdraw into themselves; (*4*) establishing ego integrity, compared to despair; being able to keep one's self-identity while relating to others and society rather than collapsing into a self-centered and isolated state. In summary, Erikson (1950) describes the teenage period as a normal phase of crisis with increased conflict characterized by fluctuations in ego strength and high growth potential. The preadolescent and adolescent are learning independence and are often in as much turmoil over these changes as their parents (Brazelton, 1992). Offer (1969) describes adolescence as a transitional period presenting adolescents with special burdens, challenges, and opportunities. Children develop personalities independent of their families, increase their self-confidence, establish a sense of comfort and strength in their own abilities, and make important decisions for their future, free of their families' influence. Elkind (1976) describes adolescents as being in a state of extreme egocentricity: everyone is watching them. Friedrich and Shaffer (1986) emphasize that adolescents are learning responsibility, independence, and heterosexual relationships. Davis (2001) emphasizes that psychologists and psychiatrists describe adolescence as a stage of development not specifically related to age. These systems do not take into account the fact that some children begin their "adolescent transition" in late childhood, before the teenage years. Others do not begin until later in their teenage or young adult years. A study of independence skills in preteenage children and teenagers using the Vineland Adaptive Behavior Scales (Sparrow et al., 1984) presents concrete data on age and acquisition of skills for independent living (S. S. Sparrow, personal communication, 2001). The study by Davis (2001) demonstrates that several independent activities are acquired by children with myelomeningocele prior to 12 years of age. The most notable of these skills are grooming of teeth, hair, and nails; personal choices when shopping; being on time for activities outside the home; knowing their own telephone number; using a telephone directory; understanding time as measured by a clock; monitoring their spending; and remembering special dates such as birthdays. Data on more intimate situations such as first sexual intercourse, on the other hand, are not well known.

Late Childhood and Preadolescence for the Child with Spina Bifida

Rutter (1980) has demonstrated that severely deprived children can overcome early childhood deprivation if provided the opportunity in later childhood. This stage of childhood development is the last opportunity to prepare the child for transition in adolescence. Davis et al. (2002) have described patients with myelomeningocele being 2 to 5 years behind same-age peers in acquiring daily living skills. Children with myelomeningocele younger than 12 years of age had developed 11 of 31 skills for independent living. In this study, the acquisition of independence skills best correlated with cognition and was not related to level of lesion or gender. The greatest discrepancies between children without disability described by Sparrow et al. (personal communication, 2001) and the delays for children with myelomeningocele involved stool and urine hygiene (Davis et al., 2002). The average age for attainment by 75% of the former was 4 years of age compared to 14 years for the latter. Participation in organized extracurricular activities declined to only 30%–40% among older teenagers. Of teenagers 18 years of age, 21% did their own laundry, 37% fixed their own meals, 49% cleaned dishes after a meal, and only 39%

managed their own money (Davis et al., 2002). Hopefully, teaching the developmental stages and using some of the suggestions previously reviewed in this chapter will properly prepare children with myelomeningocele for the period of transition discussed in Chapter 24.

Transition/Separation for the Late Childhood and Preadolescent Child with Spina Bifida

During this stage of development, the children's increase in body size and the acquisition of autonomy skills often leads those brought up in a biped ambulatory program to "retreat" into a wheelchair, despite the early childhood goal of many programs to acquire and maintain biped ambulation, as reviewed above. Children often gain sufficient weight to become obese, preventing efficient ambulation. Do those children, brought up to equate walking with success, become depressed when they fail to continue walking, withdraw into themselves, and overeat? Have these expectations placed them in a position where they are bound to fail? Like the Ogala Sioux described by Erikson (1950), they may have been presented with an unattainable goal, suppressing their initiative and becoming apathetic and depressed. A sense of despair and hopelessness will only compound underlying developmental problems (Erikson, 1950; Friedrich and Shaffer, 1986; Brazelton, 1992). If the marginal crutch and brace walker is also taught wheelchair use as a younger child, this assumption of wheelchair mobility may limit the conflict between self-concept and physique (Piaget, 1929; Anderson and Clarke, 1982; Friedrich and Shaffer, 1986). Wheelchair use should be seen as a normal method of achieving mobility, not a retreat. We suggest that during this period of development children also become oriented to independent mobility within the community using public transportation. They should also be assessed for hand control automobile driving.

Toilet Training for the Late Childhood and Preadolescent Child with Spina Bifida

Unfortunately, our data indicate that the acquisition of independent toileting skills has changed only slightly over the past 15 years (Shurtleff and Mayo, 1986; Davis et al., 2002). Only half of our patients acquired socially acceptable, independent toileting skill by 8 to 9 years of age, despite advances in urinary and bowel management. The antegrade continence enema (Ekmark and Adams, 2000; Searles et al., 2000) may contribute to easier bowel management, but it is not a solution for the noncompliant child or family. Urological advances have improved renal health but have not solved the problems of continence (Aslan and Kogan, 2002). Placing the clean intermittent catherization (CIC) catheter in the lying position and then sitting up allows better drainage of urine over the edge of the bed and reduces residual urine. We have observed significant complications, including an increase in urinary tract infections, following placement of a Mitrofanoff stoma. Having the child change from a sitting to a side-lying position with a 45° turn toward the abdomen during drainage of the urinary bladder allows urine to drain downhill via the Mitrofanoff catheter, reducing residual urine. Reducing the residual urine volume decreases the frequency of urinary tract infections (Kimura et al., 1986). Children of this age must acquire cleanliness and independent toileting; otherwise, they will enter middle or late adolescence with persistent and unacceptable stool and urine incontinence and odor. Although cleanliness has been described as being "next to godliness," we are also sure that it is a prerequisite for sexiness. At this stage of development, children tend to isolate themselves socially into like-sex activities and friendships. Both sexes begin or intensify and prolong their separation from their parents. Girls at a slightly younger age than boys become interested in heterosexual relationships. Failure to develop independence in toileting can lead to disruption of the development of these typical relationship patterns. Without independence in stool and urine toileting, these two developmental processes are severely handicapped.

Sexuality for the Late Childhood and Preadolescent Child with Spina Bifida

Children born with spina bifida, like their same-age peers without disabilities, develop an interest in intimate relationships and procreation. Their lack of mobility and socially appropriate stool and urine hygiene potentially interfere with achievement of these goals (Shurtleff and Sousa, 1977; Hayden et al., 1979; Dunne and Shurtleff, 1986; Rowley-Kelly, 1993; Sawyer and Roberts, 1999; Sarwark and Lubicky, 2001; Blackburn, 2002). We therefore recommend that teachers and medical staff bring these issues surrounding normal development and sexuality to the attention of parents of children with disabilities. When the child shows evidence of entering into puberty, we recommend discussing with them all the aspects of sexuality pertinent to any teenager. Goodwyn (1990) notes that open communication between parent and child is a psychosocial independent variable that predicts better adjustment at this age. These discussions should include the medical reasons for not participating in indiscriminate sexual intercourse to avoid pregnancy for the girl, responsibility for a child born out of wedlock for the boy, and venereal diseases for both. With girls we also discuss the complications of pregnancy, the increased frequency of urinary tract problems, and the possibility of developing herniated vertebral discs and the need for cesarean section birth. In addition, we discuss the recurrence risk of the disability in the affected child's children, prevention, prenatal diagnosis, and the prognosis for various types and degrees of neural tube defects, particularly anencephaly and different levels of myelomeningocele, as discussed above.

These suggestions terminate this chapter about toilet training, transition/separation and sexuality. The next stage of transition, launching, is discussed in Chapter 24 of this text.

REFERENCES

Anderson EM, Clarke L (eds) (1982). *Disability in Adolescence.* London: Methuen.

Arata M, Grover S, Dunne KB, Bryan D (2000). Pregnancy outcome and complications in women with spina bifida. J Reprod Med 45:743–748.

Aslan AR, Kogan BA (2002). Conservative management in neurogenic bladder dysfunction. Curr Opin Urol 12(6):473–477.

Bartonek A, Saraste H, Samuelsson L, Skoog M (1999). Ambulation in patients with myelomeningocele: a 12-year follow-up. J Pediatr Ortho 19(2):202–206.

Berry RJ, Li Z, Erickson JD, et al (1999). Prevention of neural tube defects with folic acid in China. China-U.S. Collaborative Project for neural tube defect prevention. N Engl J Med 341:1485–1490.

Blackburn M (ed) (2002). *Sexuality and Disability.* Boston: Butterworth and Heinemann.

Brazelton TB (ed) (1992). *Touchpoints: Your Child's Emotional and Behavioral Development:* "Birth–3: The Essential Reference for the Early Years." Reading, MA: Perseus Books.

Butler C, Okamoto GA, McKay TM (1984). Motorized wheelchair driving by disabled children. Arch Phys Med Rehabil 65:95–97.

Buyse GM, Inderadjaja J, vanGool JD, Verpoorten C (2002). Preserved kidneys and safe urinary continence with early-instituted therapy for the neurogenic bladder: the implementation of standards of care as a top priority. Eur J Pediatr Surg 12(Suppl 1):S54.

Carter CO, Evans K (1973). Children of adult survivors with spina bifida. Lancet 27:924–926.

Carr J (ed) (1981). *Helping Your Handicapped Child: A Step-by-Step Guide to Everyday Problems.* New York: Penguin Books.

Cass AS, Bloom BA, Luxemberg M (1986). Sexual function in adults with myelomeningocele. J Urol 136:425–426.

CDC (1992). Recommendations for the use of folic acid to reduce the number of cases of spina bifida and other neural tube defects. MMWR 41:1–7.

Chatkupt S, Skurnick JH, Jaggi M, Mitruka K, Koeneigsber MR, Johnson WG (1994). Study of genetics, epidemiology, and vitamin usage in familial spina bifida in the United States in the 1990s. Neurology 44:65–70.

Comarr AE (1976). Neurological disturbances of sexual function among patients with Myelodysplasia. In McLaurin RL (ed): *Myelomeningocele: Proceedings of a Multidisciplinary Symposium, University of Cincinnati, Cincinnati, Ohio, March 11–13.* New York: Grune & Stratton, pp. 797–808.

Davis BE (2001). Assessing the development of adolescent autonomy skills in individual with myelomeningocele. Master's thesis, University of Washington.

Davis BE, Shurtleff DB, Walker WO, Seidel K, Duguay S (2002). Age of acquisition of adult autonomy skills in individuals with myelomeningocele. Eur J Ped Surg 12(Suppl 1):560–561.

De Souza LJ, Carroll N (1976). Ambulation of the braced myelomeningocele patient. J Bone Joint Surg 58-A:1112–1118.

De Villarreal LM, Perez JZ, Vasquez PA, Herrera RH, Campos Mdel R, Lopez RA, Ramirez JM, et al (2002). Decline of neural tube defects after a folic acid campaign in Neuvo Leon, Mexico. Teratology 66(5):249–256.

Dias LS (2001). Expected long-term walking ability. In Sarwark JF, Lubicky JP (eds): *Caring for the Child with Spina Bifida.* Rosemont, IL: American Academy of Orthopedic Surgery, pp. 261–262.

Dunne KB, Shurtleff DB (1986). The adults with meningomyelocele: a preliminary report. In: McLaurin R (ed): *The Second International Symposium on the Care of Meningomyelocele.* Orlando, FL: Grune & Stratton, pp. 876–892.

Ekmark E, Adams RC (2000). The antegrade continence enema (ACE) surgical procedure: patient selection, outcomes, long-term patient management. Eur J Pediatr Surg 10(Suppl 1):49–51.

Elkind D (1976). Cognitive development and psychopathology: observations on egocentrism and ego defense. In Schapler E and Reichler RJ (eds): *Psychopathology and Child Development.* New York: Plenum Press.

Erikson EH (ed) (1950). *Childhood and Society.* New York: WW Norton.

Fay G, Shurtleff D, Shurtleff H, Wolf L (1986). Approaches to facilitate independent self-care and academic success. In Shurtleff DB (ed): *Myelodysplasias and Exstrophies: Significance, Prevention and Treatment.* Orlando, FL: Grune & Stratton, pp. 373–396.

Friedrich W Shaffer J (1986). Adolescent psychosocial adjustment. In Shurtleff DB (ed): *Myelodysplasias and Exstrophies: Significance, Prevention and Treatment.* Orlando, FL: Grune & Stratton, pp. 399–410.

Goodwyn MA (1990). A study of the biomedical and psychosocial factors that predict independence in activities of daily living, academic success, and self perceptions of children with Meningomyelocele. PhD thesis, University of Washington.

Gucciardi E, Pietrusiak MA, Reynolds DL, Rouleau J (2002). Incidence of neural tube defects in Ontario, 1986–1999. CMAJ 167(6):237–240.

Hayden PW, Davenport LH, Campbell MM (1979). Adolescents with myelodysplasia: impact of physical disability on emotional maturation. Pediatrics 64(1):53–59.

Hill ML, Shurtleff DB, Ansell JS, Chapman WH (1969). The myelodysplasia child: bowel and bladder control. Am J Nurs 69:545–550.

Hinderer KA, Hinderer SR, Shurtleff DB (1994). Myelodysplasia. In Campbell SK (ed): *Physical Therapy for Children.* Philadelphia: WB Saunders, pp. 571–619.

Hultling C, Levi R, Amark SP, Sjoblom P (2000). Semen retrieval and analysis in men with myelomeningocele. Dev Med Child Neurol 42:681–684.

Hurley AD (1993). Conducting psychological assessments. In Rowley-Kelly, Reigel DH (eds): *Teaching the Student with Spina Bifida.* Baltimore: Paul H Brookes, pp. 107–123.

Iborra J, Pages E, Cuxart A (1999). Neurologic abnormalities, major orthopaedic deformities and ambulation analysis in a myelomeningocele population in Catalonia, Spain. Spinal Cord 37(5)351–357.

Jumper BM, McLorie GA, Churchill BM, Khoury AE, Toi A (1990). Effects of the artificial urinary sphincter on prostatic development and sexual function in pubertal boys with meningomyelocele. J Urol 144:438–442.

Kimura DK, Mayo M, Shurtleff DB (1986). Urinary tract management. In Shurtleff, DB (ed): *Myelodysplasias and Exstrophies: Significance, Prevention and Treatment.* Orlando, FL: Grune & Stratton, pp. 243–266.

Laurence KM, Beresford A (1975). Continence, friends, marriage and children in 51 adults with spina bifida. Dev Med Child Neurol (Suppl)35:123–128.

Liptak GS, Shurtleff DB, Bloss JW, Baitus-Hebert E, Manitta P (1992). Mobility aids for children with high-level myelomeningocele: parapodium versus wheelchair. Dev Med Child Neurol 34:787–796.

Lutkenhoff M (ed) (1999). *Children with Spina Bifida: A Parents' Guide.* Bethesda, MD: Woodbine House.

Matsumoto S, Sato H (eds) (1999). *Spina Bifida.* New York: Springer-Verlag.

Mazur JM, Shurtleff DB, Menelaus M, Colliver J (1989). Orthopedic management of high-level spina bifida: early walking compared with early use of a wheelchair. J Bone Joint Surg 71A:56–61.

McDonald CM (2001). Mobility issues and prescribing mobility aids for children with myelomeningocele. In Sarwark JF, Lubicky JP (eds): *Caring for the Child with Spina Bifida.* Rosemont, IL: American Academy of Orthopedic Surgeons.

McManus S (1987). Neural tube defects: identification of "high risk" women. Irish Med J 80:166–168.

Miezio PM (ed) (1983). *Parenting Children with Disabilities: A Professional Source for Physicians and Guide for Parents.* New York: Marcel Dekker.

MRC Vitamin Study Research Group (1991). Prevention of neural tube defects: results of the Medical Research Council Vitamin Study. Lancet 338:131–137.

Norrlin S, Strinnholm M, Carlsson M, Dahl M (2003). Factors of significance for mobility in children with myelomeningocele. Acta Paediatr 92:204–210.

Offer D (ed) (1969). *The Psychological World of the Teenager.* New York: Basic Books.

Okamoto GA, Lamers JY, Shurtleff DB (1983). Skin breakdown in patients with myelomeningocele. Arch Phys Med Rehabil 64:20–23.

Okamoto GA, Sousa JC, Telzrow RW, Holm RA, McCartin R, Shurtleff DB (1984). Toileting skills in children with myelomeningocele: rates of acquisition. Arch Phys Med Rehabil 65:182–185.

Pasqualotto FF, Rossi-Ferragut LM, Rocha CC, Ianconelli AR, Borges E Jr (2002). Outcome of in vitro fertilization and intracytoplasmic injection of epididymal and testicular sperm obtained from patients with obstructive and nonobstructive azoospermia. J Urol 167:1753–1756.

Persad VL, Van den Hof MC, Dube JM, Zimmer P (2002). Incidence of open neural tube defects in Nova Scotia after folic acid fortification. CMAJ 167(6):241–245.

Peterson PM, Rauen KK, Brown J, Cole J (1994). Spina bifida: the transition into adulthood begins in Infancy. Rehabil Nurs 19:229–238.

Piaget J (ed) (1929). *The Child's Conception of the World.* New York: Harcourt, Brace.

Rowley-Kelly FL (1993). Social and emotional development. In Rowley-Kelly FL, Reigel DH (eds): *Teaching the Student with Spina Bifida.* Baltimore: Paul H Brookes. pp. 213–244.

Rowley-Kelly FL, Reigel D (eds) (1993). *Teaching the Student with Spina Bifida.* Baltimore: Paul H Brookes.

Rutter M (1980). The long-term effects of early experience. Dev Med Child Neurol 22:800–815.

Samuelson L, Skoog M (1988). Ambulation in patients with myelomeningocele: a multivariate statistical analysis. J Pediatr Ortho Surg 8:569–575.

Sarwark JF, Lubicky JP (eds) (2001). *Caring for the Child with Spina Bifida.* Rosemont, IL: American Academy of Orthopedic Surgeons.

Sawyer SM, Roberts KV (1999). Sexual and reproductive health in young people with spina bifida. Dev Med Child Neurol 41:671–675.

Searles JM, Roberts JP, MacKinnon AE (2000). The ACE procedure—problems behind the success. Eur J Pediatr Surg 10(Suppl 1):51–52.

Shaffer J, Friedrich WN, Shurtleff DB, Wolf L (1985). Cognitive and achievement status of children with meningomyelocele. J Pediatr Psychol 10(3):325–330.

Shurtleff DB (1966). Timing of learning in meningomyelocele patients. J Phys Ther Assoc 46:136–148.

Shurtleff DB (1986). Mobility. In Shurtleff DB (ed): *Myelodysplasias and Exstrophies: Significance, Prevention, and Treatment.* Orlando, FL: Grune & Stratton, pp. 313–358.

Shurtleff DB, Hayden PW, Chapman WH, Broy AB, Hill ML (1975). Myelodysplasia: problems of long-term survival and social function. West J Med 122:199–205.

Shurtleff DB, Mayo M (1986). Toilet training: the Seattle Experience and conclusions. In Shurtleff DB (ed): *Myelodysplasias and Exstrophies: Significance, Prevention and Treatment.* Orlando, FL: Grune & Stratton, pp. 267–284.

Shurtleff DB, Sousa JC (1977). The adolescent with myelodysplasia: development, achievement, sex and deterioration. In McLaurin RL (ed): *Myelomeningocele: Proceedings of a Multidisciplinary Symposium, University of Cincinnati, Cincinnati, Ohio, March 11–13.* New York: Grune & Stratton, pp. 809–819.

Sousa JC, Telzrow RW, Holm RA, McCartin R, Shurtleff DB (1983). Developmental guidelines for children with myelodys plasia. Phys Ther 63:21–29.

Sparrow SS, Balla D, Cicchetti DV (ed) (1984). *Vineland Adaptive Behavior Scales.* Circle Pines, MN: American Guidance Source.

Sullivan-Bolyai S, Swanson M, Shurtleff DB (1984). Toilet training the child with neurogenic impairment of bowel and bladder function. Issues Compr Nurs 7:33–43.

Taylor N, Pemberton DR (1972). Verlo orthosis for children with severe motor handicaps. Arch Phys Med Rehabil 53:534–535.

Timson J (1972). A study of the first-degree relatives of the parents of spina bifida children. Clin Genet 3:99–102.

Toriello HV, Higgins JV (1983). Occurrence of neural tube defects amongst first-, second- and third-degree relatives of probands: results of a United States study. Am J Med Genet 15(4):601–606.

Vroege JA, Zeijlemaker BY, Scheers MM (1998). Sexual function of adult patients born with meningomyelocele. A pilot study. Eur Urol 34(10):25–29.

Wald NJ, Law MR, Morris JK, Wald DS (2001). Quantifying the effect of folic acid. Lancet 358:2069–2073.

Wicks K, Shurtleff DB (1986). An introduction to toilet training, and stool management. In Shurtleff DB (ed): *Myelodysplasias and Exstrophies: Significance, Prevention and Treatment.* Orlando, FL: Grune & Stratton, pp. 203–242.

Williams EN, Broughton NS, Menelaus MB (1999). Age-related walking in children with spina bifida. Dev Med Child Neurol 41:446–449.

Wolf LS, McLaughlin JF (1992). Early motor development in infants with meningomyelocele. Pediatr Phy Ther 4:12–17.

Wright L (2002). The efficacy of bowel management in the adult with spina bifida. Eur J Pediatr Surg 12(Suppl 1):S41–S43.

26

Psychological Adjustment and Family Relationships in Children and Adolescents with Spina Bifida

RACHEL NEFF GREENLEY
GRAYSON N. HOLMBECK
JILL ZUKERMAN
COLLEEN F. BUCK

In recent years, researchers and clinicians have been interested in identifying factors associated with psychosocial adjustment among children and adolescents with spina bifida. Spina bifida is a heterogeneous condition characterized by an incomplete development of the spinal column. Subtypes of spina bifida include spina bifida occulta, identified by an abnormal spinal opening without spinal cord or nerve damage, and spina bifida cystica, characterized by the presence of a protruding fluid-filled sac that encloses the meninges (meningocele) or the meninges and spinal column (myelomeningocele). Finally, lipomeningocele is a subtype of spina bifida characterized by the presence of a fatty mass that herniates through the spinal column and attaches to the spinal cord, tethering the cord and often the associated nerve roots (Fletcher et al., 2004).

Myelomeningocele is the most common form of spina bifida occulta. It is also the most severe, resulting in neurological impairment at and below the level of the lesion. The nature of the impairment largely depends upon the level of the lesion, with thoracic level lesions indicative of the most severe impairment, lumbar lesions indicative of moderate levels of impairment, and sacral lesions associated with the mildest sensorimotor impairments. Given their neurological impairments, children with myelomeningocele typically have problems with ambulation, as well as bowel and bladder functioning. Additionally, most children with myelomeningocele have a malformation of the cerebellum and hindbrain that blocks cerebrospinal fluid flow and results in the development of hydrocephalus that necessitates shunt treatment (Fletcher et al., 2004). The majority of research to date has focused on the myelomeningocele type of spina bifida.

The clinical demands associated with a chronic illness such as spina bifida necessitate adherence to complex medical regimens and often place substantial physical, psychological, and social demands on the affected children, adolescents, and their families (Quittner and DiGirolamo, 1998). A body of research has suggested that children with spina bifida are at risk for a variety of psychosocial adjustment problems (Lavigne and Faier-Routman, 1992; Appleton et al., 1997). Parents of children with spina bifida also experience increased levels of stress compared to parents of typically developing children (Wallander et al., 1989b, 1990; Holmbeck et al., 1997).

From a developmental psychopathology perspective, the presence of spina bifida can be conceptualized as a risk factor, a variable that increases the likelihood of a negative outcome (Rolf and Garmezy, 1990). Thus, not all individuals or families of a child with spina bifida will experience negative outcomes, but across this population there exists an increased risk of maladjustment. Given variability in the degree to which children and adolescents with spina bifida and their families experience negative outcomes, investigators have attempted to isolate predictors of such variability or to suggest mechanisms that might buffer, exacerbate, or mediate the impact of a chronic pediatric condition such as spina bifida on child and adolescent adjustment outcomes (Fig. 26.1). Such predictors may include demographic factors (e.g., socioeconomic status, ethnicity), individual variables (e.g., developmental changes, coping strategies), environmental factors (e.g., levels of social support, presence of other life stressors), or family variables (e.g., quality of parenting, quality of the marital relationship). Given the important socialization role that families play throughout childhood and adolescence (Rolf and Garmezy, 1990), coupled with the tendency for children and adolescents with spina bifida to experience less exposure to extrafamilial socialization agents relative to their typically developing peers (Blum et al., 1991), the impact of family functioning on child and adolescent psychosocial adjustment has been a focus of current research. This research shares the ultimate goal of providing improved understanding of the developmental trajectories of individuals with spina bifida, and may ultimately be used to inform both researchers and health-care professionals regarding how best to prevent maladjustment in this population. Although spina bifida is clearly a developmental disorder, little research has conceptualized it in this manner, and no studies to date have attempted to identify the impact of the disorder on psychosocial and familial functioning across different developmental periods.

The goal of this chapter is to review the literature on individual and family adjustment among families of children and adolescents with spina bifida. The chapter begins with an overview of a social-ecological model of individual child and adolescent adjustment. Then the literature on the psychosocial adjustment of children and adolescents with spina bifida is summarized, followed by a review of the research on the impact of spina bifida on family functioning. The next section describes the empirical relationship between family functioning and youth psychosocial adjustment. The chapter ends with a critique of the above lines of research, followed by recommendations for researchers and health-care professionals on the basis of the existing research.

A SOCIAL-ECOLOGICAL PREDICTION MODEL OF CHILD AND ADOLESCENT ADJUSTMENT

The social-ecological model of adjustment (Bronfenbrenner, 1979) offers a theoretical framework that helps explain the various factors that impact youth psychosocial adjustment. Although this model has been applied most commonly to typically developing populations, it is also of value in understanding the adaptation of children with chronic medical conditions such as spina bifida. As

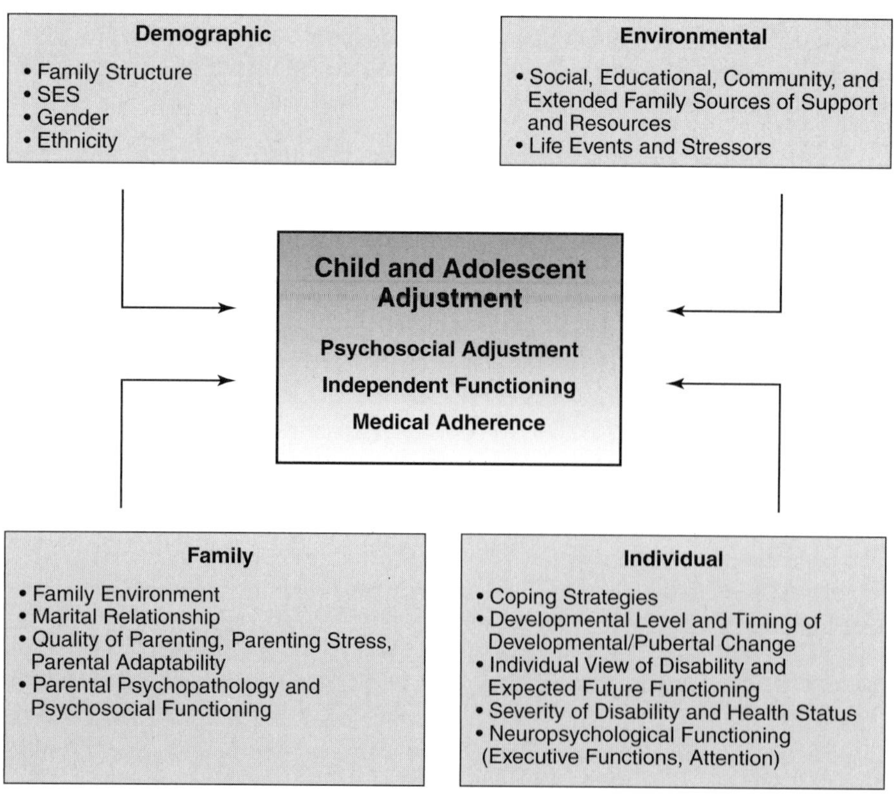

FIGURE 26.1. Social-ecological model of child and adolescent adjustment. SES, socioeconomic status.

depicted in Figure 26.1, various demographic, environmental, familial, and individual factors interact to affect child and adolescent outcomes in several domains including youth psychosocial adjustment, independent functioning, and medical adherence. More specifically, demographic factors such as the family's structure, economic background, or ethnicity may have implications for child and adolescent adjustment. Similarly, the resources available within the child's community, the extent of available support for the family, and the presence or absence of stressful life events may also impact child and adolescent adjustment. At a more proximal level, the nature of the relationships among family members, the psychosocial adjustment of the parent(s), and the childrearing strategies employed within the family may also directly influence child and adolescent adjustment. As discussed in subsequent sections, the functioning of the family system may be a particularly salient influence on youth adjustment among populations affected by spina bifida. Finally, the social-ecological prediction model calls attention to the importance of individual (i.e., child-level) factors as predictors of youth adjustment. Of particular relevance to children with spina bifida are (*1*) their neuropsychological functioning, (*2*) the timing of various developmental and pubertal changes, (*3*) the severity of the child's disability, (*4*) the child's health status, and (*5*) the child's perception of the impact of the disability on current and future functioning. In the section that follows, literature summarizing typical adjustment outcomes among children and adolescents with spina bifida is reviewed.

PSYCHOSOCIAL ADJUSTMENT OF CHILDREN AND ADOLESCENTS WITH SPINA BIFIDA

The presence of a chronic illness such as spina bifida impacts the developmental tasks of childhood and adolescence, resulting in increased vulnerability to psychosocial adjustment problems within this population. In fact, literature reviews support this contention and suggest that youth with chronic illnesses show higher rates of internalizing difficulties (i.e., emotional difficulties, feelings of depression, and symptoms of anxiety), externalizing problems (i.e., behavioral problems such as aggression and oppositionality), and lower self-concepts relative to their typically developing peers (e.g., Lavigne and Faier-Routman, 1992). As such, the presence of a chronic illness such as spina bifida may create additional challenges for psychosocial adaptation across childhood and adolescence. However, negative outcomes are not inevitable, as many children and adolescents with chronic illnesses function adaptively (Spaulding and Morgan, 1986; Van Hasselt et al., 1991; Lavigne and Faier-Routman, 1993). In the next section, the literature addressing the psychosocial adjustment of children and adolescents with spina bifida relative to their able-bodied counterparts is summarized, with attention devoted to adjustment outcomes in the following domains: (*1*) cognitive and academic functioning, (*2*) self-concept, (*3*) social functioning, and (*4*) emotional and behavioral functioning.

Cognitive and Academic Functioning

Children and adolescents with spina bifida, particularly those with shunted hydrocephalus, typically experience a pattern of cognitive impairment characterized, in part, by intellectual functioning in the low average range, with verbal domains intact relative to nonverbal (e.g., visual-motor, visual-spatial) domains (Friedrich et al., 1991; see Wills, 1993, for a review). Some research suggests that shunt status is negatively associated with intellectual functioning within this population, accounting for nearly 25% of the variance in IQ scores of youth with spina bifida in one study (Bier et al., 1997). Lesion level has also been associated with cognitive functioning, with higher lesion levels indicative of greater cognitive dysfunction (Bier et al., 1997).

In addition to impaired intellectual functioning, problems with inattention are common among children and adolescents with spina bifida, as are deficits in executive functioning (i.e., higher-order planning, mental flexibility, focused attention, ability to shift attention, working memory, and problem-solving skills), goal-directed behavior, and abstract reasoning (Landry et al., 1993; Fletcher et al., 2000; Brewer et al., 2001; Holmbeck et al., 2003b; Fletcher et al., 2004). It is important to note that measures of executive functions are not merely proxies for measures of IQ, given that group differences (e.g., hydrocephalus vs. no hydrocephalus) emerge for the former even when the latter are controlled (Dise and Lohr, 1998; Snow, 1999).

Many of the deficits manifested by children with spina bifida are consistent with the nonverbal learning disability syndrome (NLD) (Rourke et al., 2002), with roughly 50% of children with myelomeningocele exhibiting such deficits (Yeates et al., 2003). Rourke et al. (2002) have speculated that damage to cerebral white matter pathways (i.e., long myelinated fibers) that connect the frontal lobes and posterior right hemisphere (perhaps due to hydrocephalus, shunt placement, and brain anomalies in the corpus callosum, midbrain, and cerebellum; Fletcher et al., 2004) may be responsible for the deficits in executive functions (Fletcher et al., 1992a).

In addition, deficits in language pragmatics and inference-making skills are often documented among children and adolescents with spina bifida (Barnes and Dennis, 1998; Fletcher et al., 2004). *Language pragmatics* includes the ability to use language in a social and communicative manner. Children with such skills are able to understand what types of language are appropriate in which contexts, and they are more likely to know when and how to modify their language according to social demands. *Inference-making skills* include the ability to make inferences and extract meaning when reading or listening to a story and the ability to understand nonliteral language. It appears that children with spina bifida have deficits in all of these areas (Barnes and Dennis, 1998; Fletcher et al., 2004).

The aforementioned pattern of cognitive deficits has significant implications for the academic functioning of affected youth. In fact, research suggests that children with spina bifida, especially those who are shunted and from low socioeconomic backgrounds, demonstrate lower levels of scholastic competence, obtain lower grades in school, and score lower on several teacher-reported indicators of academic functioning (e.g., appropriate classroom behavior, ability to work hard in the classroom) relative to their typically developing peers (King et al., 1993; Holmbeck and Faier-Routman, 1995; Holmbeck et al., 2003b). Furthermore, most studies of children with spina bifida report academic achievement below expectation based on the child's intellectual abilities (see Wills, 1993, for a review), with performance in the areas of reading comprehension, writing, and math especially impaired (Wills et al., 1990; Fletcher et al., 1992b, 2004; Wills, 1993). Although the cognitive impairments associated with spina bifida may help to explain a number of the academic difficulties these children often have, the deficits in mathematics skills and the attention impairments characteristic of children with spina bifida seem not to be solely accounted for by group differences in intellectual functioning (Dennis and Barnes, 2002; Holmbeck et al., 2003b).

Research has identified several illness-related variables that may exacerbate the impact of spina bifida on cognitive and academic functioning including shunt status, lesion level, ambulation status, number of shunt-related surgeries, and overall illness severity (Holmbeck and Faier-Routman, 1995; Bier et al., 1997; Hommeyer et al., 1999). Findings regarding the impact of lesion level on cognitive and academic functioning are mixed, with some studies documenting poorer academic performance in children with higher lesion levels (Bier et al., 1997) and others failing to find a significant relationship between lesion level and academic functioning (Holmbeck and Faier-Routman, 1995). In contrast, shunt status has been consistently associated with cognitive and academic performance among youth with spina bifida. Specifically, children with shunts have been found to receive lower scholastic competence ratings, to earn poorer school grades, and to display more attention problems compared to unshunted children (Holmbeck and Faier-Routman, 1995; Hommeyer et al., 1999). Similarly, scholastic competence has been documented as higher for children who ambulate without assistance and have had fewer shunt-related surgeries (Hommeyer et al., 1999). Finally, Hommeyer and colleagues (1999) found that overall severity of the child's illness was negatively associated with scholastic competence and positively associated with attention problems.

The cognitive impairments associated with spina bifida not only impact child and adolescent academic functioning, but also have significant implications for the social, emotional, and behavioral functioning of children and adolescents with spina bifida. Tramontana and Hooper (1997) discuss several ways in which brain dysfunction and neuropsychological deficits may impact social, emotional, and behavioral adjustment. Specifically, they suggest that any or all of the following may occur: (*1*) abnormal brain activity may lead directly or indirectly to behavior problems or may alter an individual's personality or temperament; (*2*) children with brain dysfunction may be more likely to experience failure, frustration, and social stigma, which may produce or exacerbate already existing adjustment problems; or (*3*) family and peer reactions to neuropsychological difficulties (such as deficits in executive functions) may exacerbate levels of adjustment problems. Specific information regarding the ways in which cognitive factors influence social, emotional, and behavioral development will be discussed in each of the subsequent sections.

Self-Concept

Existing literature on the self-concepts of children and adolescents with spina bifida suggests that the presence of a physical disability such as spina bifida is a risk factor for lower perceived self-concept in several domains including athletic competence and physical appearance (Barakat and Linney, 1992; King et al., 1993; Appleton et al., 1994, 1997; Hommeyer et al., 1999; Holmbeck et al., 2003b; however, see Edwards-Beckett, 1995, for an exception to this trend). The impact of illness status on self-concept may be particularly significant for females, as results of a study by Appleton and colleagues (1997) suggest. Similarly, children with shunts to manage hydrocephalus are likely to display lower feelings of self-worth and reduced athletic competence relative to unshunted children (Holmbeck and Faier-Routman, 1995). Moreover, when adolescents believe that others view them as disabled, this may have negative implications for their own self-esteem (Wolman and Basco, 1994). Finally, the presence of peer rejection and teasing at school may exacerbate the risk of low self-worth among adolescents with spina bifida (Wolman and Basco, 1994).

In contrast, extant research has not supported a relationship between lesion level and child global self-worth (Holmbeck and Faier-Routman, 1995); however, condition severity has been negatively associated with perceived athletic competence. Additionally, certain factors may protect against the reduced self-esteem often seen among youth with spina bifida. For example, the findings of Wolman and Basco (1994) suggest that when parents treat adolescents in an age-appropriate manner and when adolescents perceive their parents as allowing them to participate in social interactions (rather than restricting their activity because of their disability), then adolescents are likely to evidence higher levels of self-esteem. Finally, as the results of a recent investigation by Appleton and colleagues (1997) suggest, perceptions of one's own physical appearance may have significant implications for symptoms of depression, and the link between physical appearance aspects of self-concept and depressed mood may be mediated by youth global self-worth. In other words, one's perception of one's physical appearance is directly associated with feelings of global self-worth, which in turn is related to symptoms of depression.

Social Functioning

Research suggests that children and adolescents with spina bifida are at increased risk of social isolation relative to their typically developing peers (Borjeson and Lagergren, 1990). Specifically, youth with spina bifida have been found to engage in less social contact outside of school (Borjeson and Lagergren, 1990; Blum et al., 1991; Kalucy et al., 1996; Holmbeck et al., 2003b), to be involved in fewer extracurricular or social activities (Blum et al., 1991; Hommeyer et al., 1999; Holmbeck et al., 2003b), to date less often (Cromer et al., 1990; Blum et al., 1991), to report more feelings of loneliness (Kazak and Clark, 1986; Lord et al., 1990; Blum et al., 1991), and to perceive themselves as less accepted in social contexts (King et al., 1993) relative to their able-bodied peers. In addition to reduced social contact, children with spina bifida often evidence impairments in their ability to interact effectively with peers. Specifically, research suggests that children with spina bifida are less socially competent than their able-bodied counterparts (Wallander et al., 1988; Lord et al., 1990; Ammerman et al., 1991; Van Hasselt et al., 1991; Nassau and Drotar, 1997; Holmbeck et al., 2003b), as well as in comparison to children with other non-central nervous system–related chronic conditions (Nassau and Drotar, 1997). Moreover, researchers have documented deficits in the ability to initiate and develop social connections among children with spina bifida (Holmbeck et al., 2003b), as well as increased levels of social immaturity within this population (Kazak and Clark, 1986; Blum et al., 1991). As the findings of King et al. (1993) suggest, deficits in adolescents' beliefs about their social skills may have important implications for their independent functioning. Although differences have been documented in the social competence of youth with spina bifida relative to age-matched controls, findings of Lemanek and colleagues (2000) suggest that the social skills of children with spina bifida do fall within the normal range of functioning when compared to normative values.

Given the differences in social skills as a function of illness status, research attention has also focused on identifying factors that may moderate this relationship. Some evidence suggests that demographic factors such as the family's socioeconomic background, when coupled with the presence of spina bifida, may constitute an additional risk factor for social difficulties even when the impact of cognitive functioning is taken into consideration (Holmbeck et al., 2003b). In contrast, demographic factors including the child's age and gender have not been consistently associated with child involvement in social activities (Kalucy et al., 1996). Attention has also been devoted to understanding the implications of medical status variables (i.e., condition severity or lesion level) for the social functioning of youth with spina bifida. In this domain, conflicting evidence exists. Whereas several studies have documented poorer social competence among children with more severe presentations (see Nassau and Drotar, 1997, for a review), others have reported no differences in children's social competence or peer activity involvement as a function of severity (Wallander et al., 1989a; Hommeyer et al., 1999) or type of spina bifida (Kalucy et al., 1996).

Some have argued that the social deficits often evident among youth affected by spina bifida may be directly related to the constellation of nonverbal cognitive deficits associated with hydrocephalus, which may inhibit a child's ability to read nonverbal cues, including facial expressions of emotion, thus negatively impacting the ability to understand fully and participate appropriately in social interactions (Rourke, 1989; Rourke et al., 2002). In addition, the ability to maintain and focus attention, employ working memory skills, monitor the impact of their own verbal and nonverbal behavior on other individuals, inhibit inappropriate social behaviors, demonstrate mental flexibility (as opposed to mental rigidity or perseverative behavior), make inferences during verbal discourse, and correctly identify and respond to the emotions of others are all expected to facilitate children's social interactions (Semrud-Clikeman and Hynd, 1991). Children who have deficits in executive functions, language skills, and emotion recognition are clearly at risk for peer rejection, given that such children likely appear impulsive, socially insensitive, and socially unskilled (Semrud-Clikeman and Hynd, 1991). Findings of a recent study by Hommeyer et al. (1999) support this contention and suggest that the relationship between shunt status and social functioning is mediated by (*1*) scholastic competence and (*2*) attention problems.

A complementary perspective, also advanced by Nassau and Drotar (1997), suggests that the physical manifestations of spina bifida (e.g., braces or assistive devices used for ambulation, unusual gait) may lead to stigmatization by peers, thus limiting the child's opportunities for age-appropriate social interaction. In support of this contention as related to individuals with spina bifida, Kalucy et al. (1996) found a significant relationship between ambulation status and number of friends; children who ambulated without assistance had significantly more friends. Similarly, Hommeyer et al. (1999) documented greater activity involvement among children with lower lesion levels, with less severe forms of spina bifida (lipomeningocele vs. myelomeningocele), and among those who ambulated either without assistance or with braces (relative to those who used wheelchairs for ambulation). Although little research has addressed the implications of social stigma on the development of social competence among children and adolescents with spina bifida, a body of research on individuals with physical disabilities suggests that children tend to display preferences for typically developing playmates compared to physically disabled ones (Nabors and Keyes, 1997; Weiserbs and Gottlieb, 2000). As such, physically disabled children have fewer opportunities to develop proficient social skills given their tendency toward social isolation. These deficient social skills, in turn, may contribute to further social isolation and peer rejection.

Emotional and Behavioral Functioning

The presence of a chronic illness, such as spina bifida, also has implications for child and adolescent emotional and behavioral adjustment. Several areas of emotional and behavioral functioning have been explored by current researchers including internalizing symptoms (e.g., depression, anxiety, somatic concerns), externalizing symptoms (e.g., oppositional behavior, aggressiveness), inattention and hyperactivity, levels of independent functioning and adaptive behavior, and assertiveness within the family context.

Regarding internalizing symptomatology, researchers have documented higher rates of depression and anxiety among children and adolescents with spina bifida (Blum, 1983; Wallander et al., 1989b; Borjeson and Lagergren, 1990; Appleton et al., 1997; Ammerman, et al., 1998; Holmbeck et al., 2003b). Specifically, youth (and particularly girls) with spina bifida have been shown to display greater symptoms of depression including increased feelings of nonspecific guilt and higher levels of suicidal ideation than their able-bodied counterparts (Wallander et al., 1989b; Borjeson and Lagergren, 1990; Appleton et al., 1997; Zurmohle et al., 1998). Similarly, increased levels of somatic concerns and other symptoms of anxiety have been documented within this population (Blum, 1983; Ammerman et al., 1998; Holmbeck et al., 2003b; however, see Zurmohle et al., 1998, for documentation of no differences in anxiety among children with spina bifida compared to their healthy counterparts).

Recent literature has suggested that apparent differences in internalizing symptoms as a function of illness status may be less salient (*1*) when examining adolescent self reports of symptoms in comparison to parent reports of symptoms (Ammerman et al., 1998), (*2*) when focusing on preadolescent populations rather than samples of adolescents (Barakat and Linney, 1992; Holmbeck et al., 2003b), and (*3*) when first accounting for the impact of cognitive ability level (Holmbeck et al., 2003b). Regarding the last point, Holmbeck et al. found that the rates of self-reported depressive symptoms among children with spina bifida were no longer significantly different from those of a demographically matched comparison sample after accounting for the impact of cognitive functioning, suggesting that the elevated scores among children with spina bifida may have been due to item misinterpretation among those at lower cognitive levels.

Despite the tendency for children and adolescents with spina bifida to display more internalizing symptoms relative to externalizing problems (Fletcher et al., 1995; Ammerman et al., 1998), a body of research suggests that youth with spina bifida also show above-average rates of externalizing problems (Wallander et al., 1989b; Van Hasselt et al., 1991; Fletcher et al., 1995; Ammerman et al., 1998; however, see Lord et al., 1990, for a contrasting perspective). For example, Ammerman and colleagues found that 13% of their sample met criteria for oppositional defiant disorder. Subclinical externalizing problems have also been documented in the literature, indicating that youth with spina bifida may be at risk for milder forms of behavioral maladjustment, such as oppositionality and aggressiveness, relative to normative comparisons (Wallander et al., 1988; however, see Lemanek et al., 2000, for a differential pattern of findings). In contrast, when compared to samples of clinic-referred youth, the behavioral functioning of children and adolescents with spina bifida appears to be less impaired (Wallander et al., 1988). Thus, as the results of Van Hasselt et al. (1991) suggest, although youth with spina bifida may display higher levels of externalizing problems in comparison to their typically developing counterparts, these problems are not typically so severe that they interfere significantly with their daily functioning. Of note is the fact that determining the prevalence of externalizing behaviors within this population is challenging, given the restrictions on mobility that many children with spina bifida experience.

Regarding symptoms of inattention and hyperactivity, children with spina bifida are reported to have higher rates of attention deficit/hyperactivity disorder (ADHD) relative to the general population. In a study by Ammerman and colleagues (1998), 33% of the children surveyed met criteria for ADHD, with symptoms of inattention endorsed more commonly than symptoms of hyperactivity or impulsivity. Similarly, Fletcher et al. (2004) found that 31% of children with average cognitive functioning displayed ADHD, the majority of whom met criteria for the inattentive type. Moreover, of those children who met criteria for the hyperactive or combined subtypes, symptoms of hyperactivity typically included verbal disinhibition or disorganization, likely reflecting difficulties with pragmatic language rather than true behavioral disinhibition (Fletcher et al., 2004).

Given the heightened risk of emotional and behavioral adjustment difficulties among children and adolescents with spina bifida, attention has been devoted to identifying factors that may protect against or exacerbate the risk of negative outcomes. With respect to internalizing symptoms, the following factors have been empirically associated with higher levels of internalizing problems: (*1*) more shunt-related surgeries (Hommeyer et al., 1999); (*2*) difficult child temperament (Lavigne et al., 1988); (*3*) greater child distractibility (Lavigne et al., 1988); and (*4*) higher levels of recent life stress (Murch and Cohen, 1989). Regarding externalizing symptoms, research suggest the following factors as demonstrating predictive utility for higher levels of behavioral dysfunction: (*1*) presence of a shunt or hydrocephalus (Holmbeck and Faier-Routman, 1995; Zurmohle et al., 1998); (*2*) lower socioeconomic status (Holmbeck et al., 2003a); (*3*) greater family psychological and material resources (Wallander et al., 1989b); (*4*) higher levels of family cohesiveness (Lavigne et al., 1988); (*5*) poorer child social skills (Lemanek et al., 2000); (*6*) greater child distractibility (Lavigne et al., 1988); and (*7*) fewer child self-coping skills (Lavigne et al., 1988). Although medical factors (i.e., the presence of a shunt to treat hydrocephalus, number of shunt-related surgeries) are risk factors unique to the spina bifida population, the aforementioned nonmedical demographic and environmental factors may also be predictive of adjustment difficulties in youth without spina bifida.

Concerning shunt status, recent research by Hommeyer and colleagues (1999) suggests that the relationship between shunt status and externalizing problems (specifically aggressive behavior) is mediated by child scholastic competence. In contrast, links between internalizing and externalizing symptomatology and (*1*) illness severity, (*2*) ambulation status, (*3*) lesion level, (*4*) child age, and (*5*) child gender are less clear, with some studies documenting no relationships between the aforementioned variables and externalizing symptoms (Holmbeck and Faier-Routman, 1995; Hommeyer et al., 1999) and others suggesting significant links (Lemanek et al., 2000). Most notably, Lemanek et al. (2002) documented significantly higher levels of maternal-reported behavior problems among children with mild spina bifida relative to children with moderately severe spina bifida, among boys relative to girls, and among older children relative to younger children.

Deficits in the independent behavior and adaptive functioning of youth with spina bifida have also been documented by researchers (Blum et al., 1991; Barakat and Linney, 1992; King et al., 1993; Holmbeck et al., 2003b). Specifically, adolescents with spina bifida have been found to display reduced levels of behavioral autonomy, which may be due, in part, to their need for parental assistance in performing illness-related tasks (Blum et al., 1991; Holmbeck et al., 2003a). Similarly, preadolescents with spina bifida evidence lower levels of intrinsic motivation and have fewer responsibilities at home in comparison to their typically developing counterparts (Blum et al., 1991; Holmbeck et al., 2003a). On observational assessments of dependent behavior, preadolescents were rated as more needy, more likely to seek physical contact, more likely to act in an immature manner, and less likely to express their own opinions in a recent study by Holmbeck and colleagues (2003a). Finally, on indices of independent behavior in the social context, adolescents with spina bifida have been shown to evidence less independence relative to their able-bodied counterparts (King et al., 1993). One factor that may help explain the deficits in independent behaviors may be poorly developed executive functioning skills. Specifically, children who are less able to exhibit planning and problem-solving abilities on tests of executive functions may be less able to develop independent functioning skills.

Moreover, within the family context, research suggests that children with spina bifida may take on a more passive role compared to their typically developing peers (Holmbeck et al., 2002a, 2003b). For example, Holmbeck et al. (2003a) found that relative to their able-bodied counterparts, preadolescents with spina bifida displayed a more passive interaction style, were less assertive in expressing their opinions during family discussions, and were less attentive to the opinions of others in an observational family interaction task, even after controlling for the impact of cognitive ability level.

Summary

Current research suggests that children and adolescents with spina bifida are at risk for psychosocial maladjustment across a number of domains. Specifically, researchers have documented cognitive and academic difficulties among this population, as well as lower levels of self-worth (particularly in athletic competence and physical appearance), reduced social contact, impaired social skills, and higher rates of emotional and behavioral difficulties. Although the presence of spina bifida constitutes a risk factor for the aforementioned negative outcomes, there exists substantial individual variability in psychosocial adjustment, such that not all children with spina bifida are expected to experience negative outcomes. Moreover, as the findings of Lemanek and others suggest (e.g., Lemanek et al., 2000), even when differences in various domains of adjustment are documented between youth with spina bifida and typically developing youth, often the functioning of children with spina bifida is within normal limits. Furthermore, several areas of psychosocial functioning (e.g., coping skills, global self-worth) may be resilient to the impact of pediatric chronic illness, as suggested by Holmbeck and colleagues (2003b). Finally, as previously reviewed, a variety of factors both intrinsic to the individual (e.g., illness-related variables, temperament) and within the larger environment (e.g., demographic factors, parental and familial functioning) may either protect against or increase the likelihood of negative outcomes (see Fig. 26.1). Just as the presence of spina bifida has implications for individual functioning, so too does it affect family adjustment. The section that follows considers the impact of spina bifida on family functioning.

FAMILY FUNCTIONING

In addition to focusing attention on the impact of spina bifida on individual psychosocial adjustment, researchers have been interested in investigating the impact of spina bifida on family functioning (see Holmbeck et al., 2003a, for a review). Several domains of family functioning have been attended to, including (*1*) the family environment or family climate, (*2*) the parenting practices a caregiver uses within the family, (*3*) the parents' martial relationship, and (*4*) the psychological functioning of the parents. With few exceptions, this body of literature has focused on identifying differences in family functioning as a result of illness status (i.e., differences between families in which a child has spina bifida compared to families in which there is a typically developing offspring). As noted by Holmbeck et al. (2003a), the extent to which differences between groups have emerged in past studies is, at least in part, a function of the number of participants surveyed. Whereas studies with larger samples have typically found between-groups differences, studies with smaller samples have often failed to document significant discrepancies, suggesting that a lack of power in many research designs may obscure important group differences. Research addressing family functioning in each of these domains will be summarized in the following sections.

Family Environment

Several aspects of the family environment have been investigated by researchers including levels of family stress, impairment, cohesion, and conflict. In general, results of such research are mixed, with some studies offering support for significant family-level differences as a function of illness status (e.g., Loomis et al., 1997; Ammerman et al., 1998) and other studies documenting an absence of noteworthy differences relative to families of a typically developing child (Spaulding and Morgan, 1986) or compared to families of children with other chronic conditions (Loebig, 1990). On a theoretical level, some have argued that caring for a child with a chronic pediatric condition such as spina bifida adds significant stress to the family system (Carr, 1991) and places the family at risk for functional impairment. In support of this contention, one study found that approximately 12% of families of youth with spina bifida fell within the clinically problematic range on a general measure of family functioning, with difficulties especially prominent in the family's ability to establish and maintain family roles and responsibilities (Wiegner and Donders, 2000; see also Kazak and Clark, 1986; Loomis et al., 1997; Ammerman et al., 1998). In contrast, other studies have found no significant differences in reports of stressful life events when comparing matched samples of families of preadolescents with and without spina bifida (Holmbeck et al., 2002a). Low socioeconomic status, ethnic minority status, and single-parent status have been documented as risk factors for higher levels of family stress among families of chronically ill children (Carr, 1991), as have child health status and available family resources to manage the child's chronic condition (McCormick et al., 1986). The moderating influence of these variables may, in part, help to explain the incongruous findings discussed above. Thus, it may be that the presence of spina bifida alone is not associated with a less optimal family climate; instead, when families are faced with rearing a child with spina bifida and are also experiencing other stressors (e.g., high levels of economic strain), family functioning may be more impaired. Similarly, the degree to which the child evidences psychological symptoms or impairments in his or her daily living skills has been found to positively predict the impact the illness has on the family, likely reflecting the increased caregiving burden present in families of children with more severe impairments (Havermans and Eiser, 1991).

In addition to an interest in discrepancies in levels of family stress and impairment as a function of illness status, investigators have attempted to assess the degree to which families affected by spina bifida evidence differences in levels of family cohesion. Holmbeck and colleagues (2002a) examined differences in levels of family cohesion in a sample of families of preadolescents with and without spina bifida using both observational and self-report measures. Their findings revealed that although families of preadolescents with spina bifida were less cohesive than families of typically developing children, the child's cognitive status mediated this relationship, such that children in the spina bifida group displayed lower levels of cognitive functioning, and lower levels of cognitive functioning were associated with lower levels of family cohesion. In a follow-up study, Coakley et al. (2002) documented a differential pattern of change in family cohesion across the adolescent transition among families of children with spina bifida and families of typically developing preadolescents. Specifically, their results suggested that levels of family cohesion increased over time in the spina bifida group (especially among those children who reached puberty early), while they decreased over time in the comparison group (especially among those children who reached puberty early).

With respect to differences in levels of family conflict as a function of illness status, research suggests lower levels of conflict among families of preadolescents with spina bifida relative to families of able-bodied preadolescents (Coakley et al., 2002). An increase in family conflict during puberty is normative, and consistent with the literature on pubertal development, typically developing preadolescents who experience early pubertal onset are at risk for heightened levels of family conflict (Coakley et al., 2002). Interestingly, families of early maturing youth with spina bifida do not show this pubertal effect, leading Coakley and colleagues to speculate that parents of children with spina bifida may be less reactive to the maturational changes in their offspring, even perhaps denying the presence of such development. Finally, among families of children with spina bifida, it seems that higher levels of child functional impairment (as evidenced by higher lesion levels) are associated with lower levels of family conflict (Holmbeck and Faier-Routman, 1995).

Parenting Behaviors

Several studies have documented differences in the childrearing strategies of parents of a child with spina bifida compared to parents of a typically developing child. Three parenting behaviors have been particularly well studied given their consistent association with psychosocial adjustment outcomes among typically developing children (Baumrind, 1991; Steinberg et al., 1992, 1994; Barber and Harmon, 2002): parental psychological control, behavioral control, and acceptance. *Psychological control* refers to parenting behavior characterized by covert and intrusive controlling of the child's emotions and behaviors, which inhibits autonomy development (Gray and Steinberg, 1999; Barber and Harmon, 2002). *Behavioral control* involves parental establishment and enforcement of age-appropriate rules and expectations for the child's behavior (Maccoby and Martin, 1983; Steinberg, 1990). *Acceptance* involves the expression of high levels of emotional support, positive evaluation, and affection toward the child (Maccoby and Martin, 1983; Gray and Steinberg, 1999).

In general, the existing body of research suggests that parents, and particularly mothers, of children with spina bifida are more likely to engage in less adaptive forms of parental control, including higher levels of overprotectiveness and psychological control relative to parents of able-bodied children (Holmbeck et al., 2002b, 2002c). Moreover, Holmbeck et al. (2002c) documented lower levels of behavioral control among fathers of children with spina bifida relative to fathers of typically developing preadolescents. Of note is the finding of Holmbeck et al. (2002b) that group differences in levels of overprotection are partially mediated by children's cognitive ability level. Thus, children with spina bifida are more likely to have lower levels of cognitive ability, and children with reduced cognitive abilities are, in turn, more likely to have parents who display high levels of overprotection (Holmbeck et al., 2002b). Anderson and Coyne (1993) have articulated a theory to help explain the process by which the child's illness status may impact parenting. According to their *miscarried helping theory,* children with chronic illnesses often require parental assistance in performing daily self-care or illness-related tasks because of the physical limitations that accompany their illness. Over time, parents' intentions to assist their children in performing illness-related tasks may generalize to other areas and can result in the use of high degrees of psychological control to gain compliance in domains outside of those directly related to the illness. Despite the tendency for parents of children with spina bifida to use less adaptive methods of control, research suggests the existence of few differences between parents of children with spina bifida and parents of typically developing children with respect to levels of parental acceptance (Holmbeck et al., 2002c) or with regard to their parenting attitudes (Spaulding and Morgan 1986).

Several variables have been found to moderate the relationship between illness status and parenting behaviors. In one study, mothers of children with higher lesion levels (i.e., lumbar or thoracic) and less functional impairment were more willing to grant autonomy to their children compared to mothers of children with lower (i.e., sacral) lesion levels (Holmbeck and Faier-Routman, 1995). The authors argued that these findings supported a *marginality hypothesis* that suggests that families of children with less severe versions of a disability may demonstrate more functional impairments because they do not clearly belong to either a chronically ill group or a typically developing group (Holmbeck and Faier-Routman, 1995). Socioeconomic status has also been associated with the parenting behaviors used within the family (Seefeldt et al., 1997). Specifically, across able-bodied and spina bifida families, parents from lower socioeconomic backgrounds may use less adaptive and less child-centered methods of control, with this effect being especially pronounced among families of a child with spina bifida from low socioeconomic strata (Seefeldt et al., 1997).

Marital Functioning

In comparison to the body of literature investigating differences in the family environment and parenting behaviors of families affected by spina bifida versus unaffected families, far less research has focused on delineating discrepancies in marital functioning across the two groups. The studies that have addressed marital functioning have generally suggested that the marital relationship is a domain that is resilient to any potentially negative effects of spina bifida. Thus, some studies have found no differences in marital satisfaction or marital adjustment between parents of children with spina bifida and parents of able-bodied children (Spaulding and Morgan, 1986; Cappelli et al., 1994; Holmbeck et al., 1997). Furthermore, Cappelli et al. (1994) suggest that mothers and fathers have similar perceptions about the marital functioning within their families. Moreover, some limited evidence suggests that rearing a child with a more severe disability can strengthen the marital relationship (Kazak and Clark, 1986; Cappelli et al., 1994).

Some authors have suggested that the quality of the marital relationship prior to the child's birth may be an important predictor of later marital adjustment. In addition, as the findings of Cappelli et al. (1994) suggest, parental stress, parental symptoms of depression, and parental perceptions of role constraints are all factors that may be negatively associated with marital quality. Interestingly, several child-level factors have also been associated with less adaptive marital functioning for mothers, including rearing a male child and parenting a preschool child (Cappelli et al., 1994).

Parental Psychological Functioning

Research investigating the adjustment of parents of youth affected by spina bifida suggests that both mothers and fathers are vulnerable to maladjustment and distress (e.g., Wiegner and Donders, 2000). Specifically, mothers have been found to have higher levels of stress, to hold less optimistic views about the future, to be more socially isolated, to evidence less adaptability to change, and to report lower levels of parenting competence and satisfaction compared to mothers of children with other medical conditions (Wallander et al., 1989; Barakat and Linney, 1995) and compared to mothers of typically developing children (Holmbeck et al., 1997). Similarly, mothers of children with spina bifida have been found to display increased psychiatric symptoms, including elevated levels of depression, anxiety, and global distress, relative to normative comparisons (Kronenberger and Thompson, 1992a). A similar pattern of findings has been documented with respect to paternal psychosocial functioning. Holmbeck et al. (1997) found that fathers of children with spina bifida displayed higher levels of psychosocial stress, lower levels of parental satisfaction, and greater symptoms of depression, anxiety, and distress compared to fathers of typically developing children (Holmbeck et al., 1997).

Although many studies have documented significant differences in parental psychological functioning across groups, this trend is not universal. In fact, Lemanek and colleagues (2000) found no significant differences in maternal ratings of psychological distress when comparing a sample of mothers of children with spina bifida to the sample on which the measure was normed. Moreover, results of this study suggested that although mothers reported less stress than fathers, levels of distress reported by both parents fell within the normal range of functioning (Lemanek et al., 2000). Similarly, Barakat and Linney (1992) documented no significant differences in levels of maternal social support or maternal psychological adjustment as a function of illness status.

Given the variability in parental psychosocial outcomes, several studies have suggested factors that may buffer against parental adjustment difficulties including the presence of strong support networks both within (Kronenberger and Thompson, 1992b) and outside of the family (Barakat and Linney, 1992; Horton and Wallander, 2001), fewer perceived life stressors (Wiegner and Donders, 2000), low levels of interfamilial conflict (Kronenberger and Thompson, 1992b), adaptive family functioning (Fagan and Schor, 1993; Wiegner and Donders, 2000), younger maternal age (Macias et al., 2001), adaptive maternal cognitive appraisal style (Kronenberger and Thompson, 1992a; Horton and Wallander, 2001), and positive marital functioning (Kronenberger and Thompson 1992b). Finally, research suggests that the level of a child's disability may impact parental psychosocial functioning in both positive and negative ways. For example, Havermans and Eiser (1991) found that although mothers of children with higher levels of disability reported more difficulties in daily living compared to mothers of children with lower levels of disability, they also evidenced higher confidence in managing the child's condition than mothers of less impaired children did.

Summary

Research supports the notion that the presence of spina bifida impacts family functioning in a variety of domains. Specifically, empirical investigations suggest that families of children and adolescents with spina bifida may be at risk for several negative outcomes including higher levels of family stress, lower levels of cohesion, more maladaptive forms of parental control, and greater impairments in parental psychological functioning. In contrast, research has also suggested that other key areas of family functioning (e.g., levels of family conflict, parental acceptance, and marital functioning) may be less negatively influenced or in some cases actually enhanced by the impact of a pediatric chronic illness. Taken together, this body of research supports a *resilience-disruption hypothesis* of family adaptation (Costigan et al., 1997) that states that families of children with spina bifida are both resilient to and disrupted by the stress associated with rearing a chronically ill child. In the next section, the focus shifts to a discussion of the relationship between family functioning and youth psychosocial adjustment within this population.

FAMILY FUNCTIONING AND CHILD AND ADOLESCENT PSYCHOSOCIAL ADJUSTMENT

The social-ecological model of adjustment (Bronfenbrenner, 1979), introduced earlier, suggests that factors in a variety of ecological domains may influence child and adolescent adaptation (see Fig. 26.1). While factors from each domain may influence child and adolescent adaptation, the impact of family factors on adjustment outcomes may be particularly important for several reasons. First, although the peer group takes on increasing salience during early and middle adolescence (Harris, 1995), many researchers still consider the family to be the primary socialization agent during this time period (Maccoby and Martin, 1983; Steinberg et al., 1995). Furthermore, research in the area of developmental psychopathology suggests that the quality of the family relationship can serve as either a protective or risk factor for child adjustment difficulties (Rolf and Garmezy, 1990). Adaptive family relationships may promote continued adaptive adjustment in children who are well adjusted or it may protect against negative adjustment outcomes in an at-risk child. Similarly, maladaptive parent–child relationships may make a well-adjusted child more susceptible to psychosocial adjustment difficulties or intensify the level of problems already present in an at-risk child. Finally, because children and adolescents with spina bifida tend to be more socially isolated than their able-bodied counterparts (Blum et al., 1991), they experience less exposure to socialization agents outside the family. For these reasons, the quality of the family environment is likely to be an especially salient predictor of adjustment among this population relative to the other social-ecological domains. In fact, a body of research has documented relationships between various domains of family functioning and child and adolescent psychosocial adjustment. In the sections that follow, research investigating relationships between various aspects of youth psychosocial adjustment and (*1*) family environment, (*2*) parenting behaviors, (*3*) marital functioning, and (*4*) parental psychosocial functioning will be summarized.

Family Environment and Youth Adjustment

Some research has suggested that the quality of the family environment can significantly impact youth psychosocial adjustment. Specifically, family cohesion has been positively associated with children's use of problem-focused coping strategies (McKernon et al., 2001) and negatively associated with internalizing and externalizing problems (Lavigne et al., 1988). Similarly, family conflict and control have been positively associated with symptoms of anxiety and depression (Murch and Cohen, 1989). In addition, low levels of family conflict and control, as well as high levels of family expressiveness, cohesion, and independence, have been linked to higher self-esteem levels among adolescents with spina bifida (Murch and Cohen, 1989). Moreover, a stress-buffering effect of low levels of family conflict and control on the relationship between negative life events and depressive symptoms has been documented in the literature, as has a stress-exacerbating effect of high levels of perceived family independence in the prediction of adolescent distress (Murch and Cohen, 1989).

Parenting Behavior and Youth Adjustment

In addition to an interest in the impact of family environmental characteristics on youth adjustment, a body of literature has examined the link between parenting behaviors and child emotional and behavioral functioning. Findings to date suggest a positive relationship between parental acceptance and children's use of adaptive coping methods including problem-focused strategies (McKernon et al., 2001), observational accounts of children's adaptive behavior (Holmbeck et al., 2002c), and teacher-reported grades (Holmbeck et al., 2002c) for youth with and without spina bifida. Negative associations between parental acceptance and preadolescent externalizing symptoms across illness contexts have also been documented (Holmbeck et al., 2002c). Findings on the relationship between parental acceptance and internalizing symptoms is less clear. Whereas evidence suggests a positive association between maternal acceptance and internalizing symptoms among preadolescents with spina bifida (particularly females), the opposite relationship has been documented regarding the impact of paternal acceptance on internalizing symptoms, particularly among males with spina bifida (Appleton et al., 1997; Holmbeck et al., 2002c).

Regarding the impact of parental monitoring and behavioral control on preadolescent adjustment, research findings are less robust. Conflicting evidence regarding the link between parental behavioral control and preadolescent externalizing symptoms emerged from a study by Holmbeck and colleagues (2002c). Whereas higher levels of mother-reported behavioral control were associated with more externalizing symptoms and lower adaptive behavior among preadolescents with spina bifida, observational assessments of maternal behavioral control were negatively associated with male externalizing behavior. Finally, a link between parental behavioral control and internalizing symptoms has been documented in the literature, with parent and child gender emerging as important moderators of this relationship. Specifically, Holmbeck et al. (2002c) documented a positive association between maternal and paternal behavioral control and female internalizing symptoms but a negative association between paternal behavioral control and internalizing symptoms for males. Across domains, maternal behavioral control was a more salient predictor than paternal behavioral control of preadolescent adjustment.

Negative associations between levels of parental psychological control and child adjustment across illness contexts have been documented (Holmbeck et al., 2002c). Specifically, increased psychological control has been associated with higher levels of internalizing and externalizing symptoms and lower levels of preadolescent adaptive behavior among children with and without spina bifida (Holmbeck et al., 2002c). In a recent study by Holmbeck et al. (2002b), the utility of a mediational model that related parental overprotectiveness (a construct similar to psychological control) to adolescent adjustment problems via parental behavioral autonomy granting was tested. Results suggested the following: (*1*) Questionnaire and observational measures of parental overprotectiveness displayed a significant negative association with measures of behavioral autonomy across both the spina bifida and comparison samples. (*2*) Questionnaire measures of maternal and paternal overprotectiveness displayed significant associations with preadolescent externalizing symptoms and depression, while maternal overprotectiveness was associated significantly with preadolescent behavioral conduct. In all cases, greater levels of parental overprotection were associated with less adaptive functioning among preadolescents with spina bifida. (*3*) Within the spina bifida group, higher levels of parental overprotection (as assessed via questionnaires) were associated with less behavioral autonomy granting. Less autonomy, in turn, was associated with more externalizing symptoms.

Finally, in a recent study by Friedman and colleagues (Friedman et al., 2004), higher levels of paternal parenting stress were both prospectively and concurrently associated with child adjustment over time among preadolescents with and without spina bifida. Specifically, in prospective analyses, paternal parenting stress predicted increasing child externalizing symptoms, while concurrent analyses suggested a positive association between paternal parenting stress and preadolescent internalizing symptoms.

Marital Functioning and Youth Adjustment

The body of literature investigating the relationship between marital functioning and youth adjustment among families affected by spina bifida is quite small, with only one study to date explicitly testing such a model. Friedman and colleagues (2004) investigated the relationship between marital satisfaction and several domains of child adjustment including internalizing symptoms, externalizing behaviors, and observed adaptive behavior. Their findings suggested that across both families of children with spina bifida and families of able-bodied children, higher levels of marital satisfaction were prospectively related to (*1*) fewer child externalizing symptoms over time and (*2*) higher levels of child adaptive functioning over time. Contrary to expectation, among families of children with spina bifida, higher levels of marital satisfaction were also associated with greater child-reported symptoms of depression over time. The researchers speculate that among families of children with spina bifida, greater attention to the marital relationship may come at the expense of too little attention to the child, resulting in greater feelings of depression among preadolescents with spina bifida.

Parental Psychological Functioning and Youth Adjustment

With respect to the relationship between parental psychological functioning and youth adjustment, research suggests a negative association between children's problem behaviors and levels of parental social support and parenting satisfaction (Wallander and Varni, 1989; Barakat and Linney, 1992; Lemanek et al., 2000), as well as a positive relationship between parenting satisfaction and youth social skills (Lemanek et al., 2000). In the same vein, Barakat and Linney (1995) documented a positive relationship between maternal use of avoidant coping strategies and child internalizing problems. In a study by Friedman et al. (2004), higher levels of both maternal and paternal psychiatric symptomatology were associated with increases in child externalizing symptoms across middle childhood, while concurrent changes in parental psychological functioning predicted changes in preadolescent internalizing symptoms. Specifically, among children with and without spina bifida, increasing parental symptomatology predicted higher rates of internalizing symptoms (Friedman et al., 2004). Finally, Edwards-Beckett (1995) found no relationship between parental expectations for child future functioning and child self-concept in a sample of 30 children with spina bifida.

Summary

Various facets of family functioning have been associated with child and adolescent psychosocial adjustment. Taken together, this body of research suggests that the presence of adaptive family environments (characterized in part by low levels of conflict and high levels of cohesiveness), the use of effective childrearing techniques by parents (i.e., high levels of acceptance and low levels of psychological control), healthy marital functioning, and the adaptive psychosocial adjustment of the child's caregivers are factors that increase the likelihood of positive adjustment outcomes among youth affected by spina bifida, findings similar to those that have emerged in studies of typically developing children. In contrast, difficulties in one or more of these areas may intensify the risk of negative child and adolescent outcomes. Despite our growing understanding of the adjustment correlates of spina bifida for both individual and family functioning, and the relationship between family functioning and individual psychosocial outcomes, this body of research is characterized by several important limitations that will be delineated in the following section.

LIMITATIONS OF PAST RESEARCH

Although researchers have begun to focus on the impact of spina bifida on individual and family processes, as well as the relationship between family functioning and youth psychosocial adjustment, these lines of research are still largely in their infancy. In this section, we highlight several limitations of the extant research in the hope of elucidating avenues for future empirical attention.

First, several key domains of psychosocial adjustment among children and adolescents have been largely neglected by past research. Specifically, relatively little attention has focused on investigating factors that impact self-esteem among children and adolescents with spina bifida. Given the relationship between low levels of self-esteem and the presence of depressive symptoms, identification of factors that positively impact self-esteem may have implications for prevention of internalizing symptoms within this population. Similarly, few observational studies of social functioning and peer relationships among youth with spina bifida have been undertaken. Efforts to conduct observational studies of social functioning within this population could provide a more ecologically valid assessment of the nature of the social deficits that children with spina bifida experience, thereby identifying targets for intervention. An additional area neglected by past research is adherence to a medical regimen. Only one study to date has investigated adherence behaviors within this population (Holmbeck et al., 1998). Given the various tasks associated with successful management of spina bifida (e.g., taking medications, catheterization, bowel programs, limb movement to avoid pressure sores), as well as the implications of poor adherence for individual and family functioning, more research in this area is needed. Finally, although the impact of chronic health issues (e.g., frequent hospitalizations, the need to take medications that negatively impact cognitive functioning, precocious puberty, and obesity in adolescence) on psychosocial adjustment is commonly addressed in clinical settings, little attention has been devoted to such factors in published research. A greater focus on the above domains would help to elucidate the wide-ranging impact of spina bifida on child and adolescent psychosocial functioning.

In addition to the need for exploration of a wider range of psychosocial adjustment outcomes, a greater focus on spina bifida as a developmental disorder with different implications for psychosocial adjustment as a function of developmental level is warranted. Much of the extant research has used samples of children and adolescents across a wide age range. Moreover, many studies to date have focused on the impact of spina bifida on individual and family functioning with samples of children, to the exclusion of adolescents and young adults (a trend also observed in studies of other chronically ill populations) (Drotar, 1997). Clearly, the developmental tasks most salient during early childhood are not the same as those of middle childhood or adolescence. Similarly, within the adolescent developmental period, substantial variability exists in the nature of peer and romantic relationships, levels of behavioral and emotional autonomy, and cognitive processes when comparing young adolescents to older adolescents. Given that spina bifida is a disorder that persists across the life span, greater research attention to changes in individual and family functioning over time is necessary.

Just as future research should expand its breadth to include the aforementioned individual psychosocial domains, greater attention should also be paid to the impact of spina bifida on more diverse family processes. As suggested by Drotar (1997), most studies to date have investigated general family processes rather than looking at illness-specific family behaviors (e.g., the role that parents play in facilitating adherence to various aspects of the treatment regimen, the impact of the child's limited mobility on levels of parental or familial stress, or the impact on well siblings of increased attention given to children with spina bifida as a result of their treatment regimen, frequent medical appointments, and recurrent hospitalizations). Moreover, little attention has focused on the relationship between family characteristics and youth cognitive functioning, academic functioning, or adherence behaviors in samples of individuals affected by spina bifida (although see Holmbeck and Faier-Routman, 1995, for an exception to this trend). Attention to such relationships could help identify family-based targets for intervention or prevention of difficulties in these domains.

In addition to the aforementioned shortcomings focused on the content domains of current research, the literature is plagued by a number of methodological limitations that threaten both the validity and generalizability of documented findings. For example, a number of studies have relied on single-method (typically questionnaire) and single-reporter (typically mother) data collection strategies, making it difficult to rule out common-method variance explanations of the findings. Moreover, some have argued that given the increased risk for psychological distress among mothers of children with spina bifida, their estimates of child functioning may be biased. Thus, greater attention to recruiting both mothers and fathers and to incorporating child, peer, and teacher perspectives would be of high value. In addition, samples used in current research are often quite small, resulting in low power to detect differences between groups (Holmbeck et al., 2003a). Also, samples are often relatively homogeneous with respect to socioeconomic status and ethnicity, failing to include diverse populations of children and families (Holmbeck et al., 2003a). The Hispanic population of children and adolescents with spina bifida is especially underrepresented in current research, and generalizability of research to this and other ethnic groups besides middle-class Caucasian populations is limited. Because spina bifida is more common among individuals from northern climates, the task of recruiting culturally diverse samples is particularly challenging, however (Ammerman et al., 1998). Many researchers to date have also employed retrospective cross-sectional research designs in which they rely on telephone or mail-in data collection strategies rather than using prospective longitudinal approaches, which allow for an assessment of individual change over time (Holmbeck et al., 2003a). Moreover, many studies have failed to include a comparison group or have failed to adequately match groups on relevant demographic factors, thus confounding group comparisons and limiting the study's internal validity (Holmbeck et al., 2003a). Finally, the samples of children with spina bifida recruited by past investigators have often been diverse with respect to level of lesion and associated neurological impairment, as well as with respect to the presence or absence of shunts to manage hydrocephalus. Inclusion of such heterogeneous groups, although a strength in terms of generalizability of findings, may introduce confounding factors into the study design, making meaningful interpretation of any findings difficult.

In addition, many researchers have failed to provide a clear theoretical or conceptual model to guide their work (Holmbeck et al., 2003a). Moreover, few investigators have tested complex theoretical models that include mediational and moderational components (Drotar, 1997). For example, few studies have addressed the mechanism by which the presence of a chronic illness impacts individual and family functioning (however, see Holmbeck et al., 2002b, for an exception to this trend). Moreover, little attention has been devoted to understanding the reciprocal manner in which family factors and youth adjustment outcomes influence each other over time (see Friedman et al., 2004, for an exception). In a related point, the pathways that lead to either negative or positive psychosocial adjustment outcomes have rarely been attended to in empirical investigations. Similarly, potential moderators of the impact of illness status on individual and family functioning have just begun to be explored. As Drotar (1997) points out, the current literature has neglected the potential interactions that exist among developmental variables, family factors, and child outcomes (e.g., if the relationship between parent willingness to grant autonomy and adolescent adjustment outcomes differs as a function of child pubertal timing). Greater attention to moderators of individual and family adjustment outcomes would help to identify subgroups of affected individuals and families that may be particularly at risk for adjustment difficulties. An understanding of the mechanisms by which predictors influence outcomes may also have significant implications for clinical interventions. For example, if the relationship between a child's illness-related knowledge and adherence behavior is explained by the child's feelings of self-worth, then educating that child about his or her disability may be a key intervention target, as it could improve the child's self-concept as well as adherence to the treatment regimen.

Finally, the majority of research has focused on the identification of risks or deficits (both individual and familial) associated with the presence of spina bifida, with far less interest in models of resiliency or predictors of positive adaptation among this population. Greater attention to factors that may protect against negative individual and family outcomes could inform efforts to prevent the development of dysfunction within this population or to enhance psychosocial functioning among well-adjusted families.

CONCLUSION AND FUTURE DIRECTIONS

Existing literature suggests important differences in the psychosocial adjustment of children with spina bifida compared to typically developing children. Taken together, this body of research indicates that children and adolescents with spina bifida appear to be at risk for various types of adjustment difficulties, and that certain characteristics of the family environment may buffer against or exacerbate this risk. Differences have also been documented with respect to the functioning of families affected by spina bifida in comparison to families not affected. Research suggests that the presence of a child with spina bifida is a risk factor for negative outcomes within several domains of the broader family context. On the other hand, many families of children with physical disabilities, such as spina bifida, appear to be resilient as they adapt to the stresses of managing a child with special needs (Holmbeck et al., 2002a). The extent to which such resilience can be supported is likely to determine whether or not members of these families exhibit adjustment difficulties in the future.

Despite the existence of a growing body of literature in the previously reviewed domains, more research is warranted to fully understand the impact of spina bifida on individual and family functioning, as well as the relationship between family factors and child and adolescent adjustment. What follows are several suggestions for future research aimed at improving our knowledge of psychosocial adjustment and family functioning among children and adolescents with spina bifida, with the ultimate goal of preventing psychosocial maladjustment and enhancing positive functioning among this population.

Suggestions for Researchers

Several avenues for future research can be suggested (Drotar, 1997; Kazak, 1997). First, researchers should enhance the external validity of extant predictive models of family influences on child/adolescent adjustment through the inclusion of ethnically, culturally, and socioeconomically diverse samples of participants in research studies. Second, investigators should move toward more specific models of family socialization in pediatric populations by attending to illness-specific family behaviors, by testing how family processes influence child adjustment over time, by researching clinically relevant and modifiable family behaviors (e.g., conflict over autonomy during adolescence), and by testing mediational, moderational, and causal processes. Third, scientists ought to document trajectories of family adaptation in response to the course of the child's illness, as well as to typical developmental transitions. Fourth, researchers should investigate study questions using a family systems perspective, attend to differences in individual and family adjustment as a function of child developmental level, and focus on areas of strength or competence to guide research. Fifth, investigators should use data from multiple respondents whenever possible. Finally, researchers should orient their work toward pediatric practice by focusing on domains of study that have implications for clinical interventions. Given the fragmented nature of much of the past research on children and families affected by spina bifida and the lack of programmatic efforts to understand psychosocial adaptation among this population (Holmbeck et al., 2003a), adherence to the above suggestions would lead to a more methodologically sound body of work and facilitate a more comprehensive understanding of the psychosocial adjustment of youth with spina bifida and their families.

Suggestions for Health-Care Professionals

In addition to building upon the existing research base as a means of ultimately promoting adaptive individual and family functioning among those affected by spina bifida, the psychosocial well-being of this population can be promoted through their ongoing relationships with health-care professionals. Several suggestions can be offered for health-care professionals who work with children and adolescents with spina bifida (Holmbeck and Westhoven, 2001). First, a child or adolescent with severe adjustment or adherence problems should be referred for professional help. Moreover, as suggested by Blum (1983), psychological counseling and support services should be used not only as a means of crisis intervention, but also as a means of preventing psychological dysfunction. Second, because youth with pediatric illnesses such as spina bifida are particularly at risk for internalizing problems (i.e., symptoms of depression, anxiety, and social withdrawal), they should be routinely screened for such difficulties and referred for psychological services whenever appropriate.

Third, given the body of research suggesting higher levels of parental overprotection and psychological control among parents of children with pediatric chronic illnesses and the negative association between high levels of overprotection and adolescent autonomous behavior, parents should be encouraged to grant developmentally appropriate levels of independence to their adolescent while maintaining a supportive emotional connection with their child. Fourth, and related to the previous point, parents should be helped to differentiate between medical and nonmedical issues with respect to granting behavioral autonomy, as high levels of parental involvement in medically related tasks may be adaptive, whereas high levels of involvement in other domains may not. Fifth, as early as possible, health-care professionals should involve children with spina bifida in treatment planning and should educate children in a developmentally appropriate manner about their medical condition. A particular area in which youth affected by spina bifida may be lacking in knowledge is their own sexual development and reproductive functioning (see Sawyer and Roberts, 1999). Health-care providers should also encourage parents to educate themselves and their children about spina bifida while modeling appropriate levels of instruction and autonomy granting.

Sixth, given the cognitive and neuropsychological correlates of spina bifida (e.g., lower intellectual functioning, impaired attentional and executive functioning processes), health-care professionals should be attentive to the fact that academic difficulties or a lack of motivation in school may be symptoms of an underlying learning disability or attentional impairment. Educational or neuropsychological testing and medication evaluation should be suggested in such instances. Seventh, because adolescents with spina bifida are particularly vulnerable to social difficulties (Blum, 1983), health-care professionals should consider referring these children to peer mentoring programs (i.e., programs in which children with spina bifida have opportunities to interact with socially competent peers with the goal of developing social skills and enhancing adaptive interpersonal functioning) that can assist them in becoming socially integrated. Moreover, medical professionals could be influential in helping families find developmentally appropriate social activities for the adolescent to promote adaptive social functioning. Eighth, because parents are also at risk for maladjustment and higher levels of psychological distress, professionals should screen parents for such symptoms and refer them for professional services as appropriate. Finally, health-care professionals should be especially attentive to potential psychosocial adjustment difficulties in children and families from impoverished economic backgrounds, given the body of research to support this relationship.

Clearly, additional programmatic efforts to understand the impact of spina bifida on individual and family functioning are warranted, as is greater attention on the part of health-care professionals to promoting healthy adjustment among this population. As indicated throughout this review, although children with spina bifida and their families are at increased risk for maladjustment, there exists considerable resilience among this population. As such, there is a pressing need for greater attention to factors that either promote or hinder psychosocial adjustment within this population.

REFERENCES

Ammerman RT, Kane VR, Slomka GT, Reigel DH, Franzen MD, Gadow KD (1998). Psychiatric symptomatology and family functioning in children and adolescents with spina bifida. J Clin Psychol Med Settings 5:449–465.

Ammerman RT, Van Hasselt VB, Hersen M (1991). Parent–child problem-solving interactions in families of visually impaired youth. J Pediatr Psychol 16:87–101.

Anderson BJ, Coyne JC (1993). Family context and compliance behavior in chronically ill children. In Krasnegor NA, Epstein L, Johnson SB, Yaffe SJ (eds): *Developmental Aspects of Health Compliance Behavior*. Hillsdale, NJ: Erlbaum, pp. 77–89.

Appleton PL, Ellis NC, Minchom PE, Lawson V, Boll V, Jones P (1997). Depressive symptoms and self-concept in young people with spina bifida. J Pediatr Psychol 2:707–722.

Appleton PL, Minchom PE, Ellis NC, Elliott CE, Boll V, Jones P (1994). The self-concept of young people with spina bifida: a population-based study. Dev Med Child Neurol 36:198–215.

Barakat LP, Linney JA (1992). Children with physical handicaps and their mothers: the interrelation of social support, maternal adjustment, and child adjustment. J Pediatr Psychol 17:725–739.

Barakat LP, Linney JA (1995). Optimism, appraisals, and coping in the adjustment of mothers and their children with spina bifida. J Child Fam Stud 4:303–320.

Barber BK, Harmon EL (2002). Violating the self: parental psychological control of children and adolescents. In Barber BK (ed): *Intrusive Parenting: How Psychological Control Affects Children and Adolescents.* Washington, DC: American Psychological Association Press, pp. 15–52.

Barnes MA, Dennis M (1998). Discourse after early-onset hydrocephalus: core deficits in children of average intelligence. Brain Lang 61:309–334.

Baumrind D (1991). Effective parenting during the early adolescent transition. In Cowan PA, Heatherington EM (eds): *Family Transitions.* Hillside, NJ: Erlbaum, pp. 111–164.

Bier JB, Morales Y, Liebling J, Geddes L, Kim E (1997). Medical and social factors associated with cognitive outcome in individuals with myelomeningocele. Dev Med Child Neurol 39:263–266.

Blum RW (1983). The adolescent with spina bifida. Clin Pediatr 22:331–335.

Blum RW, Resnick MD, Nelson R, St Germaine A (1991). Family and peer issues among adolescents with spina bifida and cerebral palsy. Pediatrics 88:280–285.

Borjeson MC, Lagergren J (1990). Life conditions of adolescents with myelomeningocele. Dev Med Child Neurol 32:698–706.

Brewer VR, Fletcher JM, Hiscock M, Davidson KC (2001). Attention processes in children with shunted hydrocephalus versus attention deficit-hyperactivity disorder. Neuropsychology 15:185–198.

Bronfenbrenner U (ed) (1979). *The Ecology of Human Development: Experiments by Nature and Design.* Cambridge, MA: Harvard University Press.

Cappelli M, McGrath PJ, Daniels T, Manion I, Schillinger J (1994). Marital quality of parents of children with spina bifida: a case-comparison study. Dev Behav Pediatr 15:320–326.

Carr J (1991). The effect of neural tube defects on the family and its social functioning. In Bannister CM, Tew B (eds): *Current Concepts in Spina Bifida and Hydrocephalus.* New York: Cambridge University Press, pp. 180–192.

Coakley RM, Holmbeck GN, Friedman D, Greenley RN, Thill AW (2002). A longitudinal study of pubertal timing, parent–child conflict, and cohesion in families of young children with spina bifida. J Pediatr Psychol 27:461–473.

Costigan CL, Floyd FJ, Harter KSM, McClintock JC (1997). Family process and adaptation to children with mental retardation: disruption and resilience in family problem-solving interactions. J Fam Psychol 11:515–529.

Cromer BA, Enrile B, McCoy K, Gerhardstein MJ, Fitspatrick M, Judis J (1990). Knowledge, attitudes, and behavior related to sexuality in adolescents with chronic disability. Dev Med Child Neurol 32:602–610.

Dennis M, Barnes M (2002). Math and numeracy in young adults with spina bifida and hydrocephalus. Dev Neuropsychol 21:145–155.

Dise JE, Lohr ME (1998). Examination of deficits in conceptual reasoning abilities associated with spina bifida. Am J Phys Med Rehabil 77:247–251.

Drotar D (1997). Relating parent and family functioning to the psychological adjustment of children with chronic health conditions: What have we learned? What do we need to know? J Pediatr Psychol 22:149–165.

Edwards-Beckett J (1995). Parental expectations and child's self concept in spina bifida. Children's Health Care 24:257–267.

Fagan J, Schor D (1993). Mothers of children with spina bifida: factors related to maternal psychosocial functioning. Am J Orthopsychiatry 63:146–152.

Fletcher JM, Bohan TP, Brandt ME, Brookshire BL, Beaver SR, Francis DJ, Davidson KC, Thompson NM, Miner ME (1992a).

Cerebral white matter and cognitions in hydrocephalic children. Arch Neurol 49:818–824.

Fletcher JM, Brookshire BL, Landry SH, Bohan TP, Davidson KC, Francis DJ, Thompson NM, Miner ME (1995). Behavioral adjustment of children with hydrocephalus: relationships with etiology, neurological, and family status. J Pediatr Psychol 20:109–125.

Fletcher JM, Dennis M, Northrup H (2000). Hydrocephalus. In Yeates KO, Ris MD, Taylor HG (eds): *Pediatric Neuropsychology: Research, Theory, and Practice.* New York: Guilford Press, pp. 25–46.

Fletcher JM, Dennis M, Northrup H, Barnes MA, Hannay HJ, Landry SH, Copeland K, Blaser SE, Kramer LA, Brandt ME, Francis DJ (2004). Spina bifida: Genes, brain, and development. In Glidden LM (ed): *Handbook of Research on Mental Retardation,* vol. 28. San Diego, CA: Academic Press, pp. 63–117.

Fletcher JM, Francis DJ, Thompson NM, Brookshire BL, Bohan TP, Landry SH, Davidson KC, Miner ME (1992b). Verbal and nonverbal skill discrepancies in hydrocephalic children. J Clin Exp Neuropsychol 14:593–609.

Friedman D, Holmbeck GN, Jandasek B, Zukerman J, Abad M (2004). Parent functioning in families of preadolescents with spina bifida: longitudinal implications for child adjustment. J Fam Psychol 18:609–619.

Friedrich WN, Lovejoy MC, Shaffer J, Shurtleff DB, Beilke RL (1991). Cognitive abilities and achievement status of children with myelomeningocele: a contemporary sample. J Pediatr Psychol 16:423–438.

Gray MR, Steinberg L (1999). Unpacking authoritative parenting: reassessing a multidimensional construct. J Marriage Family 61:574–587.

Harris JR (1995). Where is the child's environment? A group socialization theory of development. Psychol Rev 102:458–489.

Havermans T, Eiser C (1991). Mothers' perceptions of parenting a child with spina bifida. Child: Care, Health, Dev 17:259–273.

Holmbeck GN, Belvedere MC, Christensen M, Czerwinski AM, Hommeyer JS, Johnson SZ et al. (1998). Assessment of adherence with multiple informants in pre-adolescents with spina bifida: initial development of a multidimensional, multitask parent-report questionnaire. J Pers Assess 70:427–440.

Holmbeck GN, Coakley RM, Hommeyer JS, Shapera WE, Westhoven VC (2002a). Observed and perceived dyadic and systemic functioning in families of preadolescents with spina bifida. J Pediatr Psychol 27:177–189.

Holmbeck GN, Faier-Routman J (1995). Spinal lesion level, shunt status, family relationships, and psychosocial adjustment in children and adolescents with spina bifida myelomeningocele. J Pediatr Psychol 20:817–832.

Holmbeck GN, Gorey-Ferguson L, Hudson T, Seefeldt T, Shapera W, Turner T, Uhler J (1997). Maternal, paternal, and marital functioning in families of preadolescents with spina bifida. J Pediatr Psychol 22:167–181.

Holmbeck GN, Greenley RN, Coakley RM (2003a). Family functioning in children and adolescents with spina bifida: an evidence-based review. Paper presented at the Evidence-Based Practice in Spina Bifida: Developing a Research Agenda meeting, Washington, DC, May 9–10.

Holmbeck GN, Johnson SZ, Wills KE, McKernon W, Rose B, Erklin S, Kemper T (2002b). Observed and perceived parental overprotection in relation to psychosocial adjustment in preadolescents with a physical disability: the mediational role of behavioral autonomy. J Consult Clin Psychol 70:96–110.

Holmbeck GN, Shapera WE, Hommeyer JS (2002c). Observed and perceived parenting behaviors and psychosocial adjustment in preadolescents with spina bifida. In Barber BK (ed): *Intrusive Parenting: How Psychological Control Affects Children and Adolescents.* Washington, DC: American Psychological Association, pp. 191–234.

Holmbeck GN, Westhoven VC (2001). Family functioning and psychosocial adjustment in adolescents with myelomeningocele. In Sarwark JF, Lubicky JP (eds): *Caring for the Child with Spina Bifida.* Rosemont, IL: American Academy of Orthopaedic Surgeons, pp. 579–599.

Holmbeck GN, Westhoven VC, Shapera W, Bowers R, Gruse C, Nikolopoulos T, Wienke C, Davidson K (2003b). A multimethod, multi-informant, and multi-dimensional perspective on psychosocial adjustment in pre-adolescents with spina bifida. J Consult Clin Psychol 71:82–796.

Hommeyer JS, Holmbeck GN, Wills KE, Coers S (1999). Condition severity and psychosocial functioning in pre-adolescents with spina bifida: disentangling proximal functional status and distal adjustment outcomes. J Pediatr Psychol 24:499–509.

Horton TV, Wallander JL (2001). Hope and social support as resilience factors against psychological distress of mothers who care for children with chronic physical conditions. Rehabil Psychol 46:382–399.

Kalucy M, Bower C, Stanley F (1996). School-aged children with spina bifida in Western Australia: parental perspectives on functional outcome. Dev Med Child Neurol 38:325–334.

Kazak AE (1997). A contextual family/systems approach to pediatric psychology: introduction to the special issue. J Pediatr Psychol 22:141–148.

Kazak AE, Clark MW (1986). Stress in families of children with myelomeningocele. Dev Med Child Neurol 28:220–228.

King GA, Shultz IZ, Steel K, Gilpin M, Cathers T (1993). Self-evaluation and self-concept of adolescents with physical disabilities. Am J Occup Ther 47:132–140.

Kronenberger WG, Thompson RJ (1992a). Medical stress, appraised stress, and the psychological adjustment of mothers of children with myelomeningocele. Dev Behav Pediatr 13:405–411.

Kronenberger WG, Thompson RJ (1992b). Psychological adaptation of mothers of children with spina bifida: association with dimensions of social relationships. J Pediatr Psychol 17:1–14.

Landry SH, Robinson SS, Copeland D, Garner PW (1993). Goal directed behavior and perception of self-competence in children with spina bifida. J Pediatr Psychol 18:389–396.

Lavigne JV, Faier-Routman J (1992). Psychological adjustment to pediatric physical disorders: a meta-analytic review. J Pediatr Psychol 17:133–157.

Lavigne JV, Faier-Routman J (1993). Correlates of psychological adjustment to pediatric physical disorders: a meta-analytic review and comparison with existing models. J Dev Behav Pediatr 14:117–123.

Lavigne JV, Nolan D, McLone DG (1988). Temperament, coping, and psychological adjustment in young children with myelomeningocele. J Pediatr Psychol 13:363–378.

Lemanek KL, Jones ML, Lieberman B (2000). Mothers of children with spina bifida: adaptational and stress processing. Children's Health Care 29:19–35.

Loebig M (1990). Mothers' assessments of the impact of children with spina bifida on the family. Maternal-Child Nurs J 19:251–265.

Loomis JW, Javornisky JG, Monahan JJ, Burke G, Lindsay A (1997). Relations between family environment and adjustment outcomes in young adults with spina bifida. Dev Med Child Neurol 39:149–165.

Lord J, Varzos N, Behrman B, Wicks J, Wicks D (1990). Implications of mainstream classrooms for adolescents with spina bifida. Dev Med Child Neurol 32:20–29.

Maccoby EE, Martin JA (1983). Socialization in the context of the family: Parent–child interaction. In Hetherington EM, Mussen PH, Carmichael L (eds): *Handbook of Child Psychology: Socialization, Personality, and Social Development,* Vol. 4, 4th ed. New York: Wiley, pp. 1–101.

Macias MM, Clifford SC, Saylor CG, Kreh SM (2001). Predictors of parenting stress in families of children with spina bifida. Children's Health Care 30:57–65.

McCormick MC, Charney EB, Stemmler MM (1986). Assessing the impact of a child with spina bifida on the family. Dev Med Child Neurol 28:53–61.

McKernon WL, Holmbeck GN, Colder CR, Hommeyer JS, Shapera W, Westhoven V (2001). Longitudinal study of observed and perceived family influences on problem-focused coping behaviors of preadolescents with spina bifida. J Pediatr Psychol 26:41–54.

Murch RL, Cohen LH (1989). Relationships among life stress, perceived family environment, and the psychological distress of spina bifida adolescents. J Pediatr Psychol 14:193–214.

Nabors LA, Keyes LA (1997). Brief report: preschoolers' social preferences for interacting with peers with physical differences. J Pediatr Psychol 22:113–122.

Nassau JH, Drotar D (1997). Social competence among children with central nervous system–related chronic health conditions: a review. J Pediatr Psychol 22:771–793.

Quittner AL, DiGirolamo AM (1998). Family adaption to childhood disability and illness. In Ammerman RT, Campo JV (eds): *Handbook of Pediatric Psychology and Psychiatry.* Boston: Allyn & Bacon, pp. 70–80.

Rolf JE, Garmezy N (eds) (1990). *Risk and Protective Factors in the Development of Psychopathology.* Cambridge: Cambridge University Press.

Rourke BP (1989). *Nonverbal Learning Disabilities: The Syndrome and the Model.* New York: Guilford Press.

Rourke BP, Ahmad SA, Collins DW, Hayman-Abello BA, Hayman-Abello SE, Warriner EM (2002). Child clinical/pediatric neuropsychology: some recent advances. Annu Rev Psychol 53:309–339.

Sawyer SM, Roberts KV (1999). Sexual and reproductive health in young people with spina bifida. Dev Med Child Neurol 41:671–675.

Seefeldt T, Holmbeck GN, Belvedere M, Gorey-Ferguson L, Hommeyer JS, Hudson T (1997). Socioeconomic status and democratic parenting in families of preadolescents with spina bifida. Psi Chi J Undergrad Res 2:5–12.

Semrud-Clikeman M, Hynd GW (1991). Specific nonverbal and social-skills deficits in children with learning disabilities. In Obrzut JE, Hynd GW (eds): *Neuropsychological Foundations of Learning Disabilities: A Handbook of Issues, Methods, and Practice.* New York: Academic Press, pp. 603–629.

Snow JH (1999). Executive processes for children with spina bifida. Children's Health Care 28:241–253.

Spaulding BR, Morgan SB (1986). Spina bifida children and their parents: a population prone to family dysfunction? J Pediatr Psychol 11:359–374.

Steinberg L (1990). Autonomy, conflict, and harmony in the family relationship. In Feldman SS, Elliot GR (eds): *At the Threshold: The Developing Adolescent.* Cambridge, MA: Harvard University Press, pp. 355–376.

Steinberg L, Darling NE, Fletcher AC (1995). Authoritative parenting and adolescent adjustment: An ecological journey. In Moen P, Elder GH, Luscher K, Bronfenbrenner U (eds): *Examining Lives in Context: Perspectives on the Ecology of Human Development.* Washington, DC: American Psychological Association, pp. 423–466.

Steinberg L, Lamborn SD, Darling N, Mounts NS, Dornbusch SM (1994). Over-time changes in adjustment and competence among adolescents from authoritative, authoritarian, indulgent, and neglectful families. Child Dev 65:754–770.

Steinberg L, Lamborn SD, Dornbusch SM, Darling N (1992). Impact of parenting practices on adolescent achievement: authoritative parenting, school involvement, and encouragement to succeed. Child Dev 63:1266–1281.

Tramontana MG, Hooper SR (1997). Neuropsychology of child psychopathology. In Reynolds CR, Fletcher-Janzen E (eds): *Handbook of Clinical Child Neuropsychology,* 2nd ed. New York: Plenum Press, pp. 120–139.

Van Hasselt VB, Ammerman RT, Hersen M, Reigel DH, Rowley FL (1991). Assessment of social skills and problem behaviors in young children with spina bifida. J Dev Phys Disabil 3:69–80.

Wallander JL, Feldman WS, Varni JW (1989a). Physical status and psychosocial adjustment in children with spina bifida. J Pediatr Psychol 14:89–102.

Wallander JL, Pitt LC, Mellins CA (1990). Child functional independence and maternal psychosocial stress as risk factors threatening adaptation in mothers of physically or sensorially handicapped children. J Consult Clin Psychol 58:818–824.

Wallander JL, Varni JW (1989). Social support and adjustment in chronically ill and handicapped children. Am J Commun Psychol 17:185–201.

Wallander JL, Varni JW, Babani L., Banis HT, Wilcox KT (1988). Children with chronic physical disorders: maternal reports of their psychological adjustment. J Pediatr Psychol 13:197–212.

Wallander JL, Varni JW, Babani L, Banis HT, Wilcox KT (1989b). Family resources as resistance factors for psychological maladjustment in chronically ill and handicapped children. J Pediatr Psychol 14:157–173.

Weiserbs B, Gottlieb J (2000). The effect of perceived duration of physical disability on attitudes of school children toward friendship and helping. J Psychol 134:343–345.

Wiegner S, Donders J (2000). Predictors of parental distress after congenital disabilities. Dev Behav Pediatr 21:271–277.

Wills KE (1993). Neuropsychological functioning in children with spina bifida and/or hydrocephalus. J Clin Child Psychol 22:247–265.

Wills KE, Holmbeck GN, Dillon K, McLone DG (1990). Intelligence and achievement in children with myelomeningocele. J Pediatr Psychol 15:161–176.

Wolman C, Basco DE (1994). Factors influencing self-esteem and self-consciousness in adolescents with spina bifida. J Adolesc Health 15:543–548.

Yeates KO, Loss N, Colvin AN, Enrile BG (2003). Do children with myelomeningocele and hydrocephalus display nonverbal learning disabilities? An empirical approach to classification. J Int Neuropsychol Soc 9:653–662.

Zurmohle UM, Homann T, Schroeter C, Rothgerber H, Hommel G, Ermert JA (1998). Psychological adjustment of children with spina bifida. J Child Neurol 13:64–70.

27

When and How to Communicate with People with Spina Bifida and Their Families

SONYA G. OPPENHEIMER

The purpose of this chapter is to give insight to professionals who provide information at varying stages in the life of a person with spina bifida. A variety of people representing many different disciplines meet with people with spina bifida and their families at various times, including prenatally, at birth, in early childhood, adolescence, young adulthood, and older adulthood.

In the prenatal period, there is usually an obstetrician, a perinatologist, geneticist, genetic counselor, neurosurgeon, neurosurgical nurse, and at times a developmental pediatrician. At birth, patients and their parents will meet the neonatologist, neonatology nurses, neurosurgeon, orthopedist, urologist, and at times a primary care physician. In early childhood the numbers decrease to some extent and include the interdisciplinary spina bifida team, primary care doctor, and school personnel. In adolescence, they begin to meet vocational guidance personnel in addition to the same medical personnel. Once adulthood is reached, usually at 21 years of age, an entirely different group of professionals are involved, including, at times, an entire change in medical caretakers. Most pediatric units will have the person who has been followed throughout life in a pediatric setting begin to transfer to an adult setting, including both hospital and adult physicians.

This chapter will discuss examples of how to present pertinent information at these crucial times throughout the life of people with spina bifida. The specific details of the disorder itself, the complications, and medical needs will not be presented in this chapter. These can be found in the other chapters and other medical textbooks and journals.

PRENATAL PERIOD

A young couple expecting their third child had just found out that the 22-week ultrasound scan indicated that the fetus would be born with spina bifida and probably hydrocephalus because of the presence of the lemon sign. The perinatologist reviewed the basic information regarding spina bifida. Since it was the year 2003, the couple's next step was to search the Internet for all available information regarding possible treatment both prenatally and neonatally. Their next search led to various websites that indicated the locations of service providers. These, in turn, led them to a multidisciplinary spina bifida clinic for confirmation and explanation of the Internet information.

This appears to be a drastic change in the way families and professionals communicate with each other, yet the impact of how people interpret bad news and how it affects their perception and adjustment to the child's disability remains. The massive amount of written and computer-based information can confuse and overwhelm families. Computer information is not a substitute for talking with a knowledgeable, unbiased professional who can listen and respond to parental concerns.

The literature is replete with discussions of the pros and cons of how to tell bad news. Numerous attempts have been made to develop training modules for medical students and physicians in residency, yet parents still voice concerns about how physicians conducted their initial interview (Wolraich, 1982). This information is reported to shape the image that parents create of their child and his or her future, and in turn affect their attitudes toward the child and the nature of their interactions with him or her (Byrnes et al., 2003; Turner and Sloper, 1992). Krahn et al. (1993), in the article "Are There Good Ways to Give Bad News?," emphasized that the sense of loss and grief should be separated from the distress associated with how the news was given. The need for a strong physician–patient relationship is repeatedly emphasized, but in this era of medical productivity and change, short visits, and rapid turnover, this can be very difficult to achieve. It is even harder to share information with families who need to make decisions based on ultrasound pictures. The principles for sharing information remain the same (Lemons and Weaver, 1986):

- Parents want direct, honest reporting of the diagnostic information that is available.
- Parents want a physician who is knowledgeable about the natural history of spina bifida with or without treatment.
- Parents want a realistic yet not pessimistic approach to what is required to care for the infant during the early years and into adulthood.
- Parents need the overall prognosis for mortality, morbidity, and independent functioning.
- Include both parents if appropriate, as well as other family members if appropriate.
- Avoid being judgmental regarding parents' choice.
- Allow informed choice, not directive counseling based on the physician's personal belief.
- Families most likely have seen a perinatologist, a genetic counselor, and/or an obstetrician whose knowledge about spina bifida is based primarily on written rather than personal information. The professional treating children and adults with spina bifida is the ideal person to convey appropriate information if that person is available.
- The physician should be available after the initial counseling even if the parents' choice is to terminate the pregnancy.
- If the pregnancy is to be continued, make contact and be available several times during the remainder of the pregnancy.
- Give written information, lists of physicians, and phone numbers of persons who will be treating the child, as well as other support people including, if a family wishes, families who have children with spina bifida.
- Information regarding the local Spina Bifida of America Association.
- Provide, if available, a tour of the facility where the newborn child will be brought.
- Address the financial needs and costs.
- Remember to communicate with the referring obstetrician, perinatologists, neurosurgeon, and primary care physician.

BIRTH AND THE NEONATAL PERIOD

Since not all parents have had prenatal counseling, for some the birth of a baby with spina bifida is totally unexpected. The above guidelines for prenatal counseling remain essentially the same. However, when prenatal counseling has occurred, the parents and extended family members have had at least 3 to 4 months to absorb the information, read various books and articles, conduct research on the Internet, and prepare for the birth of the baby. When the birth of a baby with a malformation occurs, time is needed to process the impact of the initial shock—in other words, to go through a grieving process.

The next stage of communication occurs with the birth of the infant. This will be the first time the family is faced with the reality that their infant does indeed have a physical disability. Most of the time, once they see the new baby, they focus initially on the child's face and the fact that the baby is "a baby." Most mothers have only a glimpse of the baby until their first visit to the neonatal intensive care unit, usually at about 2 days of age if the mother has had a cesarean section. Drotar et al. (1975) describe the adaptation of parents to the birth of an infant with a congenital malformation. In their hypothetical model, separation from the infant can contribute to the feeling of estrangement, yet most mothers do develop attachment to their infants, with only a small minority evidencing overt rejection.

The physician should examine the infant in the presence of the family, again clarifying what is known about the infant's current status, the possibility for ambulation, the possibility of a shunt, and, most important, what will happen next.

The physician must be alert to the family's responses to the information. There is a fine line between enough information and too much. What are the parents really asking? Is the doctor considering where they are in the grieving process (Bristor, 1984)? As with any doctor–patient relationship, it is important to maintain communication throughout the initial hospital stay (10 days on average). Multiple care providers, neonatologists, neurosurgeons, orthopedists, urologists, nurses, social workers, and residents from all the specialties discuss various issues with the family, in an uncoordinated fashion. It is the responsibility of the primary spina bifida care team director with the appropriate support person, usually a nurse or social worker, to organize this information and remain the focal or lead person for the family. Continuity of care and personnel is needed, with the expectation that the family will become increasingly knowledgeable and comfortable with the various issues regarding spina bifida. Initially, the providers of coordinated care will be the most knowledgeable and provide advocacy for the family and child. Ideally, as the child becomes older, the child and the family will learn to assume this role.

THE FIRST YEARS

In the early developmental stages, the communication patterns established prenatally and at birth must continue. The usual mode of contact is during regular clinic visits and is not very different from good anticipatory guidance required for a child without a disability. Giving the family phone numbers where they can reach the doctor or other care providers is essential. Most families do not abuse this privilege, but it makes them feel very comfortable to know that if an emergency occurs, they will be able to reach a knowledgeable person. It is important to emphasize that the child is first a baby first who happens to have spina bifida, not a spina bifida baby. The initial fear of shunt malfunction and other medical complications diminishes toward the end of the first year, and families then begin to request information about development, initially focusing on motor skills. Though one needs to rely on literature presenting ambulation guidelines, each child must be considered individually. Predictions can be wrong if they are based only on the anatomical motor level and do not consider the child's and family's own motivations to ambulate. Realistic individual counseling is important, weighing with the family the time, cost, and physical energy sometimes required to walk independently. True independence or the ability to keep up with peers is important even for a very young child and sometimes will necessitate their use of a wheelchair even though they can learn to walk with braces and other supports.

SELF-CARE

The next major hurdle focuses on bowel and bladder control. Bowel continence is one of the most difficult areas of achievement. Families need to be periodically reminded that although all the other medical problems that occur are important, one of the most important factors for independence as the child gets older is the ability to achieve bowel control. Bowel training frequently can occur on a conditioning basis if it begins when the child is very young. However, because families assume that the child will be wearing diapers anyway, they frequently do not heed this advice. They should be reminded of this area of need at each visit. Self-catheterization is also frequently difficult for children. The nurse on the spina bifida team can be very helpful, showing the family and the child various techniques that will make this procedure easier. Catheterization can then become customary and routine.

SCHOOL INTERVENTIONS

Various support programs such as early intervention programs from birth to age 3 years, as well as preschool and kindergarten, elementary, and high school programs, require appropriate assessment of the child's developmental skills including language ability, fine motor skills, and adaptions to meet the child's total needs. Often this period can be different for families, who relive their initial concern about the child's intellectual functioning. Many children and adults with spina bifida have various learning problems, though not necessarily mental retardation, that affect their ability to function in a school environment. Today, however, appropriate adjustments can be made to help meet their individual requirements.

The spina bifida team needs to support families in their search for school interventions. A complete psychoeducation evaluation is recommended. Families require advocacy support to understand what is needed. Schools feel that once they meet the child's physical needs, they have done their job. What is needed are modifications to meet the child's learning needs.

ADOLESCENCE

The continuity of care required by people with spina bifida allows the professionals to establish a relationship with the child that should continue through adulthood. Years ago, a board member from the National Spina Association wrote a play called *Smile, Pretty Baby Jane.* It described Jane's reaction to the professionals who at each clinic visit would ask her "Where is that pretty smile?," regardless of what surgeries or medical procedures were being discussed. This question makes children think that to be accepted and praised by the professionals, they must not express their true feelings or take part in the discussions. This may be a reason that people with spina bifida are described as passive and pleasant. It is important to allow children and adults to express their true feelings and to participate actively in decision making. A 15-year-old girl who had been seen in a clinic since birth stated that she hated coming to the clinic, and hated her body. Immediately her mother looked distressed and tried to stop her from talking this way. It was soon realized that it was more important to let her verbalize these feelings and acknowledge that her situation was not fair. Helping her deal with this situation as it realistically was and allowing her to express her feelings helped her move on toward an appropriate adulthood.

ADULTHOOD

Though the older adolescent and young adult require less medical intervention than the child, young adulthood is a critical time for the person to achieve independence. Young adults must learn to care for their physical needs, avoiding decubiti, urinary problems and bowel problems, and maintaining good hygiene so that they can learn a vocation and hold a job. Lecturing is not an appropriate form of communication. Just as their parents needed accurate information, older adolescents also need information geared to their level of understanding from someone they can trust. The transition to adult services can be a stressful time since the adult medical and social service system can be difficult to access. Knowing that the people they established their initial relationships are available if needed is an excellent ongoing support. The majority of programs coordinating care for people with spina bifida provide medical help and support to the adult in a haphazard, sporadic fashion. The spina bifida clinics are in pediatric settings, with pediatric subspecialists who feel that caring for adults should be done by adult specialists; meanwhile, adult patients and their families are dependent on the people they have known for 21 years. They struggle to find the same supports they formerly enjoyed. They meet financial barriers, barriers in the lack of knowledge of adult providers concerning the subtleties of physical problems, and, most important, the lack of "maternal/paternal" support formerly provided in the pediatric setting. Pediatricians tend to want to solve problems. Adult providers expect clients to be independent and seek help when appropriate. The support system, whether provided by physicians, service coordinators, or others, must allow young adolescents to become independent adults. This requires a team of professionals that will assist them in seeking this independence rather than dependency. Physicians' feelings must also be addressed. They cannot expect to do everything and will actually provide better care if they do not always rescue the young adult. This does not mean that they abandon the family they have cared for; instead, they help the patient make an appropriate transition to the adult environment. Better training in residencies is required to understand the spina bifida population, which has very special needs starting at birth. With recognition of these issues, transition multidisciplinary clinics are being established that now include vocational guidance, sexuality support, independent living, and financial assistance. Sometimes the leader of this program is a double-boarded medicine/pediatrics physician who can make this transition easier because he or she understands the issues involved from the very beginning. Most important, however, is that the initial team must begin to let go of the patient, just as parents must begin to let go. Recently, a parent in our clinic stated that every time she sees a new baby in the clinic, it brings back all of the original feelings at the birth of her daughter. This also occurs as the family begins to face the reality that their child is entering adulthood and they have to begin the process of letting go.

Frequently, professionals forget to include the adult patient in their discussions. Recent literature from the United Kingdom describes a social model approach to counseling people with disabilities rather than using a medical and tragedy model (Swain et al., 2003). An ideal approach would be one that is holistic and gives equal emphasis to the patient's emotional and physical characteristics. This article asks whether medical professionals see people with disabilities as people first or as the disability first. Too often the physician can forget the person's role.

CARE COORDINATION

The primary coordinator of care is usually a physician who is comfortable dealing with the medical, developmental, and life span needs of a child with spina bifida and his or her family. A team of professionals who remain involved from the prenatal period through either adulthood or the transition to adulthood is important. The primary communicator will change, depending on the child's needs. The multisystem involvement required for people with spina bifida presents a challenge to the care coordinator. It is unrealistic for one person to be expected to know all the intricacies of neurosurgery, orthopedics, urology, and rehabilitation issues. What is needed is the concept of the whole child, both for the family and for the care coordinator. Every headache does not mean that there is a shunt malfunction, and not every fever indicates a urinary tract infection. However, the primary physician in the community must be aware that these are possibilities and should have a general knowledge of the symptoms seen in this population. Some primary care physicians do not feel they can manage this seemingly complex disorder. They tell the family that they will provide immunizations, and care for colds and ear infections; if there are other symptoms, they prefer to send the child to the emergency room. This is both costly and confusing to parents and to the personnel in the emergency room, who do not know the child. The contact person must be knowledgeable about treatment issues and must be available. Any child with a complex medical condition has special health-care needs and can benefit from the American Academy of Pediatrics concept of a *medical home* (see The National Center of Medical Home Initiatives for Children with Special Needs, American Academy of Pediatrics, at http://www.medicalhomeinfo.org). The medical home, contrary to many impressions, is not a place but rather a concept of coordinated, identifiable medical care that is cost-efficient and correct. Initially the concept implied that the primary care setting should be the medical home. Currently, however, it is acknowledged that medical specialists in tertiary care settings can fulfill the medical home concept. In the case of spina bifida, any medical/surgical specialists nurse practitioner could serve in that role with the recognition that primary concerns may change, depending on the specific medical needs and the age of the patient with spina bifida.

"A therapeutic model for supporting families of children with a chronic illness" described by Morison et al. (2003) appears to be an appropriate model for professionals who provide ongoing intervention for children with spina bifida and their families. This model (known as Paediatric and Adolescent Support Service [PASS]) is family centered, non-illness-oriented, specific, nonlinear, preventive, and flexible. A key statement is the belief that there is commonality to all illnesses. The following principles provide guidance to understand what subport most families want through the various stages of their child's life:

- Hope
- Empowerment to gain control
- Reconnection
- Support networks
- Coping
- Reframing that addresses the issue "why me?" and provides contact with other families coping with a child with spina bifida

The following poem summarizes how people with disabilities would like us to think of them. Having this in mind when one communicates with people about their disability is crucial.

Challenged

Submitted by Daniel Pisconte (1999)

Some say I am disabled,
But you know that isn't true.
I simply have a challenge
A little different from you.
My slight inconvenience has taught me
Things they could not know.
Each obstacle is a victory,
Enabling me to grow.
I'm not really any different,
I cry, I laugh, I snore.
I don't want to be treated
As if I'm not a person anymore.
Out of good intentions,
People are afraid to let me try.
But sometimes I have to fall,
And sometimes I need to cry.
God gives me strength and dignity,
And the courage to be all I can be.
For He doesn't see me as disabled,
He just sees me as me.

ACKNOWLEDGMENTS

This project was supported by Grant No. 5 T73 MC 00032-14 awarded by the Maternal and Child Health Bureau, Health Resources and Service Administration, DHHS, or, Grant No. 90DD0546/03, awarded by Administration on Developmental Disabilities, Administration for Children and Families, DHHS.

REFERENCES

Bristor MW (1984). The birth of a handicapped child—a wholistic model for grieving. Family Relations 25–32.

Byrnes AL, Berk NW, Cooper ME, Marazita ML (2003). Parental evaluation of informing interviews for cleft lip and/or palate. Pediatrics 112:308–313.

Drotar D, Baskiewicz A, Irvin A, Kennell J, Klaus M (1975). The adaptation of parents to the birth of an infant with a congenital malformation: a hypothetical model. Pediatrics. 55:710–717.

Krahn GL, Hallum A, Kime C (1993). Are there good ways to give bad news? Pediatrics 91: 578–582.

Lemons PM, Weaver DD (1986). Beyond the birth of a defective child. Neonatal Network 5:13–20.

Morison JE, Bromfield LM, Cameron HJ (2003). A therapeutic model for supporting families of children with a chronic illness or disability. Chid Adolesc Mental Health 8(3):125–130.

Pisconte D (1999). Challenged. Spina Bifida Association of the National Capital Area. Winter 1999 Newsletter. Available at http://www.sbanca.com/newsletters/dec99.html.

Swain J, Griffiths C, Heyman B (2003). Towards a social model approach to counseling disabled clients. Br J Guidance Counsel 31:137–152.

Turner S, Sloper P (1992). Paediatricians' practice in disclosure and follow-up of severe physical disability in young children. Dev Med Child Neurol 34:348–358.

Wolraich ML (1982). Communication between physicians and parents of handicapped children. Except Child 48:324–329.

28

Genetic Counseling and Interpretation of Risk Figures

ROBERT A. SAUL

Genetic counseling (providing genetic information, recurrence risks, and psychological support) as an activity did not begin in earnest until the twentieth century (Walker, 1998). Prior to that time, most birth defects such as neural tube defects and familial disorders such as mental retardation were attributed to external factors. These external factors included a variety of causes such as misdeeds, punishment by God, or being "marked" by some phenomenon during pregnancy. In the last category, everything from eclipses to runaway horse carts was implicated. The recognition of genetic traits, the possible transmission of those traits, and their possible recurrence was slow to evolve in the first half of the twentieth century. The second half of the century witnessed an explosion of such information. The ability to recognize genetic traits and their characteristics has led not only to the activity but also to the profession of genetic counseling.

Genetic counseling is a well-recognized component of care for individuals and families affected by neural tube defects (NTDs). The principles of genetic counseling are reviewed by Walker (1998) and include voluntary use of services, equal access, patient education, complete disclosure of information, nondirective counseling, attention to psychosocial issues, confidentiality, and privacy protection. Birth defects and genetic issues are often difficult for the affected families to understand, so health-care providers must be very adept at providing sensitive information. Harper (1998) succinctly states this dilemma as follows:

> It would be wrong to pretend that those engaged in genetic counseling never give directive advice. One's own views are likely to be expanded in the way one approaches the subject, whether the more serious or the milder aspects of a disease have been stressed and whether one holds out the possibility of future treatment. . . . Since non-directiveness has become a somewhat central tenet of genetic counselling, it is important that it should not be used as an excuse for being vague, appearing detached, or for presenting so many apparent options that it becomes difficult for those seen to reach a difficult decision. People often need support for a tentative decision; the importance of non-directiveness lies in its allowing decisions to be those of the individuals involved, not of the person giving genetic counseling. It is particularly important that couples realize that in general there is no "right" or "wrong" decision to be made, but that the decision should be the right one for their own particular situation. It is also important that those giving genetic counselling do not judge "success" or "failure" in terms of a particular outcome, and that they give support to families whatever their decisions may be.

The lynchpin in genetic counseling is providing accurate genetic information. Accurate information allows proper patient education, open discussions, and our best attempts at nondirective counseling. When information about the epidemiology of birth defects and their recurrence risks is in a state of flux, counseling is difficult, yet a reflection of the current state of affairs. We are currently in such a predicament in regard to neural tube defects.

The etiologies of NTDs (anencephaly, encephalocele, and open and closed spina bifida) are varied (Laurence, 1990; Tolmie, 2002; see Chapters 13–17). Environmental causes (infections, vascular compromise, or teratogens), syndromic associations (single gene, chromosomal, sporadic, or idiopathic), and multifactorial causation (genetic and environmental factors) have all been cited. The majority of cases of NTDs have historically been attributed to the last category, multifactorial causation. Certain geographic areas have been noted to have a higher than usual prevalence of NTDs, further evidence for environmental influences and genetic factors.

As well detailed in Chapter 29, we now know that folic acid taken prior to conception or in early pregnancy, prior to and around the time of neural tube closure, will decrease the primary occurrence of NTDs and decrease their recurrence in subsequent pregnancies. These changes are due to the pioneering work of Smithells and colleagues (1980). As a result of their work, public health recommendations have led to dietary increases in folic acid, both by supplementation and by fortification (MRC Vitamin Study Research Group, 1991; Wald 1994). These measures have been followed by a decreased prevalence of NTDs (Brent et al., 2000; Stevenson et al., 2000; Berry and Li, 2002). A decreased prevalence of NTDs should lead to reduced recurrence risks for NTDs.

In the second edition of *Principles and Practice of Medical Genetics,* Laurence (1990) provides a table for the recurrence risk for NTDs to be used for genetic counseling. That same table was adapted for the fourth edition of the same text without a significant change in the baseline recurrence risks (Tolmie, 2002). Those risk figures are shown in Table 28.1. These figures are perhaps the best current recurrence risk figures available, but they will soon need to be updated on a broad scale.

One study in South Carolina regarding NTD occurrence and recurrence in the current nutritional environment is ongoing, and preliminary figures are available. The South Carolina Birth Defects Surveillance and Prevention Project has been in place since 1992, performing NTD surveillance, prevention, and education. Over that period of time, a broad network has been established to detect new cases of NTDs and to provide appropriate evaluation and counseling for families with affected infants. This latter group has received extensive counseling regarding the importance of periconceptional folic acid use. Ongoing public health efforts have also been directed to the lay public and the health-care profession to promote the use of folic acid prior to pregnancy. Table 28.2 shows an overview of the preliminary unpublished data from 1992 through April 2003 for subsequent pregnancies in mothers of infants with NTDs. No subsequent affected infants have been detected with women using periconceptional folic acid. Three out of 50 pregnancies without folic acid use manifested NTD recurrence. A breakdown of the data for both isolated and syndromic NTDs is shown in Tables 28.3 and 28.4. Syndromic NTDs include all nonisolated NTDs such as Meckel syndrome, chromosomal abnormalities, amniotic bands, multiple congenital anomalies, and other anomalies.

These figures suggest that previously quoted NTD recurrence risks will be altered as the use of folic acid periconceptionally via supplementation (400 μg/day for previously unaffected families and 4 mg/day for affected families) or fortification increases. (Chapter 29 addresses these nutritional recommendations in further detail.) A 3%–5% risk of recurrence was previously quoted for families with isolated or nonsyndromic NTDs. Based on the preliminary South Carolina data, the recurrence risk is less than 3%–5%, but more data will be needed from broader population studies.

It is fair to say that as folic acid supplementation and/or fortification of foodstuffs increases, recurrence risk figures for NTDs will change. Genetic counseling will also be affected and will require diligent monitoring of contemporary risk figures. The principles of genetic counseling elucidated above will not change, but the impact of the information will be altered as the epidemiology of NTDs changes.

TABLE 28.1. *Recurrence Risks for Neural Tube Defects*

	Approximate Risk
Whole population occurrence risk (use local observed figure)	1:300 to 1:1000
Whole population, plus periconceptional folic acid	1:2000 or less
One affected sibling	1:25
One affected sibling, periconceptional folic acid in next pregnancy	1:100
Two affected siblings	1:8 to 1:10
Three affected siblings	1:4
One affected parents	1:25
One affected second- (aunt or uncle)	1:50
One affected third-degree relative	<1:100
Several second-/third-degree relatives	Up to 1:25 but be aware of X-linked inheritance

Source: Tolmie (2002).

TABLE 28.2. *Subsequent Pregnancies in Mothers of Infants with Neural Tube Defects (NTDs)*

Total subsequent pregnancies	331
Number taking periconceptional folic acid	281*
Spontaneous abortions (includes 4 with blighted ova)	36†
Ectopic	3
Fetal demise	9
Elective termination (trisomy 9)	1
Liveborn	219‡
In progress	17
Infants with NTDs	0
Number not taking folic acid	50
Infants with NTDs	3

*Includes four sets of twins.
†Includes one set of spontaneous abortion twins.
‡Includes three sets of liveborn twins.
Source: South Carolina Birth Defects Surveillance and Prevention Program, unpublished data, 1992–April 2003.

TABLE 28.3. *Subsequent Pregnancies in Mothers of Infants with Isolated Neural Tube Defects (NTDs)*

Total subsequent pregnancies	281
Number taking periconceptional folic acid	242*
Spontaneous abortions (includes 4 with blighted ova)	31†
Ectopic	3
Fetal demise	8
Elective termination (trisomy 9)	1
Liveborn	186‡
In progress	17
Infants with NTDs	0
Number not taking folic acid	39
Infants with NTDs	1

*Includes four sets of twins.
†Includes one set of spontaneous abortion twins.
‡Includes three sets of liveborn twins.
Source: South Carolina Birth Defects Surveillance and Prevention Project, unpublished data, 1992–April 2003.

TABLE 28.4. *Subsequent Pregnancies in Mothers of Infants with Syndromic Neural Tube Defects (NTDs)*

Total subsequent pregnancies	50
Number taking periconceptional folic acid	39
Spontaneous abortions (includes 4 with blighted ova)	5
Ectopic	
Fetal demise	1
Elective termination (trisomy 9)	0
Liveborn	33
In progress	0
Infants with NTDs	0
Number not taking folic acid	11
Infants with NTDs	2

*Includes two sets of twins.
Source: South Carolina Birth Defects Surveillance and Prevention Program, unpublished data, 1992–April 2003.

The success of a public health dietary change to significantly alter a significant birth defect is one of the true success stories in modern medicine (Brent et al., 2000; Stevenson et al., 2000). Genetic counseling can continue to herald this story on behalf of genetics and medicine in general to individual patients counseled and to population groups at large.

REFERENCES

Berry RJ, Li Z (2002). Folic acid alone prevents neural tube defects: evidence from the China study. Epidemiology 13(1):114–116.

Brent RL, Oakley GP Jr, Mattison DR (2000): The unnecessary epidemic of folic acid–preventable spina bifida and anencephaly. Pediatrics 106(4):825–827.

Harper PS (1998): *Practical Genetic Counseling,* 5th ed., Oxford: Butterworth-Heinemann, p. 14.

Laurence KM (1990). The genetics and prevention of neural tube defects and 'uncomplicated' hydrocephalus. In Emery AEH, Rimoin DL (eds): *Principles and Practice of Medical Genetics,* 2nd ed. Edinburgh: Churchill Livingstone, pp. 323–346.

MRC Vitamin Study Research Group (1991). Prevention of neural tube defects: results of the MRC vitamin study. Lancet 338:132–137.

Smithells RW, Sheppard S, Schorah CJ, et al (1980): Possible prevention of neural tube defects by preconceptional vitamin supplementation. Lancet 1:339–340.

Stevenson RE, Allen WP, Pai GS, et al (2000). Decline in prevalence of neural tube defects in a high-risk region in the United States. Pediatrics 106(4):677–683.

Tolmie JL (2002). Clinical genetics of neural tube defects and other congenital central nervous system malformation. In Rimoin DL, Connor JM, Pyeritz RE, Korf BR (eds): *Emery and Rimoin's Principles and Practice of Medical Genetics.* London: Churchill Livingstone, pp. 2975–3016.

Wald NJ (1994). Folic acid and neural tube defects: the current evidence and implications for prevention. In Bock G, Marsh J (eds.): *Neural Tube Defects.* Ciba Foundation Symposium 181. Chichester: Wiley, pp. 192–208.

Walker AP (1998). The practice of genetic counseling. In Baker DL, Schuette JL, Uhlmann WR (eds): *A Guide to Genetic Counseling.* New York: Wiley-Liss, pp. 1–26.

III

PUBLIC HEALTH ISSUES

29

Preventing All Folic Acid–Preventable Spina Bifida

GODFREY P. OAKLEY, JR.

THE PREVENTION OF FOLIC ACID–PREVENTABLE BIRTH DEFECTS IS OCCURRING TOO SLOWLY!

It is too bad that a virus is not the primary cause of spina bifida. Serious diseases caused by viruses get prevented if there are effective vaccines. As the son of a single mother in a small rural town in eastern North Carolina, I received the Salk vaccine at the county health department within a few months after the completion of the study that proved the vaccine was safe and effective. Once the scientific knowledge was available to prevent polio, there was extreme urgency and the political will to implement highly effective prevention programs because it was well known that, without the vaccinations, children would continue to become paralyzed by polio. This rapid deployment of an effective prevention program may well have prevented my sister or me from getting polio. The availability of effective vaccines against rubella and *Hemophilus influenzae* also led rapidly to effective prevention programs that each year prevents thousands of children from developing the congenital rubella syndrome and hemophilus influenza meningitis.

I had assumed that if spina bifida were shown to be a vitamin deficiency disease, there would be the rapid implementation of food fortification programs to prevent spina bifida, just as there had been the rapidly implementation of effective vaccine programs to prevent polio. By rapid, I mean that I would have expected the total prevention of folic acid–preventable spina bifida within 5 years in the developed world and in most of the world by 10 years. Unfortunately, the nutrition culture simply does not have the tradition of moving rapidly on new knowledge to implement effective prevention programs. The food and nutrition rules and regulations operational in most of the world are not structured for the rapidly implementation of population prevention programs. Perhaps the kind of nutrition intervention that has become available against disease in recent years has been the kind of intervention that requires human behavior changes that come slowly, if at all. Whatever the reason, the inertia built into the system and the bias against food fortification have not served well the people of the world. The system urgently needs to be changed so that it can and will promptly implement effective prevention programs based on food fortification.

The concern for people with acquired immune deficiency syndrome (AIDS) and cancer has led to expedited review protocols for some drugs. I suggest that food regulations acquire an expedited review process whereby the regulatory authorities would be required to make a regulatory decision within 180 days or less after a petition had been filed requesting action like mandatory fortification of flour with folic acid.

The total prevention of folic acid–preventable spina bifida will not occur until there is sufficient political will. I hope this chapter will lead those who care for children with spina bifida to create in every country the political will to prevent these birth defects from occurring in a single pregnancy. I hope the next generation of pediatricians will not see newborn babies with folic acid–preventable birth defects, just as the polio vaccine resulted in my having never seen an acute case of polio, even though I trained in a large city hospital with an infectious disease ward that a decade before had been filled by people with acute polio.

SPINA BIFIDA IS LARGELY A FOLATE DEFICIENCY DISEASE

Having a good scientific base assists the building of an effective prevention program. Folic acid–preventable spina bifida is unusual. We learned its predominant cause and prevention from a single study. Smithells and colleagues (1983) published nonrandomized controlled data suggesting that a vitamin or vitamins and minerals in a usual multivitamin would prevent the vast majority of spina bifida. While these data were very interesting, they did not provide the evidence to convince me or most birth defects scientists or policy makers that a vitamin or mineral or combination would prevent spina bifida. These data, however, made it quite plausible that spina bifida could be a vitamin/mineral deficiency disease and led to many studies.

It was, however, the results of the MRC randomized, controlled trial, led by Professor Wald, that first provided the conclusive evidence that spina bifida was primarily a folate deficiency disease, preventable by taking a pill containing synthetic folic acid before and during the early weeks of pregnancy (MRC Vitamin Study Research Group, 1991). Thus, with one study, we learned the predominant cause—folate deficiency—and the prevention—oral synthetic folic acid in a pill. The randomized, controlled trial led by Professor Czeizel soon thereafter affirmed the role of oral synthetic folic acid in preventing spina bifida and anencephaly (Czeizel and Dudas, 1992).

4000 µG OF FOLIC ACID FOR WOMEN WHO HAVE HAD A SPINA BIFIDA-AFFECTED PREGNANCY

After the publication of the MRC paper in 1991, the Centers for Disease Control and Prevention (CDC) rapidly issued a recommendation that women who had previously had an affected pregnancy should see a health-care provider and take 4000 µg or 4 mg a day of folic acid daily if they were planning a pregnancy (Centers for Disease Control and Prevention, 1991). The basis for this recommendation was that 4 mg had been the dose used in the MRC study. This recommendation still stands today. How this recommendation is implemented varies from country to country. In the United States, the only prescription folic acid is a pill with 1 mg, so women must take four of these pills a day. In some countries, a 5 mg pill is available as a prescription or over-the-counter drug. Like all women of reproductive age, women who have had an affected pregnancy should consume 400 µg of folic acid daily, even when not planning a pregnancy (see below).

RECOMMENDATION FOR ALL WOMEN OF REPRODUCTIVE AGE: 400 µg SYNTHETIC FOLIC ACID A DAY

In 1992, the CDC published the U.S. Public Health Service (PHS) recommendation that all women who become pregnant consume 400 µg of folic acid a day (Centers for Disease Control and Prevention, 1992). Although the CDC scientists assumed that it would be clear that it meant that in addition to a woman's normal diet, she should consume 400 µg synthetic folic acid in a pill or in a breakfast cereal that contains 400 µg synthetic folic acid per serving, many nutrition professionals took the recommendation to mean that the total folate consumption (natural folate from food and synthetic folic acid from pills and breakfast cereals) should be 400 µg. It is important to understand the difference because it can affect the blood level of folic acid and the amount of prevention provided.

The studies that served as the basis for the PHS recommendation were all studies in which women ate their usual diet and took a pill that provided at least 360 µg synthetic folic acid a day. The usual Western diet contains about 200 µg natural folate. This natural food folate is only about half as bioavailable as synthetic folate. Furthermore, synthetic folic acid is heat stable, while natural folate is heat sensitive and destroyed by cooking. So the PHS recommendation, if stated in terms of the natural folate equivalence, would have been 1000 µg natural folate (200 µg natural folate from food and 2 × 400 = 800 µg from synthetic folate—100 µg synthetic folate = 200 µg natural folate). To state the obvious, 400 µg natural folate is not the 1000 µg one would infer from the recommendation.

The confusion happened because in regulatory matters and in nutrition textbooks, the terms *folate* and *folic acid* are used interchangeably despite their biological differences. In 1998, the Food and Nutrition Board of the Institute of Medicine acknowledged the differences and clarified the recommendation. What is in the summary of the final report follows: "To reduce the risk of neural tube defects for women capable of becoming pregnant, the recommendation is to take 400 µg of folic acid daily from fortified foods, supplements, or both in addition to consuming food folate from a varied diet." In the body of the chapter, the recommendation text is "folate daily from supplements." It is important to know that folic acid or folate from fortified foods or supplements means synthetic folic acid. Since the report had to do with nutrition, it left out folic acid as a drug, which it is. So the statement could have included the words "from drugs," such as prenatal vitamins, but it did not.

A TOTAL FOLATE RECOMMENDATION

Since the nutrition culture likes natural folate, I propose that anyone who wants to rewrite the recommendation in terms of natural folate state the level as 1000 μg a day of natural folate. It should be understood that no experimental and very little observational data have actually tested this advice. Given that if one consumes 1000 μg natural folate, the serum folate level will be higher than if one just eats the usual 200 μg natural folate, it would be reasonable to conclude that women consuming 1000 μg natural folate would have a lower level of NTDs than those consuming only 200 μg natural folate.

FORTIFICATION AND DRUGS/SUPPLEMENTS REQUIRED FOR MAXIMUM PREVENTION OF FOLIC ACID–PREVENTABLE SPINA BIFIDA

The concept of having every woman of reproductive age consume 400 μg synthetic folic acid a day is simple. Actually doing it is difficult. The most effective way would be to have enough folic acid in a widely consumed food product so that all or almost all women consume 400 μg synthetic folic acid a day. Wheat and corn flour milled in large mills can be fortified easily and cheaply. Where this has been done, there have been remarkable increases in serum folate levels (Jacques et al., 1999; Lawrence et al., 1999; Centers for Disease Control and Prevention, 2000; Ray et al., 2002). The increases in serum folate have been high enough to virtually rid the population of folate deficiency anemia and to substantially reduce the proportion of the adult population with elevated homocysteine—a powerful risk factor for occlusive cardiovascular disease (Boushey et al., 1995). It appears that the increased serum folate level has prevented some cases of folic acid–preventable spina bifida, but far from all of it (Honein et al., 2001; Persad et al., 2002; Williams et al., 2002; De Wals et al., 2003; Oakley, 2003). The fortification experience has been studied in North America. The United States and Canada required all enriched grain products such as flour and corn meal to have enough folic acid added so that the median woman consumes an extra 100 μg synthetic folic acid. Studies postfortification have suggested that the median woman may have had a 200 μg increase in consumption of synthetic folic acid. What is not clear is how much of the increase is from the required fortification of enriched grains and how much is from the folic acid voluntarily added by manufacturers to cold breakfast cereals and selected other products. The use of a drug/supplement pill with 400 μg synthetic folic acid has not changed, so it is unlikely that such use contributed to the postfortification increase in serum folates (Erickson, 2002).

The prevalence of spina bifida and anencephaly pregnancies has decreased in both the United States and Canada. The primary question is whether or not it has decreased as much as it might. It would be helpful to know the prevalence of non-folic acid–preventable spina bifida and anencephaly pregnancies. This prevalence has yet to be determined. We have some idea of its upper limit. A large study from China showed that consuming 400 μg synthetic folic acid lowered the prevalence from either 50 or 10 per 10,000 to 6 per 10,000 (Berry et al., 1999). Giving children the benefit of the doubt and to make the math a bit easier, I conclude that the prevalence of non-folic acid–preventable spina bifida and anencephaly is no higher than 5 per 10,000. Wald and colleagues (2001) produced a model suggesting that the non-folic acid–preventable prevalence is even lower.

Realizing that the rate of non-folic acid–preventable spina bifida and anencephaly may be lower than 5 per 10,000, I will, for this discussion, conclude that it is 5 per 10,000. Stated another way, if all folic acid–preventable spina bifida and anencephaly have been prevented, the prevalence will be no higher than 5 per 10,000. The current best data to judge the effect of flour fortification in North America are from Canada. Looking at spina bifida and anencephaly prevalence today requires knowing whether or not most of the prenatally diagnosed and voluntarily terminated pregnancies have been counted. The study from Newfoundland (Persad et al., 2002) and the one from Ontario (De Wals et al., 2003) paid particular attention to collecting the data from induced abortions. The prefortification rates were about 20 per 10,000, and the postfortification rates were about 10 per 10,000—a roughly 50% reduction. Assuming that the non-folic acid–preventable spina bifida and anencephaly rate is 5 per 10,000, the data suggest that about half of the cases that could be prevented by increased consumption of folic acid have been prevented. Another conclusion is that before fortification, the rates of spina bifida and anencephaly in these two provinces were four times what they should have been. It also follows that one way to assess the folate status of a population is to determine the spina bifida and anencephaly rates. If these rates are higher than 5 per 10,000, they are too high and the population should be considered folate deficient.

400 μg FOLIC ACID FROM PILLS OR BREAKFAST CEREALS—COMPLEMENTS TO MANDATORY FORTIFICATION

The current fortification programs in the United States and Canada do not require enough folic acid to provide maximum prevention. Before folic acid fortification was implemented, the Food and Drug Administration (FDA) estimated that at the concentration it choose to require, 140 µg per 100 g grain or 1.4 parts per million, the median woman would consume 100 µg synthetic folic acid a day from fortified foods (Food and Drug Administration, 1996). Given that the China data suggest that sufficient folic acid consumption by women of reproductive age before and during the early weeks of pregnancy will reduce the spina bifida and anencephaly rates to 5 per 10,000 or less, the data from Canada suggest that after fortification, these rates are about twice what they would be if enough folic acid was required to be added to bread (Berry et al., 1999; Persad et al., 2002). If we are to achieve complete prevention of folic acid–preventable spina bifida in the United States and Canada, in the absence of an increased concentration of folic acid in flour, we must develop and implement programs that will increase the consumption of folic acid from pills or from foods voluntarily fortified by manufacturers.

Certain segments of the U.S. population have for decades consumed vitamin/food supplements available over the counter that contained 400 µg folic acid. One approach to increasing folic acid consumption is to increase the consumption of these products. So far, efforts to increase the consumption of folic acid supplements in the United States have had limited success. Only 30% of reproductive-age women consume them, and the percentage has not changed over the past decade (March of Dimes, 2003). It has been estimated that an effective supplement program would require a national program costing $100 million a year. The total amount of money allocated has been less than $10 million a year. It is possible that an adequately funded program would increase the proportion of women consuming the recommended 400 µg synthetic folic acid.

In Europe, there has been some success in increasing folic acid supplement use (Raats et al., 1998; De Walle and De Jong-Van Den Berg, 2002). These countries, however, started with use of 10% or less and have managed to rise to around 40%, similar to the use in the United States. The European experience suggests that one can increase consumption of vitamin supplements or drugs with effective health education campaigns, but these should only be used to complement fortification programs. They should not be used as a substitute for fortification programs because they will not reach as many people as do fortification programs.

In Mexico, there is a study suggesting that the weekly consumption of a 5000 µg over-the-counter drug or food supplement may be effective in preventing neural tube defects (de Villarreal et al., 2002). Perhaps in many countries a weekly program of folic acid consumption may increase the number of women consuming folic acid and make a contribution to prevention.

The combined experience in the United States, Canada, Mexico, and Europe suggests that all countries should have inexpensive vitamin supplements or over-the-counter drugs with 400 and 5000 µg folic acid, respectively. Informed women would have ready access to these products that, when consumed regularly, are effective in preventing neural tube defects.

Cold breakfast cereals are another source of synthetic folic acid. Before folic acid was known to prevent neural tube defects, only a handful of cold breakfast cereals in the United States had 400 µg per serving. Now there are over 50 kinds with 400 µg synthetic folic per serving. The contribution of these new products in raising serum folate levels is not known. Some of the increase in serum levels postfortification that has been attributed to the mandatory fortification is likely to have come from the changes in voluntary additions of folic acid to cold breakfast cereals after mandatory fortification.

In Canada and many other countries, the amount of folic acid that can be added to cold breakfast cereals is limited to about 100 µg per serving. One practical and simple way to increase consumption of folic acid would be for regulators in Canada, Europe, and elsewhere to permit these products to have 400 µg folic acid per serving.

This chapter does not allow an in-depth discussion of the programs that will be needed in countries where substantial parts of the population do not consume centrally processed foods that can be fortified. In the long run, the total prevention of folic acid–preventable birth defects will depend upon implementing effective supplement/over-the-counter drug programs or finding a way to fortify locally processed foods.

Health and nutrition professionals in all countries should encourage women of reproductive age to consume 400 µg folic acid a day from over-the-counter drugs, nutritional supplements, and food that contain synthetic folic acid. Such encouragements will help to prevent spina bifida and anencephaly.

FOLIC ACID IN ORAL CONTRACEPTIVES

A recent CDC study found that only 17% of women attending family planning clinics in Georgia were consuming vitamin supplements containing 400 µg folic acid, whereas 42% were consuming oral contraceptives (Than et al., 2002). Discussions are underway in the United States between a drug company and the FDA about marketing such a product. Such products could, without changing the behavior of women, substantially increase the proportion of young women around the world consuming the recommended 400 μg synthetic folic acid a day.

WHAT IS THE LEAST DOSE OF FOLIC ACID FOR MAXIMUM PREVENTION?

This is a very important question and the answer is not known. This is a different question from the question "What is the lowest dose of folic acid that will have some effect among women with low enough serum folate levels to have pregnancies affected with folic acid–preventable birth defects?" A study of about 50,000 nonsynthetic folic acid–consuming women showed that increasing serum folates was associated with a decreasing risk of neural tube defects (NTDs). (Daly, 1995). Wald and colleagues (2001) showed that among these women, doubling the serum folate level halved the NTD rate. Furthermore, the lower the beginning serum folate level, the bigger the absolute reduction in NTD per 100 μg increase in synthetic folic acid consumption. So we are confident that adding even a little folic acid in nonsynthetic folic acid–consuming countries will prevent some of the folic acid–preventable NTDs.

The more important question is, what is the least consumption of synthetic folic acid that is required for a population of women to have maximum prevention of folic acid–preventable spina bifida? The current recommendation that all women capable of becoming pregnant should consume 400 μg synthetic folic acid assumes that most, if not all, folic acid–preventable NTDs would be prevented by consuming 400 μg synthetic folic acid a day. Wald and colleagues (2001) have modeled data and challenged this assumption. They have produced a model suggesting that increasing the consumption of folic acid to 5000 μg a day may be required for maximum prevention.

MAXIMIZING THE PREVENTION OF FOLIC ACID–PREVENTABLE SPINA BIFIDA

Maximum fortification of centrally processed grains is an essential foundation for preventing folic acid–preventable NTDs. Folic acid is safe (Dickinson, 1995; Oakley, 2002). In the United States alone before fortification, there were more than a billion person-years of daily exposure to 400 μg synthetic folic acid by the men and women who consumed vitamin pills or breakfast cereals with this amount. Since fortification, there has been population-wide exposure to synthetic folic acid with no report of adverse effects (Mills, 2003). Quite the contrary. As mentioned above, fortification has produced marked improvement in human health. For reasons that are not data driven, food regulators have often seemed determined to limit the amount of folic acid required to be added to grains. The concentration required by the United States is too low. Chile has fortified at a level that would give the median woman 400 μg synthetic folic acid a day (Hertrampf et al., 2003). That should be the minimum goal of all fortification programs. The concentrations could vary a bit from country, to country depending upon the amount of flour eaten. A thorough review by a committee from the United Kingdom suggests fortifying at 240 μg per 100 g of grain, or about twice the 140 μg per 100 g used in the United States. [Committee on Medical Aspects of Food and Nutrition Policy (COMA) of the Department of Health, 2000]. Modeling in Australia suggested that it would safe to fortify at 280 μg per 100 g (Flood et al., 2001). I think that all countries should require centrally processed grains to be fortified at 250 μg synthetic folic acid per 100 g and adjust the level up or down with studies after the grains have been fortified. Folic acid is safe at these levels and probably at much higher levels.

Technically it is very simple to change the concentration of folic acid added to grains. A package of vitamins—called a *premix* in the trade—is added twice a day to a device (feeder in the trade) that adds the vitamins at a certain rate. To change the amount of folic acid added requires only the use of a new package of vitamins with a different concentration of folic acid. Literally, one could be fortifying at one concentration on one day and at a different concentration the next day simply by using a different vitamin premix. So changing the concentration is easy if data are generated that suggest it is needed. Using 250 μg per 100 g flour would get spina bifida prevention started much sooner than waiting for complex studies of grain consumption, followed by complicated modeling to pick a different dose. These consumption and modeling studies can take years. And while they are being done, babies will be born with spina bifida who would not have been born had fortification been done first and studies performed to adjust the dose later.

TEACH WOMEN TO CONSUME 400 μg OF FOLIC ACID FOR MAXIMUM PREVENTION

For the foreseeable future, it will be necessary to have programs that motivate women to consume 400 μg folic acid from pills or foods voluntarily fortified with folic acid. The impact and the importance will vary by country. For example, in Chile there is little use of supplements and fortification provides the median woman with 427 μg synthetic folic acid (Hertrampf et al., 2003). What is not known is how many rural women do not consume bread made from fortified flour. Preventing spina bifida among these women may depend upon an effective supplement program.

In the United States and Canada, where fortification is insufficient, it makes sense to promote both pills containing folic acid and foods voluntarily fortified with folic acid. In the United States, multivitamin supplements have 400 μg folic acid, and breakfast cereals can have 400 μg per serving. In Canada and much of the remainder of the world, multivitamins have only 200 μg folic acid and breakfast cereals are limited to 100 μg per serving. In the Netherlands, folic acid cannot be added to foods, so a pill approach is the only way.

There is a need for improved supplement programs. Although supplements do raise serum folate levels and prevent birth defects, how many women will take them? The proportion seems to plateau at 50% or less. New and more effective approaches are needed. Would a once-a-week pill with 5000 μg be effective? Would more women be willing to adopt this schedule? These remain research questions.

Pills or voluntary fortification of products are needed especially where grains are milled in small mills and where few centrally processed foods are eaten. No doubt it will be in countries with these characteristics that it will be most difficult to get all or almost all women to consume 400 μg synthetic folic acid a day.

DOES 5000 μG FOLIC ACID PREVENT MORE SPINA BIFIDA THAN 400 μg A DAY?

The very interesting modeling of Wald and colleagues (2001) suggests that consuming up to 5000 μg folic acid a day would prevent more folic acid–preventable birth defects than 400 μg a day. Wald et al. argue that, based on current evidence, the best public health policy would be to have fortification programs provide all women with 400 μg synthetic folic acid a day and that public health programs should be developed to teach as many women as possible to consume 5000 μg folic acid in a pill when they are planning a pregnancy. This seems a reasonable suggestion and gives the benefit of the doubt to preventing quite serious birth defects. The key is that neither fortification alone nor pill programs alone are sufficient; both should be done. In countries where fortification can be done and has yet to be done—all of Europe, New Zealand, and Australia—mandatory fortification of flour is long overdue and the inertia of governments has caused thousands of children each year to be born with severe and preventable birth defects.

SUMMARY RECOMMENDATIONS

1. All women of reproductive age should consume 400 μg synthetic folic acid a day.
    a. In countries where grains are centrally processed, they should be immediately fortified with 250 μg synthetic folic acid per 100 g grain (2.5 parts per million).
    b. Pills with 400 and 5000 μg folic acid should be made available over the counter in all countries.
    c. Food products, such as cold breakfast cereals, with 400 μg synthetic folic acid per serving should be available in all countries.
    d. Physicians and health-care providers should advocate for fortification and pill programs in their countries.
    e. Clinicians seeing women of reproductive age, including pediatricians seeing the children of such women, should promote folic acid consumption.
    f. Oral contraceptives should be marketed with 400 μg folic acid per pill, including the blanks.
    g. More effective pill/supplement programs should be developed.
    h. Methods to fortify foods that are processed locally in small quantities need to be developed.
2. Women who have previously had a child with an NTD should consume 4000 μg folic acid daily when planning a new pregnancy.
3. All women planning a pregnancy should be given the option of taking daily a pill with 5000 μg synthetic folic acid.

NOTE

This chapter is dedicated to all persons born with spina bifida since 1991—the year Professor Wald and his colleagues proved that taking a pill with a well-known and safe drug, the vitamin folic acid, would protect most pregnancies from being affected with spina bifida.

ACKNOWLEDGMENTS

Disclaimer: I am a coinventor with a patent that covers the addition of folic acid to contraceptive and postmenopausal hormones. If compensated for this invention, I would be compensated under the rules and regulations of the Centers for Diseases Control and Prevention, where I worked when the invention occurred. I have been a paid consultant to Ortho-McNeil on this issue.

REFERENCES

Berry RJ, Li Z, Erickson JD, Li S, Moore CA, Wang H, Mulinare J, et al (1999). Prevention of neural-tube defects with folic acid in China. China-U.S. Collaborative Project for Neural Tube Defect Prevention [corrected; erratum. N Engl J Med 341:1485–1490.

Boushey CJ, Beresford SA, Omenn GS, Motulsky AG (1995). A quantitative assessment of plasma homocysteine as a risk factor for vascular disease. Probable benefits of increasing folic acid intakes. JAMA 274:1049–1057.

Centers for Disease Control and Prevention (1991). Use of folic acid for prevention of spina bifida and other neural tube defects—1983–1991. MMWR 40:513–516.

Centers for Disease Control and Prevention (1992). Recommendations for the use of folic acid to reduce the number of cases of spina bifida and other neural tube defects. MMWR 41:1–7.

Centers for Disease Control and Prevention (2000). Folate status in women of childbearing age—United States, 1999. MMWR 49:962–965.

Committee on Medical Aspects of Food and Nutrition Policy (COMA) of the Department of Health (UK) (2000). *Folic Acid and the Prevention of Disease. Report of the Committee on Medical Aspects of Food and Nutrition Policy Reports on Health and Social Subjects*, Vol. 50. London: HM Stationery Office, pp i–xv, 1–101.

Czeizel AE, Dudas I (1992). Prevention of the first occurrence of neural-tube defects by periconceptional vitamin supplementation. N Engl J Med 327:1832–1835.

Daly LE, Kirke PN, Molloy A, Weir DG, Scott JM (1995). Folate levels and neural tube defects. Implications for prevention. JAMA 274:1698–1702.

de Villarreal LM, Perez JZV, Vazquez PA, Herrera RH, et al (2002). Decline of neural tube defects cases after a folic acid campaign in Nuevo Leon, Mexico. Teratology 66:249–256.

De Walle HE, De Jong-Van Den Berg LT (2002). Insufficient folic acid intake in the Netherlands: what about the future? Teratology 66:40–43.

De Wals P, Rusen ID, Lee NS, Morin P, Niyonsenga T (2003). Trend in prevalence of neural tube defects in Quebec. Birth Defects Res (Part A): Clin Mol Teratol 67:919–923.

Dickinson CJ (1995). Does folic acid harm people with vitamin B_{12} deficiency? QJM 88:357–364.

Erickson JD (2002). Folic acid and prevention of spina bifida and anencephaly. 10 years after the U.S. Public Health Service recommendation. MMWR Recommend Rep 51:1–3.

Flood VM, Webb KL, Smith W, Mitchell P, Bantick JM, Macintyre R, Sindhusake D, et al (2001). Folate fortification: potential impact on folate intake in an older population. Eur J Clin Nutr 55:793–800.

Food and Drug Administration (1996). Food standards: amendment of standards of identity for enriched grain products to require addition of folic acid. Fed Reg 61:8781–8807.

Hertrampf E, Cortes F, Erickson JD, Cayazzo M, Freire W, Bailey LB, Howson C, Kauwell GPA, Pfeiffer C (2003). Consumption of folic acid–fortified bread improves folate status in women of reproductive age in Chile. J Nutr 133:3166–3169.

Honein MA, Paulozzi LJ, Mathews TJ, Erickson JD, Wong LY (2001). Impact of folic acid fortification of the U.S. food supply on the occurrence of neural tube defects. JAMA 285:2981–2986.

Jacques PF, Selhub J, Bostom AG, Wilson PW, Rosenberg IH (1999). The effect of folic acid fortification on plasma folate and total homocysteine concentrations. N Engl J Med 340:1449–1454.

Lawrence JM, Petitti DB, Watkins M, Umekubo MA (1999). Trends in serum folate after food fortification. Lancet 354:915–916.

March of Dimes (2003). Folic acid and the prevention of birth defects: a national survey of pre-pregnancy awareness and behavior among women of childbearing age 1995–2003. Pub. No. 31-1784-03. Conducted by the Gallup Organization. March of Dimes, August 2003; White Plains, NY: March of Dimes.

Mills JL, Von Kohorn I, Conley MR, Zeller JA, Cox C, Williamson RE, Dufour DR. (2003). Low vitamin B_{12} concentrations in patients without anemia: the effect of folic acid fortification of grain. Am J Clin Nutr 77:1474–1477.

MRC Vitamin Study Research Group (1991). Prevention of neural tube defects: results of the Medical Research Council Vitamin Study. MRC Vitamin Study Research Group. Lancet 338:131–137.

Oakley GP Jr (2002). Inertia on folic acid fortification: public health malpractice. Teratology 66:44–54.

Oakley GP Jr (2003). Folate deficiency is an "imminent health hazard" causing a worldwide birth defects epidemic. Birth Defects Res (Part A): Clin Mol Teratol 67:903–904.

Persad VL, Van den Hof MC, Dube JM, Zimmer P (2002). Incidence of open neural tube defects in Nova Scotia after folic acid fortification. Can Med Assoc J 167:241–245.

Raats M, Thorpe L, Hurren C, Elliott K (1998). *Changing Preconceptions: Volume 2. The HEA Folic Acid Campaign, 1995–1998.* London: Health Education Authority.

Ray JG, Vermeulen MJ, Boss SC, Cole DE (2002). Increased red cell folate concentrations in women of reproductive age after Canadian folic acid food fortification. Epidemiology 13:238–240

Smithells RW, Nevin NC, Seller MJ, Sheppard S, Harris R, Read AP, Fielding DW, et al (1983). Further experience of vitamin supplementation for prevention of neural tube defect recurrences. Lancet 1:1027–1031.

Than LC, Watkins M, Daniel KL (2002). Serum folate levels among women attending family planning clinics—Georgia, 2000. MMWR Recommend Rep 51:4–8.

Wald NJ, Law MR, Morris JK, Wald DS (2001). Quantifying the effect of folic acid. Lancet 358:2069–2073.

Williams LJ, Mai CT, Edmonds LD (2002). Prevalence of spina bifida and anencephaly during the transition to mandatory folic acid fortification in the United States. Teratology 68:33–39.

30

The Half-Life of Cost-of-Illness Estimates: The Case of Spina Bifida

NORMAN J. WAITZMAN
PATRICK S. ROMANO
SCOTT D. GROSSE

Neural tube defects, which include spina bifida, are one of the most frequent and most important categories of birth defects. Accordingly, there has been considerable interest in studying the impact of spina bifida as a public health problem. This impact can be measured in various ways, including disease-specific mortality, morbidity, functional limitation or disability, and quality-of-life impairment. Each of these measures captures one component of the total burden of disease. Such measures of impact are important because they allow public health agencies, researchers, and health-care providers to understand the effects of preventive or diagnostic interventions, changes in disease incidence or prevalence, and new technologies.

In recent years, cost-of-illness estimates have been widely used. The cost of illness reflects the direct costs of providing medical care, rehabilitative care, developmental services, and special education to affected children, as well as the so-called indirect costs of reduced workforce and household productivity. All of these costs contribute to the total economic burden of spina bifida.

Generating cost-of-illness estimates is not a trivial exercise. Nearly a decade ago, we authored the most widely cited and carefully developed estimates of the cost of spina bifida and several other birth defects (Waitzman et al., 1994, 1996; CDC, 1995). This work has been widely used in economic evaluations of ultrasonography (Vintzileos et al., 1998a, 1998b, 1999; Waitzman and Romano, 1998), folic acid supplementation and fortification of foods with folic acid to prevent neural tube defects (Romano et al., 1995; Kelly et al., 1996; Postma et al., 2002), and other interventions (Randolph et al., 1996; Rouse and Stringer, 2000; Vintzileos et al., 2000; Chung et al., 2001).

Our analysis of birth defect costs involved analyzing 15 data sets over a period of 2 years and required over $200,000 in financial support from the California Birth Defects Monitoring Program, as well as support from the Agency for Healthcare Research and Quality through training grants to the first and second authors. An effort of this magnitude is unlikely to be replicated in the near future. Therefore, it is important to consider the half-life of these estimates. In other words, are the estimates that we generated nearly a decade ago still valid? Can they be adjusted in a "back-of-the envelope" fashion to reflect current prices? If so, how? If not, why not? What factors need to be considered before deciding whether to undertake a new study versus simply updating estimates from an old study?

In this chapter, we establish a simple framework for determining the continued validity of cost-of-illness estimates. We find that these estimates remain valid so long as certain conditions and assumptions do not fundamentally change. We then apply that framework to our estimates of the societal cost of spina bifida. Adjusted estimates of the cost of spina bifida per case in the United States are provided based on this exercise.

A GENERAL FRAMEWORK FOR ASSESSING VALIDITY OF COST-OF-ILLNESS ESTIMATES

Cost-of-illness estimates may grow obsolete due to factors characterized as *internal* to the disease process. Such factors include changes in treatment patterns, reimbursement, or prevalence of the condition of interest. Developments in statistics, economics, and epidemiology that establish the theoretical underpinnings and methodological approaches for estimating the cost of illness, however, can also make estimates of cost obsolete. Such *external* factors might be as rudimentary as the availability of more reliable data or as involved as the emergence of a new consensus about the disease process that reveals a misattribution of cost because co-morbidities or related conditions were previously not fully understood. Also, new analytic methods could render older estimates obsolete. For example, within economics, there is continued debate over the validity of the human capital or *livelihood* approach that has traditionally been used in cost-of-illness studies, including our own, relative to the willingness-to-pay approach, which has a firm foundation in theoretical welfare economics (Rice et al., 1990; Garber et al., 1996). New statistical techniques for estimating and predicting costs are also being developed that may be superior to their predecessors for specific purposes, such as predicting future costs (Lipscomb et al., 1998).

For the current analysis, we develop and apply a framework that relates strictly to internal factors. The methodological and theoretical underpinnings of our birth defect cost estimates are still widely accepted and applied (Luce et al., 1996; Haddix et al., 2003). An exception to such neglect of external factors in the current analysis is the integration of a new discount rate to our estimates in response to the recommendations from expert panels on the use of cost-effectiveness techniques (Lipscomb et al., 1996; Corso and Haddix, 2003).

The critical internal factors that drive change in costs include changes in treatment, transaction prices,[1] and prevalence. Patterns of treatment may be altered in response to the development and diffusion of new technologies, the acquisition and application of new information, the passage of new legislation or regulations, or other changes in the organization and delivery of services. Changes in prices will change the nominal outlays for services (direct costs, or resources used), whereas changes in labor compensation will affect the nominal level of indirect costs (resources lost due to heightened morbidity and premature mortality). Prevalence may change as a result of changes in the survival or longevity of affected individuals, introduction or diffusion of prevention strategies, or application of new screening techniques that change the incidence of the condition through higher rates of termination of pregnancy.

More formally, these three general components driving change in the cost of illness can be expressed in a simple model of prices (P), quantities (Q), and prevalence (N). The total societal cost of an illness, TC, such as spina bifida, can then be expressed as

$$TC = \Sigma_j AVG_j \times N_j \qquad (1)$$

where AVG is the average cost per case for the N number of affected individuals/cases in each jth age/demographic/severity/or other relevant category used for stratification. Furthermore, the average cost per case can be expressed as

$$AVG_j = \left[\Sigma_i P_{ij} \times Q_{ij}\right]/N_j \qquad (2)$$

where P is the transaction price, Q is the quantity of treatment used (direct costs) or productivity lost (indirect cost) for each category of cost, i, for affected individuals in each jth group above. For example, if i is the category inpatient medical care and j indicates the age category encompassing the first year of life, then the average cost of illness for this group is simply the price of services multiplied by the quantity of services provided to all infants with the condition divided by the number of such infants. This simple framework provides a straightforward way to characterize the sources of obsolescence in cost estimates, and each is addressed in turn.

Changes in Prices (P)

To the extent that costs of illness change due to changes in prices (P), cost estimates adjusted for price inflation remain valid as long as the price index used accurately captures price changes. This may be problematic because of differential rates of price inflation across goods and services and because of the inherent difficulties in separating price changes from quality changes owing to continual change in the characteristics and mix of goods and services. Furthermore, any specific price index is limited by the scope of the underlying sample that is used to generate it. For example, estimates of medical costs are often adjusted for inflation using the medical care component of the consumer price index (MCPI), as in the current study, but that index is weighted strictly by the quantity of, and transaction prices for, services that consumers pay out of pocket. The MCPI therefore ignores the substantial payments made by public entities in medical care, as well as the transaction prices paid by third-party payers.

Even without such sampling difficulties, inflation can vary dramatically among different types of medical products and services. For example, between 1988 and 2002, the overall MCPI increased by 106%, while the inpatient component of the MCPI increased by 156%. Valid estimates require that cost figures are updated using appropriate price indices that are refined enough to capture the price changes of interest. More specifically, the price index in which the price for a specific service, P_i, falls must accurately summarize and appropriately weight the change in service or cost category, i, of interest. One should not assume that even disaggregated price indices capture inflation correctly. For example, using the inpatient subcomponent of the MCPI to adjust the inpatient component of medical costs of spina bifida involves two implicit assumptions: first, that that subcomponent accurately summarized general inpatient price increases and, second, that the inpatient services generating the increase in spina bifida costs are appropriately weighted in that component of the MCPI.

Estimates of indirect costs, or productivity losses, need to be similarly updated for changes in the compensation of labor. The employment cost index (ECI), calculated by the Bureau of Labor Statistics for the civilian workforce, captures fringe benefits, including health insurance coverage, as well as wages and salaries paid by employers. Subcomponents of this index capture compensation changes for sectors of the workforce.

Changes in the Number of Affected Individuals (N)

A general change in the incidence (N) of a condition will affect total cost estimates, TC, but will leave per case estimates, AVG, unaffected. Total societal costs can therefore be accurately reestimated using AVG, as long as accurate data are available on the change in N. Per case estimates, however, will lose validity if the following three conditions are all met: the change in incidence resulted from a change in the weight of a specific stratum, N_j, within overall prevalence, N; the grouping N_j was associated with a significant variance in cost; and the original estimates of cost per case, AVG, ignored this particular jth factor. For example, location of the spina bifida lesion (thoracic/high lumbar, low lumbar, and sacral) is associated with differences in average costs, which was not formally addressed our original cost study. If mandated fortification of grains with folic acid changed the birth prevalence of spina bifida across level of lesion, then per case cost estimates could be affected. Other interventions that may have changed the birth prevalence, such as more refined prenatal diagnostic tests that led to selective termination of pregnancy based on severity, could have a similar effect.

Changes in Treatment (Q)

Our estimates of spina bifida costs were based on treatment actually delivered to persons in California rather than on some gold standard of what ought to be provided. Changes in treatment modalities will almost invariably compromise the validity of cost estimates per case, AVG, as well as estimates of total cost, TC. While an obvious source for such change is the advent and diffusion of new medical technologies, there are other important potential sources both within and outside of medicine. Within medicine, changes in the organization of medical practice under managed care, changes in reimbursement practices, and legislative changes to Medicaid and Medicare all potentially affected the incentives faced by providers over the past decade and thereby could have led to new treatment patterns for children with spina bifida. Expenditures on special education and developmental services could have changed as well due to changes in medical care, but also in response to changes in the funding and administration of such services. Changes in labor market participation by those with disabilities would similarly affect indirect cost estimates.

It is worthwhile to consider the conditions under which the validity of cost estimates is most at risk due to changes in treatment modalities (Q). If the change was strictly an add-on (a new service, i) that had no effect on other service delivery requirements, for example, then previous cost estimates need only be enhanced by estimates of costs associated with the new service. This is the case for categories of service that were neglected in the original estimates, as well as for new services that leave other treatment patterns unchanged.

Because medical care service costs represent such a large proportion of our estimated costs of congenital anomalies, and because those services affect later requirements for special education and developmental services, as well as productivity in the labor market, changes in medical care services will more drastically shorten the half-life of cost-of-illness estimates than will changes in other noncore treatment areas. Even so, this half-life may be lengthened or shortened, depending on whether or not treatment patterns change strictly for a specific jth subpopulation with the condition. If insurance status changed for a particular subgroup with the condition, such as uninsured patients, so that the treatment now received by that group more closely approximates that delivered to another subgroup, then cost estimates could potentially be adjusted without generating comprehensive new estimates, depending once again on the level of refinement of the original cost estimates.

APPLYING THE FRAMEWORK: HOW VALID ARE PRICE-ADJUSTED SPINA BIFIDA ESTIMATES?

Perhaps the most straightforward adjustments that can be applied to old cost estimates are price adjustments (P) to account for inflation. Indeed, it is general practice for researchers using cost estimates to apply some price adjustment for inflation and/or for purchasing power parity. There are other adjustments that would be fairly straightforward to incorporate, among them changes in survival, changes in the percentage with a school or work limitation, and alternative discount rates applied to future costs. But the main purpose here is to assess how valid our estimates remain when price adjustment alone is applied.

We compare our price-adjusted estimates to more recent evidence on the medical costs of spina bifida in the literature and from administrative databases. We also consider a recent estimate of special education costs for the federally designated special education category, orthopedically handicapped. Substantial differences with more recent estimates would suggest a short half-life for cost estimates. Close approximation between the estimates, on the other hand, would suggest that treatment patterns may not have changed sufficiently in the past decade to merit the generation of comprehensive new estimates.

For the consideration of price-adjusted medical care costs, we generated comparisons with three distinct sources: a Washington State study that analyzed the distribution of medical costs for certain chronic illnesses, including spina bifida (Ireys et al., 1997); estimates of inpatient costs generated from the 1997 national Kid's Inpatient Database on pediatric hospital discharges; and 1991 and 2001 claims data from a managed care organization in Utah.

Price-Adjusted Medical Costs, 1993 Evidence

A study by Ireys et al. (1997) used Washington State Medicaid data to address policy issues surrounding the distribution of medical care expenditures for children with chronic illnesses. Summary data from that study on children up to age 18 years with spina bifida are given in the first column of Table 30.1. From our estimates of birth prevalence and survival, we constructed a synthetic sample of all children with spina bifida up to 18 years of age in California in 1988 to match the subject population used in the Washington study. Summary characteristics for this synthetic sample in California are reported in the second column of Table 30.1. In terms of demographic characteristics, the average age of the two groups is nearly identical. The Washington sample had a slightly higher percentage of girls, but we have no data on the racial composition of the California sample.

In terms of cost, the reported mean Medicaid expenditure for the group in Washington in 1993 was $11,061. Our estimate for the California sample, adjusted to Medicare reimbursements, was $9924 in 1988. Price adjustments need to be made for medical care inflation between 1988 and 1993 and for differences in reimbursement between Medicare in California in 1988 and Medicaid in Washington in 1993. We adjusted reported Medicaid reimbursements in Washington to approximate Medicare reimbursement rates, as explained in the notes to Table 30.1.[2] Geographic differences in Medicare payments per beneficiary, after adjusting for differences in case severity and practice patterns, have been shown to largely reflect underlying differences in wages and costs of living (Medicare Payment Advisory Commission, 2003). We therefore adjusted the Medicare-anchored California and Washington estimates to the United States as a whole.[3] Finally, the 1988 estimate was

TABLE 30.1. *Medical Costs of Spina Bifida Taken from Washington State Medicaid Data in 1993 Compared to Adjusted California Estimates from 1988*

Study Comparative Data*	Washington	California
Sample		
Mean age (years)	8.3	8.25
% Female	56	53
% Nonwhite	32	Not available
Cost		
Raw mean ($)	11,061†	9,924†
Price and cost of living-adjusted mean	14,607‡	13,773‡

*Raw data on prevalence and survival in California from Waitzman et al. (1996) were used to generate a "synthetic" prevalent population in California to compare to the 0 to 18-year-old sample used in Ireys et al. (1997). Statistics provided in the column are from this synthetic population.

†Figures in the first column reflect actual Washington State Medicaid expenditures in FY 1993, whereas the counterparts in the second column are 1988 California estimates adjusted to Medicare reimbursement rates in that state.

‡Figures in the first column are adjusted to Washington Medicare reimbursement rates and to the United States based on cost of living data. The federal Prospective Payment Assessment Commission (1991) reported that Medicare and Medicaid reimbursed at 100% and 77% of hospital costs, respectively, in Washington in 1989. The federal Physician Payment Review Commission (1994) reported that Medicaid reimbursed physicians from 76% to 83% of Medicare fees in Washington in 1993. Figures in the second column, already adjusted to Medicare payments, are adjusted to the United States based on cost-of-living data (Berry et al., 2002) and to 1993 prices using weighted subcomponents of MCPI.

adjusted to 1993 medical care prices by applying changes in the inpatient component and "all other" components of the MCPI according to the percentage weights of such care in the original estimates. The resulting figures, reported in the final row of Table 30.1, are once again very similar to each other, $14,607 based on the Washington data and $13,773 based on our California estimates. The difference between the two estimates could be attributable to residual price differences,[4] as well as to differences in the spina bifida case mix between Washington's Medicaid program in 1993 and California's in 1988.

Price-Adjusted Medical Costs, 1997 Evidence

The Health Care Utilization Project of the federal Agency for Healthcare Research and Quality includes a national dataset on pediatric hospital discharges from 22 states, the Kid's Inpatient Database (KID). The 1997 KID was used to estimate total inpatient costs for those aged 0–1 years with spina bifida. Weights on the dataset permit national estimates. National cost-to-charge ratios for urban and rural hospitals applied to that data yielded a total national cost of $60,136,566 for discharges among children below 24 months of age for whom spina bifida was listed as a diagnosis. The Kid's Inpatient Database does not contain unique individual identifiers, so it is not possible to link discharges for the same individuals or calculate total hospital costs for an individual child.

Because no prevalence data were available from KID, a denominator had to be constructed to estimate average inpatient costs. Using a complex algorithm, Jim Robbins and Mick Tilford of the University of Arkansas for Medical Sciences calculated that the 1997 KID-weighted data covered an estimated 1387 infants with spina bifida (personal communication). Assuming a comparable number of births in the previous year and assuming 90% survival to 1 year of age (Wong and Paulozzi, 2001), we estimated that there were 2566 children less than 24 months of age with spina bifida in 1997. Using this denominator yielded an average inpatient cost of $23,436.

Our estimate of acute inpatient costs per case for the same age group in California, adjusted to 1997 using the hospital services component of the MCPI and adjusted for cost-of-living differences between California and the nation as a whole, yielded $28,151. But California inpatient care estimates from discharge data used in our study were enhanced based on our detailed analysis of a comparative subset of longitudinal data demonstrating that many hospital discharge abstracts did not list spina bifida as a primary or secondary diagnosis because the diagnosis was not made until after discharge or because the diagnosis was simply left off the hospital record. For the age group under consideration, this enhancement factor was 1.03 for California discharge data. Applying a final adjustment to our estimate due to the absence of such an enhancement factor on the 1997 national discharge data yielded $27,331, still nearly $4000 more than the corresponding estimate from the KID data.

One likely source of this $4000 discrepancy is an underestimate of the enhancement factor when applied to national data. California hospital discharge abstracts have 21 fields for diagnostic reporting, whereas nearly all other states have fewer fields. Use of discharge abstracts from such states would therefore require a larger enhancement factor than was applied to estimates based on California discharge data.

Another factor that may have contributed to the reported discrepancy between the 1997 KID estimates and the adjusted hospital cost estimates from California was the national trend between 1988 and 1997 away from inpatient care toward greater reliance on outpatient care. Note that this was not as much of a concern in the Washington/California comparison provided in Table 30.1 because that comparison was based on a comprehensive set of medical services rather than just one component of medical services. To the extent that inpatient services were substituted for by equivalent outpatient services, overall medical care estimates were unaffected. Indeed, Ireys et al. (1997) reported that 51% of medical services delivered to those with spina bifida under Medicaid in Washington in 1993 were provided on an inpatient basis. This compares with 58% in 1988 for the comparable California sample. To the extent that this difference in the locus of care reflects a real and general trend, a significant part of the $4000 discrepancy above could be attributable to that shift.

A related concern is the sensitivity of inpatient cost estimates to the choice of index for medical service price adjustment. Our adjusted estimate would be $23,945 instead of $27,331 if the general MCPI were used to inflate inpatient medical care estimates rather than the hospital services component of the MCPI. To the extent that there had been a shift in the locus of care from inpatient to outpatient services for spina bifida treatment that mirrored the general shift in locus of care in the country between 1988 and 1997 (Levit et al., 2004), the weight of the inpatient component in the overall price adjustment ought to be reduced, and the resulting estimate based on California data would be lower. As discussed below, estimates of the cost of spina bifida for 2002 given in Table 30.2 provide a sensitivity range based on different assumptions regarding the mix of inpatient and outpatient services for those with spina bifida and the correct application of corresponding medical price indices for the period 1988 to 2002.

Price-Adjusted Medical Costs, 2001 Evidence

We performed preliminary analyses of comprehensive claims made available to us on spina bifida patients in 1991 and 2001 covered by a single major insurer in Utah. These data included a detailed breakdown of all medical care services by type of service and associated billed, allowed, and reimbursed charges by age group. The relatively small number of spina bifida patients limited our ability to perform detailed analyses, particularly when restricting the sample to those enrolled in the plan continuously for an entire year. Still, certain aggregations of the data provided insights related to price-adjusted medical care estimates for spina bifida.

First, the data firmly established that the ratio of overall payments for medical care services provided for individuals with spina bifida to the subset of encounters where spina bifida was listed on claim records was consistently greater than 2.0. Furthermore, this ratio did not appear to be systematically different for outpatient versus inpatient services. This result reinforced the finding that cost estimates for spina bifida that rely strictly on the appearance of a diagnosis code in claims or discharge data, as with the estimates from the KID study, will likely underestimate the true costs of the condition.

Second, age-specific estimates of overall medical care costs from the 1991 data, when adjusted by the MCPI to 2001, fell within 10% of actual expenditures for their counterparts in the 2001 data. This suggested a lack of

TABLE 30.2. *Average Lifetime Cost per Case of Spina Bifida ($), United States, with Selected Adjustments by Cost Category*

	(A)*	(B)†	(C1)	(C2)	(C3)
Cost Category	1988, 5% Discount	1988, 3% Discount	2002, 3% Discount with Sensitivity Analysis for Medical Care Inflation‡		
Direct Costs					
Medical Inpatient (gross)	*62,359*	*76,275*	*157,127*	***161,805***	*195,264*
Medical Other (gross)	*43,421*	*54,935*	*113.166*	***123,769***	*99,982*
Medical Total (net)	89,869	107,067	220,560	**235,839**	245,511
Special education	21,089	25,836	41,337	**41,337**	41,337
Developmental services	900	1,245	2,034	**2,034**	2,034
Total direct	111,858	134,138	263,931	**279,210**	288,882
Indirect Costs					
Heightened morbidity	47,614	95,893	138,086	**138,086**	138,086
Premature mortality	74,676	151,720	218,477	**218,477**	218,477
Total indirect	122,290	247,613	356,553	**356,553**	356,553
Total Cost	234,148	381,761	620,484	**635,763**	645,435

*Figures in column A are California per case cost estimates from Waitzman et al. (1996) adjusted to the United States by dividing direct costs by a 1988 cost of living adjustment factor, 1.083 (Berry et al., 2000) and indirect costs by the ratio of average employee compensation in California to such compensation in the nation in 1988, 1.103.

†Figures in column B are those in column A applying a 3% discount rate to costs beyond the year of birth rather than 5%, as recommended by expert panels on performance of cost effectiveness analyses (Lipscomb et al., 1996; Corso and Haddix, 2003).

‡Figures in columns C1–C3 are those in Column B adjusted for price inflation to 2002 but are distinguished from each other by the adjustments for direct medical cost inflation, as described below. The medical cost figures in C1 reflect the general increase in medical care prices (MCPI) applied to all medical costs, which implicitly assumes that the inpatient/outpatient mix of medical care for treatment of spina bifida was the same as that for the delivery of medical care in general in the United States. Our analysis demonstrated that inpatient care weighed more heavily in the treatment of spina bifida than care in general, however. The medical cost figures in column C3 reflect the application of the inpatient component of the MCPI to inpatient costs and the "all other" medical care component of the MCPI to non-inpatient medical costs based on the mix of such care for those with spina bifida in our 1988 analysis. The corresponding figures in column C2, our "best" estimate, reflect the application of the same component inflation factors, but the weight of inpatient care in the mix is reduced by the general 17% shift away from inpatient care to other venues of care in the country between 1988 and 2002 (Levit et al., 2004). For all three of these columns (C1–C3), the change in various ECIs generated by the Bureau of Labor Statistics was applied to nonmedical direct costs: the ECI for primary and secondary school teachers for special education costs, the ECI for public employees in the service sector for developmental services costs, and the general ECI for civilian workers for indirect costs. For indirect costs, a 1% annual productivity adjustment factor already included in estimates of future compensation was subtracted from the general ECI.

change over time in patterns of health-care use for patients with spina bifida in a relatively homogeneous population. On the other hand, outpatient services as a percentage of total medical care services provided to each age group appeared to increase, mirroring the trend in the nation. These results are tentative for the following reasons: changes in coding conventions need to be further examined; the existence of outliers coupled with a relatively small sample made some results unstable; and the effects of dual coverage and of Medicaid managed care coverage within the system in 2001 have not yet been established.

Price-Adjusted Special Education Costs, 2000 Evidence

Orthopedic impairment is the primary category among the 11 federally designated eligibility categories to which children with spina bifida requiring special education services are assigned. Recently published data on special education costs provided from the Special Education Expenditure Project (Chambers et al., 2003) found that the average special education expenditure per pupil in the orthopedic impairment category was $14,993 (95% confidence interval, $13,398 to $16,588) for the United States in 2000. Our estimate of the average per pupil special education cost for those in the orthopedic impairment category in California was $11,110 in 1988. When adjusted for the increase in the ECI for primary and secondary schools between 1988 and 2000, and for the estimated cost-of-living difference between California and the United States in 1988, our price-adjusted estimate for the nation in 2000 was $15,288. The remarkable similarity between price-adjusted estimates from our study and estimates from later work provides support for the view that changes in spina bifida costs have been mainly attributable to price changes. In this case, the evidence suggests that students within a particular handicap category received services in 2000 similar to those in 1988. Average special education costs for children with spina bifida could still have changed since 1988 due to changes in the overall proportion of those with the condition receiving special education services or due to changes in the allocation of those receiving services across federal handicap categories, but we have no information on that.

Summary Assessment of Price-Adjusted Costs

When our 1988 medical care and special education cost estimates were carefully reconstructed to match as closely as possible available evidence from the literature and from selected databases, both before and after our estimates, and when those estimates were subjected to refined price adjustments, our adjusted estimates were remarkably similar to recent evidence. Thus, our cost estimates, when carefully subjected to price adjustments, appear to still be useful for evaluating interventions and programs that are expected to affect the incidence or prevalence of spina bifida. This conclusion is not surprising considering that the current practice of surgical closure of the spine and the placement of shunts for hydrocephalus for those born with spina bifida was also general practice in 1988, when our cost study was conducted (see Chapters 18 and 19).

Given the evidence for their continued validity, we provide price-adjusted estimates for 2002 by detailed direct and indirect cost category in Table 30.2. These figures adjust for cost-of-living differences between California and the nation applied to our original estimates (column A), the application of a 3% discount rate to costs beyond the first year of life (column B), and increases in price indices applied to the 1988 estimates in column B to arrive at a range of estimates for 2002 (columns C1–C3) based on a sensitivity analysis.

The sensitivity analysis was generated to demonstrate the adoption of different assumptions regarding the hospital/nonhospital case mix of medical care services when applying different component parts of the MCPI to medical care costs. Medical cost figures in column C1, for example, reflect the application of the increase in the overall MCPI, which implicitly assumes that the case mix for spina bifida is identical to the average mix of care in the country across all conditions. This assumption is clearly incorrect, as our data showed significantly higher inpatient use of services than average for treatment of spina bifida. But the figures are provided as an illustration because it is often general practice to price-adjust using the general MCPI, ignoring differences in mix of services. The medical care cost figures in column C3, on the other hand, reflect an assumption that the hospital/nonhospital mix of services provided for treatment of spina bifida has not changed significantly since 1988. The resultant estimate may be too high, as there has been a general shift of services from inpatient to outpatient settings since 1988, and medical care prices have risen far more for inpatient medical care services than for other medical services.

Price-adjusted medical cost figures in column C2 reflect an assumption of higher inpatient delivery of services for those with spina bifida than for the general population but a shift in venue for such treatment since 1988 equivalent to that for the nation as a whole. This represents our best estimate. The resultant per case estimate in the United States of $635,763 in 2002 using a 3% discount rate for costs beyond the first year is almost 2.75 times the original estimate for 1988 using a 5% discount rate. Most of the increase was due to price/compensation increases between 1988 and 2002. The change in discount rate disproportionately enhanced indirect cost estimates, given the prolonged period after birth before the bulk of labor market and household productivity losses are incurred.

The remainder of the current analysis is devoted to a brief discussion of potential add-ons to these cost estimates, to changes in technology that threaten to shorten the half-life of our price-adjusted estimates, and to changes in prevalence.

COSTS AND CHANGES IN TREATMENT (Q) DUE TO ADD-ONS AND CHANGES IN TECHNOLOGY

Changes in Cost Due to Q, Add-Ons

While the evidence presented thus far supports the use of price-adjusted estimates of spina bifida costs given in Table 30.2, there are add-ons that could enhance these estimates and changes in technology that potentially threaten to make such estimates obsolete. Most add-ons relate to categories of resource use that were neglected in our study rather than new treatments incorporated into practice since 1988. Perhaps the most significant neglected category was parental caregiving cost, that is, the value of additional time devoted by parents to the care of a child with spina bifida relative to that given to the average child. This cost was estimated by Lipscomb (1986) based on a survey of 104 parents of children with spina bifida conducted in North Carolina in the early 1980s showing substantial reductions in earnings due to fewer hours worked per week for both mothers (14 hours) and fathers (5 hours). These figures are likely overestimates due to the nature of the survey. They were included in the cost estimates for spina bifida reported by Kelly et al. (1996), along with figures on direct costs taken from our earlier study.

Our estimates of cost also did not include any incremental cost associated with the medical services used in the delivery of the newborn, as such costs appeared on the maternal discharge record rather than that of the infant. Some incremental costs of delivery were therefore missed, as the rate of cesarean section in 1988 was likely already higher for newborns with spina bifida than for the average newborn. Currently, delivery by cesarean section is standard practice for newborns who are diagnosed prenatally with spina bifida, so the incremental cost associated with such delivery is an appropriate add-on to our direct medical cost estimates.

The event that conditioned our cost estimates was live birth with spina bifida. Costs were assumed to be zero up to that event. Additional costs would be appropriate to include if the standard that was applied was total cost contingent on *detection* rather than *birth*. The proliferation of prenatal screening, together with more sensitive screening for congenital anomalies, has increased the prenatal detection of spina bifida. Prenatal detection has affected cost through the selective termination of pregnancy and the resulting birth prevalence of spina bifida. But to the extent that prenatal detection has led to more service delivery in preparation for live birth, including delivery by cesarean section, all such incremental prenatal services costs would be appropriate to include as an additions to our direct cost estimates of medical care.

Changes in Cost Due to New Technology

Surgical closure of the spine in utero began in 1994 on a very selective basis, and only a few hundred such surgeries have been performed, all in four hospitals in the United States (see Chapter 18). The procedure is now the focus of a 5-year randomized trial funded by the National Institute for Child Health and Human Development, underway at three centers: the University of California, San Francisco; Children's Hospital of Philadelphia; and Vanderbilt University. The potential benefits cited in the literature of such surgery are prevention of some neurological loss associated with exposure to the intrauterine environment and prevention of Arnold-Chiari II malformation of the brain with subsequent avoidance of shunts for hydrocephalus (Olutoye and Adzick, 1999). If such surgery proves to be effective and is adopted as general practice, it would likely radically alter the treatment of spina bifida and render our cost estimates obsolete. Subsequent estimates of the cost of spina bifida would also have to include the additional risks to maternal health associated with fetal surgery, which presents additional challenges with respect to data collection and estimation of both direct and indirect costs.

Prenatal screening, as noted previously, is a technology that has become more widespread. Some portion of such costs could be treated as a cost of spina bifida, but its incorporation is potentially more complicated. If prenatal detection of spina bifida results in termination of pregnancy, the cost of spina bifida is potentially affected by the ensuing cascade of events, such as a subsequent pregnancy intended to "replace" the terminated pregnancy that was affected by spina bifida (Waitzman and Romano, 1998). In addition, if prenatal care is included, it would also be logical to include public health efforts to address the impact of spina bifida, which would include folic acid fortification, promotion of supplement use during pregnancy, and surveillance and research of additional risk factors, which would not be affected in the short term by changes in the birth prevalence of spina bifida.

CHANGES IN INCIDENCE AND SURVIVAL (*N*)

Selective termination poses the problem cited in the framework provided earlier if resulting birth prevalence changes in a way that alters the composition of costs. For example, if screening resulted in an increased likelihood of termination of the most severe cases of spina bifida and cost estimates were not made according to severity, then both direct and indirect costs per case estimates would suffer some distortion because average treatment patterns changed, as did the average profile of survival and disability.

Recent data from the Metropolitan Atlanta Congenital Defects Program (MACDP) have demonstrated a steady improvement in survival among infants with spina bifida over the period 1979–1994 (Wong and Paulozzi, 2001). Survival to 1 year of age was 82.7% in the 1979–1983 birth cohort, 88.5% in the 1984–1988 birth cohort, and 91.0% in the 1989–1994 birth cohort. By comparison, our published estimates of the cost of spina bifida were based on observed 1-year survival of 80.3% in the 1983–1986 California birth cohort. Wong and Paulozzi's exclusion of infants with trisomy 13 or 18 accounts for only about 3% of the 8% difference in survival between contemporaneous birth cohorts in the MACDP and California data, suggesting that there may also have been geographic differences in patterns of care and surgical outcomes. It is not clear whether there have been any recent changes in survival beyond the first year of life. Our analysis assumed 95% survival to 5 years of age among children who survived infancy, while Wong and Paulozzi reported 92%. We suspect that these estimates are effectively equivalent, given the relatively small number of deaths upon which they are based.

Applying Wong and Paulozzi's updated estimate of 91.0% first-year survival to our earlier analysis of the cost of spina bifida would increase aggregate direct costs for medical care and special education services beyond the first year but decrease aggregate indirect costs. The close proximity of our price-adjusted cost estimates to more recent estimates suggests that these improvements in survival, to the extent that they have occurred, have not been associated with significant changes in the average level of service requirements by age.

CONCLUSION

This analysis has provided a framework for assessing the validity of cost-of-illness estimates from the vantage point of factors internal to the disease process such as treatment patterns, prices, and prevalence. Our estimates of the cost of spina bifida in California in 1988 were subjected to that framework. Evidence from this exercise suggested that price-adjusted estimates, when carefully constructed, have maintained their validity. While the continued accuracy of the adjusted estimates may be adequate, it could be significantly enhanced by estimates of certain additions, particularly caregiver costs, which were neglected in our original study. The price-adjusted per case estimates provided in Column C2 of Table 30.2 may be used with some confidence in evaluations of interventions that are likely to affect the birth prevalence of spina bifida, but such estimates are likely conservative due to the omission of certain costs.

The most profound change with respect to the societal costs of spina bifida over the past decade was the reduction in birth prevalence and subsequent cost probably due to fortification of foods with folic acid. In other words, this public health measure had a more profound impact on the total cost to society of spina bifida than did changes in medical care technology. This will not necessarily be the case in the upcoming decade, as the introduction of new technology, such as fetal surgery, may revolutionize treatment patterns for the condition. The continued development and diffusion of prenatal screening technologies also have implications related to the selective termination of pregnancy and potential alteration of the distribution of cases across severity categories. Evaluation of future interventions that affect the birth prevalence of spina bifida may therefore require greater precision with respect to some subset of cases than is possible with the adjusted per case estimates provided in Table 30.2. New estimates that more carefully account for the variation in costs according to clinical features may therefore be required even if our estimates of average cost remain valid.

NOTES

1. Transaction prices are those actually used for reimbursement. List prices, incorporated into *billed charges,* are not appropriate to apply in cost-of-illness studies, as reimbursement for medical care, often through third-party payment, is based on negotiated discount or *transaction* prices that more accurately reflect the true societal or *opportunity* costs of treatment. The myriad *transaction prices* for any given service poses a challenge for cost-of-illness investigators. Medicare reimbursement rates were adopted as the standard in our study (Waitzman et al., 1996), as such rates are widely accepted and based on detailed evaluation of underlying resource use.
2. Medicare reimbursement levels were used to approximate underlying cost (see note 1).
3. We renormalized state cost-of-living estimates from Berry et al. (2000), which were normalized to the cost-of-living in Texas in 1960, to annual national national cost-of-living averages, using intercensal state population estimates as weights. The resultant cost-of-living adjustments were .965 and 1.083 for Washington in 1993 and California in 1988, respectively.
4. Lower cost-of-living adjustments for California or higher ones for Washington would have resulted in still closer estimates. Two other sets of state cost-of-living estimates using slightly different methodologies (Nelson 1989; McMahon, 1991), generated 1988 values for California centered on the Berry et al. (2000) estimate adopted here but provided uniform support for higher Washington values.

REFERENCES

Berry WD, Fording RC, Hanson RL (2000). An annual cost of living index for the American states, 1960–1995. J Politics 62(2):550–567.

Berry WD, Fording RC, Hanson RL (2002). Cost of living index for the American states: downloads, Study 1275, Inter-university Consortium for Political and Social Research. Available at http://www.icpsr.umich.edu:8080/ICPSR-PRA/01275.xml.

CDC (1995). Economic costs of birth defects and cerebral palsy—United States, 1992. MMWR 44(37):694–699.

Chambers JG, Shkolnik J, and Perez M (2003). *Total Expenditures for Students with Disabilities, 1999–2000: Spending Variation by Disability.* Special Education Expenditure Project, Report 5. Washington DC: American Institutes for Research.

Chung A, Macario A, El-Sayed YY, Riley ET, Duncan B, ML Druzin (2001). Cost-effectiveness of a trial of labor after previous cesarean. Obstet Gynecol 97:932–941.

Corso PS, Haddix AC (2003). Time effects. In Haddix AC, Teutsch SM, Corso P (eds.): *Prevention Effectiveness: A Guide to Decision Analysis and Economic Evaluation,* 2nd ed. New York: Oxford University Press, pp. 92–102.

Haddix AC, Corso PS, Gorsky RD (2003). Costs. In Haddix AC, Teutsch SM, Corso P (eds.): *Prevention Effectiveness: A Guide to Decision Analysis and Economic Evaluation,* 2nd ed. New York: Oxford University Press, pp. 53–76.

Garber AM, Weinstein MC, Torrance GW, Kamlet MS (1996). Theoretical foundations of cost-effectiveness analysis. In Gold MR, Siegal JE, Russell LB, Weinstein MC (eds.): *"Cost Effectiveness in Health and Medicine."* New York: Oxford University Press, pp. 25–51.

Ireys HT, Anderson GF, Shaffer TJ, Neff JM (1997). Expenditures for care of children with chronic illnesses enrolled in the Washington State Medicaid Program, fiscal year 1993. Pediatrics 100(2):197–204.

Kelly AE, Haddix AC, Scanlon KS, Helmick CG, Mulinare J (1996). Cost-effectiveness of strategies to prevent neural tube defects. In Gold MR, Siegal JE, Russell LB, Weinstein MC (eds.): New York: Oxford University Press, pp. 313–348.

Levit K, Smith C, Cowan C, et al (2004). Health spending rebound continues in 2002. Health Affairs 23(1):147–159.

Lipscomb J (1986). Human capital, willingness-to-pay and cost-effectiveness analyses of screening for birth defects in North Carolina. Unpublished manuscript. Durham, NC: Duke University.

Lipscomb J, Ancukiewicz M, Parmigiani G, Hasselblad V, Samsa G, Matchar D (1998). Predicting the cost of illness: a comparison of alternative models applied to stroke. Med Decis Making 18(Suppl):S39–S56.

Lipscomb J, Weinstein MC, Torrance GW (1996). Time Preference. In Gold MR, Siegal JE, Russell LB, Weinstein MC (eds.): *Cost Effectiveness in Health and Medicine.* New York: Oxford University Press, pp. 214–235.

Luce BR, Manning WG, Siegel JE, Lipscomb J (1996). Estimating costs in cost-effectiveness analysis. In Gold MR, Siegal JE, Russell LB, Weinstein MC (eds.): New York: Oxford University Press, pp. 176–213.

McMahon W (1991). Geographical cost of living differences: an update. AREUEA J 19(3):426–450.

Medicare Payment Advisory Commission (2003). *Report to Congress: Variation and Innovation in Medicare.* Washington DC: MEDPAC.

Nelson H (1989, February). An interstate cost-of-living index. Available of www.aft.org/research/reports/col/colpape3.htm.

Olutoye OO, Adzick NS (1999). Fetal surgery for myelomeningocele. Semin Perinatol 23(6):462–473.

Physician Payment Review Commission (1994). *Annual Report to Congress.* Washington DC: PPRC.

Postma MJ, Londeman J, Veenstra M, de Jong LTW (2002). Cost-effectiveness of periconceptual supplementation of folic acid. Pharm World Sci 24(1):8–11.

Prospective Payment Assessment Commission (1991). *Medicaid Hospital Payment Congressional Report, C-91-02.* Washington DC: ProPAC.

Randolph AG, Hartshorn BS, Washington AE (1996). Acyclovir prophylaxis in late pregnancy to prevent neonatal herpes: a cost-effectiveness analysis. Obstet Gynecol 88:603–610.

Rice DP, Kelman S, Miller LS, Dunmeyer S (1990). *The Economic Costs of Alcohol and Drug Abuse and Mental Illness: 1985.* Report submitted to the Office of Financing and Coverage Policy of the Alcohol, Drug Abuse, and Mental Health Administration, U.S. Department of Health and Human Services. San Francisco: Institute for Health and Aging, University of California.

Romano PS, Waitzman NJ, Scheffler RM, Pi R (1995). Folic acid fortification of grain: do the benefits exceed the costs? Am J Public Health 85(5):667–676.

Rouse DJ, Stringer JSA (2000). An appraisal of screening for maternal type-specific herpes simplex virus antibodies to prevent neonatal herpes. Am J Obstet Gynecol 183:400–406.

Vintzileos AM, Ananth CV, Fisher AJ, Smulian JC, Day-Salvatore D, Beazoglou T (1998a). An economic evaluation of first-trimester genetic sonography for prenatal detection of down syndrome. Obstet Gynecol 91:535–539.

Vintzileos AM, Ananth CV, Fisher AJ, Smulian JC, Day-Salvatore D, Beazoglou T, Knuppel RA (1998b). An economic evaluation of second-trimester genetic ultrasonography for prenatal detection of Down syndrome. Am J Obstet Gynecol 179:1214–1219.

Vintzileos AM, Ananth CV, Fisher AJ, Smulian JC, Day-Salvatore D, Beazoglou T, Knuppel RA (1999). Cost-benefit analysis of targeted ultrasonography for prenatal detection of spina bifida in patients with an elevated concentration of second-trimester maternal serum α-fetaprotein. Am J Obstet Gynecol 180:1227–1233.

Vintzileos AM, Ananth CV, Smulian JC, Day-Salvatore DL, Beazoglou T, Knuppel RA (2000). Cost-benefit analysis of prenatal diagnosis for down syndrome using the British or the American approach. Obstet Gynecol 95:577–583.

Waitzman NJ, Romano PS (1998). Reduced costs of congenital anomalies from fetal ultrasound: are they sufficient to justify routine screening in the United States. Ann NY Acad Sci 847:141–153.

Waitzman NJ, Romano PS, Scheffler RM (1994). Estimates of the costs of birth defects. Inquiry 31(2):188–205.

Waitzman NJ, Scheffler RM, Romano PS (1996). *The Cost of Birth Defects: Estimates of the Value of Prevention.* Lanham, MD: University Press of America.

Wong L-YC, Paulozzi LJ (2001). Survival of infants with spina bifida. Pediatr Perinatal Epidemiol 15:374–378.

31

Insurance and Coverage of Care for Individuals with Spina Bifida and Other Neural Tube Defects

HOLLY GRASON
JAMIE J. PERRY

Birth of a child with a neural tube defect presents an array of medical and caregiving challenges. These vary for each individual and evolve over the life span, both medically and in relation to intellectual, social, and emotional development. While most children with a neural tube defect will require ongoing care from multiple specialists, individuals with the same diagnosis may need quite different packages of services, depending upon their age, how the condition is expressed, the presence of other chronic conditions, and family resources.

The current financing system for individuals with neural tube defects is complex, comprised of a number of *accountable* entities including public health, employers, families, the educational system, and social support systems. The financing of direct medical costs has traditionally fallen under the rubric of public and private health insurance and families. Direct medical costs include the traditional medical services used to treat individuals with neural tube defects such as inpatient care, outpatient care, drugs, laboratory tests, radiological studies, equipment, and long-term care. In contrast, nonmedical direct costs are those related to services focusing on the developmental problems and disabilities associated with the neural tube defect that cannot be addressed through medical care (Waitzman et al., 1996). Examples include special education and developmental services; these are typically publicly financed by special education and public health dollars, with families also contributing. Adding to the complexity of multiple payers is the fact that some of the services required by individuals with neural tube defects cross the boundaries between what is considered medical versus nonmedical or do not fit into one of these categories at all, which may leave inconsistencies and gaps in their funding (Perrin, 2002).

Access to the resources to help pay for needed care is also highly variable and complicated. This is particularly true in regard to health insurance. Of the approximately 25 million nonelderly disabled, 56% were privately insured in 1994 and 20% received Medicaid coverage benefits. An additional 9% were covered by Medicare only or were dually covered by Medicaid and Medicare; 15% were uninsured (Kaiser Family Foundation, 2001). Reported uninsurance rates for children with special healthcare needs vary, the most recent rate reported being 5.2% (Blumberg et al., 2004). The extent to which health insurance can assist families and individuals is dependent not only on the specific presentation of the neural tube defect, but also on individual and family circumstance. Income level, employment status, the nature of employer benefits offerings, and geographic residence are all issues that come into play in determining whether resources are available to assist families in paying for care (Silver and Stein, 2001). Many families of children with complex medical conditions such as neural tube defects struggle to find and coordinate the right mix of medical, habilitation, mental health, educational, respite, and transportation services that their children require and that change as children grow. Parents find themselves creating individualized "mini-systems" of services. Ideally, funding sources would support these systems seamlessly. However, in many cases, no one funding source covers all needed services and only partial support is available for others (Newacheck et al., 2000; Krauss et al., 2001; Perrin, 2002).

This chapter describes the general framework and the major components of health-care coverage in the current U.S. health-care system. Reference is made throughout specifically to health services for individuals with chronic conditions like neural tube defects, with a special focus on children and adolescents. Following a brief synthesis of the complexities of access and quality-of-care concerns, emerging conceptual approaches and federal legislative and administrative initiatives on the horizon are presented. The array of health-care services typically needed by individuals with neural tube defects and the general likelihood of financial support to cover their costs are detailed in the Appendix.

HEALTH-CARE SERVICES AND COVERAGE "OPTIONS"

For most children, including those with disabilities and chronic conditions, health-care coverage is procured though privately arranged and financed health insurance. Most children are covered through dependent care coverage of their parents' employer-based health plans (Kaiser Family Foundation, 2002). Children whose parents are unemployed, as well as those whose employers do not include coverage for dependents in their benefits packages, must rely on public coverage. Even when children are insured through their parents' employer-based coverage, they may need publicly financed coverage and/or services in order for their health needs to be comprehensively addressed. A recent study found that 40% of children with special health-care needs/disabilities had secondary health plan coverage, the majority of which was Medicaid. (Hill et al., 2001).

Private/Commercial Insurance

Arrangements under private insurance include traditional employer-based indemnity (fee-for-service) and managed care plans. Underinsurance, or limitation in benefits, has long been a problem for children covered under traditional indemnity plans. Because health insurance was initially conceived to protect people from catastrophic health costs, coverage under these plans has been most extensive for hospital-based care, outpatient care for acute and/or chronic conditions, and related diagnostic services such as laboratory and radiology services. As a result, gaps in employer-subsidized benefits exist for many children and adolescents with respect to preventive and primary care, but especially in regard to specialized care, such as access to medical and habilitative specialists for children with chronic health conditions like neural tube defects (Hughes et al., 1995; Short and Banthin, 1995; Newacheck et al., 2000). Traditional indemnity insurance is becoming much less common, however, and most individuals with private insurance are now enrolled in some type of managed care plan (discussed below).

Public Coverage for Low-Income Groups

Medicaid. Medicaid represents the single most important source of public health-care financing for children and individuals with disabilities. Title XIX of the Social Security Act (1965) created Medicaid, a cooperative funding venture between the federal government and the states. Broad national guidelines govern each state's provision of medical services for needy populations, but states have some discretion in defining the groups their Medicaid programs will cover and the financial criteria for eligibility. Originally, Medicaid served only very-low-income women and children receiving welfare. Expansions of the Medicaid program in the 1980s extended coverage from these welfare beneficiary families to include pregnant women and infants, to higher levels of the federal poverty level (FPL), and, as of 2001, all poor children under the age of 19. In 2000, over 21 million children and adolescents (one in four U.S. children) were covered under Medicaid (Kaiser Family Foundation, 2002).

Mandatory Medicaid eligibility groups include women and children in very-low-income families, as described above, and the aged, blind, and disabled children and adults who meet applicable Supplemental Security Income (SSI) disability, income, and resource criteria. These *categorically needy* recipients of the Medicaid program are eligible to receive inpatient and outpatient care; laboratory and X-ray services; nursing home and home health services (for those over age 21 years); early and periodic screening, diagnosis, and treatment (EPSDT); family planning services and supplies; physicians' and nurse-midwife services; and services furnished by certified family or pediatric nurse practitioners. The EPSDT program requires states to periodically screen Medicaid-eligible children under age 22 for illnesses, abnormalities, or treatable conditions, and to refer them for definitive treatment. States are required to provide any federally reimbursable service that is *medically necessary* to diagnose or treat a problem that is identified in the screening, regardless of whether that service is included in the state's Medicaid plan. Examples include prescription drugs and devices, clinic services, dental care, case management, and therapies and equipment/devices for sensory and physical impairments.

Possible pathways to Medicaid eligibility for children and adolescents with chronic conditions such as neural tube defects include both income and disability criteria.

Children from very-low-income families become eligible for Medicaid based on the financial eligibility criteria. Some families having children with chronic illnesses that incur high medical costs may also "spend down" their income to meet the financial criteria for Medicaid. Children automatically become eligible for Medicaid when they receive SSI benefits related to a disability. The severity of each child's neural tube defect and the impact on his or her day-to-day functioning will come to bear in determining whether disability criteria for SSI are met. Once a disability is determined, SSI has its own income and resource criteria. While eligibility remains complex, Medicaid is particularly important for children with medical conditions like neural tube defects. The range of services offered by this program is more extensive than that offered by private insurance and other public programs, and comprehensive benefits are essential to maintain the function of individuals with disabilities (White, 2002).

Also of relevance to the population of individuals with neural tube defects are Medicaid home and community-based service (HCBS) waivers, which afford states the flexibility to develop and implement alternatives to providing care to Medicaid-eligible individuals in institutional settings. Under Section 1915 (c) of the Social Security Act, states may request waivers of certain federal requirements in order to develop Medicaid-financed, community-based care and service alternatives. There are seven allowable services that may be financed using HCBS waivers, including case management, homemaker/home health aide service, personal care services, adult day care, habilitation, and respite care. Federal regulations permit such waiver programs to serve the elderly and persons with physical disabilities, developmental disabilities, or mental illness. States may choose to target specific populations by illness or condition and/or individuals who would otherwise qualify for Medicaid only if they were in institutional care. Currently there are 261 such programs in effect nationwide serving older and/or disabled persons, including children with special health-care needs (HCFA, 2003), some of which may serve to assist families with children with neural tube defects.

State Children's Health Insurance Program. The State Children's Health Insurance Program (SCHIP) was created as a component of the Balanced Budget Act of 1997 and was the largest single expansion of health coverage for children in more than 30 years. It provides coverage for medical expenses to children through age 18 who do not qualify for Medicaid and have no health insurance. Established as Title XXI of the Social Security Act, SCHIP allows states to provide health insurance for children in families whose income exceeds Medicaid income eligibility levels but is less than 200% of the FPL. Many of the children and adolescents enrolled in SCHIP have parents who are employed, but are unable to access insurance coverage due to absent or limited employer benefits offerings and the consequent significant expense of purchasing coverage.

States can take three major avenues to implement the law. They can expand existing Medicaid coverage, which is an option that has been pursued by 15 states and the District of Columbia. Alternatively, states can create new insurance programs with SCHIP funds or expand already existing, separate, state-run programs (16 states). Nineteen states have pursued the third option by combining both approaches. It is important to note, however, that states choosing to implement their SCHIP program through a private, non-Medicaid option are not required to offer the same extensive coverage scheme found in Medicaid. As of October 2001, SCHIP provided coverage for 4.6 million children nationwide (U.S. Department of Health and Human Services, 2002).

Managed Care

Managed care has become widespread since the late 1980s and early 1990s in response to excessive costs under traditional indemnity insurance arrangements. Managed care plans bring the functions of health insurance and health-care delivery together in a single entity (such as a health maintenance organization [HMOs] or preferred provider organization) in an effort to manage costs. These plans attempt to provide all of the medical care needed by members for a fixed cost per individual, known as *capitation*. Managed care plans accomplish this by covering individual members for a defined set of benefits, furnishing these covered services through a panel of contracted or employed providers, and using controls such as gatekeeping to manage service use. The Health Maintenance Organization Act passed by Congress in 1973 requires HMOs to provide minimum basic benefits in order to be "federally qualified." This includes physician services and referrals; hospitalizations; well-child care and immunizations; eye and ear exams for children under 18; emergency treatment; diagnostic services; inpatient and outpatient rehabilitation services; physical, occupational, and speech therapy for up to 2 months; outpatient mental health services; and home health care.

Many children with special health-care needs are now enrolled in managed care plans in both the public and private sectors. In 2000, for example, 37 state Medicaid programs enrolled children with disabilities receiving SSI payments in some form of managed care (Kaye, 2001). In theory, managed care systems offer the promise of using capitated payments to support innovative models of coordinated care for vulnerable populations (Newacheck et al., 1997; Perrin et al., 1997). By bringing the financing and delivery of care together, managed care organizations can use financial resources in a flexible manner to pay for the diverse services that a particular child requires.

In practice, however, several administrative and financial obstacles have prevented managed care companies from addressing the special needs of children with chronic health conditions or disabilities. Placing primary care physicians in the position of gatekeeper and adding economic incentives to decrease costs may limit access to services required by children with neural tube defects, even if they are covered by the plan. Limited choice of specialists within a particular managed care plan's panel of physicians may further decrease access to appropriate care (Ferris et al., 2001, 2002). In addition, personnel in many managed care plans remain unfamiliar with the patterns of costs and service needs within this population (National Policy Center for Children with Special Health Care Needs, 1999). Even employee-sponsored plans with large enrollments will have only a few children with complicated service needs or very high costs (Bethell et al., 2002). Faced with a comparatively small number of children and wide variation in need, few plans in the private sector have perceived incentives to develop special programs addressing the diverse nature and needs of this population (Wallack et al., 1996). In the absence of such attention, access to services not explicitly covered in a benefit package may depend on how well plans have structured procedures for granting "exceptions to policy" and how effectively families advocate for such exceptions.

In response to the substantial disincentives for insurers and health plans to cover and/or adequately address the needs of individuals with complex and high-cost conditions, risk adjustment methods (paying higher capitated fee rates for certain persons) have been employed to ensure that vulnerable populations are enrolled and provided with good care in a sustainable fashion (Neff and Anderson, 1995). Most state Medicaid programs that have managed care programs now use some form of risk adjustment (usually based on age, gender, and broad eligibility categories), but only a few states use methods that incorporate indices of health status (Regenstein et al., 2000). Considerable uncertainty remains regarding which of the existing health-based risk adjustment methods is most suitable for the population of children with special health-care needs (Hwang et al., 2001).

Some states have pursued special efforts within their Medicaid programs to develop managed care programs specifically for children (or in some cases children <u>and</u> adults) with special health-care needs. These models usually include assignment of a clinical case manager (usually a nurse or physician) who has specific training in the area of disabilities and chronic health conditions, access to specialized providers and services outside the benefits package, a provider panel specified for the "healthy" population, and continuity of care safeguards (Fox et al., 2000).

Other Publicly Funded Resources

Title V Children with Special Health Care Needs Program. The Maternal and Child Health (MCH) Block Grant was established in 1935 under Title V of the Social Security Act. The Children with Special Health Care Needs (CSHCN) component of the MCH Block Grant has long provided the statutory and conceptual basis for public health services for children with chronic illnesses and disabilities. State Title V CSHCN programs provide professional and policy leadership in organizing healthcare provider resources and community-level care systems addressing the broad range of services and supports needed by CSHCN and their families. At the federal level, a portion of Title V monies provides support for national leadership, resources for professional training, program innovations, and research specific to this population.

As described in the initial "crippled children's services" legislation, the purpose of the Title V CSHCN program was to "develop, extend, and improve services for locating [crippled children] and providing for medical, surgical, corrective, and other services and care and for facilities for diagnosis, hospitalization, and aftercare" (Title V Social Security Act, Public Law 74-271). The initial focus of most states' crippled children's services program centered almost exclusively on children with orthopedic conditions and fusion defects, such as neural tube defects and clefts. Over time, the program adapted to changing epidemiologic landscapes and advances in medical technology and expanded this focus. Most recently, the federal Maternal and Child Health Bureau has evolved a noncategorical, functional definition of children with special health-care needs as "those who have or are at increased risk for chronic physical, developmental, behavioral, or emotional conditions and who also require health and related services of a type or amount beyond that required by children generally" (McPherson et al., 1998).

Themes long emphasized by federal and state Title V CSHCN programs include early diagnosis and secondary prevention, a team approach to care, and organization of services to enable children and families living in rural areas to access the same scope and quality of specialty care found in large urban centers. State latitude to organize program efforts to meet the early legislation's dual intent of gap-filling (service provision or payment) and healthcare system improvements has always been present. For several decades, with no other source of public support for high-cost special services, many programs emphasized their role related to direct service provision for low-income children and families. However, passage of new federal legislation in 1989 (Omnibus Budget Reconciliation Act [OBRA] '89, Public Law 101-239) substantially revised the Title V MCH Block Grant Program. For state Title V CSHCN programs, the legislation included mandates for infrastructure building services such as family-centered, community-based systems of care and statewide needs assessment, deemphasizing direct health-care services.

Moreover, as more sources of public financing for direct medical and support services are currently available through expansions in Medicaid, creation of SCHIP, and special education dollars, Title V funds are more frequently directed to services and activities such as case management, transition planning, family support services, population monitoring, and quality assurance. In economic circumstances where commercial and public insurance enrollment and coverage shrinks, however, Title V CSHCN programs remain an important resource in helping families to secure needed services and in reducing financial hardship related to a child's disabling condition.

University Centers for Excellence in Developmental Disabilities Education, Research, and Service/ Leadership in Neurodevelopmental and Related Disabilities Programs. Also publicly funded and of relevance to individuals with neural tube defects are the University Centers for Excellence in Developmental Disabilities Education, Research, and Service (UCEDDs). These programs grew out of recommendations made in the President's Panel on Mental Retardation created by President John F. Kennedy. The UCEDDs (formerly called University Affiliated Programs) were first authorized in Title 1, Part B of Public Law 88-164, signed into law in 1963. There are now 61 centers in every state and territory, funded by the Administration on Developmental Disabilities. Located in university settings, UCEDDs facilitate the flow of knowledge between academic centers and the developmental disabilities service delivery system with the goal of encouraging independence, productivity, and inclusion of individuals with disabilities in community life. The UCEDDs are involved in training of professionals (often through the LEND programs, described below), outreach to the community with training and technical assistance, direct clinical care, research, and the dissemination of information (Association of University Centers on Disabilities, 2003).

The Leadership in Neurodevelopmental and Related Disabilities (LEND) programs are funded through federal Title V monies. These programs (36 in number) are located at major medical centers and provide graduate-level training to health professionals with the goal of producing leaders for the treatment of children with neurodevelopmental disabilities. These programs employ a coordinated multidisciplinary team approach to ensuring high-quality specialty medical care (neurology, urology, orthopedics, etc.), as well as ancillary and supportive services for individuals with neurodevelopmental disabilities and their families. The services and expertise provided by UCEDDs and LEND Programs are an important resource for many children with disabilities such as neural tube defects and their families.

The Individuals with Disabilities Education Act. The Individuals with Disabilities Education Act (IDEA) funding can be a significant source of services for individuals with neural tube defects through age 21. This act ensures that individuals with disabilities have available to them a free and appropriate public education in the least restrictive environment. It was initially signed into law in 1975 as Public Law 94-142, the Education for All Handicapped Children Act, and was most recently reauthorized and amended in 1997 in Public Law 105-17. Reauthorization negotiations were again underway in 2003 when this chapter was written. Part B of IDEA funds special education and related services designed to meet the unique needs of individuals with disabilities aged 3–21 and ultimately prepare them for employment and independent living. Related services are defined as "transportation and such developmental, corrective, and other supportive services that are required to assist a child with a disability to benefit from special education." The services included in this definition are as follows: speech-language pathology, audiology services, psychological services, physical and occupational therapy, recreation, early identification and assessment of disabilities, counseling services, orientation and mobility services, and medical services for diagnostic or evaluation purposes. Also included are school health services, social work services in schools, and parent counseling and training (34 CFR Sec. 300.24). Since 1986, a similar set of services has become available to infants and toddlers who have or are at risk for developing disabilities under Part A of IDEA (34 CFR Sec. 303.12). Services provided under these Early Intervention programs are designed to meet the needs of the child and his or her family related to enhancing the child's development.

Both Part A and Part B IDEA programs include a Child Find component, which requires school districts and states to identify potentially eligible children early and provide timely, comprehensive assessment of their developmental, educational, and related health needs. The law also establishes a rigorous standard for prompt placement and provision of services.

Most children with neural tube defects are eligible for Early Intervention services and typically receive at minimum specialized therapies and case management through this program. Many of these children also qualify for special education services as they age; however, there is considerable variability in the amount of "related services" that a child may access based on the severity and manifestations of the neural tube defect, its impact on educational opportunities, and the availability of local resources.

The Agent Orange Benefits Act. The Agent Orange Benefits Act (Public Law 104-204) was established in 1996 to address the special health needs of children of Vietnam veterans who were born with a specific neural tube defect, spina bifida, possibly as a result of exposure of one or both parents to herbicides during active service in the Republic of Vietnam during the Vietnam War era. For the purposes of this program, spina bifida is defined as all forms of spina bifida except spina bifida occulta. Benefits include lifetime health-care services for spina bifida and "any disability associated" with spina bifida, a monthly monetary allowance, and vocational training/rehabilitation services. Because services available under the act do not include health care unrelated to spina bifida, additional health insurance must be maintained (Department of Veterans Affairs, 2003).

COMPLEXITIES: CROSS-CUTTING ISSUES AND PROBLEMS

Clearly, the challenges related to health-care coverage faced by children and families impacted by neural tube defects are many. Access to health insurance may become even more challenging as children with disabilities move into adulthood. Young adults are the largest uninsured segment of the population, and young adults with disabilities are no exception. Eligibility criteria for most private and public insurance plans changes as individuals turn 18 to 23 years of age, depending on the state. Most private insurers cease to cover dependents after age 18 unless they are enrolled full-time in school. If a young person is unable to secure employment that offers affordable insurance or is not able to participate in higher education because of his or her specific medical, physical, or intellectual challenges, then the options for private health insurance coverage are few.

Public insurance (Medicaid) options depend upon a particular state's upper age limits for eligibility on the basis of family income criteria (typically somewhere between 18 and 23) and whether an individual can qualify on the basis of SSI disability criteria. When a young person with a disability turns 18 years of age, he or she must undergo a redetermination of disability based on adult criteria. Some individuals may not qualify for SSI based on the adult criteria and may therefore lose this means of obtaining health coverage through Medicaid. Also of concern to some young adults who may receive Medicaid through SSI eligibility is the disincentive to work. To receive SSI and Medicaid, the young adult must be unemployed or, if working, earn below what is called *substantial gainful activity*. As income increases, SSI benefits decrease. Some states are now allowing individuals who would not qualify for Medicaid based on earnings but do meet SSI disability criteria to buy into Medicaid (White, 2002). The Ticket to Work legislation passed by Congress in 2000 was also an attempt to allow individuals with disabilities to work without fear of losing their public health insurance benefits.

These are just some of the issues related to insurance coverage that may face individuals with chronic conditions such as neural tube defects when they transition to adulthood. Understanding the scope and complexity of both private and public insurance options and the pathways to access can be a formidable challenge for families of children with complex medical problems at any age. Even when a child or young adult is insured and particular services are "covered" there are potential barriers to obtaining needed care, especially for individuals with complex medical conditions such as neural tube defects. Particularly problematic over the years has been the geographic maldistribution of pediatric subspecialty care, with far too few specialists available in rural areas (Perloff, 1992; Schroeder, 1992). In addition, the competitive health-care market means that providers frequently move in and out of contractual arrangements with health plans, and in order to get "better value," employers often change the managed care entities with which they contract. This generates major quality-of-care concerns related to coordination and continuity of care (Stein, 2001). Insurance is becoming increasingly expensive; after a short leveling-off period between 1999 and 2001, health-care costs again began rising, causing employers to increase cost sharing by requiring employees to pay additional premium contributions or copays. Insurance coverage also is less portable than ever before due to application of extended coverage waiting periods for individuals with pre-existing conditions.

Also of importance to this discussion is the concept of *medical necessity* and how it plays into treatment and payment decisions. Many insurers use medical necessity in determining payment for services; in essence, an insurer agrees to pay for a certain service only if there is the likelihood that the service will promote resolution of or improvement in the health condition. Decisions related to medical necessity are typically made by administrative personnel or medical professionals who are not directly responsible for the patient's care and who frequently lack the highly specialized training relevant to such decisions. They must rely on generalized protocols to guide them; these protocols are often based on standards established for adults and are therefore inadequate for guiding determinations of medical necessity for complex health conditions in children, which are highly dependent on growth and developmental stage, functional implications, and family care capabilities. Services thus can be denied, though presumably covered under insurance (Ireys et al., 1999; Fox and McManus, 2001).

NEEDS AND FUTURE DIRECTIONS TO IMPROVE THE HEALTH CARE FINANCING LANDSCAPE

While the picture painted in this chapter appears bleak, encouraging shifts in thinking and action are on the horizon. Arguments for special health-care attention to children promoted over the past decade are increasingly gaining currency (Jameson and Wehr, 1993; Perrin et al., 1994; Neff and Anderson, 1995; Ireys et al., 1996; Fox and McManus, 2001; Stein, 2001). They assert that children and adolescents have health service needs distinct from those of adults, requiring different types of prevention, diagnosis, and treatment strategies; these arguments support the call for a special standard of medical necessity in children. The basis for these arguments lies in developmental vulnerability in the context of rapid growth and development, children's dependency on adults and social institutions for both financial and nonfinancial support in accessing health care, and the differential epidemiology of disease whereby health problems in children and adolescents differ in prevalence and scope from those in adults. Special standards would recognize the extent to which development influences the medical needs of children as well as the special opportunities to avoid or reduce the potential impact of disease or disability through early, aggressive, and ongoing prevention (Ireys et al., 1999).

Several other developments in the larger policy environment are creating a fertile field for the creation of innovative financing models for this population. These developments are inspired in part by responses to pressure in the private sector to provide quality care in the context of cost containment. In the public sector, the Supreme Court ruling in *Olmstead v. L.C.* and E.W. also has played a role in this regard. The Olmstead case is about L.C. and E.W., two people with mental disabilities from Georgia who had to live in a state hospital in order to receive the support services they needed. These individuals sued the state under the Americans with Disabilities Act, Title II, saying that this arrangement violated their right to services in the most integrated setting, and they won. The June 1999 Supreme Court ruling in Olmstead v. L.C. and E.W. interpreted the ADA to mean that states must provide services in the most integrated setting appropriate in order to meet the needs of qualified individuals with disabilities. It is a violation of the ADA for states to discriminate against people with disabilities by providing services solely in institutions when the individual could be served more appropriately in a community-based setting. The ruling directs states to make "reasonable modifications" in programs and activities. The Court suggested that a state could establish compliance with ADA (*1*) if it has a comprehensive, effective working plan for placing qualified people in less restrictive, integrated settings, and (*2*) if there is a waiting list for community-based services, it ensures that people can come off the list at a reasonable pace and receive services. As a result, the federal government has encouraged states to plan for reforms not only in the health arena but also in the areas of transportation, housing, education, and other social supports to fully integrate people with disabilities into the least restrictive settings.

A foundation of experience regarding consumer-directed models of service delivery is evolving (Brown and Foster, 2000; Snyder and Snyder, 2002). One of these is a major initiative based on the President's New Freedom Initiative (HCFA, May 17, 2001). As part of these efforts, in September 2001, the Centers for Medicare and Medicaid (CMS) awarded "System Change Grants for Community Living" to states for the purpose of enabling children and adults with disabilities or long-term illnesses to (*1*) live in the most integrated community setting appropriate to their individual support requirements and preferences; (*2*) exercise meaningful choices about their living environment, the providers of services they receive, the types of support they use, and the manner in which services are provided; and (*3*) obtain quality services in a manner as consistent as possible with their community living preferences and priorities. One likely impact of these grants will be to increase interest in new models of community-based systems of care for children with special health-care needs, possibly by expanding the number of child-oriented home and community-based waiver programs (LeBlanc et al., 2000).

Moreover, during the past two decades, numerous policy efforts have aimed to support collaboration between families of children with special health-care needs and health professionals in the context of a medical home and a family-centered, community-based service system. The development of quality assurance mechanisms and an integrated approach to financing and service delivery are natural extensions of these concepts. Managed care industry design of a standard quality measurement system, the Health Plan Employer Data and Information Set (HEDIS), has provided important opportunities to develop and incorporate measures specific to children with special health-care needs into the otherwise adult-oriented models for quality assurance (Kuhlthau et al., 1998; Stein, 2001; Epstein and Walker, 2002). Consumer-oriented organizations like New England SERVE and Family Voices also have capitalized on such opportunities with specific programs and publications aimed at partnerships with the insurance industry and managed care plans to implement quality-of-care strategies for children with special health-care needs (New England SERVE, 2002).

Following a different path, a group of academic researchers, family advocates, and managed care organization administrators have been working together in recent years to devise models that might be applied to address the many problems created by the structure of the current systems of care and financing (Ireys et al., 2002). The model evolving from this collaborative combines consumer choice with cost-effective benefit administration and creates incentives for families, providers, and health plans to collaborate in identifying appropriate health outcomes for the child and the services needed to achieve them. At its simplest, this approach involves a selected group of individuals meeting together to allocate a fixed amount of money for services that a child needs to achieve desired health outcomes. For example, the team might have an allocation of $2000 to spend over a period of 12 months on supportive services, associated therapies, and care coordination for a 10-year-old child who has a neural tube defect, with significant limitations in daily activities. The team can decide to use these funds to pay for transportation services to assist the child in getting to special services after school, for the pediatrician's extra time needed to write a detailed letter to the Individualized Education Plan (IEP) team at the school, or for medications. Allocations would be determined by the team's judgment regarding the child's unmet needs and what services would help to achieve specified health outcomes. The Robert Wood Johnson's Changes in Healthcare Financing and Cash and Counseling Initiatives represent important venues for supporting demonstrations of similar models of integrated health care and financing systems for persons with disabilities or chronic illness.

Finally, over the past several years, Congress has debated passage of a proposal for the Family Opportunity Act (FOA), which would allow states to create options for families with disabled children to buy into Medicaid (on a sliding fee scale) while continuing to work. Specific provisions of the pending House and Senate bills include (*1*) a new option to allow states to expand Medicaid to disabled children up to age 18 who would otherwise be eligible for SSI benefits but for their household income; (*2*) state authority to include disabled children receiving inpatient psychiatric hospital services under the state's home and community-based waiver program; and (*3*) funds to support health information centers to help families with special needs children; these centers would provide technical assistance and resource information. With substantial support as of this writing, families and advocates are very hopeful that funds for implementing the FOA will be allocated in the federal budget currently in negotiation.

Momentum nationally to address the health care and health financing needs of children and adults with chronic conditions and disabilities such as neural tube defects has, for the past several decades, been inspired by organizational advocacy. Notable among the growing number of advocacy resources is the Spina Bifida Association of America (SBAA), which was founded in 1973 to represent the specific needs of the spina bifida community. This organization provides services such public awareness campaigns, a toll-free information and referral service, newsletters, conferences and educational symposiums, and individual and systems advocacy. Another key resource of this type is Family Voices. With over 40,000 members, Family Voices serves as a national grassroots clearinghouse for information and education concerning the health care of children with any type of special health need, including those with neural tube defects. Through a network of regional and state coordinators, parents of children with chronic illnesses and disabilities share their experiences and expertise with state and national policy makers, the media, health professionals, and other families. Supported by the federal Maternal and Child Health Bureau and private foundations, Family Voices implements projects to assist families in interactions with insurers and managed care organizations to address the special needs of their children regarding access to and coverage of specialty and subspecialty health care. Given the current marketplace and policy environments of competing demands and constituencies, and the complex interactions affecting individual health needs and access to care, leadership in advocacy will remain a critical resource for individuals, families, and those who serve them.

REFERENCES

Association of University Centers on Disabilities (2003). New on our site. Available at http://www.aucd.org.

Benjamin A (2001). Consumer-directed services at home: A new model for persons with disabilities. Health Aff 20: 80–95.

Bethell CD, Read D, Stein RE, Blumberg SJ, Wells N, Newacheck PW (2002). Identifying children with special health care needs: development and evaluation of a short screening instrument. Ambul Pediatr 2:38–48.

Blumberg SJ, Osborn L, Luke JV, Olson L, Frankel MR (2004). Estimating the prevalence of uninsured children: an evaluation of data from the National Survey of Children with Special Health Care Needs, 2001. Natl Ctr Health Stat. Vital Health Stat. 136:1–38.

Brown R, Foster L (2000). *Issue Brief: Cash and Counseling: Early Experiences in Arkansas.* Princeton, NJ: Mathematica Policy Research.

Department of Veterans Affairs (2003). *Health Administration Center.* Available at http://www.va.gov/hac.

Epstein SG, Walker DK (2002). Applying the lessons learned in identifying children with special health care needs: next steps to assure quality care. Ambul Pediatr 2:26–28.

Ferris TG, Chang Y, Perrin JM, Blumenthal D, Pearson SD (2002). Effects of removing gatekeeping on specialist utilization by children in a health maintenance organization. Arch Pediatr Adolesc Med 156:574–579.

Ferris TG, Perrin JM, Manganello JA, Chang Y, Causino N, Blumenthal D (2001). Switching to gatekeeping: changes in expenditures and utilization for children. Pediatrics 108:283–290.

Fox HB, McManus MA (2001). A national study of commercial health insurance and Medicaid definitions of medical necessity: what do they mean for children? Ambul Pediatr 1:16–22.

Fox HB, McManus MA, Austrian JS (2000). *An Analysis of Safeguards for Children with Special Needs in States' Medicaid Managed Care Contracts, 1999.* Washington, DC: Fox Health Policy Consultants.

Health Care Financing Administration (2001). *Coordinated Invitation to Apply for System Change Grants for Community Living.* CFDA No. 93.779. Baltimore: Department of Health & Human Services.

Health Care Financing Administration (2003). Home and community-based services 1915(c) waivers. Available at http://cms.hhs.gov/medicaid/1915c/default.asp.

Hill I, Lutzy AW, Schwalberg R (2001). *Are We Responding to Their Needs? States' Early Experiences Serving Children with Special Health Care Needs Under SCHIP.* Occasional Paper 48. Washington, DC: Urban Institute.

Hughes RG, Davis TL, Reynolds RC (1995). Assuring children's health as the basis for health care reform. Health Aff 14:158–167.

Hwang W, Ireys H, Anderson G (2001). Comparison of risk adjusters for Medicaid-enrolled children with and without chronic health conditions. Ambul Pediatr 4:217–224.

Ireys H, Grason H, Guyer B (1996). Assuring quality of care for children with special needs in managed care organizations: roles for pediatricians. Pediatrics 98:178–185.

Ireys H, Wehr E, Cooke R (1999). *Assuring High Quality of Care for Persons with Developmental Disabilities and Other Special Health Care Needs: Specifications for a Definition of Medical Necessity.* Baltimore: Johns Hopkins University National Policy Center for Children with Special Health Care Needs.

Jameson EJ, Wehr E (1993). Drafting national health care reform legislation to protect the health interests of children. Stanford Law Policy Rev 5:152–176.

Kaiser Family Foundation (2001). *Medicaid's Role for the Disabled Population Under Age 65.* Washington, DC: Kaiser Family Foundation.

Kaiser Family Foundation (2002). *Health Coverage for Low-Income Children.* Washington, DC: Kaiser Family Foundation.

Kaiser Family Foundation (2003). *The Uninsured and Their Access to Health Care.* Washington, DC: Kaiser Family Foundation.

Kaye N (2001). *Medicaid Managed Care: A Guide for States,* 5th ed. Portland, ME: National Academy for State Health Policy.

Krauss M, Wells N, Gulley S, Anderson B (2001). Navigating systems of care: results from a national survey of families of children with special health care needs. *Children's Services: Social Policy, Research, and Practice,* 4:165–187.

Kuhlthau K, Walker DK, Perrin JM, Bauman L, Gortmaker SL, Newacheck PW, Stein RE (1998). Assessing managed care for children with chronic conditions. Health Aff 17:42–52.

LeBlanc A, Tonner C, Harrington C (2000). Medicaid 1915(c) home and community-based waivers services across the states. Health Care Financing Rev 22:159–174.

McPherson M, Arango P, Fox H, Lauver C, McManus M, Newacheck PW, Perrin JM, et al (1998). A new definition of children with special health care needs. Pediatrics 102:137–140.

National Policy Center for Children with Special Health Care Needs (1999). *Financing Workgroup: Summary of Discussion.* Baltimore. Johns Hopkins University Press.

Neff J, Anderson G (1995). Protecting children with chronic illness in a competitive marketplace. JAMA 274:1866–1869.

Newacheck PW, Hughes DC, Halfon N, Brindis C (1997) Social HMOs and other capitated arrangements for children with special health care needs. Matern Child Health J 1:111–119.

Newacheck P, McManus M, Fox H, Hung Y, Halfon N (2000). Access to health care for children with special health care needs. Pediatrics 105:760–766.

New England SERVE (2002). *Shared Responsibilities Toolkit: Tools for Improving Quality of Care for Children with Special Health Care Needs.* Boston: New England SERVE.

Perloff J (1992). Health care resources for children and pregnant women. Future Children 2:78–94.

Perrin JM (2002). Health services research for children with disabilities. Milbank Q 80:303–324.

Perrin JM, Kahn RS, Bloom SR, Davidson S, Guyer B, Hollinshead W, Richmond JB, et al (1994). Health care reform and the special needs of children. Pediatrics 93:504–506.

Perrin JM, Kuhlthau K, Walker DK, Stein RE, Newacheck PW, Gortmaker SL (1997). Monitoring health care for children with chronic conditions in a managed care environment. Matern Child Health J 1:15–23.

Regenstein M, Schroer C, Meyer J (2000). *Medicaid Managed Care for Persons with Disabilities: A Closer Look.* Washington, DC: Kaiser Family Foundation.

Schroeder SA (1992). Physician supply and the U.S. medical marketplace. Health Aff 11:235–243.

Short PF, Banthin JS (1995). New estimates of underinsured younger than 65 years. JAMA 274:1302–1306.

Silver EJ, Stein RE (2001). Access to care, unmet health needs, and poverty status among children with and without chronic conditions. Ambul Pediatr 1:314–320.

Snyder B, Snyder R (2002). Consumer choice in long-term care. In Isaacs S, Knickman J (eds): *To Improve Health and Health Care,* Vol. V. Princeton, NJ: Robert Wood Johnston Foundation, pp. 101–122.

Stein RE (2001). Challenges in long-term health care for children. Ambul Pediatr 1:280–288.

U.S. Department of Health and Human Services, Health Resources and Services Administration, Maternal and Child Health Bureau (2002). Rockville, MD: *Child Health USA 2002.* U.S. Department of Health and Human Services.

Waitzman NJ, Scheffler RM, Romano PS (1996). *The Cost of Birth Defects: Estimates of the Value of Prevention.* Lanham, MD: University Press of America.

Wallack SS, Levine HJ, McManus MA, Fox HB, Newacheck PW, Frank RG, McGuire TG (1996). Managed care for people with disabilities: caring for those with the greatest need. *Baxter Health Policy Rev* 2:351–394.

White PH (2002). Access to health care: health insurance considerations for young adults with special health care needs/disabilities. Pediatrics 110:1328–1335.

32

Assessment of Health-Related Quality of Life in Individuals with Neural Tube Defects

JIM STEVENSON
INEKE M. PIT-TEN CATE

The quality of life in people with neural tube defects (NTDs) is an important issue for clinicians and service providers. Decisions that might affect quality of life need to be informed by measurement of the quality of life of those concerned. This chapter will review what is known about the quality of life in individuals with NTDs, evaluate the different types of quality-of-life measures that are available, and highlight what has been learned from a recently conducted large-scale study of the quality of life in children and adolescents with spina bifida and/or hydrocephalus.

THE CONCEPTS OF QUALITY OF LIFE AND HEALTH-RELATED QUALITY OF LIFE

Quality of life (QOL) is a multidimensional construct that concerns physical, mental, and social well-being. When QOL is applied to areas of functioning that are directly affected by a disability/chronic illness or its treatment, this is termed *health-related quality of life* (HRQOL). The multidimensional character of QOL is reflected in the fact that several domains are included in QOL measures. Assessment of QOL in children and adolescents with serious health conditions has become more important with innovations in medical health care, resulting in higher survival rates and longer life expectancy (Spieth and Harris, 1996; Eiser, 1997).

When considering QOL measures for use with people with NTDs, it is important to first identify the domains most affected. A measure of QOL should include the following four domains: disease state and physical, psychological, and social functioning (Spieth and Harris, 1996). For persons with NTDs a QOL measure could include questions regarding the number of hospitalizations and surgeries, as well as problems with vision, hearing, bowel and bladder control, and walking. Similarly, domains of social and cognitive functioning should be included, especially for children and adolescents, such as peer relationships and school achievement.

A number of QOL measures are available, and the choice of which measure to use largely depends on the underlying aims of the assessment. To compare across disease groups or between people with and without health conditions, a generic questionnaire would be appropriate. On the other hand, if the interest is in the specific impact of a treatment, a disease-specific measure may be more sensitive (Spieth and Harris, 1996; Eiser, 1997).

AGE-RELATED CHANGES IN HEALTH-RELATED QUALITY OF LIFE

It is expected that HRQOL will change with age. The impact of a given condition on HRQOL will be different for a 6-year-old, a 16-year-old, and a 60-year-old. The range of activities and their salience will be different at different stages of the life cycle. This means that any conclusion about the impact of NTDs on HRQOL needs to be qualified by the age range that is being considered. In this chapter, we will concentrate on the impact of NTDs on the HRQOL of children and adolescents.

AVAILABLE MEASURES OF HEALTH-RELATED QUALITY OF LIFE

Spieth and Harris (1996) reviewed the available measures of HRQOL for children and adolescents. They conclude that psychometrically sound HRQOL measures are lacking in the area of pediatric psychology. Five years later, in a review, Eiser and Morse (2001) concluded that the situation had not changed markedly and that only a few QOL measures showed acceptable psychometric properties. Specifically, they found that only three generic measures—the Child Health Questionnaire (CHQ-CF87, Landgraf and Abetz, 1997), the Pediatric Quality of Life Inventory (PedsQL; Varni et al., 1999), and the Health Utilities Index (Feeny et al., 1998) measures—showed acceptable reliability and validity.

The CHQ-CF87 can be used for children aged 4–19 years (parent report) or 10–19 years (child report) and covers 12 domains. This measure was developed in the United States but has several translations in United Kingdom English and German. The PedsQL is a brief measure that assesses the child's and parent's perceptions of HRQOL and can be used for children aged 2–18 years. The measure consists of 15 core items of global QOL and 8 supplemental modules assessing specific symptoms or treatment domains. Finally, the Health Utilities Index is a 7-item measure covering seven domains and can be completed by parents of children aged 6–18 years. The measure is focused on core attributes of health status and on the capacity of an individual to function with respect to these attributes. Neither the review or Speith and Harris (1996) nor that of by Eiser and Morse (2001) included a NTD specific measure.

In the study on HRQOL in children and adolescents with NTD reported below, the child health-related quality of life measure was used (CHRQOL; Graham et al., 1997; Stevenson, 1997). This instrument was designed to provide a core set of dimensions (15 plus an overall rating) on which QOL could be rated for children with a wide variety of physical and mental illnesses. The measure has parent- and child-rated versions suitable for children aged 8–16 years, so ratings can reflect both parent and child perspectives across the 15 domains. Each dimension is rated for level of functioning compared to that of other children of the same age. The test-retest reliability for the combined function score (aggregated across the 15 domains) was .64. Internal consistency alpha coefficients ranged from .81 to .87. The predictive and construct validity have also been established (Graham et al., 1997).

The dimensions are also rated for the degree of satisfaction and emotional upset for the child arising from this level of functioning. In general, the function, satisfaction, and upset scores are highly correlated. Although this three-component evaluation of each dimension is valuable when individual children are considered, at the group level the results for function, satisfaction, and upset are very closely related. In the results to follow, only those for the function scores are reported.

The following are two illustrative items form the CHRQOL—Child Questionnaire:

2. Doing things for yourself

Possible problems include: Cannot do up buttons or laces: cannot use a knife to cut food: needs help with feeding; difficulties in washing or dressing: totally unable to look after self

Over the past month how well have you been able to do these things?

Better than children of the same age . . . . Totally unable to look after self

[a 7-point scale with the extremes labeled as above]

How upset have you been by not being able to do these things?

Extremely upset. . . . . Not upset at all

[a 7-point scale with the extremes labeled as above]

How satisfied have you been with the way you do these things?

Very satisfied. . . . . Not satisfied at all

[a 7-point scale with the extremes labeled as above]

6. Friends

Possible problems include: No special friends; a lot of arguing and bickering; few close friends; often teased or bullied; no friends at all.

Over the past month how well have you got on with you friends?

Better than children of the same age . . . . No friends at all

[a 7-point scale with the extremes labeled as above]

How upset have you been by the way you get on with other children?

Extremely upset. . . . . Not upset at all

[a 7-point scale with the extremes labeled as above]

How satisfied have you been by the way you get on with other children?

Very satisfied. . . . . Not satisfied at all

[a 7-point scale with the extremes labeled as above]

For the full versions of these CHRQOL measures see Stevenson (1997).

One of the problems identified by Eiser and Morse (2001) is the limited availability of disease-specific measures. For children with NTDs we could only identify one measure, the HRQOL instrument, for use in children with spina bifida (Parkin et al., 1997). This measure contains 44 and 47 items for children and adolescents, respectively. Items cover 10 domains: social, emotional, intellectual, financial, medical, independence, environmental, physical, recreational, and vocational. Items are scored on a 5-point Likert scale (1 = only a little, 5 = a lot). Higher scores reflect better HRQOL. Data have been presented to support reliability and predictive and construct validity of this measure.

There have been a number of studies of HRQOL in people with NTDs. This will be reviewed in the next section.

STUDIES OF HEALTH-RELATED QUALITY OF LIFE IN PEOPLE WITH NEURAL TUBE DEFECTS

Spina Bifida

The effect of spina bifida on the child's functioning depends on the level of the lesion and the nerve damage involved. Associated problems include varying degrees of lower extremity motor impairment, sensory loss, and bowel and bladder dysfunction. It has been found that spina bifida and hydrocephalus affect cognitive functioning. The level of cognitive ability may also have important implications for HRQOL. In general, children with spina bifida and hydrocephalus function within the low average range of intelligence. The performance of these children on verbal tasks is better than their performance on tasks that require visual and spatial awareness (e.g., Dennis et al., 1981; Donders et al., 1991; Fletcher et al., 1992; Wills, 1993; Brookshire et al., 1995). Data from a longitudinal study by Fletcher and colleagues (Fletcher et al., 1992; Brookshire et al., 1995) suggested that differences between verbal and nonverbal performance do not seem to reflect the motor demands of the nonverbal tasks. However, the differences may be attributable to neuropsychological deficits associated with white matter abnormalities (Donders et al., 1991). A study by Dise and Lohr (1998) provided further evidence that children with spina bifida have deficits in higher-order cognitive abilities. They reported that subjects with spina bifida aged 10 to 23 years experienced problems in at least one domain of executive functioning, that is, mental flexibility, processing efficiency, conceptualization, or problem solving, regardless of their lesion level or IQ.

For children with spina bifida, lesion level is associated with cognitive functioning; higher (thoracic) lesion levels are associated with lower IQ scores, especially on visual-motor tasks. This finding may be due to the fact that hydrocephalus is also more common with higher lesion levels (Wills, 1993). The etiology of hydrocephalus may also be important in this context. Larger discrepancies between verbal and nonverbal performance are noted in children with hydrocephalus associated with aqueduct stenosis than in children with hydrocephalus associated with spina bifida or prematurity (Dennis et al., 1981; Fletcher et al., 1992). Early-developing obstructive hydrocephalus, such as hydrocephalus due to Arnold Chiari malformation, may affect visual-spatial and visual-motor performance specifically, with limited effect on language abilities, whereas later-developing hydrocephalus, such as hydrocephalus associated with intraventricular hemorrhage, yields low scores on both nonverbal and verbal tasks. In general, the more complications associated with the cause of hydrocephalus, the poorer the outcome on cognitive functioning for that diagnostic group (Wills, 1993).

In addition to having low average IQ levels, children with spina bifida and hydrocephalus often display academic problems involving arithmetic, spelling, and reading comprehension (see Wills, 1993, for a review). These learning problems may arise from impairments in other cognitive functions. For example, children with shunted hydrocephalus of different etiology were more likely to display cognitive visual problems, concerning object recognition and orientation, for example, than children without cerebral pathology, with most affected children having multiple cognitive visual problems (Houliston et al., 1999). Furthermore, children with hydrocephalus are at risk for discourse and pragmatic impairments. A study analyzing the development of narrative content of language suggested that children with hydrocephalus have content-poor language. Compared to those of matched controls, the narratives of children with hydrocephalus were characterized by impaired textual rhetoric—less cohesive, less clear, and less coherent (Dennis et al., 1994).

Neural tube defects may also contribute to disrupted social relationships such as decreased opportunities for peer relationships, prolonged dependency on parents, and decreased community acceptance (Kirpalani et al., 2000). Repeated findings of psychopathology and low self-esteem have been reported for children and adolescents with spina bifida and hydrocephalus (Dorner, 1975; Hayden et al., 1979; Kazak and Clark, 1986; Thompson et al., 1989; Appleton et al., 1994; Ammerman et al., 1998; Williams and Lyttle, 1998).

A further mechanism whereby NTDs can impinge on QOL is via an increased likelihood of psychological difficulties. Estimates of the prevalence of emotional and behavioral disorders among children with hydrocephalus range from 24% to 44% (Donders et al., 1991). Young people with spina bifida, especially girls, have been found to be at greater risk for social isolation, depressive mood, lower self-worth, and suicidal ideation (Dorner, 1975;

Appleton et al., 1994). In addition to observed social isolation, the social interaction patterns of children with spina bifida differ qualitatively from those of nonaffected peers, often interacting with fewer people for longer periods and having less contact with peers of the opposite sex (Tin and Teasdale, 1985).

Results of a study by Dorner (1975) suggested that impaired mobility is associated with both social isolation and feelings of depression in the adolescent with spina bifida. However, in more recent studies, elevated levels of behavior and social competence problems were not associated with disability parameters such as level of lesion, ambulatory status, or bladder function (Ammerman et al., 1998).

It should be noted that not all aspects of self-esteem may be affected by NTDs. Appleton et al. (1994) reported that although children with spina bifida scored significantly lower on athletic and scholastic competence and peer acceptance than able-bodied peers, their ratings of physical appearance, behavioral conduct, and global self-worth were similar. Hommeyer et al. (1999) examined the relationship between severity of condition and psychosocial functioning in children with spina bifida, thereby differentiating between proximal functional status and distal adjustment outcomes. Proximal functional status outcomes were defined as functional consequences of specific disability-related symptoms such as physical and cognitive outcomes. In contrast, distal adjustment outcomes do not clearly represent functional limitations associated with the disability, such as mental health and social functioning. As predicted, condition severity was associated with the proximal functional status outcomes (i.e., scholastic competence, athletic competence, attention problems and degree of involvement in activities) but not with distal outcomes (i.e., behavioral problems and social competence) (Hommeyer et al., 1999).

The above studies suggest that there are many aspects of spina bifida and of hydrocephalus that can affect functioning. These may or may not influence HRQOL. The distinction here is between functioning, which refers to characteristics that are open to external validation, and HRQOL, which centers on the individuals' self-reported reactions to their perceptions of the functional limitations caused by their condition. There are other NTDs that may affect HRQOL even more markedly. Encephaloceles are protrusions of the brain and meninges through a defect in the skull. When they are small and cystic, the prognosis following closure is good. There have been no studies of QOL for people with this condition. However, when the encephalocele contains a large volume of brain tissue, the rest of the brain is often small, poorly developed, and severely hydrocephalic, in which case a much poorer outcome is expected. In a study of a cohort of 83 children born with encephalocele, survival over a 20-year period was evaluated (Siffel et al., 2003). Most children (79%) had isolated posterior or anterior defects. Twenty-five children died of the condition, most on the first day of life. The survival probability to 1 or 20 years of age was quite similar (71% and 67%, respectively). Factors associated with increased mortality included low birth weight, presence of multiple defects, and ethnicity, with African American children being more at risk than Caucasian children.

Summary of Level of Health-Related Quality of Life in Persons with Neural Tube Defects

Compared to Other Conditions. In a review, Lavigne and Faier-Routman (1993) concluded that children with physical disorders, especially those with sensory and neurological impairments, are at increased risk for psychological adjustment problems and decreased self-esteem. Quality of life is relatively poor in neurological conditions, renal disease, and musculoskeletal disorders (Sprangers et al., 2000). There is an emerging pattern of results suggesting that spina bifida and other conditions involving the central nervous system are likely to present particular threat to QOL.

Are Some People More Prone to a Poor Health-Related Quality of Life Than Others? Children with spina bifida and hydrocephalus typically have additional brain abnormalities; for example, the corpus callosum is often malformed or missing, further affecting neuropsychological functioning (Wills, 1993). Chauvel (1991) uses criteria defined by Lorber (1971) to determine the prognosis of a child with spina bifida: (*1*) the degree of paralysis, (*2*) the presence of hydrocephalus, (*3*) the presence of kyphosis/scoliosis, and (*4*) the presence of associated gross congenital anomalies or perinatal trauma. The prognosis is poorer if the level of the lesion is higher, hydrocephalus and pathological spinal curvature of the spine are present at birth, and the child suffered birth injury or has congenital organ system anomalies. There may, however, not be a simple relationship between severity of disability and QOL. In a study involving 12 adolescents with spina bifida, results showed that although disability was inversely related to the physical aspects of QOL, for the mental aspects less disability was associated with greater psychological distress. More specifically, subjects with fewer physical problems displayed more emotional symptoms, which in turn affected their ability to perform daily activities (Padua et al., 2002).

The effects of hydrocephalus on functioning vary considerably among children and depend on the areas of the brain most affected. The varying neurobehavioral outcomes reflect the influence not only of hydrocephalus, but also of other congenital neuropathological processes and environmental, sociocultural, and emotional factors (Fletcher et al., 1996). They can include impairment in fine motor skills, executive functioning, learning, attention, and behavior (Tew, 1991).

Child or parental adjustment may further affect the HRQOL of children with disabilities. Viemero and Kraus (1998) reported that the person's ability to cope with everyday life had a bigger impact on QOL than the nature of the disability. Aspects of family resources, such as hope and instrumental support, are predictors of HRQOL in children with spina bifida (Rudeberg et al., 1995; Kirpalani et al., 2000). A study by Kirpalani et al. (2000) showed that although physical limitations explained a significant proportion of the variance in self-reported QOL in children with spina bifida, an additional 19%–24% of variance was explained by "parental hope," as measured by the Miller Hope Scale (Miller and Powers, 1988).

The question of QOL in children with spina bifida and/or hydrocephalus was investigated in a recently completed study by the authors—the Child Health and Development Study (CHADS). The study was designed to establish the extent to which QOL was affected by NTDs, which aspects of QOL were most affected, and the characteristics of children and adolescents with NTDs that made them more vulnerable to adverse effects on QOL. The results of this study will be presented in the next section.

FINDINGS FROM THE CHILD HEALTH AND DEVELOPMENT STUDY ON HEALTH-RELATED QUALITY OF LIFE

The findings on a postal sample of children and adolescents with spina bifida ($n = 62$), hydrocephalus ($n = 354$), and spina bifida plus hydrocephalus ($n = 128$) identified via a UK national register have already been published (Pit-ten Cate et al., 2002) and will be briefly reviewed below. Subsequently, a further, more intensively studied sample was identified, and the findings on this group of children and adolescents are presented in the following section.

Quality of Life in a Postal Sample

Parents completed the CHRQOL, a family needs survey, and a caregiving self-efficacy scale (CSES). There were no overall significant differences in CHRQOL (see Total in Table 32.1). The Total CHRQOL was over 1 SD lower than that obtained previously for children with a range of physical disabilities and chronic illnesses (Graham et al., 1997). The children's CHRQOL was not related to either gender or age.

The three groups did differ on specific aspects of CHRQOL. Children with spina bifida had poorer CHRQOL scores on self-care, continence, and mobility/activities while those with hydrocephalus had poorer scores on school activities, sight, and communication (see Table 32.1). Associations were found between overall CHRQOL and problems discernible at birth as well as epilepsy, but the presence of shunts was not related to overall CHRQOL.

Quality of Life in the Intensively Studied Sample

A second stage of the CHADS study was conducted on an additional sample of children and adolescents aged 6 to 18 years of age living in the South of England. It included participants with spina bifida ($n = 28$), hydrocephalus ($n = 51$), spina bifida plus hydrocephalus ($n = 36$), and healthy controls ($n = 56$). In this sample, we could test more directly the difference between the CHRQOL scores for the condition groups and the control group. The controls were identified in schools from the same area as the condition groups, were of the same age, and had a gender ratio similar to that of the condition groups. As can be seen in Table 32.2, with the exception of Family relationships, the condition groups had poorer CHRQOL than the control group. In addition, all three condition groups fared less well than the healthy controls on the individual aspects of CHRQOL with the exception of Sight and Eating (where the spina bifida group was not significantly different from the controls) and Communication and Sleep. Here the spina bifida plus hydrocephalus group was not significantly different from the controls, although the mean was lower for Communication.

For those participants aged 12 and over, self-reported QOL was obtained on the CHRQOL. The means for the CHRQOL items and the Total score are presented in Table 32.3. The pattern of results was similar to that based on parents' reports of their child's QOL. For example, post-hoc tests show that the mean Total score for the adolescents with spina bifida is significantly worse than that of the controls. There were fewer significant differences between the healthy controls and the three condition groups. This was partly due to the smaller number of subjects in these analyses of self-reported CHRQOL and partly to the higher scores (lower QOL) reported by the control adolescents compared to their parents (see below). There were no significant differences between the three condition groups.

The correlation between the parent and adolescent reported CHRQOL was significant ($r = 0.53$, $p < .001$) but was higher for controls ($r = 0.60$, $p < .001$) than for the NTD groups ($r = 0.34$, $p < .03$). Adolescents rated their QOL as less good than did their parents. The mean Total CHRQOL reported by adolescents was 43.62 compared to 38.22 as rated by the parents (paired-$t = 3.11$, $df = 68$, $p < .004$). This effect was most marked for the controls ($M = 37.11$ vs. 27.34, paired-$t = 3.98$, $df = 25$, $p < .001$) and was not significant for the three NTD groups ($M =$

TABLE 32.1. *Parent-Rated Child Health-Related Quality of Life (Functioning) in a Postal Sample*

	Spina Bifida $n = 63$		Hydrocephalus $n = 348$		Spina Bifida and Hydrocephalus $n = 124$		One-Way ANOVA			Post-Hoc		
Variable	Mean	SD	Mean	SD	Mean	SD	F	df	p	SB vH	SB v SB + H	H v SB + H
Getting about	3.26	1.30	3.34	1.38	3.87	1.52	6.72	2,520	<.002	ns	<.02	<.003
Doing things for self	3.06	1.66	3.76	1.74	3.98	1.65	6.20	2,532	<.003	<.009	<.003	ns
Soiling/wetting	4.56	2.18	2.83	1.96	5.43	1.73	89.30	2,528	<.001	<.001	<.02	<.001
School	2.70	1.46	3.45	1.47	3.23	1.38	7.41	2,531	<.002	<.001	<.05	ns
Out-of-school activities	3.42	1.65	3.80	1.78	4.24	1.81	4.94	2,532	<.008	ns	<.01	<.05
Friends	3.13	1.69	3.52	1.80	3.08	1.57	3.69	2,534	<.05	ns	ns	<.05
Family relationships	3.25	1.99	2.97	1.93	2.52	1.78	3.84	2,534	<.03	ns	<.05	ns
Discomfort	3.15	1.77	3.23	1.86	3.18	1.87	0.08	2,524	ns	ns	ns	ns
Worries	3.13	1.85	3.62	1.86	3.61	1.87	1.91	2,523	ns	ns	ns	ns
Depression	2.81	1.60	2.62	1.65	2.71	1.61	0.41	2,523	ns	ns	ns	ns
Sight	1.90	1.18	2.96	1.60	2.22	1.28	20.38	2,532	<.001	<.001	ns	<.001
Communication	2.24	1.47	2.98	1.65	2.37	1.49	10.35	2,532	<.001	<.003	ns	<.002
Eating	2.95	1.84	3.19	1.93	3.16	1.93	0.41	2,533	ns	ns	ns	ns
Sleep	2.54	1.68	3.01	1.77	2.70	1.68	2.79	2,531	ns	ns	ns	ns
Appearance	2.57	1.46	2.53	1.38	2.85	1.52	2.32	2,530	ns	ns	ns	ns
Total	44.05	15.16	47.32	15.67	49.21	14.44	2.15	2,530	ns	ns	ns	ns

TABLE 32.2. *Parent-Rated Child Health-Related Quality of Life (Functioning) in an Intensively Studied Sample*

	Spina Bifida $n = 28$ (a)		Hydrocephalus $n = 51$ (b)		Spina Bifida and Hydrocephalus $n = 36$ (c)		Controls $n = 56$		One-Way ANOVA $df = 3{,}167$		
Variable	Mean	SD	Mean	SD	Mean	SD	Mean	SD	F	p	Contrast vs. Control*
Getting about	3.50	1.35	2.96	1.51	3.83	1.50	1.50	0.69	30.70	<.001	a b c
Doing things for self	2.64	1.28	3.08	1.64	3.33	1.71	1.44	0.60	19.43	<.001	a b c
Soiling/wetting	4.64	2.04	2.47	1.80	4.44	2.27	1.42	0.97	33.06	<.001	a b c
School	2.50	1.32	2.73	1.31	2.81	1.17	1.73	0.92	8.92	<.001	a b c
Out-of-school activities	3.61	1.71	3.02	1.68	3.58	1.48	1.61	0.97	19.58	<.001	a b c
Friends	3.00	1.87	2.90	1.79	3.00	1.51	1.79	0.78	7.85	<.001	a b c
Family relationships	2.64	1.99	2.76	1.72	2.53	1.59	2.18	1.33	1.26	ns	—
Discomfort	3.46	2.04	2.76	1.76	3.03	1.80	1.84	1.29	7.20	<.001	a b c
Worries	3.18	1.76	3.16	1.75	3.47	1.89	1.95	1.28	8.29	<.001	a b c
Depression	2.82	1.56	2.39	1.52	2.56	1.32	1.80	1.08	4.37	<.01	a b c
Sight	2.39	1.40	2.49	1.33	3.05	3.44	1.69	0.93	3.96	<.01	b c
Communication	2.32	1.31	2.71	1.47	2.08	1.18	1.71	0.95	5.97	<.01	a b
Eating	2.50	1.52	2.63	1.79	2.83	1.75	2.00	1.28	2.43	ns	b c
Sleep	2.93	1.80	2.59	1.55	2.61	1.90	1.96	1.36	2.74	<.05	a b
Appearance	2.57	1.48	2.59	1.40	3.08	1.27	1.77	0.85	9.15	<.001	a b c
Total	44.71	14.59	41.24	15.49	46.25	12.98	26.41	8.82	23.46	<.001	a b c

*Letter for group significantly different from that of controls at $p < .05$.

TABLE 32.3. *Adolescent Self-Rated Health-Related Quality of Life (Functioning) in an Intensively Studied Sample*

	Spina Bifida $n = 12$ (a)		Hydrocephalus $n = 16$ (b)		Spina Bifida and Hydrocephalus $n = 20$ (c)		Controls $n = 26$		One-Way ANOVA $df = 3,74$		Contrast vs. Control*
Variable	Mean	SD	Mean	SD	Mean	SD	Mean	SD	F	p	
Getting about	4.00	1.20	3.38	1.15	3.89	1.15	2.46	1.30	6.50	<.001	a b c
Doing things for self	2.37	1.30	2.81	1.72	3.57	1.64	2.00	1.06	4.63	<.006	c
Soiling/wetting	4.00	1.41	2.31	1.85	3.94	1.61	1.77	1.37	9.24	<.001	a c
School	3.50	1.20	3.06	1.64	3.21	1.40	2.31	1.44	2.20	ns	—
Out-of-school activities	3.25	1.49	3.41	1.54	3.74	1.41	1.85	1.05	8.71	<.001	a b c
Friends	2.88	1.88	3.06	1.81	2.37	1.16	2.11	0.99	1.83	ns	—
Family relationships	2.88	1.55	2.25	1.18	3.00	1.53	2.65	1.26	.95	ns	—
Discomfort	3.50	1.07	3.31	2.12	3.36	1.57	2.69	1.59	0.91	ns	—
Worries	2.75	1.98	3.31	1.74	3.21	1.36	2.35	1.20	1.92	ns	—
Depression	3.31	1.46	2.94	1.39	3.00	1.29	2.73	1.40	0.24	ns	—
Sight	2.88	1.64	3.19	1.60	3.05	1.22	2.69	1.91	0.35	ns	—
Communication	3.00	1.51	3.00	1.59	2.84	1.30	2.30	1.29	1.13	ns	—
Eating	3.37	1.19	3.25	1.95	3.47	1.17	2.85	1.38	0.77	ns	—
Sleep	3.25	1.67	2.50	1.93	3.47	1.43	3.11	1.93	0.91	ns	—
Appearance	3.25	1.67	2.88	1.26	3.68	1.42	3.23	1.41	0.97	ns	—
Total	52.67	13.19	44.62	13.13	48.80	14.40	37.15	15.32	4.15	<.01	a

*Letter for group significantly different from that of controls at $p < .05$.

47.56 vs. 44.79, paired-$t = 1.21$, $df = 42$, ns). This suggests that it is important to obtain the young person's ratings of QOL in addition to those from parents whenever this is developmentally appropriate.

Factors within Spina Bifida and Spina Bifida Plus Hydrocephalus Related to Poor Health-Related Quality of Life in the Intensively Studied Sample

Clinical Condition Features. Children with spina bifida were divided into those with high (cervical, thoracic, and upper lumbar) lesions ($n = 15$), middle (lower lumbar) lesions ($n = 20$), and low (sacral and coccygeal) lesions ($n = 21$). The aggregated CHRQOL Total score was compared between these groups. Although the high lesion group (mean = 51.47, SD = 9.54) rated QOL as less good than either the middle (mean = 43.10, SD = 17.70) or the lower (mean = 44.15, SD = 12.29) lesion groups, these differences were not significant ($F(2,52) = 1.76$, ns).

Similarly dividing the children with spina bifida into those with occulta ($n = 8$), meningocele ($n = 17$), and myelomeningocele ($n = 37$) did not identify significant differences in QOL. The parents of children with spina bifida occulta reported better CHRQOL (mean = 42.25, SD = 10.44) than those with meningocele (mean = 45.29, SD + 15.01) and with myelomeningocele (mean = 47.42, SD = 13.74), but these differences were not significant ($F(2,58) = 0.51$, ns).

Significant relationships were found between overall QOL and parental ratings of severity of disability and functional impairment (parent-rated QOL: $r = 0.55$ and $r = 0.65$; child-rated QOL: $r = 0.34$ and $r = 0.34$ for severity of disability and functional impairment, respectively). Severity of disability was defined in terms of the child's ability to walk, urinary and bowel function, weight, and the occurrence of pressure sores. This measure was adapted from the scheme used by Dorner (1975). Functional limitations were measured using six questions regarding the child's difficulties with activities of daily life, that is, washing, dressing, eating, continence, finding one's way, and walking ordinary distances. These results indicate that children with more functional impairment have a poorer QOL.

Two other features of the children's development were investigated for their relation to CHRQOL. The first was IQ. When all children (including the controls) were pooled together, the overall correlation between IQ and aggregated total CHRQOL was significant ($r = -0.39$, $p < .001$). However when the condition groups were separated, the correlation with IQ dropped substantially, and in none of the condition groups or the control group was the correlation significant. The apparent correlation with IQ arises because the condition groups differ from the controls in CHRQOL and in IQ.

The situation was different for behavioral difficulties. Here the overall correlation with CHRQOL was larger

($r = 0.56$) and remained significant within each of the condition groups. The inclusion of worries and depression in the CHRQOL measure makes it possible that there is a spurious correlation between the total SDQ score and the CHRQOL, since these aspects of psychological distress are included in the CHRQOL measure. It is important to note, therefore, that the same pattern of correlations was seen when the behavior scores was restricted to conduct problems. This suggests that behavioral problems arise in children who experience a poorer QOL. It is also possible that behavior disorders adversely affect QOL.

Age. In the intensively studied sample, there were few dimensions in which parental ratings of function were significantly correlated with age. The same was true within the condition groups. To illustrate this lack of change in QOL with age across the 6–16-year age group, the correlation with age for the aggregated Total CHRQOL score was $r = 0.04$ (ns). The same was found for the postal sample ($r = 0.07$, ns).

Gender. To investigate whether the child's gender was related to QOL, a 2 (Gender) by 4 (Condition Group) ANOVA was conducted on the Total Aggregated CHRQOL score of parent's ratings of function. The main effect of Condition Group was highly significant ($F(3,163) = 23.13, p < .001$), but neither the main effect of Gender ($F(1,163) = 0.93$, ns) nor the Condition Group by Gender interaction ($F(3,163) = 0.11$, ns) was significant.

Family and Social Factors. There is no evidence that the education of either fathers ($r = 0.56$, ns) or mothers ($r = .09$, ns) is related to aggregated Total HRQOL. Dividing fathers' occupations into manual (mean = 35.46, SD = 10.07) and nonmanual (mean = 35.56, SD = 14.62) did not produce significant differences in aggregated total HRQOL ($t = 0.04$, $df = 167$, ns). It would appear from these results that QOL was not related to broad indicators of social disadvantage.

PLACE OF MEASUREMENT OF HEALTH-RELATED QUALITY OF LIFE IN THE CLINICAL MANAGEMENT OF NEURAL TUBE DEFECTS

The assessment of QOL can serve several functions related to the clinical management of chronic illness and disability. Assessment of QOL can be used to evaluate differential changes in morbidity and the relative efficacy of medical interventions, to identify acute or residual dysfunction secondary to illness or treatment, and to identify patient subpopulations at risk for psychological or behavioral problems. Assessment of QOL can facilitate the estimation of health-care needs, clinical decision making, and the evaluation of medical care (Spieth and Harris, 1996). In other words, QOL assessment provides information that can form the basis for the planning of medical and psychological care; it can help clinicians focus on the areas that are most important to the child and family, as well as the evaluation of treatment. Although several generic and disease-specific QOL measures are available, it is important that the clinician choose a measure that is reliable and valid, easy to administer, and provides norms. Using a disease-specific measure ensures that all potentially affected domains are covered and that children/adolescents can be compared with other people suffering from the same condition (within-group comparison). The use of a generic measure can give insight into a person's functioning in general QOL domains and can be used for comparison with people without health problems or those suffering from other conditions. Both within- and between-group comparisons can give the clinician valuable information. For example, within-group comparison gives insight into the extent of primary and secondary problems in relation to others suffering from the same condition. Scores that deviate from the norm give an indication of decreased/increased vulnerability. Between-group comparison provides information on the extent of the problems compared to those of people with other conditions or no health problems. Deviations from the norm give insight into the extent to which the condition affects specific areas and QOL overall.

Incorporating measures of QOL into the care of patients is important because it focuses on the patient's own experience of his or her condition. The concept is embedded in the personal appraisal of life circumstances. This appraisal may be substantially different from assessments made by clinicians. When dealing with young children, the appraisal of QOL is obtained by proxy using parents as informants. Nevertheless, the principle is the same, namely, that an appraisal is made about the child's personal experiences.

It is important not to assume that the QOL reported is determined solely by the impact of the condition. In the same way as in the general population, QOL is determined by a wide range of factors. Some of these are related to personal characteristics, such as temperament and aptitudes, and others to social factors, such as family relationships and social support. It must be remembered that this same range of factors will operate for people with NTDs. The consequences of the condition for QOL act as influences on QOL in addition to this broader range of factors.

It is also the case that variation in QOL within groups of people with NTDs is not a simple function of clinical severity or complexity of their condition. Many personal characteristics operate to moderate the impact of features of the condition on QOL. These include personality characteristics, expectations about lifestyle, and personal preferences for different activities. For example, limitations on social contacts may distress some people greatly and detract from QOL, whereas for others this may be a much less salient feature of their preferred activities.

These considerations mean that clinicians have to be aware of individuals' own reports of their QOL. The measure developed by Graham et al. (1997) allows children and parents to report on what they both consider the child's level of functioning in aspects of QOL. A separate rating is made of how satisfied the child is about his or her perceived level of functioning. A third rating allows children to report how upset they are about their level of functioning. This allows at least partial dissociation between these aspects of QOL. This is an important feature of QOL measurement in that it allows children, for example, to report on a level of functioning that they see as less good than that of others and with which they are dissatisfied without being unduly upset. It also allows children to identify aspects of QOL that are creating distress for them. The use of systematic QOL appraisal allows children with NTD to identify areas where support and interventions can occur that will benefit them as individuals.

From the above, it has become clear that QOL assessment can serve several functions. Unfortunately, QOL measures are not yet routinely integrated into pediatric care. Although the relevance of QOL assessment for individual treatment planning and evaluation has been recognized, routine assessment often does not include QOL, and to date little information is available about the application of QOL assessments in intervention work. Most literature focuses on group comparisons and fails to specify how QOL assessment can serve individuals and their families.

It is essential that approaches to the assessment of QOL do not assume that people with NTD will necessarily have a poorer QOL than others. For both persons with NTDs and their families, there may be positive gains arising from the experience of the NTD. Chernoff and colleagues (2001) asked mothers to identify the positive impact and potential benefits associated with raising a child with a chronic illness. Almost 90% of the mothers reported feeling better about themselves by learning to manage their child's condition, 70% reported increased family strength, and 80% reported that their family had benefited from the experience. For example, mothers reported increased family cohesion, increased awareness, sensitivity, and tolerance, and enhanced self-esteem.

In a substudy of CHADS, 20 parents of children with spina bifida and/or hydrocephalus (randomly selected from the CHADS sample) were interviewed using open-ended questions for parents to describe positive and negative experiences associated with raising their children. Positive events focused on the child's achievements, peer relationships, social-physical activities, and family involvement. Negative events included medical treatments and incontinence, child behavior problems, academic and physical incompetence, problems with peer relationships, and difficulties related to social-physical activities. Most of the events seemed to reflect powerful experiences, indicating strong emotional associations, and most experiences were said to have had an effect on daily life and on life in the long term. Most interestingly, the long-term effect of both positive and negative experiences was rated positively; families were able to cope with the adverse situations such that the long-term outcome was positive (Pit-ten Cate, 2003).

Measures of QOL are potentially useful in evaluating treatments and interventions. However, it is not yet common practice to include these measures in clinical trials (Eiser, 1997). In addition to the aid provided to planning the care of individuals, the routine inclusion of QOL measurements would contribute to the monitoring of services. An advantage of using a generic QOL measure is that services for different conditions can be compared on the same metric.

To conclude, the incorporation of QOL assessments as part of the routine care of people with NTD will enhance both the delivery of services tailored to the needs of the individual and the development of more demonstrably efficacious interventions.

ACKNOWLEDGMENT

The study from which findings are presented in this chapter was funded by research grants awarded by the Association for Spina Bifida and Hydrocephalus (ASBAH). We are grateful to ASBAH, and to the families and the children who took part in out studies, for their enthusiastic support of our work.

REFERENCES

Ammerman RT, Kane VR, Slomka GT, Reigel DH, Franzen MD, Gadow KD (1998). Psychiatric symptomatology and family functioning in children and adolescents with spina bifida. J Clin Psychol Med S 5:449–465.

Appleton PL, Minchom PE, Ellis NC, Elliott CE, Boll V, Jones P (1994). The self-concept of young people with spina bifida: a population based study. Dev Med Child Neurol 36:198–215.

Brookshire BL, Fletcher JM, Bohan TP, Landry SH, Davidson KC, Francis DJ (1995). Verbal and nonverbal skill discrepancies in children with hydrocephalus—a 5 year longitudinal follow-up. J Pediatr Psychol 20:785–800.

Chauvel PJ (1991). Spina bifida and hydrocephalus. In AJ Capute, PJ Accardo (eds): *Developmental Disabilities in Infancy and Childhood.* Baltimore: Paul H Brookes, pp. 383–393.

Chernoff, RG, List DG, DeVet KA, Ireys HT (2001). Maternal reports of raising children with chronic illnesses: the prevalence of positive thinking. Ambul Pediatr 1:104–107.

Dennis M, Fitz CR, Netley CT, Sugar J. Harwood-Nash DCF, Hendrick EB, et al (1981). The intelligence of hydrocephalic children. Arch Neurol-Chicago 38:607–615.

Dennis M, Jacennik B, Barnes MA (1994). The content of narrative discourse in children and adolescents after early onset hydrocephalus and in normally developing age peers. Brain Lang 46:129–165.

Dise JE, Lohr ME (1998). Examination of deficits in conceptual reasoning abilities associated with spina bifida. Am J Phys Med Rehab 77:247–251.

Donders J, Rourke BP, Canady AL (1991). Neuropsychological functioning of hydrocephalic children. J Clin Exp Neuropsychol 13:607–613.

Dorner S (1975). The relationship of physical handicap to stress in families with an adolescent with spina bifida. Dev Med Child Neurol 17:765–776.

Eiser C (1997). Children's quality of life measures. Arch Dis Child 77:350–354.

Eiser C, Morse R (2001). A review of measures of quality of life for children with chronic illness. Arch Dis Child 84:205–211.

Feeny D, Furlong W, Barr RD (1998). Multiattribute approach to the assessment of health-related quality of life: health utilities index. Med Pediatr Oncol Suppl 1. 54–59.

Fletcher JM, Brookshire BL, Landry SH, Bohan TP, Davidson KC, Francis DJ, et al (1996). Attentional skills and executive functions in children with early hydrocephalus. Dev Neuropsychol 12:53–76.

Fletcher JM, Francis DJ, Thompson NM, Brookshire BL, Bohan, TP, Landry SH, et al (1992). Verbal and nonverbal skill discrepancies in hydrocephalic children. J Clin Exp Neuropsychol 14:593–609.

Graham P, Stevenson J, Flynn D (1997). A new measure of health related quality of life for children: preliminary findings. Psychol Health 12:655–665.

Hayden PW, Davenport SLH, Campbell MM (1979). Adolescents with myelodysplasia: impact of physical disability on emotional maturation. Pediatrics 64:53–59.

Hommeyer JS, Holmbeck G, Wills KE, Coers S (1999). Condition severity and psychosocial functioning in pre-adolescents with spina bifida: disentangling proximal functional status and distal adjustment outcomes. J Pediatr Psychol 24:499–509.

Houliston MJ, Taguri AH, Dutton GN, Hajivassiliou C, Young D (1999). Evidence of cognitive visual problems in children with hydrocephalus: a structured clinical history-taking strategy. Dev Med Child Neurol 41:298–306.

Kazak AE, Clark MW (1986). Stress in families of children with myelomeningocele. Dev Med Child Neurol 28:220–228.

Kirpalani HM, Parkin PC, Willan AR, Fehlings DL, Rosenbaum PL, King D, VanNie AJ (2000). Quality of life in spina bifida: importance of parental hope. Arch Dis Child 83:293–297.

Landgraf JM, Abetz LN (1997). Functional status and well-being of children representing three cultural groups: initial self-reports using the CHQ-CF87. Psychol Health 12:839–854.

Lavigne JV, Faier-Routman J (1993). Correlates of psychological adjustment to pediatric physical disorders: a meta-analytic review and comparison with excisting models. J Dev Behav Pediatr 14:117–123.

Lorber J (1971). Results of treatment of myelomeningocele. Dev Med Child Neurol 13:279–303.

Miller JF, Powers MJ (1988). Development of an instrument to measure hope. Nurs Res 37:6–10.

Padua L, Rendeli C, Rabini A, Girardi E, Tonali P, Salvaggio E (2002). Health-related quality of life and disability in young patients with spina bifida. Arch Phys Med Rehabil 83:1384–1388.

Parkin PC, Kirpaliani HM, Rosenbaum PL, Fehlings DL, VanNie A, et al (1997). Development of a health-related quality of life instrument for use in children with spina bifida. Qual Life Res 6:123–132.

Pit-ten Cate IM (2003). Family adjustment to disability and chronic illness in children. Unpublished doctoral dissertation, University of Southampton, UK.

Pit-ten Cate IM, Kennedy C, Stevenson J (2002). Disability and quality of life in spina bifida and hydrocephalus. Dev Med Child Neurol 44:317–322.

Rudeberg A, Donati F, Kaiser G (1995). Psychosocial aspects in the treatment of children with myelomeningocele: an assessment after a decade. Eur J Pediatr 154:S85–S89.

Siffel C, Wong LYC, Olney RS, Correa A. (2003). Survival of infants diagnosed with encephalocele in Atlanta 1979–98. Paediatr Perinat Epidemiol 17:40–48.

Spieth LE, Harris CV (1996). Assessment of health related quality of life in children and adolescents: an integrative review. J Pediatr Psychol 21:175–193.

Sprangers MAG, de Regt EB, Andries F, van Agt HME, Bijl RV, de Boer JB, et al (2000). Which chronic conditions are associated with better or poorer quality of life? J Clin Epidemiol 53:895–907.

Stevenson J (1997). Health and illness in childhood. In Sclare I (ed): *Child Psychology Portfolio.* Windsor, UK, NFER-Nelson Publishing Company, pp. 1–73.

Tew B (1991). The effects of spina bifida and hydrocephalus upon learning and behaviour. In Bannister CM, and Tew B (eds): *Current Concepts in Spina Bifida and Hydrocephalus: Clinics in Developmental Medicine* No. 122. London: MacKeith Press, pp. 158–179.

Thompson RJ, Kronenberger WG, Johnson DF, Whiting K (1989). The role of central nervous system functioning and family functioning in behavioral problems of children with myelodysplasia. J Dev Behav Pediatr 10:242–248.

Tin LG, Teasdale GR (1985). An observational study of the social adjustment of spina bifida children in integrated settings. Br J Educ Psychol 55:81–83.

Varni JW, Seid M, Rode CA (1999). The PedsQL (TM): measurement model for the pediatric quality of life inventory. Med Care 37:126–139.

Viemero V, Krause C (1998). Quality of life in individuals with physical disabilities. Psychother Psychosom 67:317–322.

Williams J, Lyttle S (1998). Mother and teacher reports of behaviour and perceived self-competence of children with hydrocephalus. Eur J Pediatr Surg 8:5–9.

Wills KE (1993). Neuropsychological functioning in children with spina bifida and/or hydrocephalus. J Clin Child Psychol 22:247–265.

33

Ethics at the Forefront: Moral Decisions and Responsibility When Confronted with Spina Bifida

MARK J. BLITON

INTO THE TWENTY-FIRST CENTURY WITH PRENATAL DIAGNOSIS

The refinements and use of obstetric ultrasound and other imaging modalities to identify fetal conditions that may require neurosurgical intervention present a crucial set of recurrent moral issues regarding parental decision making and informed consent. These advances also create a new kind of ethical complexity because perinatal obstetrics and pediatric neurosurgery may share the task of counseling a pregnant woman and her partner (Wilcox et al., 1993: 1282). For instance, when neurosurgeons are invited to consult with pregnant women carrying fetuses diagnosed with spina bifida and myelomeningocele, they may encounter complicated challenges traditionally associated with the roles assumed by obstetricians, genetic counselors, and perinatologists (Cromblehome et al., 1996; Madsen et al., 1998: 49). Thus, collaborative efforts and interdisciplinary cooperation among these various specialties are required to help pregnant women and their families understand and cope with difficult and agonizing decisions (Nichols and Bianchi, 1996).

The moral complexities inherent in these consultations take place in social and moral environments shaped by the volatile convergence of two deeply contested themes in contemporary American public life—abortion and disability. A woman's pregnancy is now often framed by the advances in genetic screening and genetic manipulations, in addition to increasingly powerful methods for fetal visualization and diagnosis. Many women who receive routine prenatal care undergo diagnostic screening with obstetric ultrasound and serum or amniotic fluid alpha fetoprotein (AFP) testing (Meany et al., 1993). As a result, additional and patently qualitative distinctions are being introduced into women's pregnancies because prenatal diagnosis exceeds the current therapeutic reach of perinatal medicine. Prenatal diagnosis identifies conditions for which no treatment is available, leaving termination of pregnancy or giving birth to an affected infant—possibly with changes in obstetric management such as cesarean section for spina bifida—as the only options.

However, at the point in pregnancy where a diagnosis of spina bifida is generally made, between 16 and 20 weeks gestation, very few women have much prior knowledge about or experience with the condition (Roberts et al., 2002). Furthermore, discussions about compromised fetuses are filled with conflicting beliefs. The public debate is typically couched in impassioned arguments about reproductive rights that create a challenging context for personal decisions. Likewise, the influence of social attitudes toward disability and termination of pregnancy is experienced at many levels in personal and social life (Luker, 1984; Callahan, 1986; Parens and Asch, 2000).

Numerous studies document the various ways that medical access to and images of a fetus via ultrasound influence the emotional and bodily perceptions of pregnant women (Petcheskey, 1987; Duden, 1993; Gregg, 1995). Ultrasound provides a visual window into the pregnant woman's uterus, where often, if she has an opportunity to watch, the ultrasound images become blended into a woman's experience of the pregnancy (Sandelowski, 1994). Those images evidently evoke deeply ingrained emotive, valuational, and intellectual responses by the woman (frequently by her partner as well), which shape and guide the choices and actions that follow (Rapp, 1997).

Thus, when the ultrasound examination results in a diagnosis of a fetal anomaly, clinicians may be confronted with a pregnant woman's and her partner's shock, confusion, loss, anxiety, and dread. Although muted by both the degree of pervasive uncertainty and the strained expression of emotions typical in clinical settings, when fetal anomalies like spina bifida are diagnosed by ultrasound, a very trying and potentially devastating experience is shaped for pregnant women and their partners (Manchester et al., 1988: 74).

Perhaps most significantly, because these obstetric imaging technologies have led to an uncoupling of biological and social birth (Morgan, 1996) couples' experiences during an ultrasound consultation can now become analogous to those emotional disturbances encountered when, prior to the routine use of diagnostic obstetric ultrasound, infants were born with such anomalies. For example, instead of the hoped-for feeling of relief that the fetus is apparently normal, the initial responses frequently include those of intense crisis. Many times numbness, grief, disgust, waves of helplessness, rage, and disbelief are felt: the expected perfect child is lost, and the feared damaged fetus is identified with a spinal defect. Pregnant women and their partners may wish at first to "get rid" of the fetus, followed by feelings of guilt, self-blame, and intense anxiety (Bentovim, 1972; Matthews, 1990).

Indeed, what confronts parents of a newborn, or prospective parents newly told of the diagnosis of spina bifida, confronts us all in that deep vein of social unease and wariness directed toward birth defects, physical disabilities, and especially neurological deformities of any kind. As a result, the anxiety, uncertainty, and wariness of disability manifested by pregnant women and their partners can be intensified by feelings of grief, loss, and guilt. These become likely factors explaining the fact that, according to the available (although incomplete) data, the *prevalence* of spina bifida at birth is less—by a range of 20% to almost 65%—than the *incidence* of spina bifida as a prenatal diagnosis.[1]

Prenatal screening for severe neurological defects and the option of termination of pregnancy provides prospective parents an opportunity to selectively prevent an outcome that they may reasonably want to avoid. However, the moral environment and ethical issues pertinent to the legally acceptable options can be relevantly different, depending on whether the fetus is previable or viable (Bliton, 2003).[2] Best estimates indicate that many times decisions to terminate the pregnancy are made within a rushed time frame in those few weeks remaining after the initial ultrasound diagnosis and before the 24th week of pregnancy, without benefit of adequate counseling about spina bifida (Freeman, 1998; Press et al., 1998).

This narrow time frame poses an important challenge to counseling. Limited on one side by the ability to detect metabolic changes resulting from an open neural tube defect and on the other side by viability, these time constraints are unlikely to change much. In response, physicians and other care providers need to develop strategies for optimizing informed decision making within these time constraints.

In this context, parents confront the potent uncertainties that accompany the wide range of predicted outcomes in the prognoses about what life will be like for the child and for the family. Parents understandably tend to focus intensely on the long-term outcomes and the uncertainties that may influence the quality of life of their child. When a myelomeningocele is diagnosed with a more severe range of potential outcomes, parents and physicians are challenged with choices about the "least worst" or perhaps "lesser evil" (Shelp, 1987), between terminating the perhaps wanted pregnancy or continuing the pregnancy in the face of potentially devastating compromise for the child. Similarly, many women who have had insufficient prenatal care, or prenatal care late in the third trimester, and deliver an infant with a myelomeningocele are likely to experience a range of feelings similar to those described above.

The diagnostic and prognostic uncertainties inherent in such choices permeate the moral uneasiness that suffuses the recent history of medical management of spina bifida with myelomeningocele and hydrocephalus. To help illustrate several of the difficult and prominent ethical implications associated with that history, this chapter will address factors associated with parental decision making and treatment decisions for fetuses and infants with spina bifida and myelomeningocele. Because attempts to develop ethical strategies to medically manage myelomeningocele chart an important and influential history for clinical ethics, this chapter provides a brief summary of that history. There are additional reasons for undertaking this review. The primary ethical point is to identify and emphasize the importance of parental responsibility and involvement in decision making. Also, a historical perspective illustrates that the more extensive moral issues, such as justice and fairness to potentially handicapped newborns, do not fall under the purview of any one profession or discipline. For this reason, a multidisciplinary team approach is advised for the management of fetal and infant myelomeningocele.

SETTING THE STAGE: REGARDING NEW TECHNOLOGY AND UNRESOLVED QUESTIONS

Reading the recent history of medical ethics through the lens of the infant with spina bifida—specifically, the ethical questions about whether and how to treat infants with myelomeningocele—can help to make explicit what is implicit in the fiercely contested moral issues found there. For example, an idea often proposed is that our high-technology medicine has created new ethical issues, particularly those posed by development of newer technologies (e.g., the invention of silicone, development of the Holter valve and ventriculoperitoneal shunting, mechanical ventilation for premature infants, dialysis). Likewise, it was anticipated that enhanced applications of ultrasound imaging and the array of techniques for prenatal diagnosis would provide the means and the more precise information needed to reduce the uncertainty and controversies that accompany neonatal compromise.

However, the ethical matters raised seem to rest, in turn, on a more basic question: What is the nature and limit of the ethical obligations to aggressively diagnose and treat perinatal and neonatal disease and injury? Of course, what is so unsettling is that this question leads to two still more fundamental ones: What is it about infants that grounds such ethical obligation? What is the moral status of the newborn infant? And, to what extent do such obligations and moral status exist for fetuses, given that prenatal diagnosis is primarily designed to provide information and choices to pregnant women and their partners?

In particular, the moral status of malformed infants has for centuries been a source of not merely diverse, but passionately contested views (Amundssen, 1987; Post, 1988). Our society in general and medical culture more particularly have inherited a plurality of passionately held and contentious views, and thus continue to wrestle with the resultant moral controversies. Crucial to note, however, is that this divergence of multiple viewpoints so prominent in our society was not caused by advanced high-technology medicine, even though new technologies surely have complicated the discussions. This does not mean that newly developed medical technologies do not create frustrating results. However, much of that frustration is stimulated by our impatient anticipation that new, enhanced applications of those technologies will provide both the means and more precise information needed to reduce deeply troubling uncertainty and controversies. Still, increased technical precision does not resolve the more extensive moral issues embedded in the multiple viewpoints at issue. From that vantage point, new technologies are probably better understood as compounding the moral ambiguities that are already present. As a result, it is not so much that our moral and ethical sensibilities have been outstripped by technology; rather, these issues, which have always been confounding and uncertain, have become perhaps even more so (McCullough and Myser, 1987: 217).

THE NEED FOR INFORMED CHOICES

In an article published in 1998, John Freeman, a neurologist who has contributed greatly to the discussion about the ethics involved in selective withholding of treatment for spina bifida, identified this confounding uncertainty when reviewing his own interaction with that history. Looking back, he says, "I discovered that what was considered ethical at one time in my career was considered unethical or at least unacceptable at another. I discovered how far I had come in this ethical journey and what a tortuous road I had traveled. Much to my surprise, I found that I had returned close to where I had begun in 1972" (1998: 302).

Two considerations that frame contemporary decision making regarding fetuses and infants with spina bifida will help focus the historical review of the ethical issues. First, Freeman reports that after ultrasound diagnosis, "decisions to carry the baby to term rarely are informed, and although some may be based on religious beliefs or feelings about abortion, many are made without information" (305). On the basis of his experience with medical management of spina bifida and its ethical implications, Freeman asks, "Is an uninformed decision to continue to carry the baby to term a more ethical decision than an uninformed decision to terminate the pregnancy?" (305).

A second, associated ethical question occurs in David McLone's recent discussion about standard repair of myelomeningocele, and invites consideration of still unresolved clinical and societal questions. He notes, "if the problem is corrected and the newborn survives, he or she is likely to have varying degrees of handicap. The significant question is not, 'can the child survive?'; with surgery, he or she can. Rather the question is 'what if the child survives?' " (1998: 111).

At a minimum, these questions from Freeman and McLone implicate societal dimensions of significant ethical issues regarding prenatal diagnosis of fetal myelomeningocele. First, such social factors, including biases toward the physically and cognitively impaired, influence moral justifications proposed for choices about whether to continue a pregnancy. Given that prenatal screening and termination of pregnancy currently allow prospective parents to selectively prevent an outcome that they may want to avoid, Retsinas writes that "the mother of a disabled child confronts a society that may have little sympathy with her and her child—especially if that society sees the child's birth as her choice, not as an unforeseen accident" (1991: 90). Second, in the face of such pervasive social attitudes, practical ethical questions arise regarding what counts as sufficient information about the medical, economic, and especially psychosocial (regarding functional abilities and disabilities) prognosis needed to satisfy the requirement for informed consent on the part of prospective or new parents (Bier et al., 1996, Press et al., 1998).

An additional factor is found in a subtle (or not so subtle) attitude adopted as a component of professionalism. Care providers may expect disabled children and their families to live up to idealized norms regarding attitudes and responses to disability. It is important that physicians and other care providers recognize and appreciate the existential attributes of personal suffering that occur in encounters with disability (Saetersdal, 1997).

Of course, the influence of such attitudes can run in contrasting directions. For example, one inference of Freeman's question about uninformed decisions reflects the ways in which the weight of ethical support shifts toward making apparently uninformed choices because those choices seem to match up with socially accepted attitudes. Broadly speaking, a decision to terminate a pregnancy (before 23 weeks gestation) after a prenatal diagnosis of spina bifida is a legally permissible and private decision (Steinbock, 2000). It also matches up with a social view, admittedly incomplete, that clearly attaches negative values to the developmental and cognitive impairments of spina bifida (Darling, 1979; Saxton, 1987).

McLone's question sharpens the point, albeit in a contrasting direction. This factor concerns the elements necessary for a parental choice to be an informed choice. Although the choice to continue the pregnancy based on religious beliefs might go against one set of generally accepted social attitudes, if a woman finds out at 16 to 20 weeks gestation that her fetus has spina bifida, and makes the decision not to terminate the pregnancy, then for all practical purposes she has by that very act decided at the same time to treat, to repair the lesion. That is, for those women choosing to continue the pregnancy, the decision to treat—in appropriate ways—most likely has already been made. And, it must be emphasized, that decision is often made without full awareness of *all* that is implied by a lifetime of "treatments" (Freeman, 1998).

One clinical and ethical issue, therefore, is that while a prognosis about any newborn's functional abilities (or deficits) may be more accurate than prenatal evaluations—due to the ability to physically examine and clinically evaluate the severity of the defect—that prognosis remains limited in its technical ability to accurately predict the full extent of deficits (Steinbok et al., 1992; Cochrane et al., 1996; Liptak, 1998; Jacobs et al., 2001). Botto et al. state that "medical problems may result from the neurologic defect or from its repair (e.g., paralysis, hydrocephalus, Arnold-Chiari type II malformation, endocrine abnormalities, tethered cord, syringomelia, and syringobulbia) or may be sequelae of the neurologic deficit (e.g., deformations of the limbs and spine; bladder, bowel, and sexual dysfunction; and learning disabilities)" (1999: 1511). These deficits and problems are related to the spinal cord level of the lesion and the degree of damage to the cord itself during the pregnancy, the delivery, and the neonatal period. Clinical evidence suggests that a cumulative pattern of physical and cognitive deterioration can continue over time (Liptak, 1998; Jacobs et al., 2001). Thus, parental choices to treat, whether made during the prenatal period or after the infant is born, are most often made with insufficient understanding of what is actually entailed by that lifetime of treatments.

By contrast, what we can predict is that the decision to continue a pregnancy after prenatal diagnosis of a sacral-lumbar myelomeningocele (and higher on the fetal spine) complicated by fetal ventriculomegaly means that the family will face significant economic costs, and emotional and marital stresses, as well as social challenges and obstacles (Botto et al., 1999). What we cannot predict is the actual, experienced meaning of those costs, stresses, challenges, and obstacles for any specific family. In addition, McLone notes that severe mental retardation requiring some form of custodial care is the likely fate of 10% to 15% of these infants. Also, 10% to 15% of these children will die, despite aggressive medical care, before they reach first grade (McLone, 1998: 112; see Steinbok et al., 1992). Mortality can approach 35% for children with more severe symptoms related to brainstem dysfunction secondary to the Arnold-Chiari malformation (Worley et al., 1996).

ONGOING PROBLEMS

Nonetheless, once an infant is born, the presumption to treat is the standard of care in contemporary medical management (McLone, 1998; Botto et al. 1999). Influenced by the availability of prenatal diagnosis (which is assumed to afford the opportunity to terminate the pregnancy or prepare for the necessary treatments), that presumption corresponds with improved treatment methods and the prevailing opinions about the infant's best medical interests. With the increased prevalence and sensitivity of routine prenatal ultrasound surveillance of pregnancy, and with that presumption to treat, an inability or reluctance to use such testing means that the infants (and parents) who present with myelomeningocele after little or no prenatal care are most likely to receive, as a matter of standard practice, surgical coverage of the defect and shunt placement.

A clinical study published by Bell and colleagues (1996) illustrates both sides of this complex scenario. Over a 40-month period, this group diagnosed 37 singleton pregnancies with neural tube defects. Of those, five were anencephalic and one had an encephalocele. Of the remaining 31 fetuses with myelomeningocele and associated hydrocephalus, 18 (58%) were terminated prior to the age of viability. Whether those numbers are generally representative is difficult to determine. They do correspond with reports published by teams at other high-risk perinatal centers, which in some cases document even higher rates of termination for pregnancy with fetal spina bifida (Grevengood et al., 1994; Forrester et al., 1998). That issue aside, there is the equally significant fact that during that same time span, at the same medical center, there were 25 neonates with myelomeningocele that presented postnatally. Although left unaddressed in study by Bell et al., presumably those infants were treated in accord with standard practice, and no mention was made otherwise. Difficult ethical questions about the "accident of birth" permeate such circumstances (Spiegelburg, 1986). For example, is the mother who would have terminated the pregnancy of a fetus with spina bifida, had she known this, now obligated to provide lifelong care for a possibly severely handicapped child (Freeman, 1998)? This most difficult question continues to confront us. The remainder of this chapter will outline prominent ethical concerns inherent in this challenging question.

CLINICAL CONTEXT FOR ETHICAL DECISION MAKING

The extensive and complex scope of the issues mentioned above has been detailed and thoroughly documented throughout the preceding chapters of this book. Not only can important questions be raised in discussions about the moral issues inherent in the medical knowledge about and treatment of spina bifida—including genetic, fetal, and infant conditions, clinicians' evaluations and research, and parental attitudes—but also raised are issues of the appropriate process and methods by which to address these substantial questions. Of particular significance for this chapter is the evolving picture of psychological adjustment and relationships for families with infants and children with spina bifida (Holmbeck and Faier-Routman, 1995; Hommeyer, et al., 1999), as well as attempts to clarify the influence of factors such as hope and social support, and the roles these might play in the adaptability of families (Horton and Wallander, 2001).

In that context, this chapter proposes that clinical ethics, in practice, provides a means to articulate, examine, and respond to those possible meanings most prominently evoked within specific circumstances (Baylis, 1994: 27–28; La Puma and Schniedermayer, 1994: 20; Ten Have, 1994: 126–127). Frequently, such practice involves identifying the problems perceived by individuals confronted with a clinical decision, and entails gathering the viewpoints of many different participants included in that decision. Clinical ethics provides assistance not only to patients and families but to health professionals as well. The aim is to help each individual do what is, for most of us, neither habitual, native, nor easy: to look into one's own basic sense of worth that has becomes challenged by the potential outcomes of spina bifida—to find ways, as Zaner says, to talk about "this core of what is held to be most worthwhile as fully and fairly as circumstances permit" (1993a: 26–27). People are typically not prompted to think about spina bifida; even when they do, it is likely not pursued to any great depth. Yet, the threat of injury (whether congenital or from social circumstances) to their child from spina bifida creates situations that require serious in-depth thinking about what is most worthwhile to parents and their families.

For instance, the need to discuss this "core of what is held to be most worthwhile" is underscored by the issues regarding parental and social attitudes entailed in the social circumstances, beliefs, attitudes, and values that compose what Kitcher (1997: 196–200) calls "laissez-faire eugenics." Identifying the idea of fairness, Kitcher illustrates the point:

> If laissez-faire eugenics is to accord with the advertisement that it promotes individual reproductive freedom, our societies will have to combine attempts to bring into the world children whose lives are not sadly restricted with public commitment to assist those who are born to realize the highest possible degree of development. Disability activists already fear that the spread of prenatal tests will erode the tenuous systems of support that have made it possible for many people to go far beyond the limits once foreseen for them. If those systems decay, prospective parents will experience ever more relentless pressure to eliminate those whom their society views as "defective." (200).

Thus, regarding the issue of parental choices, Kitchner says, "only if they are assured that all people have a serious chance of receiving respect and the support they need can prospective parents decide on the basis of their own values" (1997: 200).

Similar concerns are voiced by many in the disability rights movement who oppose the underlying premise of *quality of life* employed in the prevailing medical models of prenatal testing, diagnosis, and termination of pregnancy (Saxton, 2000), "with its concern with functional impairment, negative perceptions of the experience of life with disability, and its rhetoric about the 'prevention of suffering' " (Wyatt, 2001: 17).

However, as Adrienne Asch, an advocate for disabled persons and their families, writes, "Seeking to avoid the experience of raising a disabled child is no crime or callous, selfish statement, as some may claim. It is an honest, understandable, if perhaps misinformed, response to the fears that a disabled child will not fulfill what many women seek in mothering—to give ourselves a new being who starts out with the best we can give, and who will enrich us, gladden others, contribute to the world, and make us proud" (1989: 86). Honest and understandable, perhaps these choices are not so misinformed, as no less a sparkling and esteemed intellectual than Stephen Jay Gould wrote shortly before his own death, "for I live this life every day, that nothing can be harder than the undesired responsibility for raising a child with severe handicaps" (2002: xii–xvii).

There are other disconcerting factors to consider in this context. For example, in preparation for writing his 1998 article, Freeman spoke with two young adults with spina bifida who had been patients of his. Both exhibited good intelligence, had graduated from high school, and held government jobs. Both had high paraplegia, were in wheelchairs, and had undergone many surgical procedures. In their discussion about the ethics of treatment and decision making for spina bifida, Freeman recalled, "One said that she was Catholic and therefore did not believe in abortion. She went on to say that, nevertheless, she wished she had not been born and would advise parents to terminate an affected fetus" (1998: 305). As Minchom et al. (1995) report, "it is incorrect to assume that the psychological impact is less in the mildly disabled young person" (see also; Holmbeck and Faier-Routman, 1995).

Discussion of the ethical dimensions of such appraisals about unacceptable lives (and suffering) is often difficult among relative strangers. When such discussion occurs, it often does so furtively under differing estimations of or differing strategies regarding quality of life (Arras, 1987). For care providers, these ethical difficulties experienced within a professional role are perhaps compounded by their encounter with real limits on their ability to change either clinical outcomes or social attitudes. For example, although the complications associated with ventricular shunting are well documented, Dias and McLone suggest that "one complication of shunting that has not been emphasized is the psychologic burden shunting places on the neurosurgeon, patient, and family" (1993: 719). On the other hand, that lack of ability and the presence of real limitations do not mitigate the responsibility to fulfill other obligations that are relatively clear, including an obligation not to create circumstances where infants are left to suffer because of conditions that are accidental and undeserved.

In this way, all involved continue to be confronted by the ethical considerations discussed decades earlier by John Freeman and others, in which decision making regarding "each child, and each family is a unique problem. Blanket rules that every child should be operated upon are easier for the physician to live with, for they evade the ethical and moral dilemmas and necessity for decisions" (Freeman, 1974: 15). Perhaps "blanket rules" might diminish the perception of dilemmas, but they should not be allowed to diminish the fact that extraordinary moral commitments are involved when deciding to care for such a child. Thus, for anyone participating in a discussion of the ethical considerations regarding a fetus or newborn with myelomeningocele, there is the extremely important need never to take the nature and source of one's own of values for granted. Instead, the factual data and moral perceptions on which decisions are based must be constantly identified and reevaluated. Clinical uncertainty and questions about the factual reliability of a prognosis need to be distinguished from far-reaching moral implications regarding whether the infant can achieve a meaningful life, and whether those considerations should ever count in a family's decision making.

We cannot avoid considerations about the connections between a meaningful life and quality of life because we cannot avoid issue of harm to other people, specifically to parents and families of multiply compromised infants and children (Strong, 1983). Furthermore, while more sophisticated approaches concerned with the factors that contribute to the successful adaptation of some families whose children are disabled continue to develop (Ferguson, 2002), it remains quite unclear just what factors could reliably predict the relation between condition severity and psychosocial functioning (Hommeyer et al., 1999) and good family adaptation, not to mention what processes might need to be developed for evaluating and supporting adaptive parental attitudes during the prenatal period and infancy.

Accordingly, clinical ethics in decision making about myelomeningocele should serve not only as "a reminder of that need for deliberation about deeply serious issues," but should also strive "to serve as an affirmation of that need and the significance of those issues and the profound feelings they evoke" (Zaner, 1993a: 147). Each clinical participant in such situations needs to remember that one's own values are involved in considerations about the many issues that bear on these decisions. Beliefs regarding human uniqueness, quality of life, autonomy, privacy, and the moral fabric of society can all come into play. It is also important to be aware that others' values have developed from their own religious, cultural, and societal backgrounds—including what Duff and Campbell refer to as an individual's *moral community* composed of family intimates and advisors (Duff and Campbell, 1987: 276).

When trying to understand the issues in any clinical situation, one immediately encounters a highly complex set of autobiographical situations, for each of which the meaning emerges by way of tangled communication in the complex environment of the hospital or clinic. The moral work is to identify, weigh, deliberate, and eventually reach judgments about the multiple aspects of this complex set of issues (Zaner, 1988).

This careful and deliberative process seems necessary to discover what and whose issues need attention. What many cases require is careful questioning about the complicating factors of the situation, attentively listening to the answers given, all the while seeking to make explicit what is otherwise implicit, yet potentially significant.

THE INFANT WITH MYELOMENINGOCELE: A PROTOTYPE FOR ETHICAL DELIBERATION

Many of the social attitudes and medical responses evident in the 1970s continued to underscore the public understanding and policies regarding decision making for compromised infants over the next 20 years and are still influential today. In the effort to make explicit what is otherwise implicit, a specific milestone in the history of medical ethics and medical management of spina bifida deserves a careful look. This milestone occurred in 1971 when John Lorber proposed a set of criteria specifically to address the quality of life for infants with severe myelomeningocele. Lorber argued that it was possible to establish clinical criteria to distinguish between infants whose severity of spina bifida allowed the prospect of meaningful lives and infants for whom the severity of spina bifida doomed them either to years of tragic suffering if treated or the likelihood of death in the first year of life if left untreated. On that basis, he argued for a policy of selective nontreatment as a means to spare infants with a poor prognosis the burden of irredeemable suffering (Lorber, 1971, 1972).

Guided by the apparent belief that death is preferable to life under circumstances like profound impairments, repeated and only partially successful operations, paralysis, and retardation, especially when these conditions are predictable following surgery, Lorber's proposals generated a maelstrom of controversy. And yet, there were those, like Freeman, who acknowledged this dilemma and described the decision as caught "between the Scylla of treating all children with meningomyeloceles with the resultant increase in the number of survivors with severe handicapping conditions, and the Charybdis of not treating some children and permitting nature to take its often long, lingering course" (Freeman, 1972: 904). However, in response, Freeman directed the discussion unflinchingly to one of its unsettling implications: "Having seen children with unoperated meningomyeloceles lie around the ward for weeks or months untreated, waiting to die, one cannot help but feel the highest form of medical ethic would have been to end the pain and suffering, rather than wishing the patient would go away" (905).

In these early attempts to identify a moral compass by which to survey and navigate the perilous, remarkably complex, and deeply unsettling issues roiling out of the growing controversy, Freeman rightly forecast the ramifications of the advances in prenatal diagnosis. He asked, "if there were mechanisms for the diagnosis of myelomeningoceles at 20 to 24 weeks of gestation, would we not encourage parents to request termination of pregnancy?", followed by the jarring inference: "If it is permissible to kill a fetus at 20 to 24 weeks, should it not also be permissible to kill an infant at 40 weeks gestation?" (904).

Moral slogans quickly developed: that every child should be surgical treated because it has a right to life, or that physicians and parents should not make judgments about a child's potential quality of life, while at the same time, physicians, families, and the trusted advisers to both, as well as ethicists and legal experts, grappled with the far-ranging and complicated issues. The complex medical, familial, economic, and social issues, as well as the disturbing ethical questions characteristic of spina bifida, were thought to make it a *prototype* for discussions about decisions to medically treat or withhold treatments from what were considered severely defective newborns. Significant at that time, therefore, were other studies suggesting that a life defined as intolerable by physicians might come to be defined in a very different manner by parents. Thus, there were calls to identify a range of social factors that correlated with parental acceptance of handicaps, such as religion, social class, parenting other (normal) children, and the presence of supportive friends and relatives (Darling, 1977).

In the search for guidance about ethically permissible and medically appropriate decision making, and to address the need for extensive public discussion, a conference was organized in 1977 by Chester Swinyard to discuss "decision making and the defective newborn" (Swinyard, et al., 1978). This conference was attended by Lorber (1978), Freeman et al. (1978), and other well-known commentators like Paul Ramsey, Raymond Duff (1978), Norm Fost (1978), Warren Reich (1978), John Robertson (1978), and John Fletcher (1978), all of whom (except Ramsey) contributed papers to the discussion.

INFLUENTIAL ATTITUDES TOWARD DEFECTIVE NEWBORNS IN THE 1970S

Early in 1974, Richard McCormick presented a moral position on the preservation of life, arguing that "the meaning, substance, and consumation of life is found in human relationships" (1974: 174) and that "life is a value to be preserved only insofar as it contains some potentiality for human relationships" (175). Other views, like those of Paul Ramsey, suggested that decision makers should concentrate on the medical indications for treatment. Deliberations about treatment, Ramsey held, should emphasize "the *equality* of particular lives regardless of their state or condition" (1978: 241–243).

Given that such attitudes depict the outlines of what can become deep and grievous moral conflicts, with the potential for dividing health-care providers from one another and from parents or prospective parents, they merit more than a cursory look. In that regard, it will be helpful to revisit the conference organized by Swinyard. In his presentation there, John Fletcher grappled with the complex task of documenting and describing what he took to be the "general attitudes towards the defective newborn with spina bifida and myelomeningocele that emerge from the literature and published discussions on the subject" (1978: 283). We can reasonably assume that in practice then, as now, such attitudes overlapped and intersected in various ways, yielding an unsettling and problematic ambiguity. Indeed, Fletcher noted that as a matter of practice, policies for selection tended to be unstated and varied. Furthermore, he explained, "there had not been a concerted effort to refine criteria for nontreatment in the United States, probably due to the extraordinary ethical pluralism that obtains, as well as the precarious legal situation" (1978: 297).

This assessment was supported by a lawyer, John Robertson, who explained this "precarious legal situation" and asserted that infants born with potentially severe cognitive and physical disabilities had the same right to be treated as anyone else. On Robertson's (1975) own assessment, it was primarily the nonenforcement of existing criminal laws that granted parents and physicians effective discretion to decide the fate of an infant born with a range of defects.

Due to their extraordinary moral complexity, it is important to consider the extent to which these tensions are still prominent, and thus influence the moral outlines of the discussions that accompanied the medical developments in the decades that followed. Accordingly, what follows is a brief summary of the two sets of general attitudes Fletcher reported.

The first set of attitudes he defined was concerned with the idea of fairness. More specifically, Fletcher noted that special emphasis was placed on the need for fairness in the evaluation of children born with myelomeningocele. This viewpoint suggested that fairness dictates that each child be provided with adequate treatment sufficient to stimulate and develop individual attributes in organized attempts to compensate for serious disability (Fletcher, 1978: 285).

The second set of attitudes he defined was concerned with the effort to integrate the individual diagnosis with overall social responsibility. These issues were generated in part by the increasing technological sophistication and clinical effectiveness of life-sustaining interventions. Thus, a key task for the physician was to select for treatment only those infants who, according to the established clinical criteria for selection, would survive with a reasonable degree of independence and cognitive capacity (Fletcher, 1978: 294).

Commensurate with the differences among these two sets of attitudes, the social role of medicine takes on significantly different responsibilities. The role of medicine in relation to the first set of attitudes was to focus exclusively on the individual care of the physician's patient. That focus was to be steadfastly maintained, and not qualified or complicated by the potential suffering and inconvenience caused to families and society. Likewise, the role of the family in the decision-making process was considered susceptible to the emotional trauma of having a defective child, potentially compromising the quality of parental participation in the decision to treat or not to treat. Given the extent of uncertainty in the ability to predict a therapeutic outcome in any individual case, it was thought better to pursue the least irreversible strategy of offering corrective interventions compared to selecting for nontreatment (Fletcher, 1978).

The role of medicine in relation to the second set of attitudes was to consider and evaluate the treatment of an individual patient in terms of an estimation of the consequences for the patient, the patient's family, and society. The rationale was that medicine should not be segregated from other aspects of social and political life. Following the rationale of Lorber's criteria, it was considered possible to predict the "*minimum degree of future handicap* in an individual even if *it is impossible to forecast the maximum degree of disability*, which he may suffer, if he survives" (1971: 300). These predictions were claimed to be sufficiently accurate to make selection for treatment rationally compelling. Clinical pessimism, more than optimism, was justified when thinking about the future of severely compromised infants, including those born with spina bifida, because surgical treatments could not ensure a satisfactory quality of life (Fletcher, 1978: 292).

The concluding ethical issue that Fletcher raised was this: given the gravity of such decisions, new parents not only deserved to play a major part in the decision to treat or not to treat, but their participation required that they possess information about the outcome of sufficient quality to provide *informed* consent to the decision (Fletcher, 1978: 291). In that regard, the sociological and psychological literature of the 1970s that evaluated the influence of a child with spina bifida was not encouraging for parents, with findings supporting the notion that the family with a disabled child was a disabled family (Tew et al., 1974; Singh 2003). Furthermore, Fletcher maintained that decisions about "the injustice of prolonging life" should be made by "those most involved with the suffering." And yet, as Fletcher urged, "their best decisions must finally be challenged in the ethical debate beyond the decisions made in anguish, passion, and uncertainty, even in the face of the certainty of predictable suffering" (1978: 296).

A principal difficulty in the ethical debate was that the tensions among these clinical and social roles reflected the commitments of divergent moral stances. As described by Hauerwas, both stances are directed by the desire to prevent suffering. The first is primarily guided by the ethical imperative to always treat individuals as ends and not as means for the benefit of others. The second is guided by the maxim of acting in ways that produce the least amount of suffering for the largest number of human beings with spina bifida (1977: 243–244). Because these imperatives and maxims entail the fundamental assumptions that individuals hold about moral life, especially for the parents of affected infants, these two rationales, each justifiable in terms of its own premises, remained inadequate for clinical application in specific circumstances because of insufficient attention to the elements of parental decision making and responsibility.

CONTROVERSIAL 1980S: FEDERAL REGULATIONS AND ETHICAL PLURALISM

Ranked among the major ethical issues in the 1970s, these controversies and their accompanying disputes escalated through the early 1980s. The twin elements of the legalization of abortion in the 1973 *Roe v. Wade* decision and the increased prevalence of clinical applications for obstetric ultrasound imaging intensified controversies about the medical ability to diagnose fetal defects and increased the focus on the ways new technologies affected attitudes toward handicapped newborns (Retsinas, 1991). Fueled by fervent discussions about the effects of prenatal diagnosis and abortion on social attitudes toward handicapped infants, the controversies surrounding the clinical judgments became more publicly visible and intense (Ramsey, 1978; Reiser, 1986: 202–203). The bristling edges of these issues increasingly confronted each other in clinical and research practices shaped by equally public efforts to modify the tendencies of paternalism in medical decision making and a specific focus on creating a more robust, legally enforced notion of informed consent (Annas et al., 1977). Patients (and parents) had the moral right to medical information and to decide what was the most appropriate medical course to take based on that information and their own values.

By the late 1970s, the ethical issues had been clarified to the extent that clinicians acknowledged that "one must be acutely aware of one's own biases, the background and attitudes of the family, the legal and social elements, and yet somehow make decisions that are primarily in the best interest of the infant" (McLaughlin and Shurtleff, 1979: 474). Thus, medical management developed with an equal focus on the medical indications and improved techniques in surgical repair, as well as projected outcomes for the treatment of myelomeningocele. As result, "by the late 1970s in the United States, Lorber's selection criteria had been largely rejected and most children with spina bifida we operated on shortly after birth, regardless of the level of the lesion" (Freeman, 1998: 304). Improved diagnostic techniques such as computed tomography and ultrasound, as well as better knowledge about how to use shunts, the earlier identification of infections, and a greater number of antibiotics to treat infection added support to the decision to treat most affected infants.

However, a report published in *Pediatrics* by Gross and colleagues in 1983 described their 5-year effort (July 1, 1977–June 30, 1982), using Shurtleff's criteria for selective nontreatment (Shurtleff et al., 1974) to evaluate 69 infants. This group used a multidisciplinary group in a process that resulted in a recommendation to the infant's parents and family. For 36 infants, the team decided to recommend "active vigorous treatment" and for 33 infants to inform the parents that the team did not consider the parents obligated to pursue treatment. Of those 33, only 28 couples (families) accepted the recommendation for "supportive care" only. Of those 28, 1 family moved and was lost to follow-up, and 3 other infants received delayed treatment at the request of parents, leaving 24 infants who received supportive care only (Gross et al., 1983: 452–453).

Each infant in the treatment group was provided all medically indicated treatments, including surgical covering of the spinal lesion and placement of a shunt to drain cerebrospinal fluid from the brain, and all survived. The 24 infants who did not receive vigorous intervention also did not receive active treatment for infection, and "sedatives were not routinely administered." None of the 24 survived, and the article noted: "The 'untreated survivor' has not been a significant problem in our experience" (Gross et al., 1983: 455).

Freeman's acute response in *Pediatrics* observed that "the mere fact that a team can be put together, can assure compliance, can reach consensus not to treat half the infants, and can get the infants to die quickly, hardly makes it as the best available alternative for the management of infants with myelomeningocele" (1984: 566). The 24 infants who died "might also have done well, as in many series walked with assistive devices, gone to regular school, been of normal intelligence, and achieved bowel and bladder control" (566). "Indeed," Freeman went on, "the sole difference between those treated and those given supportive care may be that the latter are more likely to end up in a wheelchair or with more bracing" (566).

The *Pediatrics* report prompted an unprecedented number of letters in response, almost all of which were critical of the approach taken (Freeman, 1984: 162–167; Weir, 1985). It ignited another round of clinical debate in the medical literature (Charney et al., 1985; McLaughlin et al., 1985; Gross, 1985) as well as an immediate and intense public response (Weir, 1985).

Looking back, it may be hard to remember (or to imagine) just how intense and sustained these controversies were. The outcry about ethics and the lack of reliable and medically clear answers to questions about the harms and benefits of pursuing treatment for such severely affected infants had already raised public and governmental concerns to an unprecedented level (Paige and Karnofsky, 1986; Pence, 1990). At the forefront of those concerns were questions about whether diagnostic or therapeutic interventions were being arbitrarily withheld from these as well as other medically compromised newborns. Following the American predilection to appeal to the law to resolve uncertainties and fears about medical neglect, the uproar that accompanied earlier and similar controversies led to efforts spearheaded by Surgeon General C. Everett Koop to develop a federal policy and regulations to guide decisions for compromised infants (Gardell and Engelhardt, 1987; Moss, 1987).

Created to curtail the perceived reliance on a parent's inevitable concern with the infant's real or imagined quality of life or with expected resources, these regulations asserted that the basis for decisions must be solely "the individual's medical condition" (Department of Health and Human Services, 1984: 1622). While the authority of parents to make decisions for their children has never been absolute, historically they have been recognized as their children's principal decision makers (Shelp, 1986: 26–49). However, in the early days of this very public discussion of so-called Baby Does, this authority was severely questioned by some groups who claimed that parents could not be entrusted with such difficult decisions. Also important to note was the American Medical Association's comment that "quality of life is a factor to be considered in determining what is best for the individual. Life should be cherished despite disabilities and handicaps, except when prolongation would be inhumane and unconscionable" (Department of Health and Human Services, 1984: 1629).

The final result was the 1985 Amendment to the Child Abuse Prevention and Treatment Act and the accompanying Department of Health and Human Services (DHHS) regulations, commonly known as the *Baby Doe Regs.* A new category of child abuse was defined: failure to provide appropriate medical and surgical treatments for multiply compromised infants with life-threatening conditions. In the end, however, these legislative mechanisms proved far too rigid and too vague to apply with any precision to bedside judgments about the extent of appropriate therapies. As a result, these regulations proved to be ineffective and unenforceable, although concerns about how best to interpret the standards may have influenced decision making by physicians and parents (Kopelman et al., 1988; Todres et al., 1988).

Even so, and perhaps more significantly, it was not until this final DHHS rule that the parent's right to make decisions was formally acknowledged: "The decision to provide or withhold medically indicated treatment, except in highly unusual circumstances, is made by parents or legal guardian" (Department of Health and Human Services, 1985: 14880). Earlier versions of these regulations did not recognize this parental right.

Indeed, the premise of the regulations seemed flawed from the start, for it excluded systematic examination of many crucial matters in the many interactions that occur in clinical circumstances—such as how patients, families, and health professionals think and feel about the problems they face, their work, themselves, and their relationships with one another, as well as much less broad issues such as justice or those posed by the science and technologies they use (Duff, 1987: 249). Those issues seemed to be relevant to the various studies in the literature at that time, which indicated that parents of children with spina bifida, especially mothers, continued to experience certain negative effects—increased financial problems, excessive time demands on the mother, and a decrease in family opportunities (Singh, 2003).

ETHICAL PLURALISM AND THE NEED FOR "CLOSE-UP" ETHICS

On the other hand, academic (if not systematic) philosophical arguments in the medical ethics literature were dominated by language about infants (and fetuses) as *persons,* and thus about *rights* and corresponding obligations of care providers (Ramsey 1975, 1978; Weir, 1984; Engelhardt, 1986). This language and its prevalence were intended to address two crucial questions: Is the infant born with potentially devastating medical complications a person? If so, is such an infant thus entitled to full moral status, with full rights and protections? Echoing the *ethical pluralism* John Fletcher reported, the ethics literature became swollen with arguments addressed to such moral questions about personhood and rights (Warren, 1975; Murray, 1985; Shapiro and Barthel, 1986). Several different justifications were given in those arguments. Although many if not most people would grant that infants are endowed with moral status as persons, for some philosophers like Engelhardt, only full persons (i.e., self-conscious, rational, capable of language) are entitled to full moral status (Engelhardt, 1986; Shelp, 1986). For others, while acknowledging that all human beings may not be persons, the understanding is that human beings acquire their particular moral status from those who are (Solomon, 1983; Whitbeck, 1983). Decisions about these not-yet-full-persons can and must be made by others, who should focus on the medical indications, which turns out to have considerable importance for the best interests for an infant.

These arguments remain unresolved and continue to shape the discussions about decision making for infants. Thus, what Alasdair MacIntyre argued decades ago continues to be accurate: that "it is impossible in our culture now to find a systematic way of using such words as 'ethical' and 'moral' which does not already embody not merely a particular morality, but a particular contentious morality which is at war with its rivals" (MacIntyre, 1978: 10–13). In a pluralistic society like ours, there are not only many different ethical viewpoints, but these are deeply at odds with each other: while each of them may be perfectly self-consistent, each starts from quite different basic premises that rival others.

One result is that few clinical discussions can cause more consternation than those substantively involving ethics. This is especially the case if, while trying to decide what is the right, just, or merely best action to take regarding an imperiled fetus or newborn, primary decision makers are encouraged to assume an *objective* attitude. This tendency reflects the fact that many discussions in the ethics literature use the abstract language of principles and autonomy (Churchill and Simán, 1986). That assumption adopts a potentially distorting yet predominant image of individuals, both patients and physicians, as somehow equal and independent partners to an agreement, and where patients suffer no imbalances of vulnerability, dependency, or power. Such a view is severely inadequate as a description of clinical situations, especially with respect to parents suffering grief and shock. Nonetheless, this view is often adopted to subdue the possibly conflictual, and dynamic, character of ethical engagement in clinical decision making.

Unfortunately, the abstraction inherent in such standard accounts make "alienation the central moral virtue" by insisting that we "learn to view our desires, interests, and passions as if they could belong to anyone . . . that we view our own projects and life as if we were outside observers" (Burell and Hauerwas, 1977: 122). By contrast, responding to the actual circumstances, people, and compelling moral issues surrounding decisions about infants with poor prognoses requires that the traditionally *distant ethics* of predominantly academic methods of analysis be replaced by a more clinically oriented and experientially based *close-up* ethics (Duff, 1987).

The moral recognition commensurate with the experiential basis of clinical, or close-up, ethics was reported by Duff, exemplified in a note by Minnich. She noted that when faced with such compelling circumstances, people "want no abstraction, no neutrality, no generalizations to help them" (in Duff, 1987: 250). In an eloquent summary that could stand as a touchstone for close-up ethics, she reports about individuals facing the limits of medical interventions: "They want help finding out what decision they can live with, what their own deepest values and needs are. They were insistent that decisions must be personal, and that they cannot be imposed but, rather, discovered. They want to think things through . . . through the thickest parts, until they find their own way. They do not think 'ethics' has to do with universal principles: they think it has to do with uncertainty, risk, individual commitment and, strongly so, with the deepest emotions" (in Duff, 1987: 250–251).

The point is that every ethical view makes demands on our lives, our actions, and our commitments. It may well turn out that there is no one correct sort of ethics, but in fact many different options through which to possibly resolve morally complex circumstances. Thus, we need to develop counseling and decision-making processes that identify factors generated by deep emotions, personal opinions, and ethical complexity, factors that continue to characterize clinical decisions about whether to selectively not treat severely compromised infants and potentially compromised fetuses.

The ethical task is not to try to determine which, if any, of the competing views seems best (if that can even be done conceptually). Rather, the real task is to examine a situation in all of its complexity to figure out what is specifically at issue—and why—and what can be done about it without compromising the evident commitments held by individuals in that situation. That kind of clarification especially needs to be accomplished by interacting with the people who make the decisions and must live with the aftermath (Zaner, 1988).

Physicians, nurses, and other health professionals do and must play an important role when medical treatment decisions are made for infants compromised by severe spina bifida. The experience of these professionals is crucial to assist parents in identifying and sorting through possible treatment options and their outcomes. Most crucially, perhaps, they can participate in, and thus review, parental decisions to withhold or provide treatment when ethical issues arise regarding whether such options are consistent with current medical thinking about the medical (or best) interests of the infant (Caplan and Cohen, 1987: 19).

PARENTAL RESPONSIBILITY FOR MAKING DECISIONS

What needs to be highlighted in the brief history reviewed above is the clear need to identify and emphasize the importance of parental involvement in decision making. Clearly, there has been increased awareness and integration of shared decision making between parents and clinicians. In the decades following the Baby Doe regulations, there has been ongoing support for the idea that parents should play a significant role in these decisions (Jellinek et al., 1992; Harrison, 1993). Primarily negotiated around the legislation of patients' rights, proxy decision making, and increased medical knowledge about the efficacy of treating infants with myelomeningocele, consensus has resulted from the clarification of good reasons for emphasizing the primacy of parents' role in making decisions about their own infants. Earlier, the President's Commission for the Study of Ethical Problems in Medicine and Biomedical and Behavioral Research addressed this issue directly: "Given that parents are usually present, concerned, willing and able to be informed, and cognizant of the values of the culture in which they intend to raise a child, they are best situated to have the primary place in making decisions about their infant's care" (1983: 214–215).

Perhaps equally important is that society confers upon parents the responsibility to care for their children, a responsibility that in part stems from the fact that whether or not the parents voluntarily initiated the pregnancy, over time they continuously reaffirmed the decision to become parents (since the pregnancy, at least within certain limits, could have been terminated). Underlying this is a moral ought: one ought to recognize and assume responsibility or one's choices, including whatever can be reasonably foreseen to result from that choice (most of all bearing, birthing, and rearing children). That one can, as implied above, deny, betray, or refuse to assume this responsibility only underscores the moral point.

CONDITIONS FOR PARENTAL RESPONSIBILITY FOR DECISIONS

Parental responsibility extends beyond providing the physical necessities of life. Perhaps most basically, it involves promoting and safeguarding the newborn's moral status as a person—to enable the infant to become a full moral agent within the surrounding moral community—however the criteria for this status may be viewed (Magnet and Kluge, 1985: 149–150). The relevant feature to note is the decision-making authority embedded in the obligation to safeguard an infant and administer to his or her needs. As Magnet and Kluge say, "Those who assume the obligation of care for the neonate *qua* person also assume the obligation to act as surrogate decision-maker to protect the child's rights" (150).

The authority to make decisions for one's child therefore has as its ground whatever is required to allow parents to fulfill their moral responsibility to care for the child. The point is, the moral status of parenting (with its network of responsibilities and obligations) cannot be fulfilled except on the condition that parents are accorded the moral authority to make decisions on behalf of their children (Magnet and Kluge, 1985: 150)—an authority that may, of course, be defeated by one's own or others' action or failure to act.

From the moral authority of the parents emerges a second condition. Given the correlation between decisional authority and moral responsibility to care for one's own children, there is a corresponding obligation on the part of anyone else who has a legitimate role in caring for these children—including physicians and nurses. While such professionals may serve as major advisors to parents who must make difficult decisions, their primary responsibility is to ensure that parents are as fully informed as possible about their child's condition—that is, to ensure that parents understand the medical problems and prospects as accurately as possible. As primary decision makers, parents must have as much information, knowledge, and understanding as possible (within the obvious constraints of situation, personal circumstances, and abilities) about the specific facts and treatments for the child's medical conditions and the probable outcomes of treatments, as well as the overall prognosis.

QUALITY OF LIFE: THE MOST UNSTABLE AND CONTROVERSIAL NOTION

The shared responsibility of parents and physicians raises a crucial issue. Although certainly linked, the variable and clinically uncertain considerations about medical conditions, probable outcomes, and prognoses raise one set of questions about the quality of life for the child the fetus may become, another set for a newborn with myelomeningocele, and still more questions regarding the family (Zaner, 1986). Taken together, these remain the most far-reaching and controversial set of unresolved issues. Some have proposed that quality of life is equivalent to a list of qualities or capacities for meaningful life (intellectual function, social interaction, and so on) (Fletcher, 1974); others focus on the relational potential possessed in a capacity for becoming human in relationships with others (McCormick, 1974); and still others believe that "quality" is best understood as the *sacredness* of life (Ramsey, 1978). Precisely what quality of life means remains at the crux of the controversy, although one distinction that seems consistently included emphasizes *social* human functioning in contrast to custodial, *biological* human functioning.

Thus, not only is the meaning of the term *quality of life* variable, but the moral passions evoked by the reduction of humanity to biological functioning themselves rest on a profound set of issues. As argued by others noted above, especially Ramsey, Carl Elliott recognizes that we are "inheritors of a strong tradition of rights and equality" and thus are "reluctant to withhold treatment from a person on the grounds of her intelligence or disabilities" that might result from severe neurological compromise (2003: 20).

Focusing here specifically on decisions made about infants born with myelomeningocele—and distinguishing these from those made prenatally about fetuses—we remain confronted by the deeply unsettling issues left unresolved in the controversies summarized above. Many times a crucial factor in an evaluation of the potential severity of a handicap for the infant includes a prospective assessment about the future mental status/cognitive ability of the infant. Specific questions focus on the extent or degree of cognitive impairment that can be reasonably expected to result from the severity of a neurological defect and the severity of the indicated hydrocephalus. Not only are the sequelae of these two factors exceedingly difficult to predict, but there are other considerations. Zaner poses a key question regarding the assumed connection between cognitive capability and quality of life: "does being mentally retarded or compromised diminish the quality of life of the person with retardation and if so, precisely how?" (1986: 89).

Furthermore, while serious studies (Holmbeck and Faier-Routman, 1995; Pit-ten Cate et al., 2002) have attempted to assess the variety of combined factors that constitute the quality of life for individuals living with spina bifida, these are neither adequately nuanced nor specific enough to answer such ethical questions. Perhaps quality of life does not merely refer to the cognitive capacity of the impaired individual, because such studies do indicate that there are underlying cultural, environmental, and hence moral factors that affect individuals with spina bifida and their families. These factors include familial and social resources, attitudes of others, and the presence or modification of physical and social barriers to persons with disabilities (Pit-ten Cate et al., 2002; Simeonsson et al., 2002). Additional factors are also pertinent. Mothers with children who have spina bifida rely on denial of disability and other problems, possibly as way to manage the stresses generated by the uncontrollable and chronically stressful life events associated with spina bifida (Holmbeck et al., 1997). For many children—and adults—with spina bifida, most if not all of these societal factors contribute influence the individual's quality of life and are just as significant as their physical handicaps.

However, in consideration of the overwhelming compromise of physical and cognitive abilities that can result from the severest forms of neural tube defects, the Elliott's plain statement captures the issue of a "meaningful life" for families faced with such circumstances. We "see that the lives of these children have deep significance for their families," he says. "Yet on the other hand, we recognize that these lives fail to meet the criteria by which we count our own lives as meaningful. We try to convince ourselves that we should protect vulnerable lives, but we cannot imagine this as a life we would want to continue living" (2003: 20).

Regarding neurological devastation in infants, Jan Van Eys realizes a correlative point. He incorporates the arguments regarding *personhood* in way that emphasizes the intertwined social characteristics and mutuality entailed in a meaningful life. Van Eys suggests that what, or who, is considered abnormal is related to the degree to which it becomes legitimate to exclude them from the web of social interactions and concerns. Thus, he says, "we all create our limit of 'unacceptable exceptionality,' the boundary beyond which a child or adult cannot cope." Van Eys explains, "there are indeed such severely brain-damaged babies that all will say, 'this is an unacceptable life.' " "What is meant," he goes on to say, "is that society cannot accept that child without major adjustments that we are unwilling to make" (2001: 11). That individual will not be able to participate in social interactions in the ways necessary to maintain the social fabric or in ways minimally necessary for human relationships.

In short, if an infant or child is likely to benefit from treatments, then there are sound medical arguments for providing them. There has been, however, extensive and sometimes polarized debate about whether simple existence, with the human biological experience limited to eating, sleeping, and warmth, demands moral protection. However, decision makers must rely on their values, which also may represent, in one form or another, societal values, as noted by Minnich, Elliott, and Van Eys. And the views adopted often reflect McCormick's considerations about possessing a *relational capacity* (McCormick, 1974).

Of course, the great variance in severity—and potential suffering—of those with myelomeningocele is precisely the issue that continues to makes decisions for infants with severe spina bifida so troubling and difficult. The relevant boundaries are exceedingly difficult to determine. However, while those distinctions among simple sentience and relational capacities are far from precise, they provide guidelines for a relevant maxim—"even though a line is not drawn in nature, it may well be needed in practice" (Bok, 1978: 277)—because in those cases where the involved decision makers interpret that the infant lacks even the potential for basic personal capacities, talk of "medical interests" and "best interests" becomes problematic (Arras, 1987). Finally, if being born with spina bifida is unfair, on the basis of an entire array of social attitudes toward the disabilities associated with spina bifida, then, as pointed out by Van Eys, it is because we make it so.

The issue then is not merely that persons—parents, physicians, and other care providers, policy makers, legislators, theologians, educators, and so on—contribute to decisions about what is to be considered valuable about other human beings. The basis for the strength of the moral appeal to quality of life—as a *meaningful life*—is its connection to the power of the real, and more profound, dimensions of human responsibility, especially parental responsibility, as considered above. This means that the ability to protect an infant's rights requires both the moral authority and the means to support the meaningful content associated with rights. And, in consideration of circumstances in which the compromised infant will not have a meaningful life, parents are faced with the need to determine whether that life represents an existence worse than death.

Therefore, equally significant is the requirement that decisions about compromised fetuses and infants include consideration of the needs of the parents and the potential harms to the family, as well as other social consequences (Strong, 1983, 1984). These factors gain legitimacy primarily because parents are not obligated to make decisions on the basis of the imagined rights of infants who are so medically damaged that they would never be able to claim such rights (Fletcher, 1979). However, because parents and physicians in fact share responsibilities in decision making, a collaborative approach should be used in discussions of the ethical issues specific to the clinical situation.

AT THE FOREFRONT: CAREFUL AND THOROUGH PRENATAL COUNSELING OF PREGNANT WOMEN, PARENTS, AND FAMILIES

The discussion immediately above about meaningful lives for severely compromised newborns reinforces the need for more information for pregnant women, new parents, and their families. We have previously separated decisions made about infants from those made about affected fetuses in order to focus on the issues concerning parental responsibility. This section will distinguish between prenatal counseling and neonatal counseling in order to focus on the more recent and less well documented complexities of prenatal counseling. As stated earlier, the time constraints that exist in the prenatal setting are unlikely to disappear, so strategies need to be designed for practical and effective interactions within those constraints that enhance informed decision making on the part of pregnant women and their partners.

To review the issues raised at the beginning of this chapter, advances in prenatal diagnosis mean that the complex and ethically challenging task of counseling pregnant women and their partners is becoming more common. A multidisciplinary approach is advised (Wilcox et al., 1993; Crombleholme et al., 1996; Madsen et al., 1998). The actual composition of the team may depend on the specific characteristics and needs of each patient and family. For many families, their pediatrician or primary care physician is an important and familiar resource. In addition, the array of specialties available should include (but not be limited to) those involved in clinical care (e.g., pediatric neurosurgeons, pediatric surgeons, perinatologists, and neonatologists), as well as the supporting services (such as ultrasonography, genetics, and genetics counseling). Staff from social work, clinical and surgical nursing (both obstetrical and neonatal), and financial counseling should be available as needed. Ethics consultation and chaplains should also be included to ensure effective discussion about and careful attention to the moral issues that may arise in specific circumstances.

For example, in the recent experience with elective open-uterine fetal repair of spina bifida, many couples reported that the initial counseling they received after their initial ultrasound examination from their own obstetrician was slanted—both against disability and toward terminating the pregnancy—while their own convictions directed them to continue the pregnancy. What they remembered was how the initial obstetric consultation portrayed as grim a picture as possible of their future child's prognosis. Their immediate sense of desperation was thus evoked in response to the challenges of disability. Their fears were about mental deficits, mental retardation, paralysis, and doubts about their own ability to manage those obvious challenges (Bliton, 2001). Thus, one difficulty faced by obstetricians and perinatologists is not knowing whether or exactly how a pregnant woman's predisposition to treat or to terminate might be influenced, or even exacerbated, by talk of termination and/or disability.

To promote the pregnant woman's ability to make an informed decision based on her beliefs, values, and goals, all of the options, including termination of the pregnancy, should be presented in a nondirective fashion. The involvement of pediatric neurosurgeons is therefore crucial for at least three practical reasons. First, the information provided to prospective parents is presented by a physician knowledgeable about the care of infants and children with the condition. Second, the family gets to meet the neurosurgeon. Finally, discussions about the timing and route of delivery, as well as considerations for surgery after birth, can occur, with the parents given time to think and consult with other trusted advisors (Madsen et al., 1998).

A list of the actions to be taken in counseling parents and families with affected fetuses includes the following:

- Assisting the prospective parents in understanding (within the obvious constraints of situation, personal circumstances, and abilities) the facts about treatments for the child's medical conditions and probable outcomes of treatment, as well as the overall prognosis. Videotapes and pamphlets can be provided to enable couples to digest the information at their own pace.
- Ensuring that sufficient time and assistance are provided to help women and their partners address the many questions they may have about the diagnostic indications regarding the location and severity of the fetal defect.
- Providing them with sufficient information about hereditary and embryonic factors in neural tube defects.
- Identifying the number of options available to them and asking them to consider which course of action seems appropriate to their specific circumstances.
- Discussing clinical uncertainty. In some instances, the diagnosis of the fetal condition will be uncertain. Even when the diagnosis is assured, specific steps for follow-up may remain unclear or require refinement. Clear discussions about the details and goals of subsequent treatment (e.g., urinary and orthopedic), and about the influence of clinical uncertainties—such as prediction of psychosocial and linguistic functions—on decision making must take place.

- Reiterating information is essential if distraught couples are to fully understand their situation (Wilcox et al., 1993). Each stage in the consultation with and counseling of pregnant women and their partners needs to include opportunities for candid discussion about their understanding of spina bifida and myelomeningocele, the option of terminating the pregnancy, the surgical options (both in utero, whether available under research protocols or electively, and postnatally), and the likely outcomes associated with each option.
- Encouraging couples to ask questions also requires allowing sufficient time for such meetings so that adequate time can be given to the especially sensitive and difficult matters regarding parental fears and hopes.

Pregnant women, as well as prospective and new parents, will need assistance when confronting and considering the life-transforming issues they will invariably encounter. With variations designed to address specific circumstances, this format for discussions with pregnant women and their partners contributes essential components needed for informed understanding and decision making.

NOTES

1. Cragan and Khoury (2000) note that estimates of the prevalence of neural tube defects indicate that, depending on the region and on variance across different ethnic populations, up to 50% of all pregnancies with any neural tube defect and up to 80% of those with anencephaly may be electively terminated. However, due to a variety of factors, including the fact that such terminations may occur outside the hospital, discrepancies can result from the exclusion of pregnancies for which spina bifida was prenatally diagnosed and pregnancies were electively terminated. Comparing the *prevalence* of spina bifida *at birth* with the reported *incidence* of spina bifida as a *prenatal diagnosis*—that is, the number of babies with spina bifida actually born compared to the reported number of fetuses diagnosed with it—the best surveillance data during the years most recently reported by the Centers for Disease Control, 1985–1994, reveals that one-fifth to one-third of the pregnancies diagnosed with spina bifida were terminated (Cragan et al., 1995). In a separate study from Velie and Shaw (1996) for California during 1989–1991 the percentages were similar: 247 infants were born with spina bifida out of 352 pregnancies that were diagnosed prenatally—indicating that 30% of these pregnancies were terminated.

   At high-risk obstetric centers during that same general time period, the numbers were smaller and the percentage of terminations was generally higher. Bell et al. (1996) reported that during 1990–1993, 18 (58%) out of the 31 fetuses diagnosed with meningomyelocele and associated hydrocephalus were electively terminated. Grevengood et al. (1994) report that during from 1987 to 1992, 21 of 27 (77.8%) of the women carrying fetuses with spina bifida elected to terminate their pregnancies. Forrester et al. (1998) reported that during 1987–1996, 58 cases of spina bifida were diagnosed and 28 (48.3%) of these pregnancies were terminated. Taking the data from the Department of Health Services in California as at least representative of trends in a diverse population, the more recent numbers from 1996–1999 tell more of the story: 277 instances of fetal spina bifida were registered, and 175 (63%) of these pregnancies were terminated (G. C. Cunningham, personal communication, 2000).
2. Additionally, for a newborn, the issue of legal protections and options becomes more prominent (Heimer and Staffen, 1998). To pursue those issues further would require an explication for each one. Given the focus of this chapter on parental responsibility and decision making, these issues must be left for another time.

REFERENCES

Amundsen DW (1987). Medicine and the birth of defective children: approaches of the ancient world. In McMillan RC, Engelhardt, HT Jr, Spicker SF (eds): *Euthanasia and the Newborn: Conflicts Regarding Saving Lives.* Dordrecht, the Netherlands: D Reidel, pp. 3–22.

Annas GJ, Glantz LH, Katz BF (1977). *Informed Consent to Human Experimentation; the Subject's Dilemma.* Cambridge, MA: Ballinger.

Arras JD (1987). Quality of life in neonatal ethics: Beyond denial and evasion. In Weil WB, Benjamin M (eds), *Ethical Issues at the Outset of Life.* Boston: Blackwell Scientific, pp. 151–186.

Asch A (1989). Reproductive technology and disability. In Cohen S, Taub N (eds): *Reproductive Law for the 1990s.* Clifton, NJ: Humana Press.

Baylis FE (1994). A profile of the health care ethics consultant. In Baylis FE (ed): *The Health Care Ethics Consultant.* Totowa, NJ: Humana Press, pp. 29–44.

Bell WO, Nelson LH, Block SM, Rhoney JC (1996). Prenatal diagnosis and pediatric neurosurgery. Pediatr Neurosurg 24:134–138.

Bentovim A (1972). Emotional disturbances of handicapped pre-school children and their families—attitudes to the child. Br Med J 3:579–581.

Bier J-AB, Liebling JA, Morales Y, Carlucci M (1996). Parent's and pediatrician's views of individuals with meningomyelocele. Clin Pediatr 35:113–117.

Bliton MJ (2001). Over the cutting edge: how ethics consultation illuminates the moral complexity of open-uterine fetal repair of spina bifida and patient's decision making. J Clin Ethics 12(4): 346–360.

Bliton MJ (2003). Ethics: "life before birth" and moral complexity in maternal-fetal surgery for spina bifida. Clin Perinatol 30:449–464.

Bok S (1978). Death and dying: euthanasia and sustaining life: ethical views. In Reich W (ed): *Encyclopedia of Bioethics.* New York: Free Press, pp. 268–277.

Botto LD, Moore CA, Khoury MJ, Erickson JD (1999). Neural tube defects. N Engl J Med 341:1509–1519.

Burrell D, Hauerwas S (1977). From system to story: An alternative pattern for rationality in ethics. In Engelhardt HT Jr, Callahan D (eds): *Knowledge, Value and Belief,* Vol. II, *The Foundations of Ethics and its Relationship to Science.* Hasting-on Hudson, NY: Institute of Society, Ethics and Life Sciences, pp. 111–152.

Callahan D (1986). How technology is reframing the abortion debate. Hastings Center Rep 16(1):33–42.

Caplan A, Cohen CB (eds) (1987). Imperiled newborns. Hastings Center Rep 17(6):5–32.

Charney EB, Weller SC, Sutton LN, et al (1985). Management of the newborn with myelomeningocele: time for a decision-making process. Pediatrics 75:58–64.

Churchill LR, Simán JJ (1986). Principles and the search for moral certainty. Social Sci Med 23:461–468.

Cochrane DD, Wilson RD, Steinbok P, Farquharson DF, Irwin B, Irvine B, et al (1996). Prenatal spinal evaluation and functional outcome of patients born with myelomeningocele: information for improved prenatal counseling and outcome prediction. Fetal Diagn Ther 11:159–168.

Cragan JD, Roberts HE, Edmonds LD, Khoury MJ, et al (1995). Surveillance for anencephaly and spina bifida and the impact of prenatal diagnosis: United States 1985–1994. MMWR CDC Surveill Summ 44:1–13.

Cragan JD, Khoury MJ (2000). Effect of prenatal diagnosis on epidemologic studies of birth defects. Epidemiology 11:695–699.

Crombleholme TM, D'Alton M, Cendron M, Almen B, et al (1996). Prenatal diagnosis and the pediatric surgeon: the impact of prenatal consultation on perinatal management. J Pediatr Surg 31:156–163.

Darling RB (1977). Parents, physicians and spina bifida. Hastings Center Rep 7(4):10–14.

Darling RB (1979). *Families Against Society: A Study of Reaction to Children with Birth Defects*. Vol. 88, Sage Library of Social Research. Beverly Hills, CA: Sage.

Department of Health and Human Services (1984, Jan. 12). Nondiscrimination on the basis of handicap; procedures and guidelines relating to health care for handicapped infants. Fed Reg 45 CFR (Pt 84):1622–1654.

Department of Health and Human Services (1985, Apr. 15). Child abuse and neglect prevention and treatment program: final rule. Fed Reg (45 CFR Pt 1340):14878–14901.

Dias MS, McLone DG (1993). Hydrocephalus in the child with dysraphism. Neurosurg Clin North Am 4:715–34.

Duden B (1993). *Disembodying Women: Perspectives on Pregnancy and the Unborn*. Cambridge, MA: Harvard University Press.

Duff RS (1978). A physician's role in the decision-making process: a physician's experience. In Swinyard CA (ed): *Decision Making and the Defective Newborn: Proceedings of a Conference on Spina Bifida and Ethics*. Springfield, IL: Charles C Thomas, pp. 194–219.

Duff RS (1987). "Close-up" versus "distant ethics": deciding the care of infants with poor prognosis. Semin Perinatol 11:244–253.

Duff RS, Campbell AGM (1987). Moral communities and tragic choices. In McMillan RC, Engelhardt HT Jr, Spicker SF (eds): *Euthanasia and the Newborn: Conflicts Regarding Saving Lives*. Dordrecht, the Netherlands, D. Reidel, pp. 273–289.

Elliot C (2003). Attitudes, souls, and persons: children with severe neurological impairment. Ment Retard Dev Disabil Res Rev 9:16–20.

Engelhardt HT Jr (1986). *The Foundation of Bioethics*. New York: Oxford University Press.

Ferguson PM (2002). A place in the family: an historical interpretation of research on parental reactions to having a child with a disability. J Special Ed 36:124–130.

Fletcher JF (1974). Four indicators of humanhood—the enquiry matures. Hastings Center Rep 4:4–7.

Fletcher J (1978). Spina bifida with myelomeningocele: a case study in attitudes towards defective newborns. In Swinyard CA (ed): *Decision Making and the Defective Newborn: Proceedings of a Conference on Spina Bifida and Ethics*. Springfield, IL: Charles C Thomas, pp. 281–303.

Fletcher J (1979). Prenatal diagnosis, selective abortion, and the ethics of withholding treatment from the defective newborn. In Capron AM, Lappé M, Murray RF, et al (eds): *Genetic Counseling: Facts, Values and Norms*. Birth Defects: Original Article Series, Vol. XV, No. 2. New York: Alan R Liss, pp. 239–254.

Forrester MB, Merz RD, Yoon PW (1998). Impact of prenatal diagnosis and elective termination on the prevalence of selected birth defects in Hawaii. Am J Epidemiol 148:1206–1211.

Fost N (1978). How decisions are made: a physician's view. In Swinyard CA (ed): *Decision Making and the Defective Newborn: Proceedings of a Conference on Spina Bifida and Ethics*. Springfield, IL: Charles C Thomas, pp. 220–230.

Freeman JM (1972). Is there a right to die—quickly? J Pediatr 80:904–905.

Freeman JM (1974). To treat or not to treat. In Freeman JM (ed): *Practical Management of Meningomyelocele*. Baltimore: University Park Press, pp. 13–22.

Freeman JM (1984). Early management and decision making for the treatment of myelomeningocele: a critique. Pediatrics 73:564–566.

Freeman JM (1998). Changing ethical issues in the treatment of spina bifida: a personal odyssey. Ment Retard Dev Disabil Res Rev 4:302–7.

Freeman JM, Shulman K, Reinke W (1978). Decision making and the infant with spina bifida. In Swinyard CA (ed): *Decision Making and the Defective Newborn: Proceedings of a Conference on Spina Bifida and Ethics*. Springfield, IL: Charles C Thomas, pp. 95–110.

Gardell MA, Engelhardt HT Jr (1987). The Baby Doe controversy: an outline of some points in its development. In McMillan RC, Engelhardt, HT Jr, Spicker SF (eds): *Euthanasia and the Newborn: Conflicts Regarding Saving Lives*. Dordrecht, the Netherlands: D Reidel, pp. 293–299.

Gould SJ (2002). Introduction: to open a millennium. In Atwan R (series ed), Gould SJ (ed): *Best American Essays, 2002*. Boston: Houghton Mifflin, pp. xiii–xvii.

Gregg R (1995). *Pregnancy in a High-Tech Age: Paradoxes of Choice*. New York and London: New York University Press.

Grevengood C, Shulman LP, Dungan JS, et al (1994). Severity of abnormality influences decision to terminate pregnancies affected with fetal neural tube defects. Fetal Diagn Ther 9:273–277.

Gross RH (1985). Newborns with myelodysplasia—the rest of the story. N Engl J Med 312:1632–1634.

Gross RH, Cox A, Tatyrek R, Pollay M, Barnes WA (1983). Early management and decision making for the treatment of myelomeningocele. Pediatrics 72:450–458.

Harrison H (1993). The principles for family-centered neonatal care. Pediatrics 92:643–650.

Hauerwas S (1977). Selecting children to live or die: an ethical analysis of the debate between Dr. Lorber and Dr. Freeman on the treatment of meningomyelocele. In Horan DJ, Mall D (eds): *Death, Dying and Euthanasia*. Washington, DC: University Publications of America, pp. 228–247.

Heimer CA, Staffen LR (1998). Responsibility as a joint enterprise: the role of the state in the NICU and the home. In *For the Sake of the Children: The Social Organization of Responsibility in the Hospital and Home*. Chicago: University of Chicago Press, pp. 137–177.

Holmbeck GN, Faier-Routman J (1995). Spinal lesion level, shunt status, family relationships, and psychosocial adjustment in children and adolescents with spina bifida myelomeningocele. J Pediatr Psychol 20:817–832.

Holmbeck GN, Gorey-Ferguson L, Hudson T, Seefeldt T, Shapera W, Truner T, Uhler J (1997). Maternal, paternal, and marital functioning in families of preadolescents with spina bifida. J Pediatr Psychol 22:167–181.

Hommeyer JS, Holmbeck GN, Willis KE, Coers S (1999). Condition severity and psychosocial functioning in pre-adolescents with spina bifida: disentangling proximal functional status and distal adjustment outcomes. J Pediatr Psychol 24:499–509.

Horton TV, Wallander JL (2001). Hope and social support as resilience factors against psychological distress of mothers who care for children with chronic physical conditions. Rehabil Psychol 46:382–399.

Jacobs R, Northam E, Anderson V (2001). Cognitive outcome in children with myelomeningocele and perinatal hydrocephalus: a longitudinal perspective. J Dev Phys Disabil 13:389–405.

Jellinek MS, Catlin EA, Tordes ID, Cassem EH (1992). Facing tragic decisions in the neonatal intensive care unit: clinical perspectives. Pediatrics 89:119–122.

Jonsen AR (2000). A chronicle of ethical events: 1940s to 1980s. In *A Short History of Medical Ethics*. New York: Oxford University Press, pp. 99–114.

Kitcher P (1997). *The Lives to Come: The Genetic Revolution and Human Possibilities*. New York: Touchstone.

Kopelman, LM, Irons TG, Kopelman AE (1988). Neonatalogists judge the "Baby Doe" regulations. N Engl J Med 318(11):677–683.

LaPuma J, Schniedermayer D (1994). *Ethics Consultation: A Practical Guide*. Boston: Jones and Bartlett.

Liptak GS (1998). Controversies in the treatment of neural tube defects wit neurological deterioration. Ment Retard Dev Disabil Res Rev 4:296–301.

Lorber J (1971). Results of treatment of myelomeningocele: an analysis of 524 unselected cases, with special reference to selection for treatment. Dev Med Child Neurol 13:279–303.

Lorber J (1972). Spina bifida cystica: results of treatment of 270 consecutive cases with criteria for selection for the future. Arch Dis Child 47:854–873.

Lorber J (1978). Ethical concepts in the treatment of myelomeningocele. In Swinyard CA (ed): *Decision Making and the Defective Newborn: Proceedings of a Conference on Spina Bifida and Ethics*. Springfield, IL: Charles C Thomas, pp. 59–67.

Luker K (1984). *Abortion and the Politics of Motherhood*. Berkeley: University of California Press.

MacIntyre A (1978). How to identify ethical principles. *The Belmont Report: Ethical Principles and Guidelines for the Protection of Human Subjects of Research*. DHEW Pub. No. (OS) 78-0013, Vol. I, 10:1–41. Washington, DC: U.S. Government Printing Office.

Madsen JR, Estroff J, Levine D (1998). Prenatal neurosurgical diagnosis and counseling. Neurosurg Clin North Am 9:49–61.

Magnet JE, Kluge E-HW (1985). *Withholding Treatment from Defective Newborn Children*. Cowanville, Quebec: Brown Legal Publications.

Manchester D, Clewell W, Manco-Johnson M, Pretorius D, Meier P (1988). Management of pregnancies with suspected fetal anomalies: clinical experience and ethical issues. In Nimrod C, Griener G (eds): *Biomedical Ethics and Fetal Therapy*. Waterloo, CA: Wilfrid Laurier University Press, pp. 65–79.

Matthews AL (1990). Known fetal malformations during pregnancy: a human experience of loss. In Fine BA, Gettig E, Greendale K, Leopold B, Paul NW (eds): *Strategies in Genetic Counseling: Reproductive Genetics and New Technologies*. Birth Defects: Original Article Series 26. White Plains NY: March of Dimes Birth Defects Foundation, pp. 168–175.

McCormick RA (1974). To save or let die: the dilemma of modern medicine. JAMA 229:172–176.

McCullough LB, Myser C (1987). Recent developments in perinatal and neonatal medical ethics: a U.S. perspective. Semin in Perinatal 11:216–223.

McLaughlin JF, Shurtleff DB, Lamers JY, Stuntz JT, Hayden PW, Kropp RJ (1985). Influence of prognosis on decisions regarding the care of newborns with myelodysplasia. N Engl J Med 312:1589–1594.

McLone D (1998). Care of the neonate with myelomeningocele. Neurosurg Clin North Am 9:111–120.

Meany FJ, Riggle SM, Cunningham GC (1993). Providers and consumers of prenatal genetic testing services: what do the national data tell us? Fetal Diagn Ther 8(Suppl 1):18–27.

Minchom PE, Appleton PL, Lawson V, Boll V, Jones P, Elliot CE (1995). Impact of functional severity on self-concept in young people with spina bifida. Arch Dis Child 73:48–52.

Morgan LM (1996). Fetal relationality in feminist philosophy: an anthropological critique. Hypatia 11:47–70.

Moss K (1987). The "Baby Doe" legislation: its rise and fall. Policy Studies J 15(4):629–651.

Murray TH (1985). Why solutions continue to elude us. Social Sci Med 20:1103–1107.

Nichols VG, Bianchi DW (1996). Perinatal pediatrics: traditional subspecialty definitions no longer apply. Pediatrics 97:729–732.

Paige C, Karnofsky EB (1986). The antiabortion movement and Baby Jane Doe. J Health Politics Policy Law 11(2):255–269.

Parens E, Asch A (eds) (2000). *Prenatal Testing and Disability Rights*. Washington, DC: Georgetown University Press.

Pence GE (1990). The Baby Jane Doe case. In *Classic Cases in Medical Ethics: Accounts of the Cases That Have Shaped Medical Ethics with Philosophical, Legal, and Historical Backgrounds*. New York: McGraw-Hill, pp. 136–163.

Petchesky RP (1987). Foetal images: the power of visual culture in the politics of reproduction. In Stanworth M (ed): *Reproductive Technologies: Gender, Motherhood and Medicine*. Minneapolis: University of Minnesota Press, pp. 57–80.

Pit-ten Cate IM, Kennedy C, Stevenson J (2002). Disability and quality of life in spina bifida and hydrocephalus. Dev Med Child Neurol 44:317–322.

Post SG (1988). History, infanticide and imperiled newborns. Hastings Center Rep 18(4):14–17.

President's Commission for the Study of Ethical Problems in Medicine and Biomedical and Behavioral Research (1983). *Deciding to Forego Life-Sustaining Treatment: A Report on the Ethical, Medical, and Legal Issues in Treatment Decisions*. Washington, DC: Author.

Press N, Browner CH, Tran D, Morton C, Le Master B (1998). Provisional normalcy and "perfect babies": pregnant women's attitudes toward disability in the context of prenatal testing. In Franklin S, Ragoné H (eds): *Reproducing Reproduction: Kinship, Power, and Technological Innovation*. Philadelphia: University of Pennsylvania Press, pp. 46–65.

Ramsey P (1975). *The Ethics of Fetal Research*. New Haven, CT, and London: Yale University Press.

Ramsey P (1978). *Ethics at the Edges of Life: Medical and Legal Intersections*. New Haven, CT, and London: Yale University Press.

Rapp R (1997). Real-time fetus: the role of the sonogram in the age of monitored reproduction. In Downey GL, Dumit J (eds): *Cyborgs and Citadels: Anthropological Interventions in Emerging Sciences and Technologies*. Santa Fe, NM: School of American Research Press, pp. 31–48.

Reich WT (1978). Quality of life and defective newborn children: an ethical analysis. In Swinyard CA (ed): *Decision Making and the Defective Newborn: Proceedings of a Conference on Spina Bifida and Ethics*. Springfield, IL: Charles C Thomas, pp. 489–511.

Reiser SJ (1986). Survival at what cost?: Origins and effects of the modern controversy on treating severely handicapped newborns. J Health Politics Policy 11:199–213.

Retsinas J (1991). The impact of prenatal technology upon attitudes toward disabled infants. In: Wertz DC. *Research in the Sociology of Health Care, Vol. 9*. Greenwich, CT: JAI Press Inc., pp. 75–102.

Roberts CD, Stough LM, Parrish LH (2002). The role of genetic counseling in the elective termination of pregnancies involving fetuses with disabilities. J Special Ed 36:48–55.

Robertson JA (1975). Involuntary euthanasia of defective newborns: a legal analysis. Stanford Law Rev 27:213–269.

Robertson JA (1978). Legal issues in the nontreatment of defective newborns. In Swinyard CA (ed): *Decision Making and the Defective Newborn: Proceedings of a Conference on Spina Bifida and Ethics*. Springfield, IL: Charles C Thomas, pp. 359–383.

Saetersdal B (1997). Forbidden suffering: the pollyanna syndrome of the disabled and their families. Family Process 36:431–435.

Sandelowski M (1994). Separate, but less equal: fetal ultrasonography and the transformation of expectant mother/fatherhood. Gender Society 8:230–245.

Saxton M (1987). Prenatal screening and discriminatory attitudes about disability. Women Health 13:217–224.

Saxton M (2000). Why members of the disability community oppose prenatal diagnosis and selective abortion. In Parens E, Asch A (eds): *Prenatal Testing and Disability Rights*. Washington, DC: Georgetown University Press, pp. 147–164.

Shapiro RS, Barthel R (1986). Infant care review committees: an effective approach to the Baby Doe dilemma? Hastings Law J 37:827–862.

Shelp EE (1986). *Born to Die?: Deciding the Fate of Critically Ill Newborns*. New York: Free Press, 1986.

Shelp EE (1987). Choosing among evils. In McMillan RC, Engelhardt HT Jr, Spicker SF (eds): *Euthanasia and the New-born: Conflicts Regarding Saving Lives*. Dordrecht, the Netherlands: D Reidel, pp. 211–231.

Shurtleff DB, Hayden PW, Lowser JD, et al (1974). Myelodysplasia: decision for death or disability. N Engl J Med 291:1005–1011.

Simeonsson RJ, McMillen JS, Huntington GS (2002). Secondary conditions in children with disabilities: spina bifida as a case example. Ment Retard Dev Disabil Res Rev 8:198–205.

Singh DK (2003). Families of children with spina bifida: A review. J Dev Phys Disabil 15:37–55.

Solomon RC (1983). Reflections on the meaning of (fetal) life. In Bondeson WB, Engelhardt HT Jr, et al (eds.): *Abortion and the Status of the Fetus*. Dordrecht, the Netherlands, and Boston: D Reidel, pp. 209–226.

Spiegelberg H (1986). "Accident of birth": a non-utilitarian motif in Mill's philosophy. In *Steppingstones Toward an Etics for Fellow Existers: Essays 1944–1983*. Dordrecht, the Netherlands: Martinus Nijhoff, pp. 107–129.

Steinbock B (2000). Disability, prenatal testing and selective abortion. In Parens E, Asch A (eds): *Prenatal Testing and Disability Rights*. Washington, DC: Georgetown University Press, pp. 108–123.

Steinbok P, Irivine B, Cochrane DD, Irwin BJ (1992). Long-term outcome and complication of children born with meningomyelocele. Child's Nerv Syst 8:92–96.

Strong C (1983). Defective infants and their impact on families: ethical and legal considerations. Law Med Health Care 11(4):168–172, 181.

Strong C (1984). The neonatologist's duty to patient and parents. Hasting Center Rep 14(4):10–16.

Swinyard CA, ed (1978). *Decision Making and the Defective New-born: Proceedings of a Conference on Spina Bifida and Ethics*. Springfield, IL: Charles C. Thomas, Publisher.

Ten Have H (1994). The hyperreality of clinical ethics: a unitary theory and hermeneutics. Theoret Med 15:113–131.

Tew BJ, Payne H, Laurence KM (1974). Must a family with a handicapped child be a handicapped family? Dev Med Child Neurol 16(Suppl 32):95–98.

Todres DI, Guillemin J, Grodin MA, Batten D (1988). Life-saving therapy for newborns: a questionnaire survey in the state of Massachusetts. Pediatrics 81(5):643–649.

Van Eys J (2001). Commentary: humanity and personhood. Pharos Alpha Omega Honor Med Soc 64(2):11.

Velie EM, Shaw GM (1996). Impact of prenatal diagnosis and elective termination on prevalence and risk estimate of neural tube defects in California, 1989–1991. Am J Epidemiol 144:473–479.

Warren MA (1975). On the moral and legal status of abortion; with A postscript on infanticide. In Wasserstrom R (ed): *Today's Moral Problems*. New York: Macmillian, pp. 120–136.

Weir R (1984). *Selective Nontreatment of Handicapped Newborns*. New York and Oxford: Oxford University Press.

Weir R (1985). Selective nontreatment—one year later: reflections and a response. Social Sci Med 20:1109–1117.

Whitbeck C (1983). The moral implication of regarding women as people: new perspectives on pregnancy and personhood. In Bondeson WB, Engelhardt HT Jr, et al (eds): *Abortion and the Status of the Fetus*. Dordrecht, the Netherlands, and Boston: D Reidel, pp. 247–272.

Wilcox DT, Karamanoukian HL, Glick PL (1993). Antenatal diagnosis od pediatric surgical anomalies: counseling the family. Pediatr Clin North Am 40:1273–1287.

Worley G, Schuser JM, Oakes WJ (1996). Survival at 5 years of a cohort of newborn infants with myelomeningocele. Dev Med Child Neurol 38:816–822.

Wyatt J (2001). Medical paternalism and the fetus. J Med Ethics 27(Suppl II):ii15–ii20.

Zaner RM (1986). Soundings from uncertain places: difficult pregnancies and imperiled infants. In Dokecki PR, Zaner RM (eds): *Ethics of Dealing with Persons with Severe Handicaps*. Baltimore and London: Paul H Brookes, pp. 71–92.

Zaner RM (1988). *Ethics and the Clinical Encounter*. Engelwood Cliffs, NJ: Prentice Hall.

Zaner RM (1993a). *Troubled Voices: Stories of Ethics and Illness*. Cleveland: Pilgrim Press.

Zaner RM (1993b). Voices and time: the venture of clinical ethics. J Med Philos 18:9–31.

Index